Index of Suspicion in
TREATABLE DISEASES

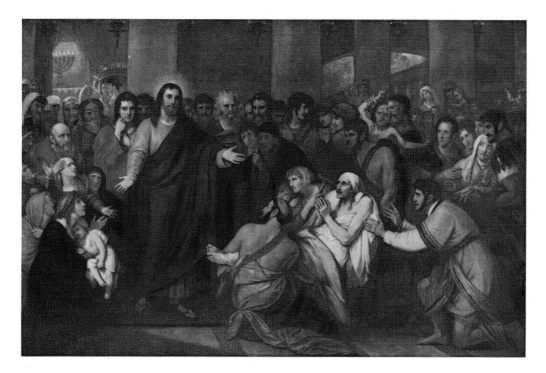

Benjamin West's superb picture of Christ Healing the Sick in the Temple hangs in all its majesty inside the entrance to the Pennsylvania Hospital. Included among his patients are a woman and an infant, a mother and a rickety child, a blind girl, a palsied woman, a blind man, and a lunatic boy. He could cure, help and comfort all who believed in him, and many who did not. Our scope is more limited, but by asking the greatest use of the gifts God has given us we can do much.

Associate Editors

Peter F. Binnion

> Associate Professor of Medicine, Associate Professor of Pharmacology
> University of Pennsylvania
> Staff Cardiologist, Pennsylvania Hospital

Frank Elliott, M.D.

> Professor of Neurology, University of Pennsylvania
> Consultant Neurologist, Pennsylvania Hospital

George Ross Fisher, III

> Assistant Clinical Professor of Medicine, University of Pennsylvania
> Associate Physician to Pennsylvania Hospital

Frank H. Gardner, M.D.

> Professor of Medicine, University of Pennsylvania
> Director of Medicine, Presbyterian Hospital—University
> of Pennsylvania Medical Center

Robert J. Gill

> Assistant Clinical Professor of Medicine, University of Pennsylvania
> Physician to Pennsylvania Hospital
> Head, Section of Vascular Disease and Hypertension, Pennsylvania
> Hospital

C. William Hanson, Jr.

> Assistant Professor of Medicine, University of Pennsylvania
> Director of Emergency Services, Hospital of the University of Pennsylvania

Francis Sterling

> Assistant Professor of Medicine, University of Pennsylvania

Index of Suspicion in
TREATABLE DISEASES

ORVILLE HORWITZ, M.D.

Professor of Medicine, University of Pennsylvania School of Medicine
Physician to the Pennsylvania Hospital
Consultant to Bryn Mawr Hospital

JOSEPH H. MAGEE, M.D.

Assistant Professor of Medicine, University of Pennsylvania School of Medicine
Assistant Physician to the Pennsylvania Hospital

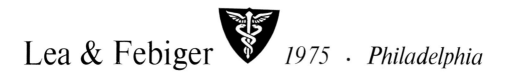

Lea & Febiger   1975 · *Philadelphia*

Library of Congress Cataloging in Publication Data

Horwitz, Orville, 1909–
    Index of suspicion in treatable diseases.

    1. Diagnosis. 2. Therapeutics. I. Magee, Joseph H., joint author.
II. Title. [DNLM: WB141 H824i] RC71.H78 1975   616.07′5
74-32256   ISBN 0-8121-0505-2

Published in Great Britain by Henry Kimpton Publishers, London

PRINTED IN THE UNITED STATES OF AMERICA

This book is dedicated to our teachers and associates, who believe in trying to diagnose something satisfactorily treatable, to Drs. Francis C. Wood, Hugh Montgomery, and Henry A. Schroeder, who have imparted wisdom and encouragement to many patients, physicians, and students, and particularly to the patients themselves, some of whom we hope will be helped by this book.

Preface

When asked why he robbed banks, Willie Sutton replied, "Because that's where the money is."

Many Professors of Medicine believe that their schools should try to teach their students to list differential diagnoses in order of satisfactory treatability rather than in order of frequency of occurrence. This philosophy has evolved in the middle third of the twentieth century, since before 1920 therapeutics was a much more limited field. In fact, fifty years ago less than 10% of the conditions mentioned in this book were amenable to more than purely symptomatic treatment. At the turn of the century pathology was the basic science of the internist, and his skill was measured by his ability to predict postmortem findings. Physiology, Pharmacology, Biochemistry, and Molecular Biology then developed rapidly and became the necessary basic sciences of the practicing physician and led to the present age of therapeutics. So, asked today, why we should have a high index of suspicion of treatable disease, we might paraphrase Willie Sutton : "Because those are the diseases in which we may be of the greatest help to those who are afflicted by them."

This book is based on a course entitled "Specifically Treatable Diseases" given under the auspices of the American College of Physicians. The stated object of the course was to "deal specifically with treatable diseases confronting the internist and the general practitioner regardless of the rarity or the vulgarity of the lesion" and to include "the illnesses which all diagnosticians hope never to miss." This obviously provides no strict line of demarcation between treatable and untreatable disease.

Of course, we found ourselves dealing with a spectrum, which is so often the case when dealing with the classification of biological phenomena. At one end of the spectrum are conditions so obviously diagnosable and treatable that it would be absurd to include them in the discussion. A list of such maladies would include such conditions as a foreign body in the eye, epistaxis, and carbuncle on the buttock. At the other end of the spectrum are harbored such monsters as carcinoma of the esophagus with metastasis and amyotrophic lateral sclerosis, which may in some instances be difficult to diagnose, but are presently almost impossible to cure. Between these two extremes are the conditions to be considered in this book.

The actual goal of the book then has become somewhat less like the *stated* goal of the course upon which it was based, and probably more like the *actual* goal of the course in which satisfactorily treatable disease rather than specifically treatable disease was discussed. It would be pleasant if there were a specific remedy for all ailments (or would it?). However, we must compromise in some cases with partial success or amelioration in dealing with certain disorders, and we believe that these should also be included in our thesis. There is no merit in missing any diagnosis, but missing the diagnosis of a serious condition in which the pathophysiological process may be halted or retarded by therapy can be disastrous.

Ultimately this book concerns itself with those conditions which, if properly diagnosed, can be either eradicated or controlled in such a manner that immediate suffering, permanent crippling, or death can be satisfactorily averted, and not merely held "awhile at arms end" as stated by Orlando in Shakespeare's "As You Like It."

In order to make a diagnosis at least three elements must be present in the mind of the diagnostician. First, he must be aware of the existence of the disorder with which he is confronted. Second, he must become suspicious that one or more of the conditions of which he is aware might be the disorder he is attempting to diagnose. Third, he must know enough to match his knowledge of the clinical picture with his knowledge of the disease process.

So often do we hear, "The diagnosis was really easy, once you thought of it." This is true for many of the conditions mentioned in this book for which there is a specific test, therapeutic or otherwise, which will confirm the diagnosis once the index of suspicion has been elevated to the proper height. Conditions of this sort require little discussion. However, there are other disorders, particularly among the endocrine and renal dysfunctions, which require considerable knowledge of pathochemicophysiology in order to suspect their presence or even to become truly aware of their existence. For these reasons there is necessarily great disparity in the amount of space devoted to different topics.

Sometimes the diagnosis may become evident by process of elimination. Under these circumstances it is encouraging to remember that as Sherlock Holmes said in "The Sign of the Four," "When you have eliminated the impossible, whatever remains, however improbable, must be the truth."

The format adopted for each condition, and adhered to throughout, minimally contains the following:

> Name of Condition
> Cause
> Early Manifestations
> Treatment
> Possible Dire Consequences Without Treatment
> Reference(s)

Sometimes the name alone is enough to suggest and actually to make the diagnosis. Certainly if the cause is known, the diagnosis will be soon forthcoming. A proper history should contain a statement concerning positive or negative exposure to a possible cause.

Early manifestation, which hopefully raise indices of suspicion, must now be divided into two categories: (1) data obtained from history and physical examination (those which actually bring most sick people to doctors) and (2) routine laboratory and roentgen studies often included in periodic health examinations. As early manifestations, both must be considered. Although most of our listed early manifestations are symptoms and signs, some are listed by such appellations as "high serum calcium," "hyponatremia," or "hypokalemia." Unfortunately, there are manifestations which, at an early date, can only be detected by apparatus such as the electrocardiogram or the flame photometer.

Treatment and possible dire consequences without treatment are necessary for the reader to be able to figure out whether or not the treatment is worse than the disease. We believe that we have included only conditions in which the risk/benefit ratio is not too high, but it is surely the privilege of our readers to disagree.

A few conditions are mentioned in which the treatment is deemed to be unsatisfactory. The purpose of this is either to compare them with similar diseases in which the treatment is satisfactory or to advise against treatment under such circumstances.

We have attempted to include at least one recent and comprehensive reference for each condition. Sometimes this has not been possible and many references have been listed. The soundness of the knowledge of a disease seems to vary inversely to the amount of literature concerning it.

We have undoubtedly omitted conditions which should have been included and vice versa. We would be glad to receive nominations for either inclusion or rejection.

During the construction of this book it has been assumed that it is usually not too difficult to recognize the system or systems involved in most disease processes. Exceptions are mentioned in the introductions to various chapters throughout the text.

Infections as a group are presently the most satisfactorily treatable of all conditions. It is probable that they are declining numerically, although many patients with them are not hospitalized any more in western countries and therefore do not become statistics. Some of the infections mentioned are extremely rare, but others are among the world's commonest diseases and/or killers: malaria, schistosomiasis, and hookworm. Many are easily enough diagnosed once the observer thinks of them.

Bacteria may cause kidney disease directly from the blood stream or the lower urinary tract or indirectly from streptococcal infection usually of the upper respiratory tract. Both are amenable to treatment. Other renal disorders are now treatable, thanks to the great strides forward in this field since the advent of the flame photometer.

We also felt that a sound physiological basis was necessary to properly understand the definitive diagnosis and treatment of hypertensive diseases.

Some discussions of allergy are scattered throughout the book, but allergy itself, as exemplified by the duo of hay fever and asthma, is not included. These two conditions are usually obvious.

Megavitamin therapy is not mentioned, since it still appears to be of questionable therapeutic value in spite of its champions.

In the March 27, 1974, issue of *Medical Tribune* is the headline: "Leading Cancer Specialists Dismayed by Inept Treatment." Particularly cited are acute lymphatic leukemia, cancer of the ovary, and Hodgkin's disease. A most promising but so far unpublished treatment, we understand now, has been developed for reticulum cell carcinoma. Another volume written a few years hence on treatable disease will probably require a chapter on cancer and possibly one on chemically treated psychiatric conditions.

The contents of this book have not been accumulated with the thought that they will be of particular help to specialists trying to know more about their particular field. Rather the book may be useful to internists, to general practitioners, to students, to nurses, to paramedical personnel, and to specialists seeking knowledge outside of their specialty.

Finally, the purpose of this book may best be expressed by a dictum to the healing profession apparently anonymously propounded in fifteenth century France or earlier: "To cure sometimes, to relieve often, to comfort always." ("Guérir quelquefois, soulager souvent, consoler toujours.") The "cure" and "relieve" are partially covered in this book. The "comfort" is still the most important and is not only in the province of the medical profession, but in the province of all mankind.

Philadelphia, Pennsylvania   ORVILLE HORWITZ
                                                                       JOSEPH H. MAGEE

Acknowledgements

We wish to thank: John F. Spahr and Samuel A. Rondinelli of Lea and Febiger for advice and assistance, our associate editors and authors for their scholarship, Mr. Orville H. Bullitt and Mr. William White for counsel, Mr. Morris Cheston, Mr. M. Todd Cooke, Mr. H. Robert Cathcart, the Board of Managers of the Pennsylvania Hospital, and the Foundation for Vascular-Hypertension Research for support, and our families for educating us in the first place.

We are especially grateful to Mrs. Virginia A. Faugl for typing the whole book —more than once, for correcting most of our errors, and for preserving a working relationship between editors and authors.

Contributors

Baggenstoss, Archie H.
Professor of Pathology, Mayo School of Medicine, University of Minnesota

Banerjee, Chandra M.
Professor of Physiology, Southern Illinois University

Billings, F. Tremaine, Jr.
Clinical Professor of Medicine, Vanderbilt University

Binnion, Peter F.
Associate Professor of Medicine
Associate Professor of Pharmacology, University of Pennsylvania

Bornstein, Donald L.
Associate Professor of Medicine, State University of New York

Brown, Robert K.
Associate Clinical Professor of Surgery, University of Colorado

Burns, William
Associate Professor of Ophthalmology, University of Pennsylvania

Coffman, Jay
Professor of Medicine, Boston University

Cohen, Sidney
Associate Professor of Medicine, University of Pennsylvania

Conn, Hadley L. Jr.
Professor of Medicine, Rutgers University

Deren, Julius J.
Associate Professor of Medicine, University of Pennsylvania

Duncan, Theodore G.
Assistant Clinical Professor of Medicine, University of Pennsylvania

Ehrlich, George E.
Professor of Medicine and Rehabilitation, Temple University

Elliott, Frank
Professor of Neurology, University of Pennsylvania

Eshleman, John D.
Clinical Assistant Professor of Medicine, University of Rochester Medical School

Fisher, George Ross, III
Assistant Clinical Professor of Medicine, University of Pennsylvania

Gardner, Frank H.
Professor of Medicine, University of Pennsylvania

Gill, Robert J.
Assistant Clinical Professor of Medicine, University of Pennsylvania

Goldwein, Manfred
Assistant Professor of Medicine, University of Pennsylvania

Gorshein, Dov
Assistant Professor of Medicine, University of Pennsylvania

Gross, Paul
Assistant Professor of Dermatology, University of Pennsylvania

Hanson, C. William
Assistant Professor of Medicine, University of Pennsylvania

Harrison, Frank S., Jr.
Clinical Assistant Professor of Medicine, Thomas Jefferson University

Horwitz, Orville
Professor of Medicine, University of Pennsylvania

Israel, Harold
Professor of Medicine, Thomas Jefferson University

Johnson, Lois H.
Assistant Professor, University of Pennsylvania

Johnson, William T. M.
Professor of Chemistry, Lincoln University
Research Associate in Medicine, University of Pennsylvania

Kastor, John A.
Associate Professor of Medicine, University of Pennsylvania

Keller, Wayne W.
Cardiologist, Bryn Mawr Hospital

Kershbaum, Kenneth
Clinical Associate in Medicine, University of Pennsylvania

Kunin, Calvin M.
Professor of Medicine, University of Wisconsin

Long, Edwin T.
Associate Professor of Surgery, University of Pennsylvania

Mac Neal, Perry S.
Associate Clinical Professor of Medicine, University of Pennsylvania

Mc Brearty, Frank X., Jr.
Resident Physician in Pathology, Pennsylvania Hospital

Mc Clenahan, John
Clinical Associate Professor of Medicine, Thomas Jefferson University

Magee, Joseph H.
Assistant Professor of Medicine, University of Pennsylvania

Makous, Norman
Assistant Clinical Professor of Medicine, University of Pennsylvania

Marvel, James P., Jr.
Assistant Clinical Professor of Orthopedic Surgery, University of Pennsylvania

Montgomery, Hugh
Emeritus Professor of Medicine, University of Pennsylvania

Morris, David
Assistant Professor of Medicine, Rutgers University

Moulder, Peter
Professor of Surgery, University of Florida

Murphy, Scott
Assistant Professor of Medicine, University of Pennsylvania

Parry, Carolyn
Associate in Radiology, University of Pennsylvania

Paskin, David
Assistant Professor of Surgery, University of Pennsylvania

Randall, Eileen
Associate Clinical Professor of Pathology, Northwestern University

Roberts, Brooke
Professor of Surgery, University of Pennsylvania

Robert, Victor
Instructor of Neurology, State University of New York

Rockower, Steven
Medical Student, Temple University School of Medicine

Root, Richard K.
Associate Professor of Medicine, University of Pennsylvania

Rothman, Richard H.
Associate Professor in Orthopedic Surgery, University of Pennsylvania

Rush, Alexander
Associate Clinical Professor of Medicine, University of Pennsylvania

Sack, John
Senior Resident in Orthopedic Surgery, Pennsylvania Hospital

Schless, Guy L.
Assistant Clinical Professor of Medicine, University of Pennsylvania

Schoenfield, Leslie J.
Professor of Medicine, University of California, Los Angeles

Schutta, Henry S.
Professor of Neurology, State University of New York

Simeone, Frederick A.
Associate Professor in Neurosurgery, University of Pennsylvania

Soloway, Roger D.
Assistant Professor of Medicine, University of Pennsylvania

Stainbach, William C.
Professor of Surgery, Thomas Jefferson University

Sterling, Francis
Assistant Professor of Medicine, University of Pennsylvania

Summerskill, W. H. J.
Professor of Internal Medicine, Mayo School of Medicine, University of Minnesota

Swenson, Robert
Associate Professor of Medicine
Associate Professor of Microbiology, Temple University

Wagner, Joseph
Assistant Clinical Professor of Medicine, University of Pennsylvania

Wesson, Lawrence G., Jr.
Professor of Medicine, Thomas Jefferson University

Williams, William
Professor of Medicine, State University of New York

Wood, J. Edwin
Professor of Medicine, University of Pennsylvania

Contents

Chapter I

Hematologic Diseases

Introduction

It seems doubtful that any of the subspecialities of medicine has produced a wider variety of specific treatments for disease than has Hematology during the last fifty years. These treatments include the use of the following: folic acid, vitamin B_{12}, iron, splenectomy, hormones (particularly cortico-steroids), transfusions, withdrawal of drugs (salicylates in particular), withdrawal of antibiotics, phlebotomy, cancer chemotherapeutic agents, ^{32}P, plasmapheresis, cytotoxic agents, radiotherapy, factor VIII, factor IX, and surgical measures to stop bleeding.

Hematologic disease is also probably characterized by a wider assortment of complaints than is any other group of diseases. Among the possible early manifestations are weight loss, chills, night sweats, fatigue, malaise and lassitude, weakness, general loss of strength, headache, paresthesias, bleeding gums, confusion, impairment of consciousness, olfactory hallucinations, sore tongue, ulceration, dryness of the mouth, dysphagia, dyspnea and palpitation, cough, tenderness of the sternum, abdominal fullness, belching or discomfort, abdominal pain, gastrointestinal bleeding, hematemesis or melena, constipation, impotence or bladder dysfunction, arthritis or arthralgia, petechiae and ecchymoses, excoriation, cyanosis, and splenomegaly.

Weakness and bleeding are probably the most common complaints for which patients seek medical attention.

The available therapeutic agents mentioned exceed the number of diseases discussed in this chapter. Some conditions require more than one agent and some agents are useful in the treatment of more than one condition.

Other conditions which may present as hematological disease, but are in fact diseases originating in other systems are: peptic ulcer, cancer of the ascending colon, bleeding from aortic aneurysm, cranial arteritis, retroperitoneal bleeding from excessive anticoagulation, chronic nephritides, chronic infections, infectious mononucleosis and other leukemoid reactions.

1. Folic Acid Deficiency Disease

Frank H. Gardner

Cause: Deficiency of folic acid, one of the vitamins of the B complex group that is essential in biochemical transfer of one-carbon fragments in synthesis of proteins—especially purines.

Early Manifestations: Associated with nonspecific symptoms of malaise and anorexia as well as pallor, evidence of wasting of tissue, and skin pigmentation. Primarily seen in patients with poor diet, dietary faddism, and alcoholism.

Treatment: Oral folic acid.

Possible Dire Consequences without Treatment: Progressive anemia and death.

The discovery of folic acid allowed the physician to understand the macrocytic anemias that have been observed in younger patients, and to separate this nutritional deficiency from pernicious anemia (vitamin B_{12} deficiency). Folic acid is not synthesized by man, who is dependent for supply on green leafy vegetables, citrus fruits, and organ meats (kidney, liver). At any one time the body has only a three- to four-month store of folate available if intake ceases. The main site of absorption is in the upper third of the small intestine and the process is an active one that deconjugates complex glutamates into mono-triglutamyl forms. Dietary faddism and especially alcoholism appear to be the main cause of deficiency, but malabsorption (adult celiac disease) must be considered.

Patients with increased bone marrow activity associated with chronic hemolytic anemias such as thalassemia and hemoglobinopathies (sickle cell anemia and hemoglobin C disease) require extra folic acid to compensate for excessive erythropoiesis. Indeed, increased metabolic demands of hyperthyroidism, myeloid metaplasia, and lymphomatous disease increase the utilization of folic acid. Malabsorption of folic acid in the small bowel may be associated with anti-epileptic therapy (Dilantin).

Diagnosis is dependent upon the history of poor diet and awareness of alcoholism. The patient should manifest findings of a macrocytic anemia associated with hypersegmented neutrophils and megaloblastic erythropoiesis. An associated iron deficiency may lessen the apparent macrocytosis and diminish the megaloblastic appearance of the bone marrow. Serum folate levels are low and can be measured if there is any doubt of the diagnosis (less than 3 ng./ml. versus normal value of 6 to 20 ng./ml.). Serum iron levels are elevated, with increased saturation of iron-binding protein. Often the serum lactic dehydrogenase activity is high; indeed values over 600 units may be expected.

Treatment consists of oral folic acid, 1 mg. daily for several weeks. Careful correction of diet and elimination of alcohol are imperative to prevent recurrence. Patients with chronic hemolysis should receive 1 mg. folic acid twice weekly indefinitely. Such supportive therapy is of special concern in the growing child to achieve maximum hemoglobin levels. Similar chronic therapy is useful for the metabolic demands of myeloid metaplasia and lymphoproliferative disease.

References

Gough, K. R., Read, A. E., McCarthy, C. F., and Waters, A H.: Megaloblastic anaemia due to nutritional deficiency of folic acid. Quart. J. Med., *32*:243, 1963.

Herbert, V.: Minimal daily adult folate requirement. Arch. Intern. Med., *110*:649, 1962.

Johns, D. G., and Bertino, J. R.: Folates and megaloblastic anemia. A review. Clin. Pharmacol. Ther., *6*:372, 1965.

Lindenbaum, J., and Lieber, C. S.: Hematologic effects of alcohol in man in the absence of nutritional deficiency. New Eng. J. Med., *281*:333, 1969.

Lindenbaum, J., and Klipstein, F. A.: Folic acid deficiency in sickle-cell anemia. New Eng. J. Med., *269*:875, 1963.

Oliner, H. L., and Heller, P.: Megaloblastic erythropoiesis and acquired hemolysis in sickle-cell anemia. New Eng. J. Med., *261*:19, 1959.

Rose, D. P.: Folic acid deficiency in leukemia and lymphomas. J. Clin. Path., *19*:29, 1966.

2. Vitamin B$_{12}$ Deficiency

Frank H. Gardner

Cause: Impaired absorption of vitamin B$_{12}$ from the gastrointestinal tract. There is no intrinsic source of vitamin B$_{12}$ synthesis in man, and he is dependent entirely on food intake for supply.

Early Manifestations: Similar to those of folic acid deficiency, primarily anemia. The lassitude and weakness may be associated with neurosensory defects as well. When first seen the patient may complain of neurosensory symptoms.

Treatment: Parenteral injections of crystalline vitamin B$_{12}$.

Possible Dire Consequences without Treatment: Progressive anemia, with or without neurologic complications (combined system disease), leading to cardiac collapse and death.

The understanding of vitamin B$_{12}$ deficiency evolved from the classic studies leading to the definition of the malabsorption of B$_{12}$ intrinsic factor complex in pernicious anemia. The physiologic description of intrinsic factor initiated a prolonged study to define the specific material in liver extract that has been found to complex in the stomach with intrinsic factor to promote absorption of the vitamin in the ileum. Microbial synthesis is the only source of vitamin B$_{12}$ available to man.

This deficiency is a genetic disorder found predominantly in North Europeans and is associated with gastric atrophy. Vitamin depletion initiates all of the symptoms of megaloblastic anemia that have been described for folic acid deficiency. It is of great clinical significance that neurologic changes related to vitamin B$_{12}$ deficiency have been called subacute combined degeneration disease, involving the dorsal and lateral columns of the spinal cord. The mechanism of these neurologic complications is not known; they may be observed before the megaloblastic anemia is noted. It is imperative to treat these changes quickly, while they are still reversible.

Vitamin B$_{12}$ deficiency should always be diagnosed with care, since replacement therapy is required indefinitely in all patients. Prior to or during therapy, gastric analysis can be done without discomfort to demonstrate achylia, which can be correlated with low serum vitamin B_{12} if a Schilling test is not immediately available. Careful radiologic examination should be done to exclude blind loop syndrome from previous surgery, diverticula, or strictures.

Parenteral vitamin B_{12} is the only therapy. Although large pharmacologic doses of oral vitamin B_{12} (1 mg. tablets) have been used, the physician should see the patient regularly and not prescribe oral medication. Initially the anemic patient should receive 100 μg. daily for two weeks. Thereafter this dosage should be given weekly for the next six weeks and monthly forever. If there are neurologic changes, 100 μg. weekly should be given for six months and then every two weeks indefinitely. Most patients can be trained to give themselves injections without a specific program to see a physician, except for three-month intervals in the first year, and twice yearly thereafter. Although hydroxycobalamin is less rapidly excreted than cyanocobalamin, there would appear to be no significant difference in the parenteral preparations. There is *no* acceptable oral preparation of vitamin B_{12} combined with intrinsic factor.

Some elderly anemic patients (less than 5 gm. hemoglobin) should have transfusions of sedimented red cells given slowly, each 250 ml. given over a three-hour interval. Presence of cardiac failure does indicate that the physician should plan to give blood as an exchange transfusion. Hence, 50 ml. can be removed and replaced with the same amount of sedimented red cells (hematocrit 85%). Although some improvement with corticoid therapy has been reported, this never can be used as a substitute for vitamin B_{12} replacement.

References

Castle, W. B.: A century of curiosity about pernicious anemia. Trans. Amer. Clin. Climatol. Assoc., *73*:54, 1961.
Lindenbaum, J., and Lieber, C. S.: Hematologic effects of alcohol in man in the absence of nutritional deficiency. New Eng. J. Med., *281*:333, 1969.
Schloesser, L. L., Deshpande, P., and Schilling, R. F.: Biologic turnover rate of cyanocobalamin (vitamin B_{12}) in human liver. A.M.A. Arch. Int. Med., *101*:306, 1958.

3. Iron-Deficiency Anemia or Hypochromic Anemia

FRANK H. GARDNER

Cause: Inadequate iron replacement in adults, in most instances from blood loss, not infrequently from bleeding hemorrhoids. Less commonly it is associated with malabsorption from the gastrointestinal tract.

Early Manifestations: Fatigue, headache, palpitation, dyspnea, and pallor. Less commonly observed are spoon nails, stomatitis, and pedal edema.

Treatment: Iron salts orally. Rarely, parenteral iron is indicated.

Possible Dire Consequences without Treatment: Continued symptoms that rarely are fatal.

Iron deficiency continues to be the major cause of anemia in the United States. Without adequate dietary replacement, young adults after adolescent growth will have depleted iron stores. Women with menorrhagia have continued loss of iron with mild anemia that they may accept as normal. Chronic blood loss in both sexes can be related to excessive use of aspirin associated with gastritis. Although in rare cases blood loss from gastritis may be massive, in most instances the chronic oozing is not known to the patient. The use of analgesics with meals or of soluble aspirin products can diminish gastrointestinal mucosal irritation. If hypochromic anemia cannot be attributed to menorrhagia, careful radiologic evaluation of the gastrointestinal tract is necessary to exclude hiatal hernia and malignancy; examination for hemorrhoids also is indicated.

Initially iron stores are lost from the bone marrow, as the body seeks to ensure adequate maintenance of the circulating red cell mass. Continued iron deficiency causes microcytosis of the erythrocyte without hypochromia. Further iron loss is reflected in the classic blood film of pale small erythrocytes with variation in size and shape. The mean corpuscular hemoglobin concentration (MCHC) has been the most useful guide to assess severe iron deficiency quickly. Serum iron measurements are becoming available to most physicians, and can be used as confirmatory evidence. The percentage of iron saturation of the total iron-binding protein should be used, since absolute values of serum iron vary in different laboratories. With the formation of small hypochromic red cells, excess protoporphyrin is present, since iron is not available to synthesize heme. Heretofore, laboratory techniques for measuring erythrocyte protoporphyrin levels have been cumbersome, but newer methods have made this study more useful and reproducible, causing it to replace serum iron ratios as the initial confirmatory measurement. Usually serum iron values below 20% saturation are observed in iron deficiency. Early stages of iron deficiency can be diagnosed accurately by the determination of stainable iron in the bone marrow. It is important to make such judgment on fixed smears of bone marrow particles, since decalcification may leach stainable iron particles to give false-positive evidence. With progressive severity of the anemia, a normoblastic hyperplasia also is noted in the bone marrow aspirate.

In most instances the condition responds to oral iron salts. Despite the profusion of iron preparations, most physicians can expect excellent response with ferrous sulfate and gluconate preparations. Usually 300 mg. given before each meal proves a satisfactory schedule. It is difficult to accept patients' complaints of intolerance to iron salts. Such symptoms of bowel irritation can be solved easily by the use of liquid iron (elixir of ferrous sulfate). Small doses (by drops if necessary) can be prescribed initially with anticipation that adult dosage can be achieved in weeks. Women might well have the habit of taking two iron tablets daily during each menstrual period until menopause. There is no need to encourage use of multivitamin mixtures with iron salts.

Should the physician prescribe parenteral iron? There is some minor risk of allergic reactions with all preparations. Patients who have malabsorption from sprue, rapid transit time following subtotal gastrectomy or inadequate small bowel as a result of surgical resection, or regional enteritis may benefit from intramuscular iron dextran. The rare patient who is unable or unwilling to follow instructions or accept oral medication can benefit from a calculated replacement of 3 to 4 gm. of elemental iron by intramuscular injection. Parenteral iron is not used effectively by the bone marrow and is retained in the reticuloendothelial system with a slower release than we can expect from oral iron salts. The increments of hemoglobin levels achieved with intramuscular iron are similar to values observed with oral iron salts.

Severe anemia of 9 gm. or less exhibits reticulocytosis within five days of oral iron therapy, and shows a peak in ten days. In mild anemia hemoglobin values gradually return to normal within a two- to three-month interval. The physician should at all times discourage casual use of iron salts by men with normal hemoglobin levels.

References

DeLeeuw, N. K. M., Lowenstein, L., and Hsieh, Y.: Iron deficiency and hydremia in normal pregnancy. Medicine, *45*:291, 1966.

Fairbanks, V. F., Fahey, J. L., and Beutler, E.: Clinical Disorders of Iron Metabolism. 2nd Ed. New York, Grune & Stratton, 1971.

Hilal, H., and McCurdy, P. R.: A pitfall in the interpretation of serum iron values. Ann. Intern. Med., *66*:983, 1967.

Jacobs, A., and Butler, E. B.: Menstrual blood-loss in iron-deficiency anemia. Lancet, 2:407, 1965.

Kasper, C. K., Whissell, D. Y. E., and Wallerstein, R. O.: Clinical aspects of iron deficiency anemia. J.A.M.A., *191*:359, 1965.

Scott, D. E., and Pritchard, J. A.: Iron deficiency in healthy young college women. J.A.M.A., *199*:897, 1967.

Taymor, M. L., Sturgis, S. H., and Yahia, C.: The etiological role of chronic iron deficiency in production of menorrhagia. J.A.M.A., *187*:323, 1964.

4. Hereditary Spherocytosis and Elliptocytosis with Significant Hemolysis

ORVILLE HORWITZ

Cause: Autosomal dominant defect (spherical erythrocytes).

Early Manifestations: Most common hereditary hemolytic defect (1:5000 population). Anemia, jaundice, splenomegaly.

Treatment: Splenectomy if discovered before age fifty.

Possible Dire Consequences without Treatment: Gallstones, chronic hemolytic anemia, possibly hemachromatosis.

This most common hereditary hemolytic defect (1:5000 population) is also the most easily treatable cause of hereditary hemolytic anemia. It is important to make this diagnosis for two reasons: (1) The patient will be saved from cholelithiasis and chronic anemia and (2) the diagnosis may result in further contribution to the science of hematologic genetics. Diagnosis has been made in patients ranging in age from one day to ninety years.

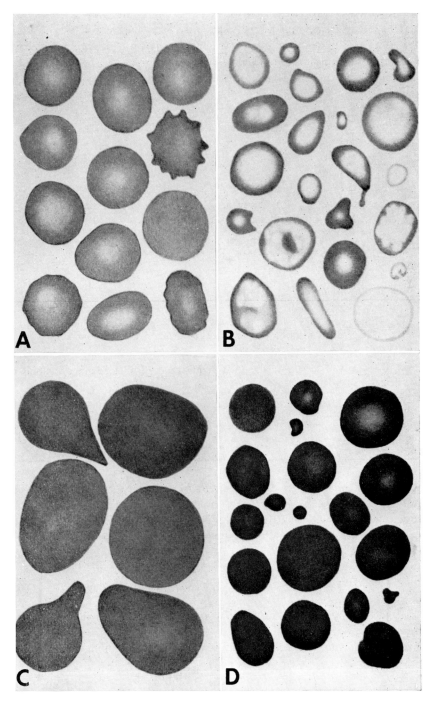

Fig. I–1. A. Normal blood cells. B. Iron Deficiency Anemia. C. Pernicious Anemia.
D. Spherocytosis.

The disorder results in a hyperactive bone marrow which enables the hematocrit to be maintained at about 30%. Eventually the bone marrow can become over-worked and lose its race against hemolysis.

It should be suspected particularly in younger patients who show moderate anemia and bleeding from the gastrointestinal tract.

Reference

Cooper, R. A., and Jandl, J. H.: Hereditary spherocytosis. *In* Hematology. Edited by W. J. Williams, E. Beutler, A. J. Erslev, and W. R. Rundles. New York, McGraw-Hill Book Co., 1972.

5. Aplastic Anemia and Erythroid and Megakaryocyte Aplasia

ORVILLE HORWITZ

Cause: Unknown 50%. Drugs, particularly chloramphenicol, sulfonamides, benzene, Dilantin, isoniazid, and para-aminosalicylic acid. Thymoma and post-hepatitis.

Early Manifestations: Depressed red cell count and platelet count, symptoms of anemia, and bleeding.

Treatment: Transfusions, long-term platelet support, hormones, and vitamin B_{12}. Folic acid *not* useful. Salicylates contraindicated. Thymectomy.

Possible Dire Consequences without Treatment. Profound anemia, hemorrhage, death.

The object of the supportive treatment is to allay serious symptoms of anemia and/or bleeding. Efforts should be made to keep the hematocrit greater than 25%.

It should be noted, when concentrated platelet transfusions are given, that platelets from a single unit of whole blood will only raise the platelet count by about 8,000 per cubic millimeter. It is not surprising then that 10 to 20 units daily for two to four days often may be necessary for controlling bleeding. Then too the short survival time (T1/2 < 4 days) is an additional limitation. Practical platelet typing at this time is difficult. Few laboratories are equipped for this.

Prolonged therapy by male hormone and corticosteroids, in spite of the disagreeable side effects and toxicity, is also indicated in erythroid aplasia and aplastic anemia. Male hormone acts mostly on the erythropoietic system, corticosteroids on the "marginal pool" of marrow leukocytes.

The use of chloramphenicol, unless definitely found to be an offender, should not be withheld if urgently needed at a future date to combat a Salmonella infection. Salicylates, however, are contraindicated during and after an attack. Since bleeding and infection are the usual causes of death, these patients should be "covered" by large doses of kanamycin sulfate and sodium cephalothin, which are the antibiotics of choice until a definite organism has been identified.

References

Scott, J. L., Cartwright, G. E., and Wintrobe, M. M.: Acquired aplastic anemia. Medicine, *38*:119, 1959.

Wallerstein, R. O., Condit, P. K., Kasper, C. K., Brown, J. W., and Morrison, F. R.: State-wide study of chloramphenicol therapy and fatal aplastic anemia. J.A.M.A., *208*:2045, 1969.

6. Polycythemia Vera

Dov Gorshein

Cause: Unknown. Considered to be a chronic disorder of hematopoietic proliferation and, as such, belongs to the group of myeloproliferative disorders. An extra C-group chromosome is present in 10% of cases.

Early Manifestations: May or may not occur. Can be insidious and nonspecific or acute and related to a major or minor vascular accident.

Treatment: Phlebotomy, ^{32}P, chemotherapy.

Prognosis: If properly treated, patient can maintain comfortable life with median survival of thirteen years.

Possible Dire Consequences without Treatment: Circulatory disturbances manifested by cerebrovascular, peripheral vascular, or cardiac malfunction.

Of prime importance is the demonstration of increased red cell mass with normal arterial oxygen saturation. Since many polycythemic patients tend to bleed (most commonly from upper gastrointestinal tract), documentation of high red cell mass (and hematocrit) may not be easy.

Symptoms vary considerably and may include the following complaints: splenomegaly with abdominal fullness; thromboembolic phenomena with major accidents in cerebral, cardiac, or other vessels; bleeding which, if from upper gastrointestinal tract, may be related to the increased frequency of peptic ulcer compounded by platelet function abnormalities; increased nucleoprotein turnover with hyperuricemia and uric acid nephropathy (5 to 10% actually develop secondary gout); excessive histamine released from basophils induces pruritus and hemorrhagic gastritis.

Treatment

Emergency phlebotomy is indicated when major hazards are imminent, such as impending vascular occlusion (e.g., transient ischemic cerebral attacks, anginal syndrome). Ideally, however, polycythemia should be controlled for a few months to reduce the risk of operation.

Myelosuppressive therapy is indicated by the presence of active hematopoiesis which requires frequent phlebotomy; signs of myeloid metaplasia (hepatosplenomegaly and peripheral blood with signs of either extramedullary hematopoiesis or cytopenia secondary to splenic sequestration); symptoms related to hyperhistaminemia and/or hyperuricemia not relieved by phlebotomy.

The specific therapeutic agents are ^{32}P and alkylating compounds. Radioactive phosphorus is initially given intravenously, 3 to 5 mC; occasionally a second dose of 2 to 3 mC is required two to three months later, depending on blood counts. Four out of five patients respond favorably with remissions lasting one-half to two years.

Alkylating agents used are busulfan, 4 to 6 mg. daily for one month, then maintenance of 2 mg./day or intermittently repeated courses; chlorambucil, 6 to 8 mg. for four to five months, then maintenance of 2 mg./day; cyclophosphamide, 100 to 150 mg. daily for four months, then 50 mg./daily. Any therapy should be monitored by blood counts. The possible connection of the treatment of polycythemia vera with the induction of acute leukemia is unresolved at present. It is possible that the latter is an integral part of the natural course of polycythemia vera. It is also possible that irradiation and myelosuppressive agents have leukemogenic effects, and thus increase the incidence of acute leukemia.

Reference

Glass, J. L., and Wasserman, L. R.: Primary polycythemia. *In* Hematology. Edited by W. J. Williams, E. Beutler, A. J. Erslev, and R. W. Rundles. New York, McGraw-Hill Book Co., 1972.

7. Primary Macroglobulinemia

Dov Gorshein

Cause: Unknown. Possible contributing factors are same as cited for multiple myeloma.

Early Manifestations: May simulate chronic lymphatic leukemia or slowly developing lymphoma.

Treatment: Plasmapheresis, cytotoxic agents.

Prognosis: Difficult to define because of possible heterogeneous group of diseases designated as primary. Symptoms may not be severe for a number of years.

Possible Dire Consequences without Treatment: Cerebrovascular accidents, loss of vision, hemorrhages.

Primary macroglobulinemia is a syndrome caused by proliferation of IgM producing plasma (or plasma-like) cells and characterized by anemia, bleeding, and hyperviscosity phenomena.

The anemia is multifactorial in its genesis (decreased production, increased destruction, and dilutional factors). Bleeding is attributed to agglutination of platelets, or the interference in function of coagulation factor by the abnormal protein.

Infections and renal damage, although possible, are not as common and severe as in multiple myeloma.

Treatment

Symptoms related to hyperviscosity (central nervous system symptoms, visual disturbances) constitute a medical emergency. Plasmapheresis of 10 to 20 ml./kg. body weight is initiated and may be repeated two to three times a week for a few weeks. The patient should be carefully observed for possible signs of volume depletion. Chlorambucil, 8 to 10 mg./day, also is given for that period of time. Maintenance dose is 2 to 4 mg./day. Continuous therapy is recommended. Some objection to the use of cytotoxic agents has been voiced lately in view of the uncertainty in the natural course of macroglobulinemia and the possible dire effects of cytotoxic therapy.

Reference

McCallister, B. D., Bayrd, E. D., Harrison, E. G., and McGuckin, W. F.: Primary macroglobulinemia. Amer. J. Med., *43*:394, 1967.

8. Chronic Lymphatic Leukemia

ORVILLE HORWITZ

Cause: Unknown

Early Manifestations: Usually no early symptoms. Diagnosed by routine count.

Treatment: None at first. Later, anti-malignancy measures.

Possible Dire Consequences without Treatment: None at first. Following the diagnosis, many patients live for more than ten years. Median survival of patients with newly discovered disease is five years.

Although this disease eventually causes bone pain, fever, anemia, lymphadenopathy, splenomegaly, and death in possibly half of all cases, it is possible for some patients to remain symptom-free for perhaps the best part of two decades. In the latter situation, an attitude of extreme optimism should prevail. The possibilities for proper treatment before the onset of lymphadenopathy, anemia, thrombocytopenia, or splenomegaly are as follows:

1. Not mentioning it to the patient at all.
2. Telling the patient that he (or she) has a white cell condition that may cause trouble much later.
3. Telling the patient that leukemia exists but that the name is wrongly used by the profession and that the condition is actually benign. After all, it is sometimes referred to as benign lymphatic leukemia.
4. Not making the diagnosis in the first place.

The drug of choice for treatment, when started, is chlorambucil.

Reference

Dameshek, W.: Chronic lymphocytic leukemia—an accumulative disease of immunologically incompetent lymphocytes. Blood, *29*:566, 1967.

9. Multiple Myeloma

Dov Gorshein

Cause: Unknown. Possible association with multiple factors including chronic inflammation or infection, irradiation, or chromosomal abnormalities.

Early Manifestations: May be a chance finding of M-type protein in plasma, high sedimentation rate, and proteinuria.

Treatment: General management—proper hydration, antibiotics if necessary, analgesics, and orthopedic support. Specific treatment—chemotherapeutic drugs (melphalan, cyclophosphamide), steroids, irradiation.

Prognosis: Uniformly fatal, remissions in 60 to 70%, median survival three years.

Possible Dire Consequences without Treatment: Renal failure, infections, pathologic fractures, and death.

This is the most common form of plasma cell dyscrasia. The incidence of multiple myeloma is roughly equal to that of Hodgkin's disease (25 cases per million). Its clinical manifestations include (1) infections, which commonly result from leukopenia associated with bone marrow replacement of tumor tissue or induced by chemotherapy, as well as specific immunoglobulin deficiency; (2) kidney failure, with Bence Jones protein precipitates in tubular cells, and such manifestations as nephrotic syndrome, adult Fanconi syndrome, hypercalcemia, hypercalciuria, hyperuricosuria, and rapid dehydration with rising BUN; and (3) bone lesions, the most frequent manifestation, which can "start out" as diffuse osteoporosis and evolve into the common lytic lesions. Lesions can be very destructive, causing shorter stature following collapse of vertebrae; rarely blastic lesions occur.

A slew of neurologic symptoms also are possible: mental changes secondary to hypercalcemia, infiltration of peripheral nerve with accompanying amyloidosis, direct pressure due to collapsed vertebrae and multiple leukoencephalopathy, hemorrhagic thrombocytopenia resulting from marrow replacement, and specific coagulation factor deficiency induced by abnormal protein.

Diagnosis

The suggestion is most commonly made by the clinical manifestation. The serum or urine contains abnormal protein in almost 100% of cases. Plasmacytosis of bone marrow may require repeated aspiration for its demonstration.

Treatment

Treatment is directed toward preventing renal failure and infection. Good orthopedic care with early mobilization is advised. Hypercalcemia, commonly observed, is associated with obligatory diuresis which, if untreated, terminates in dehydration and acute renal failure. The urinary output should be at most 30 ml./hour. Severe hypercalcemia can be rapidly controlled by intravenously administered saline or sodium sulfate (38.9 gm./1000 ml. water). Infections are common and are due to a specific humoral type of immunologic defect in multiple myeloma. They are pneumococcal more often than bacterial. The proper antibiotic should be given. The value of routine administration of γ-globulin has yet to be established. Chemotherapy employs mainly one of two alkylating agents: cyclophosphamide or melphalan. Treatment with the first is initiated by 200 mg./daily for one week, after which the dose is cut by $\frac{1}{2}$ or $\frac{1}{4}$. Proper hydration after cyclophosphamide administration may help prevent hemorrhagic cystitis. Melphalan is started with 10 mg./day for one week. Maintenance dose thereafter is 2 mg./day. This drug is somewhat unpredictable in its capacity to induce profound myelosuppression. Careful follow-up is required with either regimen. Useful criteria for evaluation of response are both subjective and objective. Subjective symptomatic improvement may occur within 24 hours, but this is difficult to define. Objective criteria are: (1) decrease in serum M-type protein, (2) decrease in urinary Bence Jones protein, (3) increase in hematocrit, and (4) regression of tumors (plasmacytoma).

References

Alexanian, R., Haut, A., Khan, A. U., Lane, M., McKelvey, E. M., Migliore, P. J., Stickey, W. J., and Wilson, H. E.: Treatment of multiple myeloma. J.A.M.A., *208*:1680, 1969.
Carbone, P., Kellerhouse, L. E., and Gehan, E. A.: Plasmacytic myeloma. Amer. J. Med., *42*:937, 1967.

10. Idiopathic Thrombocytopenic Purpura (ITP)

Scott Murphy

Cause: Circulating immunoglobin or immunoglobulin-containing material (antiplatelet factor) which sensitizes platelets for removal from circulation by spleen and reticuloendothelial system.

Early Manifestations: Easy bruising, menorrhagia.

Treatment: Corticosteroids, splenectomy.

Possible Dire Consequences without Treatment: Exsanguinating hemorrhage, intracranial hemorrhage.

Although ITP occurs in both sexes and in all age groups, it is more prevalent in young women. The onset is gradual, and the patient gives a history of chronic illness. Easy bruising and menorrhagia are the most common symptoms. Occasionally the disease has a stormy, acute onset with widespread purpura and mucous membrane bleeding.

All patients with these manifestations should have a quantitative platelet count so that the disease will not be overlooked. In addition to thrombocytopenia, the patient may have anemia from blood loss. The white and differential counts are normal and there is no lymphadenopathy or organomegaly. In most instances, a patient with thrombocytopenia should undergo one marrow aspiration and biopsy as part of his initial evaluation to exclude infiltrative disease. In ITP, the marrow is normal save for megakaryocytic hyperplasia. Unfortunately, there is no reliable *in vitro* assay for the circulating antiplatelet factor responsible for the thrombocytopenia in this disease.

Faced with this clinical picture, the clinician must question the patient carefully to rule out recent ingestion of drugs that might cause isolated thrombocytopenia. Quinidine, quinine, sulfonamides, thiazide diuretics, gold salts, Dilantin, and digitalis preparations are the more common offenders. Occasionally, an ITP-like condition can be inherited; therefore, a detailed family history is important. The much rarer condition, thrombotic thrombocytopenic purpura, occasionally mimics ITP, but these patients usually have at least one of the following: hemolytic anemia with poikilocytosis in the peripheral blood smear, neurologic abnormalities, fever, renal failure. Finally, both lymphosarcoma and systemic lupus erythematosus are associated with thrombocytopenia, occasionally indistinguishable from ITP. Lymphadenopathy or organomegaly should suggest these two diagnoses. However, the diagnosis often is not made until the characteristic pathologic features are found in the resected spleen.

ITP, then, is a clinical diagnosis made by excluding the possibilities reviewed above. Symptomatic patients should be treated with corticosteroids, the equivalent of 40 to 60 mg. prednisone daily. Once a remission has been induced, the dosage hould be tapered and maintained at the minimum required to control symptoms. We have arbitrarily continued this temporizing therapy for three months because some patients, albeit the minority, undergo spontaneous remission. If after three months, steroids are still required to control thrombocytopenia, the spleen should be removed. Approximately 60% of patients experience complete remission, and others continue asymptomatic, with moderate thrombocytopenia. Immunosuppressive agents such as azathioprine and cyclophosphamide are helpful in those few patients who remain symptomatic after operation.

Splenectomy merely removes that portion of the reticuloendothelial system that removes from the circulation the platelets sensitized by the antiplatelet factor. The antiplatelet factor continues to circulate. It is capable of crossing the placenta and causing neonatal thrombocytopenia even when the mother is in full remission after splenectomy.

Reference

Baldini, M.: Idiopathic thrombocytopenic purpura. New Eng. J. Med., *274*:1245, 1966.

11. Aspirin-Induced Platelet Dysfunction

SCOTT MURPHY

Cause: Ingestion of aspirin, which interferes with platelet function.

Early Manifestations: Easy bruising.

Treatment: Discontinuing drug.

Possible Dire Consequences without Treatment: Life-threatening hemorrhage from lesions such as peptic ulcer which might otherwise remain asymptomatic. Aggravation of bleeding tendency in patients with clotting factor deficiencies such as hemophilia and patients on oral anticoagulants.

When a vessel is injured or interrupted, flowing blood is exposed to subendothelial connective tissue. Platelets adhere to connective tissue and release their granular pool of adenine nucleotides, which then cause aggregation of platelets at the site. This formation of a plug of platelets is one of the body's first defenses against hemorrhage. The release reaction is partially inhibited by aspirin in very low doses. Because of this effect, a modest prolongation of the bleeding time can be demonstrated for 48 to 72 hours after the ingestion of only 600 mg. aspirin by normal subjects.

At any point in time, it is estimated that one quarter to one half of the population have recently ingested enough aspirin to show this effect. A large number of these individuals are unaware of their aspirin intake, since the drug is present in so many "over-the-counter" drug combinations. Of course, the vast majority of people are not affected deleteriously by aspirin, but a few otherwise normal individuals exhibit minor but definite bleeding tendencies while taking the drug. Easy bruising may stop completely when aspirin ingestion is discontinued.

Of greater import is the danger of serious hemorrhage that aspirin can produce in patients with underlying hemorrhagic tendencies or potential bleeding lesions. For example, if aspirin-induced platelet dysfunction is added to the clotting factor deficiencies of hemophiliacs or patients taking oral anticoagulants, the defect in hemostasis is worsened. It is known that the use of aspirin is dangerous in patients with peptic ulcer disease. Some of this effect is related to local mucous membrane irritation, but the systemic effect on platelet function may be at least equally important.

Aspirin is a useful drug, but should be avoided in patients with hemorrhagic manifestations or potential hemorrhagic manifestations. Propoxyphene hydrochloride (Darvon) or acetaminophen (Tylenol) does not affect platelet function and can be substituted for aspirin in these patients.

References

Weiss, H. T., Aledort, L. M., and Kochwa, S.: The effect of salicylates on hemostatic properties of platelets in man. J. Clin. Invest., 47:2169, 1968.

Kaneshiro, M. M., Mielke, C. H., Jr., Kasper, C. K., and Rapaport, S. I.: Bleeding time after aspirin in disorders of intrinsic clotting. New Eng. J. Med., 281:1039, 1969.

12. Lymphosarcoma (LSA) and Reticulum Cell Sarcoma (RCS)

Manfred Goldwein

Cause: Unknown. Malignancy of the lymphatic tissues characterized histologically by neoplastic lymphocytes or reticulum cells.

Early Manifestations: Lymphadenopathy, hepatosplenomegaly, abdominal complaints, anemia, bone pain.

Treatment: Radiotherapy, chemotherapy.

Possible Dire Consequences without Treatment: Progressive disability and death.

Lymphosarcoma (LSA) and reticulum cell sarcoma (RCS) are characterized by neoplastic proliferation of lymphocytes or reticulum cells with varying degrees of differentiation. The present scheme of classification is as follows:

1. Lymphosarcoma
   a. Well-differentiated type
   b. Poorly differentiated type
   c. Mixed (histiocytic-lymphocytic) type
2. Reticulum cell sarcoma
3. Malignant lymphoma, undifferentiated Burkitt type

Since all forms except malignant lymphoma may have a follicular pattern, the designation "follicular lymphoma" is no longer used. Rather, each type is subclassified as nodular or diffuse.

Unlike Hodgkin's disease, these diseases are multifocal, as evidenced by their tendency to occur simultaneously at anatomically distant sites and to recur in unpredictable regions with relapse. Prognosis, all else being equal, depends to some degree on the histologic type, the well-differentiated or small-cell LSA having the best prognosis. In approximately 50% of cases, peripheral adenopathy is the first manifestation. However, disease may first manifest itself by involvement of bone, bone marrow, spleen, abdominal viscera, or deep lymph nodes, in which cases early symptoms signify which sites are involved and often pose a diagnostic challenge. Definitive diagnosis is made by examination of biopsy specimen of involved tissue.

Treatment

Because of the tendency of multifocal involvement, staging, as outlined in the section on Hodgkin's disease, is of only limited value. Nevertheless an accurate assessment of the extent of disease is necessary for proper therapy. Again, unlike the treatment of Hodgkin's disease, a clearcut program has not been devised. Megavoltage roentgen therapy at doses of 3,500 to 4,000 rads to involved regions in stages I and II of the disease (see staging in discussion of Hodgkin's disease, p. 17) often effects a prolonged unsustained remission, especially in LSA. The success of radiotherapy in RCS is much less predictable, since this tumor is often radio-resistant. Intensive local radiotherapy is of particular value in localized RCS of bone and in LSA confined to one area of the gastrointestinal tract, in which five- to ten-year "cures" are not uncommon.

Disseminated disease is best treated by chemotherapy. The drugs outlined in the section on Hodgkin's disease, namely the mustards, adrenal steroids, vinca alkaloids, procarbazine, and BCNU, all have significant activity. Used singly or in combination, they frequently produce prolonged remissions, especially in LSA. RCS more often is resistant to all forms of chemotherapy. Unfortunately, because the bone marrow is frequently involved early during the course of the disease, intensive combination chemotherapy is often not possible. However, patients with aggressive disease who have an adequate marrow reserve should be treated with cyclic intensive combination therapy, such as the "MOPP" regimen (see Hodgkin's disease) or combinations of cyclophosphamide, prednisone, and vincristine. Preliminary results of such treatment regimens have shown significant improvement of remissions and longevity over single-drug therapy.

In summary, the methodology of therapy in the non-Hodgkin's lymphomas is, as of now, not as clearcut as that in Hodgkin's disease. In general, LSA responds well to radiotherapy in confined disease, to single cytotoxic agents in nonaggressive disseminated disease, and to cyclic combination chemotherapy in aggressive disease. Response to all agents in RCS, except with single-bone involvement, is much less satisfactory.

References

Hoogstraten, B., Owens, A. H., Lenhard, R. E., Glidewell, O. J., Leone, L. A., Olson, K. B., Harley, G. B., Townsend, S. R., Miller, S. P.., and Spurr, C. L.: Combination chemotherapy in lymphosarcoma and reticulum cell sarcoma. Blood, *33*:370, 1969.
Rosenberg, S. A., Diamond, H. D., and Craver, L. F.: Lymphosarcoma: the effects of therapy and survival in 1,269 patients in a review of 30 years' experience. Ann. Intern. Med., *53*:877, 1960.
Rundles, R. W.: Lymphosarcoma. *In* Hematology. Edited by W. J. Williams, E. Beutler, A. Y. Erslev, and R. W. Rundles. New York, McGraw-Hill Book Co., 1972.
Rundles, R. W.: Reticulum cell sarcoma. *In* Hematology. Edited by W. J. Williams, E. Beutler, A. Y. Erslev, and R. W. Rundles. New York, McGraw-Hill Book Co., 1972.

13. Hodgkin's Disease

MANFRED GOLDWEIN

Cause: Unknown. Malignancy of the lymphatic tissues characterized histologically by an intermingling of neoplastic and reactive elements and the presence of Reed-Sternberg cells.

Early Manifestations: Inadvertent findings on chest roentgenogram. Peripheral lymphadenopathy—most often in the cervical region; less commonly and with worse prognosis, systemic symptoms such as weight loss, fever, malaise, pruritus, hepatosplenomegaly.

Treatment: Radiotherapy, chemotherapy.

Possible Dire Consequences without Treatment: Progressive tumor involvement, disability, and death.

The diagnosis of Hodgkin's disease is in most cases easily made by biopsy of involved tissue. At times, however, the histology is atypical, despite the presence of characteristic clinical features. Re-biopsy or multiple biopsies usually establish the definite diagnosis in these situations.

Staging

In contrast to other lymphatic malignant disease, Hodgkin's disease seems to have a unifocal origin in many patients, particularly those with the following characteristics:

1. Younger age group
2. More "benign" histology
3. Absence of systemic symptoms
4. Disease confined to adjacent or nearly adjacent chains of lymph nodes

Since it has been demonstrated that such patients have an excellent chance for cure by intensive radiotherapy, cases are "staged" both histologically and clinically according to the criteria outlined in Table I–1.

Significant correlation exists between histologic type, clinical stage, and prognosis. Stage I and II, for example, are more likely to occur with lymphocytic predominance or nodular sclerosis and good prognosis, whereas, stages III and IV correlate more often with mixed cellularity or lymphocytic depletion and poor prognosis. Nodular sclerosis is by far the most common histologic type and can be present in all four stages. The prognosis in this histologic type depends mostly on the clinical stage. The presence of systemic symptoms (substage B) in all stages bespeaks a less favorable prognosis.

TABLE I–1

STAGING, HISTOLOGIC CLASSIFICATION, AND PROGNOSIS
IN HODGKIN'S DISEASE

Clinical Stage		Prognosis for "Cure"	Histologic Type
I (A & B)	Disease confined to one or two contiguous chains of lymph nodes on the same side of the diaphragm	Excellent	Lymphocytic predominance
II (A & B)	Disease in more than two noncontiguous chains of nodes on the same side of the diaphragm	Intermediate	Nodular sclerosis
III (A & B)	Disease on both sides of the diaphragm, but limited to lymph nodes, spleen, or Waldeyer's ring	Poor	Mixed cellularity
IV (A & B)	Disease involving any tissue other than those mentioned in III, including skin, lung, bone marrow, and liver		Lymphocytic depletion

Note: Substage A or B refers to absence (A) or presence (B) of systemic symptoms, which include fever, weight loss of greater than 10%, night sweats, and pruritus.

METHODOLOGY OF STAGING

Complete clinical staging requires, in addition to the usual history and physical examination, the following procedures:

1. Complete blood count, including platelet count
2. Roentgenograms of chest and bones
3. Lymphangiogram
4. Liver function tests
5. Bone marrow biopsy
6. Laparotomy with splenectomy, liver biopsy, and biopsies of retroperitoneal nodes

In a number of medical centers every patient with Hodgkin's disease is subjected to the complete staging routine, including laparotomy. It must be emphasized that *routine* laparotomy is as yet an experimental procedure, designed to characterize the disease more completely in all its facets. Treatment dictated by findings on routine laparotomy has not yet been shown to improve the prognosis in a significant proportion of patients. It is our custom to perform laparotomy only when it seems necessary to the choice of treatment. Thus we *do not* perform laparotomy in patients with lymphocytic predominance or nodular sclerosis, stage I or II_A, who have normal liver function tests, unequivocally normal lymphangiograms, and normal-size spleens. Patients with proven stage III_B or IV disease also are spared this procedure. In our practice, laparotomy is performed in (1) patients with stage I or II_A disease who are under the age of 50, with either equivocal or abnormal lymphangiograms, splenomegaly, or abnormal liver function tests and (2) patients with stage III_A disease who are under the age of 50, with nodular sclerosis, in whom we consider radical radiation therapy.

Treatment

Vera Peters' classic observation in 1950 and subsequent studies by Kaplan have demonstrated that confined Hodgkin's disease has an excellent chance for cure by means of intensive radiotherapy. Furthermore, the recent introduction of combination chemotherapy has produced prolonged maintained remissions in a significant proportion of patients with disseminated disease. There is tentative evidence that sequential radiotherapy and combination chemotherapy further improve prognosis.

Radiotherapy is used for stage I and stage II disease. Megavoltage therapy at dosages of 3,500 to 4,000 rads to all node-bearing areas on the side of diaphragm affected is given over a four- to five-week period. In many centers upper abdominal nodes and the splenic area also are irradiated routinely when the disease is above the diaphragm.

In some centers total nodal irradiation is given for stage III_A disease. Its superiority over chemotherapy in this instance has not been established. Careful shielding of lung parenchyma, heart, kidneys, and liver is mandatory.

Chemotherapy is given to patients with disseminated disease (stage III or IV), or those who have developed radioresistant disease. Aggressive combination chemotherapy is now the treatment of choice for patients who can tolerate it, since prolonged unmaintained remissions and possible cures have been produced in a significant number of cases. Agents known to be effective are listed in Table I–2. These agents

TABLE I–2
AGENTS EFFECTIVE IN THE TREATMENT OF HODGKIN'S DISEASE

1. Alkylating agents
   Nitrogen mustard
   Cyclophosphamide
   Chlorambucil

2. Vinca alkaloids
   Vinblastine
   Vincristine

3. Methylhydrazine derivatives
   Procarbazine

4. Adrenal corticosteroids

5. Nitrosourea compounds
   BCNU

used singly produce partial and sometimes complete remissions in a majority of cases but relapse after a brief time is the rule after a single course. The use of single agents or combinations of two agents is now generally reserved for elderly patients or patients who have low tolerance to more intensive therapy by reason of marrow damage due to previous therapy. Maintenance therapy with one or two agents in these situations frequently results in prolonged remissions.

Aggressive multi-agent therapy, first reported in depth by De Vita *et al.*, represents a significant advance in drug therapy in disseminated disease. In the original study, 35 of 43 previously untreated patients developed complete remissions. Seventeen of these remained in remission at forty-two months after conclusion of therapy. Many regimens are in use. A modification of De Vita's "MOPP" regimen, as outlined below, is as efficacious as any:

1. Nitrogen mustard, 6 mg./m.^{2} ⎫
                                      ⎬ IV days 1 and 8
2. Vincristine, 1.4 mg./m.^{2} ⎭
3. Procarbazine, 100 mg./m.^{2}/day PO, days 1 through 10
4. Prednisone, 40 mg./m.^{2}/day PO, days 1 through 10

This combination is given every four weeks for an optimal period of six months. Dosages are reduced when significant side effects become evident, especially leukopenia, thrombocytopenia, or peripheral neuropathy.

References

De Vita, V. T., Jr., Serpick, A. A., and Carbone, P. P.: Combination chemotherapy in the treatment of advanced Hodgkin's disease. Ann. Intern. Med., *73*:881, 1970.

Frei, E., Luce, J. K., Gamble, J. F., Coltman, C. A., Jr., Constanzi, J. J., Talley, R. W., Monto, R. W., Wilson, H. E., Hewlett, J. S., Delaney, F. C., and Gehan, E. A.: Combination chemotherapy in advanced Hodgkin's disease. Ann. Intern. Med. *79*:376, 1973.

Kaplan, H. S.: Role of intensive radiotherapy in the management of Hodgkin's disease. Cancer, *19*:356, 1966.

Lukes, R. J., and Butler, J. J.: The pathology and nomenclature of Hodgkin's disease. Cancer Res., *26*:1063, 1966.

Peters, M. V.: A study of survivals in Hodgkin's disease treated radiologically. Amer. J. Roentgenol., *63*:299, 1950.

14. Hemophilia A, Classic Hemophilia, and Factor VIII Deficiency

WILLIAM WILLIAMS

Cause: An inherited deficiency of factor VIII activity in the plasma. The condition is sex-linked, and therefore is limited to males, for all practical purposes.

Early Manifestations: Excessive bleeding following trauma, or bleeding occurring "spontaneously." The bleeding tendency is usually manifested in childhood, but in mild cases may not become evident until adult life, thus presenting diagnostic problems for internists.

Treatment: Local measures to stop bleeding, and replacement of the deficient factor VIII activity with normal factor VIII. Drugs that interfere with platelet aggregation, such as aspirin, must be avoided in patients with hemophilia.

Possible Dire Consequences without Treatment: Continuing hemorrhage, with the possibility of exanguination if free bleeding occurs, or damage to normal structures if the hemorrhage is internal, e.g., in the brain or, more commonly, in a joint space.

Hemophilia A, or classic hemophilia, was long attributed to a failure of synthesis of factor VIII, but more recent evidence points to synthesis of a functionally inactive, but immunologically reactive, factor VIII molecule as the cause (Hougie, 1972; Stites *et al.*, 1971; Zimmerman, *et al.*, 1971). The bleeding manifestations correlate reasonably well with the level of factor VIII activity demonstrable in the plasma (Hougie, 1972). Severe manifestations occur with factor VIII activity of 1% (or less) of normal; moderate manifestations occur with factor VIII activity of 1 to 5%; and mild manifestations occur with factor VIII activity of greater than 5%. Thus, hemarthroses, the classic manifestations of hemophilia, occur commonly with factor VIII activities of less than 1%, but are unusual in patients with factor VIII levels of greater than 5%.

Effective therapy requires that the deficient factor VIII activity be replaced with fresh frozen plasma or a concentrate of factor VIII (Johnson et al., 1972). Epsilon-aminocaproic acid has been advocated as a useful agent in the treatment of hemophilia, but conflicting reports on the efficacy of this agent have appeared in the literature. Replacement therapy in bleeding disorders is complicated, and requires considerable individualization for each patient, although certain general principles apply. This discussion is limited primarily to these general concepts.

Factor VIII activity is expressed in arbitrary units, with one unit defined as the activity present in 1 ml. of normal human male plasma. The factor VIII activity in patient's plasma is often expressed as a percentage of normal, assuming that normal plasma has 100% activity. These two notations cause some confusion, although they are readily convertible. Thus, factor VIII activity of 100% is the same as 1 unit/ml., activity of 50% is the same as 0.5 unit/ml. and so on. Since one usually estimates the concentration of factor VIII necessary for hemostasis in terms of per cent, and then calculates the dosage to be given in terms of units, some care is necessary to keep the decimal point in the right place.

The level of factor VIII to be achieved and maintained in a patient with hemophilia is determined from the clinical estimate of the severity of the bleeding or risk of bleeding which is present. Thus, serious bleeding such as occurs with extensive trauma, or major surgery, usually can be controlled by maintaining the level of factor VIII above 25% of normal. With less severe bleeding, such as hemarthroses, levels of factor VIII of 15 to 20% will suffice.

For effective replacement therapy, one must determine the dosage of factor VIII, the frequency of administration, and the duration of therapy. The dosage of factor VIII which must be given to achieve a predetermined plasma level may be calculated by multiplying the difference between the patient's factor VIII level and the desired level by the plasma volume, and then multiplying this quantity by 1.25 in order to compensate for the fact that the yield of factor VIII in the circulating plasma is only about 80% of the administered dose. The plasma volume may be assumed to be 4% of the body weight. The following formula is useful:

> Dose of factor VIII (units) = (body weight in kg. × 40) × (desired factor VIII level [units/ml.] − Pretreatment factor VIII level [units/ml.]) × 1.25.

> The expression (body weight in kg. × 40) yields the plasma volume in milliliters. The factor VIII level in units/ml. is obtained by dividing the factor VIII level in per cent by 100 (*i.e.*, 50% is 0.5 units/ml.).

Thus, if one decides it is necessary preoperatively to raise the factor VIII level to 60% in a severely afflicted 70 kg. patient with less than 1% of factor VIII, the initial dosage required would be 2100 units, calculated as follows: 2100 = (70 × 40) × (0.6–0) × 1.25.

Subsequent doses of factor VIII are lower than the initial dose because the pretreatment factor VIII level at the time of the next dose will be increased to a level depending on the interval between doses. This interval is the second variable to be considered. The frequency of administration of factor VIII replacement is determined by the duration of the factor VIII activity in the circulating plasma. The disappearance curves of plasma coagulation factors from the circulation are complex, involving at least two components. The first component is rapid and is due in part to diffusion out of the vascular compartment, whereas the second component is slower and due to metabolism of the factor. In patients receiving replacement therapy, the first component of the disappearance curve becomes slower with continued therapy, possibly because of equilibration of the extravascular pools with the circulation, although this is not clearly established. Whatever the mechanism, the practical point is that with continued therapy it is possible to increase the time interval between doses and still expect to maintain the desired factor levels. The metabolic half-life of factor VIII is about nine to eighteen hours, but the initial phase of the disappearance curve has a considerably shorter half-time. Experience has shown that satisfactory levels of factor VIII may be maintained in patients with severe bleeding by administration of factor VIII at intervals of eight hours for the first twenty-four hours, and then at intervals of twelve hours. In patients with minor bleeding, factor VIII administered every twelve hours will usually suffice.

As noted above, the dose necessary to maintain the plasma level is less than that required initially, and usually one administers one-half of the initial dose for maintenance. Thus, in the example used above (70-kg. man with severe hemophilia undergoing major surgery), the maintenance dose would be 1000 units. This is based on the assumption that in eight hours the factor VIII level will have fallen to 30% (0.3 units/ml.), and the additional 1000 units will return the level to 60% (0.6 units/ml.). Since the goal of replacement therapy is maintenance of the factor VIII level above a minimum hemostatic level, and there is a continuous fall in factor VIII, it is essential that each dose raise the level considerably above the desired minimum.

Ideally the response to factor VIII therapy is monitored by assay of factor VIII levels. However, this assay often is not available, and one may obtain some idea of the factor VIII level by measuring the activated partial thromboplastin time, recognizing that the levels of factor VIII of about 30% of normal will give normal results in this test.

The duration of therapy depends on the severity of the bleeding, and the response of the patient. Thus, in patients with minor bleeding and a prompt response to therapy, the replacement need be continued only for twenty-four hours after bleeding stops. For more severe bleeding it is wise to maintain therapy for five to seven days after bleeding has stopped; with major surgery one must often continue therapy for two weeks or more. In these latter instances therapy should be maintained until complete healing has occurred and sutures are removed. The levels of factor VIII required in the later stages of healing are less than those necessary for initial hemostasis, and the dosage and frequency can therefore be reduced.

A convenient form of concentrated factor VIII is the so-called cryoprecipitate, which may be prepared from fresh frozen plasma in the usual hospital blood bank. Quite satisfactory commercial preparations of factor VIII are also available. The concentration of factor VIII in the commercial preparations is determined by assay of the factor VIII activity of each batch, and is indicated on the label. When using fresh frozen plasma or cryoprecipitate, one must estimate the content of factor VIII because of the obvious problem of assaying each unit. A reasonable estimate is that the yield of factor VIII in fresh frozen plasma is 80%, the yield in cryoprecipitate is 40%. Thus 200 ml. of fresh frozen plasma would usually be considered to contain 160 units of factor VIII, while the cryoprecipitate prepared from 200 ml. of fresh frozen plasma would be considered to contain 80 units.

Replacement therapy in patients with inhibitors of factor VIII activity is more complex, and requires estimation of the inhibitor level and careful and frequent monitoring of the effect of administered factor VIII (Johnson *et al.*, 1972). Prophylactic therapy with factor VIII preparations has been successful in some instances, and is being evaluated in a number of centers. These topics are beyond the scope of this article.

The principal hazard of replacement therapy is hepatitis. The risk of contracting this disease is high, since patients usually require repeated therapy, and the commercial material is prepared from large plasma pools. Thus far no effective means of preventing hepatitis has been developed.

References

Hougie, C.: Hemophilia and related conditions—congenital deficiencies of prothrombin (factor II), factor V, and factors VII to XII. *In* Hematology. Edited by W. J. Williams, E. Beutler, A. J. Erslev, and R. W. Rundles. New York, McGraw-Hill Book Co., 1972.

Johnson, A. J., Aronson, D. L., and Williams, W. J.: Clinical use of plasma and plasma fractions. *In* Hematology. Edited by W. J. Williams, E. Beutler, A. J. Erslev, and R. W. Rundles. New York, McGraw-Hill Book Co., 1972.

Kasper, C. K., Dietrich, S. L., and Rapaport, S. I.: Hemophilia prophylaxis with factor VIII concentrate. Arch. Intern. Med., *125*:1004, 1970.

Stites, D. P., Hershgold, E. J., Perlman, J. D., and Fudenberg, H. H.: Factor VIII detection by hemagglutination inhibition: Hemophilia A and von Willebrand's disease. Science, *171*:196, 1971.

Zimmerman, T. S., Ratnoff, O. D., and Powell, A. E.: Immunologic differentiation of classic hemophilia (factor VIII deficiency) and von Willebrand's disease. J. Clin. Invest., *50*:244, 1971.

15. Hemophilia B, Christmas Disease, Factor IX Deficiency

WILLIAM WILLIAMS

Cause: An inherited deficiency of factor IX activity in the plasma. The condition is sex-linked, and therefore is limited to males, for all practical purposes.

Early Manifestations: Same as for hemophilia A.

Treatment: Same as for hemophilia A, except that normal factor IX is used for replacement therapy.

Possible Dire Consequences without Treatment: Same as for hemophilia A.

As with hemophilia A, hemophilia B was initially considered to be due to a failure of synthesis of factor IX, but more recently the situation has been shown to be more complex (Hougie, 1972). Some patients with hemophilia B appear to synthesize a functionally inactive but immunologically reactive factor IX molecule. Abnormalities in the one-stage prothrombin time have been found in some patients with the immunologically reactive, functionally inactive factor IX, and it has been suggested that the abnormal factor IX has an inhibitory role in these patients. However, other patients have been found who have the abnormality of the prothrombin time without demonstrable nonfunctional factor IX. Other variants have also been described. Further work is obviously needed to clarify this problem.

Therapy of hemophilia B follows the same principles as outlined for hemophilia A in the preceding section. Therapy is effected with fresh frozen plasma or commercial concentrates containing factor IX (Johnson *et al.*, 1972). Cryoprecipitate does *not* contain factor IX. The units of factor IX are defined as for factor VIII; *i.e.*, one unit is the activity in 1 ml. of normal plasma.

Two significant differences exist between factor IX and factor VIII with regard to replacement therapy. First, the *in vivo* recovery of factor IX is only 30 to 50%, which means larger doses are required. Second, the half-life of factor IX is longer, about twenty-four hours, so that therapy may be repeated less frequently.

In practice one calculates the initial dose of factor IX using the formula presented on page 22, except that the correction factor for yield should be 2 instead of 1.25. The interval between maintenance doses may be either twelve or twenty-four hours. If twelve hours are chosen, one administers approximately one-fourth of the loading dose, and if twenty-four hours are chosen one administers approximately one-half of the loading dose. The concepts determining the duration of therapy are the same as those used for hemophilia A.

Acquired inhibitors of factor IX occur much less frequently than do those of factor VIII, but present the same problems in therapy when they do occur. Prophylactic therapy of hemophilia B with factor IX is theoretically easier than with hemophilia A because of the longer half-life of factor IX. This form of therapy is presently under study in several centers.

References

Hougie, C.: Hemophilia and related conditions—congenital deficiencies of prothrombin (factor II), factor V, and factors VII to XII. *In* Hematology. Edited by W. J. Williams, E. Beutler, A. J. Erslev, and R. W. Rundles. New York, McGraw-Hill Book Co., 1972.

Johnson, A. J., Aronson, D. L., and Williams, W. J.: Clinical use of plasma and plasma fractions. *In* Hematology. Edited by W. J. Williams, E. Beutler, A. J. Erslev, and R. W. Rundles. New York, McGraw-Hill Book Co., 1972.

16. Von Willebrand's Disease

WILLIAM WILLIAMS

Cause: Von Willebrand's disease is an inherited disease characterized by a prolonged bleeding time, abnormal platelet adhesiveness, and a deficiency of factor VIII. It is inherited as an autosomal dominant disorder. It may be due to a deficiency of a plasma factor.

Early Manifestations: Excessive bruising and epistaxis are common early manifestations. Since the disease appears frequently in women, menorrhagia is common. Bleeding after trauma or surgery may be the first manifestation.

Treatment: The administration of fresh frozen plasma or certain plasma derivatives, e.g., cryoprecipitate, can correct the abnormal bleeding time, platelet adhesiveness, and factor VIII deficiency, and thus provides specific treatment. As with other hemorrhagic disorders, drugs that interfere with platelet aggregation, such as aspirin, must be avoided in order not to aggravate the bleeding tendency.

Possible Dire Consequences without Treatment: In severe cases, continuing hemorrhage with the result dependent on the site and extent of the bleeding.

The exact cause of von Willebrand's disease is unknown. It may be due to a deficiency of a plasma factor, as is suggested by the observed correction of all aspects of the hemostatic defect by administration of large amounts of plasma derivatives to patients with the disease.

The factor VIII deficiency differs from that in hemophilia A in two important respects: first, the deficiency appears to be due to a lack of synthesis of factor VIII, rather than to synthesis of an immunologically reactive but functionally inactive molecule (Stites, 1971; Zimmerman, 1971); second, the administration of plasma or certain plasma fractions causes the factor VIII level to rise much higher than would be expected from the factor VIII content of the administered material (Nilsson et al., 1957). The ability to stimulate factor VIII "production" is found in fresh frozen plasma, cryoprecipitate, and some of the more concentrated factor VIII preparations.

The diagnosis of von Willebrand's disease may be difficult (Weiss, 1972). Abnormalities in the bleeding time, platelet adhesiveness, or factor VIII level should be demonstrated, in addition to a history and/or physical findings indicating abnormal bleeding. Various combinations of the three laboratory abnormalities have been observed. Further, there may be marked variations in the degree of abnormality of any of the tests, and in a particular patient any one, or all, may be normal at one time and grossly abnormal another time. Therefore repeat testing may be required to establish the diagnosis.

The best means of treatment of von Willebrand's disease has not been established (Johnson et al., 1972; Weiss, 1972). The two variables that have received the most attention are the bleeding time and the factor VIII level. It has been stated that correction of the factor VIII level corrects the hemostatic defect sufficiently to bring about the cessation of bleeding, but it appears more likely that correction of the bleeding time is required as well. In patients with a normal bleeding time, obviously attention must be centered on correction of the factor VIII level.

Both the factor VIII level and the abnormal bleeding time can be corrected by fresh frozen plasma or by cryoprecipitate (Bennett and Dormandy, 1966; Perkins, 1967). The latter material has proved quite satisfactory in my experience.

Correction of the factor VIII deficiency is more readily accomplished in von Willebrand's disease than in hemophilia A because of the secondary rise in factor VIII levels that occurs in nearly all patients. The few patients who appear to have von Willebrand's disease and do not show this secondary rise must be treated as though they have hemophilia A. Usually the factor VIII deficiency is mild in patients with von Willebrand's disease, but levels in the range of 1 to 5% are encountered.

If the goal of replacement therapy is correction of the factor VIII level, this can be accomplished by administration of fresh frozen plasma, cryoprecipitate, or other factor VIII concentrates which are known to contain the material necessary for the secondary rise in factor VIII activity.

The half-life of the essential component of the replacement agents is unknown, and the replenishment of factor VIII is independent of the half-life of factor VIII. Thus, cryoprecipitate administered in an initial dose of 1 bag (70 to 100 units of factor VIII) per 10-kg. body weight, and at the same maintenance dose daily or every other day, should be sufficient to maintain the factor VIII level above 25% in patients with factor VIII deficiency due to von Willebrand's disease. This level should be sufficient for hemostasis in patients with severe bleeding. However, in patients with serious acute bleeding the initial dosage should be calculated as for a patient with hemophilia A, and the maintenance dosage for the first day or two be similarly calculated in order to provide sufficient factor VIII prior to full induction of the secondary rise. Smaller maintenance doses may then be given. In patients undergoing surgery, therapy should be started two days preoperatively, if possible, in order to permit full development of the secondary rise before operation. It is important to monitor the factor VIII levels in patients with von Willebrand's disease because the secondary rise in factor VIII level may vary somewhat in time of onset and extent of increase, and it is obviously important to ascertain that factor VIII activity is indeed sufficient to ensure hemostasis.

Correction of the bleeding time in patients with von Willebrand's disease is more difficult than restoration of the factor VIII level since the corrective effects of administered cryoprecipitate, for example, may last only two to four hours. The Duke bleeding time (ear lobe) is more readily corrected than is the Ivy bleeding time (forearm, with increased venous pressure induced with a blood pressure cuff). However, the small size of the ear lobe precludes use of this site for repeated testing, and it is usually necessary to use the Ivy method. Initially both methods may be profitably employed to determine the patient's response to therapy. The bleeding time may be normalized temporarily by the dosage described above for correction of the factor VIII level, but larger amounts of replacement therapy may be required, and it will be necessary to give the replacement therapy at shorter intervals than once daily in order to maintain the correction of the bleeding time. In initiating therapy the bleeding time (Ivy and/or Duke) should be determined prior to the first dose. The initial dose calculated, as for correction of the factor VIII level (*i.e.*, 1 bag per 10 kg.), is administered as rapidly as possible. The bleeding time is repeated shortly after the end of the infusion, and at intervals of two hours thereafter, to determine the extent of correction and the duration of the effect. Further therapy, in terms of both dosage and frequency, can be projected from these data.

The above discussion is not intended to provide the reader with a specific therapeutic regimen, since it is obvious that the best approach to the treatment of von Willebrand's disease remains to be developed. Repeated determination of the effects of therapy on the bleeding time and factor VIII level is essential for proper management of these patients. For the present the best course appears to be to provide sufficient replacement therapy to correct the bleeding time, if this is possible, especially in a patient whose response to therapy has not been evaluated previously. This disease is being studied actively in a number of centers and hopefully we shall have better-defined modes of therapy in the near future.

References

Bennett, E., and Dormandy, K.: Pool's cryoprecipitate and exhausted plasma in the treatment of von Willebrand's disease and factor-XI deficiency. Lancet, 2:731, 1966.

Johnson, A. J., Aronson, D. L., and Williams, W. J.: Clinical use of plasma and plasma fractions. *In* Hematology. Edited by W. J. Williams, E. Beutler, A. J. Erslev, and R. W. Rundles. New York, McGraw-Hill Book Co., 1972.

Nilsson, I. M., Blomback, M., and von Francknr, I.: On an inherited autosomal hemorrhagic diathesis with antihemophilic globulin (AHG) deficiency and prolonged bleeding time. Acta Med. Scand., *159*:35, 1957.

Perkins, H. A.: Correction of the hemostatic defects in von Willebrand's disease. Blood, *30*:375, 1967.

Stites, D. P., Hershgold, E. J., Perlman, J. D., and Fudenberg, H. H.: Factor VIII detection by hemagglutination inhibition: Hemophilia A and von Willebrand's disease. Science, *171*:196, 1971.

Weiss, H. J.: Von Willebrand's disease. *In* Hematology. Edited by W. J. Williams, E. Beutler, A. J. Erslev, and R. W. Rundles. New York, McGraw-Hill Book Co., 1972.

Zimmerman, T. S., Ratnoff, O. D., and Powell, A. E.: Immunologic differentiation of classic hemophilia (factor VIII deficiency) and von Willebrand's disease. J. Clin. Invest., *50*:244, 1971.

Chapter II

Arthritis

Introduction

Modern methods of medical and surgical treatment have greatly reduced the crippling effects of arthritis. Seldom do we see the stiff pretzel-like fingers and the extreme in rigidity of other joints that were all too common about thirty years ago. The diagnosis of arthritic conditions usually is not difficult, but the choice of medical and surgical treatment may be problematic.

Other conditions which may present as arthritic disease, but are in fact diseases originating in other systems: Autoimmune reactions. Lupus erythematosus. Hemophilia. Temporal arteritis.

1. Gout

F. Tremaine Billings, Jr.

Cause: A genetic abnormality of purine metabolism or excretion ordinarily identifiable by hyperuricemia, which must be differentiated from secondary hyperuricemias due to antihypertensive, antineoplastic, and other agents.

Early Manifestations: Acute inflammatory arthritis or tendonitis associated with microcrystalline sodium urate deposits in these areas.

Treatment: Colchicine is still the most effective drug in the treatment and prevention of the acute attack. Uricosuric agents, such as probenemid, and allopurinol, a xanthine oxidase competitive inhibitor, provide the most satisfactory method for long-term management of gout.

Possible Dire Consequences without Treatment: Recurrent incapacitating episodes of acute inflammatory arthritis, chronic deforming arthritis, tophaceous deposits in and around joints, tendons, and cartilages, uric acid nephrolithiasis, and gouty renal disease.

Gout is a well-known disease with a long historical background. As a cause of joint aches, pains, and inflammation, the diagnosis can be missed repeatedly if gout is not considered and uric acid serum levels determined. Examination of joint fluid with identification of needle-shaped birefringent crystals of sodium urate in leukocytes and a dramatic response to colchicine help to establish a diagnosis.

3

Gout may be primary and thus related to the genetic purine metabolic disorder. On the other hand, it may be secondary to increased uric acid serum levels associated with renal insufficiency, or with malignant disease such as myeloid leukemia or other blood dyscrasia. Hyperuricemia sufficient to precipitate acute attacks of gout may occur with prolonged use of chlorothiazides. Proper management of gout depends on appropriate differential diagnosis.

References

Hollander, J. L., and McCarty, D. J., Jr. (Eds.): Arthritis and Allied Conditions. 8th Ed., Philadelphia, Lea & Febiger, 1972.
Wyngaarden, J. B., Stanbury, J. S., and Fredrickson, D. S. (Eds.): Gout. *In* The Metabolic Basis of Inherited Disease. 2nd Ed. New York, McGraw-Hill Book Co., 1966.

2. Rheumatoid Arthritis

GEORGE EHRLICH

Cause: Unknown. Viral initiation is suspected. Proliferative synovitis of joints and tendon sheaths is accompanied by systemic features.

Early Manifestations: Symmetrical joint pain and swelling, often migratory; prolonged stiffness after rest; early fatigability.

Treatment: Early: analgesics and anti-inflammatory agents.
Progressive: gold salts (antimalarials, or systemic or local corticosteroids indicated in some cases; immunosuppressive agents used experimentally).
Physical measures: early surgery or reconstructive procedures.
Attention to psychosocial features.

Possible Dire Consequences without Treatment: Crippling and disability, inanition, death from complications of prolonged bed rest and chronic illness.

Rheumatoid arthritis may represent the overt expression of more than one underlying cause. In its early stages, its manifestations may be relatively evanescent or migratory, although a fixed symmetrical polyarthritis is also possible. Characteristically, pain of aching nature occurs in involved joints, accompanied by generalized stiffness. This stiffness is pronounced in duration, degree, and distribution in the morning, but also follows any period of rest (gelling). The joint manifestations are the result of localized synovitis and thus include swelling, tenderness, pain on motion, and to some extent, redness and heat. It is at this early stage that rheumatoid arthritis is eminently treatable and, at the same time, demands a holding action to see which direction the disease will take, before a long-term management program is begun. In common with most viral arthritis (following chicken pox, mumps, measles, German measles, and infectious hepatitis), early rheumatoid arthritis frequently is self-limited. In many cases evidence of active disease disappears in six months to one year, leaving few or no residua. In the remainder, several courses are possible. Some patients experience remissions and exacerbations, in a step-wise pattern, but remissions rarely restore the patient to the pre-exacerbation status. In other patients, progression is slow but steady. In the minority of patients, progression is rapid and inexorable.

Systemic features complicate the course of most patients whose disease becomes progressively worse. These systemic features include the development of rheumatoid nodules at pressure points, usually on the extensor surfaces of the forearms, the back of the skull, the lower end of the spine, and the back of the heel. Rheumatoid nodules also may form internally, in the lungs and meninges. In a large proportion of patients, the features of Sjögren's syndrome supervene, including dryness of the eyes and mouth, dry tracheitis, atrophic vaginitis, proctitis, patchy alopecia, pulmonary fibrosis, pleuritis, pericarditis, splenomegaly, and lymph node enlargement. In rare instances, tubular acidosis develops. Erythrocyte sedimentation rate generally reaches high levels, concurrent with development of anemia. Leukocytosis is frequent, although patients who have complicating Sjögren's features may have leukopenia. Dysproteinemia develops, with elevations of $alpha_2$ and gamma globulins, the latter a polyclonal gammopathy. Secondary amyloidosis as a sequel is encountered less frequently than was previously reported. Peripheral neuropathy (especially mononeuritis multiplex), peripheral skin ulcers, and a febrile course often characterize diffuse vasculitis, which may develop late in the course in some patients, and earlier in those treated with corticosteroids.

At the joints, early synovitis, through pannus formation and increased joint fluid, frequently leads to instability and deformity of synovial joints. As the disease progresses, arthritis may be mutilating, leading to shortening of bones because of cartilaginous and juxta-articular bone destruction; in some patients, fibrous ankylosis occurs instead, followed by bony ankylosis and resulting in joints that are immobile while deformed.

A multitude of serologic abnormalities can occur. Rheumatoid factor, as tested by latex fixation, is positive in titers of 1:80 or higher in about 70% of patients bearing this diagnosis. Positive lupus erythematosus preparations are found in 15% of the total, usually patients who also have positive rheumatoid factor tests. With the development of Sjögren's syndrome, other autoantibodies, including antinuclear antibodies, in some cases anti-DNA antibodies, antithyroid antibodies, and a variety of antimucosal antibodies can be discovered. Serologic tests for syphilis may register false positives in about 10% of these patients. Complement levels in the serum are normal or high, although reduced complement may be found in joint fluid. Rheumatoid joint fluid contains a large number of white blood cells, especially polymorphonuclear cells, usually above 5000/cm. Viscosity is poor, the fluid dropping like water. The fluid is turbid, and the mucin clot test shows dispersion of the material.

While the direction the disease will take is still obscure, analgesic and anti-inflammatory medications will provide comfort. As soon as progressive rheumatoid arthritis becomes apparent, administration of gold salts should be considered. These compounds become effective within three or four months of initiation of therapy. In a large proportion of patients, they seem to induce total remission. In a similar proportion, remission is not achieved, but the course appears to be slowed. In a minority of patients, perhaps 10%, there is a lack of effectiveness, and in a similar proportion, untoward toxic manifestations interdict continuation of this treatment. Antimalarial compounds appear to be weak in effecting remission, and the risk of retinal toxicity limits their use except in conjunction with careful and frequent ophthalmologic supervision. Intra-articular administration of corticosteroids after aspiration of excessive fluid provides approximately three weeks of relief at a given joint, and is especially indicated as part of a complete treatment program during the initiation of long-term management. Too frequent or too repetitious administration of corticosteroids into the joint should be avoided. Oral or parenteral steroid therapy now appears indicated in a minority of patients in whom the course is inexorable and defies the standard measures.

Hospitalization early in the course is recommended to initiate physical and occupational therapy, teach joint conservation techniques, investigate psychosocial factors and attempt environmental manipulation, and supervise the early stages of treatment. In selected patients who have rapidly progressive disease, immunosuppressive therapy may be offered under careful control, following peer review and elaboration of a searching protocol. Before destructive changes have occurred at a joint, synovectomy may slow or halt the progression of arthritis; reconstructive surgery, especially the newer total joint prostheses, can restore function and provide pain relief at joints already destroyed by the disease. The systemic features of rheumatoid arthritis rarely require separate management, often responding satisfactorily to standard therapeutic regimens.

References

Ehrlich, G. E. (Ed.): Total Management of the Arthritic Patient. Philadelphia, J. B. Lippincott, 1972.

Hollander, J. L., and McCarty, D. J., Jr. (Eds.): Arthritis and Allied Conditions. 8th Ed., Philadelphia, Lea & Febiger, 1972.

Sharp, J. T., Calkins, E., Cohen, A. S., Schubart, A. F., and Calabro, J. J.: Observations on the clinical, chemical, and serological manifestations of rheumatoid arthritis. Medicine, *43*:41, 1964.

3. Inflammatory Osteoarthritis

GEORGE EHRLICH

Cause: Unknown. Familial history and onset in women about the time of menopause suggest hereditary and hormonal complicity.

Early Manifestations: Symmetrical joint pain and swelling, especially in the interphalangeal joints of the fingers.

Treatment: Analgesic and anti-inflammatory medications. Surgery.

Possible Dire Consequences without Treatment: Greater discomfort.

Inflammatory osteoarthritis afflicts a significant minority of those patients in whom degenerative joint disease is diagnosed. It is characterized by the abrupt onset of pain, tenderness, swelling, and marked redness at interphalangeal joints of the fingers. While generally afflicting women between the ages of forty-five and fifty-five, earlier onset seems to be provoked by artificial menopause or strong familial history, and later onset is also possible. Men may develop inflammatory osteoarthritis, but the onset is generally later in life, and the proportion of men to women seen with this condition is rather small. Both the distal and proximal interphalangeal joints of the fingers are the sites of the earliest lesions, the interphalangeal and metacarpophalangeal joints of the thumbs sharing this predilection. However, other metacarpophalangeal joints may occasionally take part in this syndrome, and the carpometacarpal joint at the base of the thumb characteristically is involved, with squaring of the thenar eminence. Concurrent involvement of cervical spine, knees, and hips is frequent, though it is by no means a certainty that these lesions are etiologically related.

The disease is symmetrical, and painful only during a self-limited period lasting from a few months to about five years. Characteristic osteophytic development at joint margins leads to knobby deformities, and erosive lesions can be seen on roentgenography. Erosive osteoarthritis is the usual end result, leading to deformities that rarely disable the patient except when they afflict the knees, consistent with continued function but cosmetically unacceptable.

Standard anti-inflammatory medication helps to relieve the symptoms in the acute phases, but surgical correction is the only recourse once permanent deformities have become established. Unless there is marked impairment of joint function, such surgical intervention is probably not indicated. Physical measures, including the wearing of stretch gloves overnight, can help to relieve the stiffness and associated symptoms and discomforts that plague patients during the chronic phase of the disease.

On the whole, functional prognosis is good.

Reference

Ehrlich, G. E.: Inflammatory osteoarthritis. J. Chronic Dis., *25*:317, 1972.

4. Osteoarthritis of the Hip

JAMES P. MARVEL, JR.

Cause: Idiopathic, possible biochemical causes.

Early Manifestations: Progressive pain in hip often presenting as referred pain to the medial aspect of the knee.

Treatment: Arthroplasty

Possible Dire Consequences without Treatment: Continued severe pain and disability.

Osteoarthritis of the hip is perhaps the most common cause of gait disturbances in the aging patient. Often the complaints of the patient will progress over a period of years being primarily involved with pain in the lateral aspect of the hip and groin with radiation to the medial aspect of the knee. This pain is usually progressive in nature and begins as pain aggravated by activity and weight bearing. As time progresses this pain becomes of a more constant nature and eventually will be present even at rest. Typically the patient will present with an antalgic type of gait.

The most common type of osteoarthritis is that which is referred to as idiopathic or for which no specific cause can be found. Other causes of osteoarthritis of the hip involve the secondary changes associated with rheumatoid arthritis, previous trauma with damage to the joint resulting in irregularity of the joint surfaces, predisposing congenital dysplasia of the hip, and secondary changes occurring associated with avascular necrosis. Associated with the progressive pain and limp is a progressive restriction of the active and passive range of motion of the hip.

Patients presenting with the earliest form of osteoarthritis are best treated by conservative measures which include protection of weight bearing, active exercise program for muscle strengthening of the structures about the hip, salicylates or anti-inflammatory medications such as the phenyl butazone group, and the intra-articular injection of steroids.

Once the patient has reached the point where pain is present during all stages of weight bearing and/or at rest surgical measures should be contemplated. Surgical measures may include the use of osteotomy, femoral endoprosthesis or total hip replacement. Within the past few years there has been a definite increase in the use of the total hip replacement in the United States with uniformly gratifying results in regard to osteoarthritis of the hip. Osteoarthritis of the hip remains the prime indication for the use of total hip replacement.

The following references will give further specific information in regard to osteoarthritis of the hip.

References

Campbell, R. E. and Rothman, R. H.: Chainley low-friction total hip replacement. Am. J. Roent. Ras. Ther. and Nuc. Med. CXIII, 1971.

Charnley, J.: The long-term results of low-friction arthroplasty of the hip performed as a primary intervention. J. Bone Joint Surg. (Br.) 54:61, 1972.

De Palma, A. F., Rothman, R. H., and Klemek, J. S.: Osteotomy of the proximal femur in degenerative arthritis. Clin. Ortho. No. 73, Nov.–Dec. 1970.

Stinchfield, F. E. and White, E. S.: Total hip replacement. Ann. Surg. 174:655, 1971.

Tronzo, R. G.: Surgery of the Hip Joint. Philadelphia, Lea & Febiger, 1973.

Chapter III

Eye Diseases

Introduction

There is a bare minimum of diseases which the practitioner of all branches of medicine may encounter frequently. For instance, certain drugs, such as corticosteroids and parasympathomimetic preparations, are associated with cataracts.

The subject of Red Eye is of importance to all physicians and surgeons. Most frequently this is caused by conjunctivitis. However, the possibility of its being either iridocyclitis or glaucoma is always present.

1. The Red Eye

WILLIAM BURNS

Cause: Usually conjunctivitis, iridocyclitis, or acute glaucoma.

Early Manifestations: Various degrees of pain, lacrimation, decreased visual acuity.

Treatment: Depending on the condition.

Possible Dire Consequences without Treatment: Anything from prolonged irritability to loss of vision and/or eye.

In the absence of trauma or foreign body, the possibility of one of the above three conditions should be considered. A diagnosis is important in order to estimate the seriousness of the condition and to plan the proper treatment.

TABLE III–1. DIAGNOSES IN RED EYE

	Conjunctivitis	*Iridocyclitis*	*Acute Glaucoma*
Location vision	Usually bilateral, normal or slightly blurred because of secretions	Usually unilateral, normal to extremely blurred	Usually unilateral, greatly impaired
Intraocular tension	Normal	Normal	Increased
Redness (see plates)	Away from cornea in cul-de-sac area	Adjacent to cornea	Marked infection throughout
Pupils	Normal	Usually constricted due to ciliary spasm	Semi-dilated and fixed.
Cause	Bacteria, allergy, virus	Inflammatory process	Changes in eye causing increased intraocular pressure
Photophobia	None	Severe	None
Pain	Radiating to forehead and temple, worse at night	Severe in and about eyes to the extent of causing nausea	Discomfort, but no real pain
Treatment	Cycloplegia, local heat, rest, try to find cause (possibly steroids)	Medical miosis with 1% pilocarpine Surgical: iridectomy, possibly enucleation	Rest, compresses, 10% sulfacetamide, ointment, search for exact cause

Reference

Allen, J. H.: May's Diseases of the Eye. 24th Ed. Baltimore, The Williams & Wilkins Co., 1968.

Chapter IV

Skin Diseases

Introduction

Thanks to the advent of new pharmaceutical preparations, notably corticosteroids, certain diseases of the skin can now be specifically treated. Patients with ghastly conditions, such as pemphigus and mycosis fungoides, may now be helped or even cured, whereas previously they could only be comforted. On the other hand, one should always remember how frequently the skin is adversely affected by various pharmaceutical preparations, some of which have been in constant use for many years.

1. Dermatitis Herpetiformis

Paul Gross

Cause: Unknown.

Early Manifestations: Symmetrical pruritus; urticarial bullous rash over shoulder, back, buttocks, and extremities.

Treatment: Sulfapyridine and sulfones.

Possible Dire Consequences without Treatment: Chronic pruritus with discomfort.

This rare condition is characterized by the development of extremely pruritic vesicular skin lesions. Occasionally urticarial and bullous forms are recognized. The mucous membranes, particularly of the small bowel, are sometimes involved. The eruption tends to be grouped and symmetrically distributed over the shoulders, back, buttocks, and extremities. It may last a lifetime or disappear after several years. The cause is unknown, though many patients have an associated gluten-sensitive enteropathy. However, treatment of the small bowel disease does not affect the skin, nor does improvement in the skin relieve the gastrointestinal problems. Histopathol gically, blisters develop in a subepidermal location, at the tips of the dermal papillae. Though the condition may respond to administration of systemic steroids, characteristically it is dramatically improved with sulfapyridine or sulfones. The response to treatment is so striking that these agents may be used as a therapeutic diagnostic test. Since other antibiotics, including sulfonamides, are not effective,

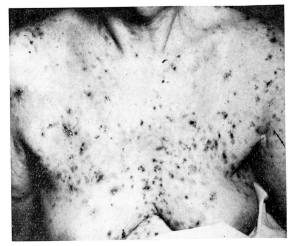

Fig. IV–1. Dermatitis herpetiformis

these agents are probably not working through an antibacterial mechanism. Usually one starts with a dose of 2.0 gm. sulfapyridine per day and gradually reduces the dose, as the disease comes under control. As much as 4.0 gm. per day may be required. When the rash abates, the doses are gradually reduced to maintenance levels, which may be as low as 0.5 gm. per day. Sulfapyridine can cause leukopenia, and so the white blood cell count should be determined periodically. Approximately every six months the medication should be discontinued to see whether the disease is still active. Occasionally, patients are not relieved by sulfapyridine, and in such cases diaminodiphenylsulfone may be employed. This is a more toxic drug and may induce methemoglobinemia and hemolytic anemias even in patients with normal levels of glucose-6-phosphate dehydrogenase. It also produces headaches and nausea. Again, the smallest possible dose that controls the rash is recommended.

Reference

Domonkos, A. N.: Dermatitis herpetiformis (Dhuring's disease). *In* Diseases of the Skin. 6th Ed. Edited by G. C. Andrews and A. N. Domonkos. Philadelphia, W. B. Saunders Co., 1971.

2. Bullous Pemphigoid

PAUL GROSS

Cause: Generally idiopathic, but may be drug induced.

Early Manifestations: Bullae, smaller than in pemphigus and less frequently seen in mucous membranes.

Treatment: Steroids and immunosuppressive agents, in smaller doses than in pemphigus vulgaris.

Possible Dire Consequences without Treatment: Mortality lower than in pemphigus vulgaris.

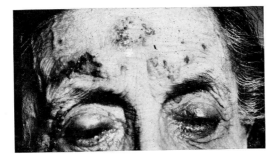

Fig. IV–2. Bullous pemphigoid.

This condition may be confused with pemphigus. It occurs mainly in elderly patients, may be idiopathic, drug-induced, or related to occult malignancy. These patients develop cutaneous blisters, but usually *no* mucosal ulcerations. The bullae are usually smaller, more tense, and rupture less easily. It does *not* lead to rapid demise if untreated. Here, the blisters form in a subepidermal location, and acantholysis is not observed histologically. These patients also may show circulating immuno-globulins, but they are directed against the basement membrane at the dermal-epidermal junction. The disease responds to elimination of causal factors, if possible. It also may be controlled with systemic steroids, though usually the heroic doses required in pemphigus are not needed. Here, too, immunosuppressant agents can be used with good effect (see under Pemphigus Vulgaris).

Reference

Domonkos, A. N.: Bullous pemphigoid. *In* Diseases of the Skin. 6th Ed. Edited by G. C. Andrews and A. N. Domonkos. Philadelphia, W. B. Saunders Co., 1971.

3. Pemphigus Vulgaris

Paul Gross

Cause: An autoimmune process seems likely.

Early Manifestations: Flaccid or tense bullae with little tendency to heal.

Treatment: Huge doses of corticosteroids and immunosuppressive agents.

Possible Dire Consequences without Treatment: Death.

This serious blistering disease was formerly universally fatal. Contrary to early beliefs, it occurs in all races, both sexes, and in patients of all ethnic origins. The blisters involve the mucous membranes as well as the skin. Erosions and secondary infection are common. The classic cutaneous sign is the Nikolsky phenomenon, in which gentle pressure applied to the skin produces a blister or causes the extension of a blister that is already present.

Histopathologically, one sees within the epidermis a blister that has formed by acantholysis. This is a peculiar breaking up of cellular connections, which is confirmed by electromicroscopy as a dissolution of the tonofilament-desmosomal complexes at the epidermal cellular junctions. Recently, immunofluorescent techniques have demonstrated the presence of circulating antibodies in the sera of these patients. These antibodies localize at the cellular membranes, the site of the pathologic process. Additional evidence for an autoimmune process is the high correlation of other immunologic abnormalities, such as the association with lupus erythematosus in some cases, the presence of antinuclear antibodies, and the occasional association with thymoma.

Systemic steroids are life-saving, and are given in doses high enough to control the blistering process (prednisone, 500 mg. [or more] daily). Since long-term therapy is required, all measures must be taken to reduce steroid side effects. It has been found that a single daily dose of steroids may be as effective as several smaller doses. This may prevent many complications. Alternate-day therapy also can be tried after control has been achieved. Additional precautions are prophylactic antacids and a bland diet to prevent peptic ulceration. Hypertension is to be expected and should be treated when it develops. Diabetes almost always develops, but it is nonketotic and is likely to be insulin-resistant; therefore, it often is not treated. Calcium, estrogens, and androgens together may prevent steroid-induced osteoporosis. Isoniazid may be given prophylactically to prevent any reactivation of tuberculosis.

Unfortunately, although many patients survive their pemphigus, a large number die of infections, gastrointestinal bleeding, or other steroid-related complications. Lately, it has been most gratifying to use immunosuppressive agents to allow us to reduce the steroid dosage more rapidly: methotrexate in weekly doses of 50 to 100 mg. IM or IV and/or cyclophosphamide 100 to 150 mg. per day. Appropriate checks of the hematologic, hepatic, and renal systems must be performed. It remains to be seen whether long-term usage of immunosuppressants leads to the development of lymphomas and other malignancies in these patients.

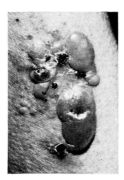

Fig. IV–3. Pemphigus vulgaris.

Reference

Anderson, H. J., Newcomer, V. D., Landau, J. W., and Rosenthal, L. H.: Pemphigus and other diseases. Arch. Derm., *101*:538, 1970.

4. Erythema Multiforme— Stevens-Johnson Syndrome

PAUL GROSS

Cause: Hypersensitivity reactions to drugs and infections.

Early Manifestations: Macular or papular urticaria, bullae, conjunctivitis.

Treatment: Huge doses of steroids and treatment of infection.

Possible Dire Consequences without Treatment: Panophthalmia, blindness, nephritis, carditis, death.

These cutaneous hypersensitivity reactions are characterized by widespread skin lesions, which may be urticarial, macular, papular, or bullous. Most characteristic is the lesion in the iris. The cause is usually found to be a drug reaction. Sulfonamides are the most serious offender, but virtually any drug may be responsible. Other causes include streptococcal infections, viral infections (especially herpes), deep fungal infections (such as histoplasmosis), or internal malignant disease.

The most severe form of this disease is known as Stevens-Johnson syndrome, in which bullous and ulcerative mucous membrane lesions predominate. There may be severe stomatitis and vulvovaginitis. The eyes are almost always involved with conjunctivitis, keratitis, or panophthalmitis, which can lead to blindness. Secondary septicemia accounts for the high mortality rate. Stevens-Johnson syndrome is a medical emergency, and high doses of systemic steroids are required along with supportive measures. Uusally, systemic antibiotics are given prophylactically. The doses of steroids (100 to 200 mg. prednisone per day) are often required for several weeks. If patients do not improve rapidly, the dosage of steroids should be doubled every one or two days until the proper levels are obtained. The dosage is then reduced slowly over several weeks. Early ophthalmologic consultation is highly desirable.

Reference

Coursin, D. B.: Stevens-Johnson syndrome: nonspecific parasensitivity reaction? J.A.M.A., *198*:113, 1966.

5. Porphyria Cutanea Tarda

Paul Gross

Cause: Rarely genetic, usually secondary to liver disease.

Early Manifestations: Pigmentation, hirsutism, fragility and blistering in areas exposed to sunlight.

Treatment: Phlebotomy, abstinence from alcohol and other contributing drugs, sodium bicarbonate.

Possible Dire Consequences without Treatment: Continued morbidity and death, probably from hepatic disease.

This is another somewhat unusual syndrome with cutaneous and systemic manifestations. Though there are rare genetic forms of the disease, most are acquired and are secondary to liver disease (such as hepatoma, alcoholic cirrhosis) or drug-induced. Barbiturates, sulfonamides, and estrogens are most often responsible. Patients usually have impaired liver function tests associated with the photosensitivity reaction. The skin changes are pigmentation, hirsutism, and fragility and blistering in areas exposed to sunlight, such as the face, back of the hands, and back of the neck. It is not to be confused with acute intermittent porphyria, in which patients have abdominal crises, neurologic signs, and high excretion rates of porphobilinogen (detected by a positive Watson-Schwartz test). Patients with porphyria cutanea tarda have high fecal and urinary excretion of coproporphyrins and uroporphyrins. If a urine sample is acidified and exposed to a black light, typical red fluorescence is demonstrated. There is an extremely rare condition known as porphyria variegata, in which the signs and chemical abnormalities of both acute intermittent porphyria and porphyria cutanea tarda are present simultaneously.

Treatment of porphyria cutanea tarda consists of abstinence from alcohol, and from any drugs that are believed to be contributory. Specifically, the most effective therapeutic modality is phlebotomy. In these patients, high hemoglobin and hematocrit levels generally exist, but not polycythemia. The serum iron levels are often elevated, with increased saturation of the iron-binding capacity. However, even in patients with normal iron, improvement is effected by bleeding. Usually, 500 cc. of blood is drawn weekly until the urine is no longer fluorescent, at which point hemoglobin levels are reduced to the level of 10 or 12%. The patients become asymptomatic and remissions may be permanent. Occasionally, repeated courses of treatment may be required if symptoms recur after several months or years.

References

Dean, G.: The Porphyrias. London, Pitman Medical Publishing Co., 1963.
Wirgand, S. E., Copeman, P. W. M., and Perry, H. O.: Metabolic alkalinization in porphyria cutanea tarda. Arch. Derm., *100*:544, 1969.

6. Mycosis Fungoides

PAUL GROSS

Cause: Not understood.

Early Manifestations: Pruritus and eczematous rashes; later discrete plaque formation; and still later tumors.

Treatment: Topical nitrogen mustard solution.

Possible Dire Consequences without Treatment: Tumor stage, disseminated lymphomata, death.

This rare cutaneous reticulosis classically has three distinct stages.

Stage 1. For years the patient may have only pruritus and nondescript erythematous rashes. The histopathology at this time is not diagnostic.

Stage 2. Gradually discrete plaques develop at which time the diagnosis can be made.

Stage 3. The final stage is one of painful ulcerating cutaneous tumors, with eventual demise being due to secondary infection or inanition.

In some cases, there may be transition to other lymphomas including Hodgkin's disease and monocytic leukemia.

Initially, patients are helped by steroids, locally at first, then systemically. X-ray and superficial radiation (grenz ray, electron beam therapy) may give temporary relief. Systemic chemotherapeutic agents such as methotrexate also may be employed as the disease progresses.

Of recent extreme interest is the finding that the patients can be completely cleared of the disease in the early stages by topical treatment with nitrogen mustard solution. Although this is a potent sensitizing agent and some patients develop severe contact dermatitis precluding further use, some subjects realize complete clearing of the disease without systemic toxicity. Certainly long-lasting remissions have been induced. However, it remains to be seen whether these patients are actually cured. This form of treatment is most effective in Stage 1 or Stage 2, before tumors develop. The solution must be prepared freshly each day and applied to the entire surface of the skin. It may lead to rather intense pigmentation, but this is a small price to pay. Experimental work, involving pretreatment with cyclophosphamide, is under way to develop a program whereby immunologic tolerance can be induced to such an extent that these patients do not become allergic to the compound.

References

Epstein, E. H., Jr., Levin, D. L., Croft, J. D., Jr., and Lutzner, M. A.: Mycosis Fungoides. Medicine, *51*:61, 1972.

Pillsbury, D. W., Shelley, W. B., and Kligman, S. M.: Dermatology. Philadelphia, W. B. Saunders Co., 1955.

Taswell, H. F., and Winklemann, R. K.: Sézary syndrome—a malignant reticulemic erythroderma. J.A.M.A., *177*:465, 1961.

7. Angioneurotic Edema

ORVILLE HORWITZ

Cause: Allergy to drugs, frequently to penicillin; often a psychosomatic condition in patients with allergic background.

Early Manifestations: Localized edema. May present as partial or very rarely complete esophageal or intestinal obstruction. Also may present as laryngeal edema.

Treatment: Adrenalin or corticosteroids.

Possible Dire Consequences without Treatment: Usually nothing more than temporary discomfort and embarrassment, but high mortality from laryngeal obstruction in familial type.

This disease may be a debilitating condition in which local edema may cause closure of the eyes, gross enlargement of the tongue, partial (and occasionally complete) obstruction of the larynx or esophagus, and generalized giant urticaria.

There are apparently three types:

1. Following drug therapy as an allergy, often to penicillin.
2. Idiopathic and recurring, often triggered by trauma or an insect bite.
3. Hereditary angioneurotic edema (HANE) associated with absence of serum inhibition of C'1-esterase.

Types 1 and 2 usually respond well to low doses of corticosteroids or to epinephrine, 0.5 ml. of 1:1000 solution subcutaneously.

Type 3 does not respond as well to these pharmaceutical preparations. Prophylaxis by epsilon-aminocaproic acid (EACA) is far from satisfactory at this time.

References

Donaldson, V. H.: Therapy of "the neurotic edema." New Eng. J. Med., *286*:835, 1972.

Frank, M. M., Sergent, J. S., Kane, M. A., and Alling, D. W.: Epsilon aminocaproic acid therapy of hereditary angioneurotic edema: a double-blind study. New Eng. J. Med., *286*:808, 1972.

Chapter V

Neurologic Diseases

Introduction

Until recently, certain infections, certain benign tumors, and vitamin B$_{12}$ deficiency were the only neurologic conditions for which there was adequate treatment. Because of new pharmaceutical preparations and greatly improved techniques in vascular and neurologic surgery, we have been able to add many more to this list. It is hoped that this material will help the internist and general practitioner to recognize these diseases.

Other conditions which may present as neurological disease, but are in fact diseases originating in other systems: Vitamin B$_{12}$ deficiency. Hypertension. Arteriosclerosis. Multiple myeloma. Meningitides. Central nervous system, Lues. Delirium tremors. Polycythemia. Sickle cell anemia. Beriberi. Psychoses. Insulin porphyria. Macroglobulin anemia. Temporal arteritis. Emboli. CO poisoning.

1. Transient Ischemic Attacks

FRANK ELLIOTT

Cause: Commonly due to microembolism, less often to episodes of arterial hypertension in patients with carotid or vertebral-basilar stenosis, or to constriction of diseased carotid or vertebral arteries by head turning in patients with cervical spondylosis.

Early Manifestations: Episodes of focal cerebral dysfunction lasting from five minutes to several hours.

Treatment: Anticoagulants, aspirin(?), surgical correction of stenosed arteries, control of factors thought to accelerate atherosclerosis and its complications, removal of osteophytes compressing vertebral arteries.

Possible Dire Consequences without Treatment: Stroke; continued symptoms.

The term "transient ischemic attack" applies to brief episodes of cerebral dysfunction of vascular origin which are not followed by persistent neurologic deficit. Symptoms last a few minutes to several hours. As ordinarily understood, the term does not include symptoms resulting from reduced cerebral blood flow secondary to failure of the systemic circulation—as in fainting, severe hemorrhage, myocardial infarction, Stokes-Adams syndrome, tussive syncope, carotid sinus sensitivity, or severe postural hypotension. However, an episode of hypotension or hypoglycemia can cause a brief neurologic deficit in patients with carotid or vertebral-basilar stenosis.

In most cases, the condition is associated with occlusive vascular disease. Small fragments of blood clot, or microemboli composed of fused platelets or atheromatous material, break off from atheromatous plaques and are swept upward to become impacted in small intracranial or intraocular vessels. Emboli from the heart also may cause transient ischemic attacks, but are more apt to produce massive infarction.

The clinical features of transient ischemic episodes in the carotid system include unilateral weakness, numbness on one side of the body, aphasia, disturbance of thinking, monocular blurring of vision, brief impairment of memory, disorientation of time and place, and—perhaps—focal epileptic seizures.

In the vertebral-basilar system the symptoms are more diverse. They include vertigo, diplopia, transient paralysis of gaze, homonymous hemianopia, cortical blindness, scintillating visual hallucinations, memory lapses (including global amnesia), numbness down one side of the body or on one side of the face, bilateral weakness, alternating weakness on the two sides of the body, dysarthria, dysphagia, impaired hearing in one ear, attacks of vertigo, episodes of staggering, sudden drop attacks without unconsciousness, and a curious sense of lightheadedness without vertigo.

The prognosis is variable. In a fifteen-year follow-up of patients with transient ischemic attacks, conducted at the Mayo Clinic, 50% died of cardiac disease and 36% died of stroke. Morbidity and mortality rates are adversely affected by increasing age, heart disease, and hypertension.

Treatment

Long-term treatment with anticoagulants is effective in reducing the number and severity of transient attacks. Anticoagulants are contraindicated in the very elderly, in diabetics, and in the presence of uncontrolled hypertension. Recent experience suggests that the type of transient ischemic attack caused by platelet emboli can be controlled by the administration of 300 mg. aspirin twice a day; the drug inhibits platelet stickiness and their tendency to aggregate. This treatment is under evaluation at the present time.

Patients with stenosis of the internal carotid or vertebral arteries should be considered for surgical reconstructive operations, but surgery is contraindicated in the presence of severe persistent neurologic deficit, occlusive arterial disease involving multiple cranial and peripheral arteries, or associated with myocardial infarction or congestive heart failure.

The patient in whom transient ischemic attacks are induced by head turning should wear a Thomas collar. There is some evidence that removal of osteophytes that compress the vertebral arteries may be beneficial (Smith et al., 1972).

All these forms of treatment, however, are short-term measures and must be reinforced by such measures as may retard the advance of the underlying disease, atherosclerosis.

Prospective studies carried out in Framingham, Mass., Evans County, Ga., Los Angeles, and Hiroshima, have identified risk factors which appear to increase liability to stroke. The same risk factors apply to coronary thrombosis. They are hypertension, hypercholesterolemia, diabetes, a hematocrit in the upper range of normal, and the cigarette habit. It is generally believed that hypertriglyceridemia and severe emotional stress also contribute to both strokes and myocardial infarction. Strokes are also more liable to occur in patients with arteriosclerotic heart disease.

Evidence is accumulating that careful control of hypertension, the hyperlipidemias, the hematocrit, diabetes, and obesity, together with avoidance of cigarettes and the reduction of stress can significantly affect the prognosis in patients with cerebral vascular disease. Elliott and Leonberg have treated a group of 102 patients who had survived a thrombotic cerebral infarction for an average period of five years. This model was chosen because its natural prognosis is known. Several studies have found that such patients die at the rate of 10 to 12% per year, usually from another stroke or from a myocardial infarction. For treated patients in the series, the mortality was 3.8% per year.

Hypertension, defined as a blood pressure (in the office) of 160/100, is treated on traditional lines. Diabetes is strictly controlled by diet with or without insulin or oral agents. Blood cholesterol and triglycerides are maintained below 250 and 150 mg. % respectively, by diet, supplemented in some cases by clofibrate. However, whether the fasting lipids are elevated or not, all patients are prescribed a diet low in fat and sugar because the alimentary lipemia induced by a rich meal produces conditions favorable to the deposition of mural thrombi—shortening of coagulation time, increased platelet stickiness, and a sharp reduction in fibrinolytic activity.

An hematocrit of 50% or more is treated by phlebotomy, which is repeated as often as necessary. This reversion to eighteenth century medical practice is based on the observation that modest elevations of the hematocrit within the range of what is usually considered normal appear to predispose to stroke and myocardial infarction. Second, when the hematocrit approaches 50%, capillary blood flow is retarded, as can readily be seen in the bulbar conjunctival vessels. Since the increase of viscosity associated with these modest elevations of the hematocrit is insufficient to affect blood flow through arteries the size of the coronary and cerebral vessels, the impact of an elevated hematocrit must be on the microcirculation, including the vasa vasorum. A study currently in progress in New York may provide the answers as to whether the regular reduction of the hematocrit by phlebotomy (in blood donors) will reduce the incidence of stroke and myocardial infarction.

Cigarette smoking should be banned.

Stress is a part of modern life which is difficult to assess and control. Clinical experience provides many examples of a stroke or a myocardial infarction following a period of severe emotional stress. Acute stress, even if pleasurable, increases the blood pressure and causes an elevation of free fatty acids and catecholamines. The latter increases platelet stickiness. Furthermore, continuous stress can produce an elevation of the hematocrit, the blood pressure, and free fatty acids.

Much can be done to reduce stress by alterations of working habits and by the judicious use of mild sedatives, but there are situations (and personalities) which defy adjustment; for such, Taggart and Carruthers suggest that beta adrenergic blocking agents, such as Oxprenolol, may prove useful because they suppress stress-induced elevations of free fatty acids, blood glucose and tachycardia.

Regular surveillance is necessary in order to identify elevations of blood pressure, departures from the prescribed diet, escape from diabetic control, unexpected increases of the hematocrit, and episodes of stress. Patients should be seen at regular intervals, from every two weeks to every three months, depending on the circumstances.

References

Elliott, F. A. and Leonberg, S. C.: A Program for Stroke Prevention. Proceedings of the 53rd Annual Session of the American College of Physicians, Apr. 1972, Atlantic City.

Smith, D. R., Vanderark, G. B. and Kempe, L. G.: Cervical Spondylosis Causing Vertebral Basilar Insufficiency: A Surgical Treatment. J. Neurol. Neurosurg. & Psychiatry, *34*:388, 1971.

Taggart, P. and Carruthers, M.: Suppression by Oxprenolol of Adrenergic Response to Stress. Lancet, *2*:256, 1972.

2. Herpes Zoster (Shingles)

FRANK ELLIOTT

Cause: A virus that is closely related to that of chicken pox.

Early Manifestations: Pain in the distribution of one or more sensory nerve roots, is followed within one to five days by a herpetic rash in the cutaneous distribution of the affected roots.

Treatment: Prompt administration of large doses of steroids.

Possible Dire Consequences without Treatment: Persistent and untreatable postherpetic neuralgia; occasionally, muscular paralysis.

The virus attacks one or more sensory ganglia, usually on one side of the body but sometimes on both. The inflammatory process can extend inward to the meninges and into the root entry zone of the spinal cord; occasionally it involves the ventral horns, resulting in lower motor neuron paralysis of more or less segmental distribution. The related peripheral nerve or nerves are involved by a true inflammatory neuritis. Encephalitis and myelitis occasionally occur in debilitated subjects.

The earliest symptom is pain in the distribution of the affected root or roots— around the trunk, or as a linear strip on the upper or lower limb, or in one or more divisions of the trigeminal nerve. It involves the pinna, external auditory meatus, and anterior pillar of the fauces in geniculate herpes. In rare instances the disease is painless. The skin of the affected zone is hyperesthetic even before the rash appears. If muscular paralysis appears, it is not always within the area of the rash, and it may become evident one to two weeks after the rash has appeared. Such paralysis is uncommon except in the case of geniculate herpes, which is usually accompanied by facial paralysis resembling Bell's palsy.

Postherpetic neuralgia is a common sequel, particularly in patients over fifty. The pain is persistent, and is usually aggravated by emotion and fatigue. The skin is at first sensitive to touch, but after a year or two this sensitivity disappears.

In the pre-eruptive stage, the pain can lead to a mistaken diagnosis of thoracic or abdominal disease. The possibility of herpes should be considered in all cases of thoracic or abdominal pain of a relatively rapid onset in which no other cause can be found. Rarely, the eruption is so slight that it is missed, and if this happens in a patient reporting with a rapid onset of muscular weakness of segmental distribution accompanied by fever for a few days, it is possible to make an erroneous diagnosis of poliomyelitis. Every case of Bell's palsy should be closely scrutinized for evidence of herpetic vesicles. In ophthalmic herpes there is special danger to the eye, which may be secondarily infected by bacteria. This can lead to panophthalmitis, and even if this does not occur, corneal opacities or glaucoma can result from the herpes itself. Partial third nerve palsies and primary optic atrophy have been described.

In most cases, herpes zoster arises in otherwise healthy individuals; in a minority, it occurs against a background of lymphoma, leukemia, carcinoma, radiation therapy, or the use of immunosuppressive drugs. Under these circumstances, the treatment of herpes by steroids is contraindicated because it may lead to generalization of the infection.

Herpes zoster occurring in otherwise healthy persons should be treated by *large doses* of steroids as soon as the rash appears. The *minimum* dose is 60 mg. a day for a week, 30 mg. a day for the second week, and 10 mg. a day for the third week. An antacid should be given between meals. Provided treatment is started in *the first four or five days* of the rash, the pain disappears in twenty-four to seventy-two hours and never returns. Postherpetic neuralgia does not occur when steroids are used promptly and in sufficient doses; moreover herpetic paralysis subsides within weeks, as opposed to months in untreated cases.

When steroids have not been administered and postherpetic neuralgia is present, there is no entirely satisfactory method of treatment. X-ray therapy, alcohol injection of the affected roots, division of sensory roots, and ultrasound are, in my opinion, a waste of time. It has been reported that the application of a vibrator to the affected area of the skin for twenty minutes several times a day is helpful. Attempts to abolish the pain by stereotaxic operations on the thalamus are being made at the present time.

References

Elliott, F. A.: Treatment of herpes zoster with high doses of prednisone. Lancet 2:610, 1964.
Russell, W. R.: Treatment of Post-Herpetic Neuralgia. Lancet 1:242, 1957.

3. Tic Douloureux (Paroxysmal Trigeminal Neuralgia)

FRANK ELLIOTT

Cause: Unknown.

Early Manifestations: Paroxysms of lancinating pain occurring in one or more divisions of the trigeminal nerve, in the absence of objective signs of neurologic disease in the face or elsewhere.

Treatment: Carbamazepine (Tegretol) is effective in 90% of all cases; surgical measures are necessary for the remainder.

Possible Dire Consequences without Treatment: Continued symptoms.

Tic douloureux occurs at any age after puberty, but four-fifths of all patients are between forty and seventy years of age. It is more common in women than in men. The pain usually involves the second or third division of the nerve, or both, and it may spread to all three, but it is seldom confined to the first division. It is usually unilateral, but can be bilateral. Pain occurs in recurrent bouts which last days, weeks, or months, with intervals of complete freedom. During each bout the pain is intermittent, but as time goes on it tends to become persistent and more severe, with fewer and shorter intermissions.

The pain is described as knife-like, red hot needles under the skin, or painful electric shocks. The face may suddenly screw up as the result of pain, hence the term "tic." The pain often can be induced by a light touch to trigger areas within the territory of the affected division, and may also be caused by talking or eating, or by a cold draft. It is characteristic of the condition that the pain is more easily evoked by light stimuli than by strong ones. Unilateral lacrimation and reddening of the eye can occur, and salivation is not unknown.

There is no sensory loss. There may be graying of the hair and coating of the tongue on the affected side. The spinal fluid is normal in all respects.

Precisely similar pain, unaccompanied by sensory loss or other objective neurologic findings, occasionally occurs during the early development of tumors and aneurysms in the cerebellopontine angle, multiple sclerosis, persistence of the embryonal trigeminal artery, glioma of the pons, and syringobulbia. Frontal and maxillary sinusitis occasionally causes a stabbing pain with tic-like periodicity. The same is true of neoplasms of the maxilla and nasopharynx and disease of the temporomandibular joint, but generally speaking the pain caused by these conditions is more constant than tic douloureux, and there are usually accessory symptoms and signs that make the diagnosis clear. Postherpetic neuralgia and other continuous pains in the face are so different from the recurrent shooting spasms of tic douloureux that they should not cause confusion.

The condition tends to worsen with advancing years and is apt to undermine both health and morale. If the second and third divisions are involved, the patient ultimately becomes afraid to eat, and this can cause a severe degree of inanition.

The treatment of tic douloureux has been revolutionized by the introduction of carbamazepine, which suppresses the pain though it does not cure the disease. The oral administration of 200 mg. three times a day, one hour before meals, is effective in the majority of cases. Sometimes a single dose taken in the morning protects the patient from pain throughout the day; in resistant cases it may be necessary to give as many as 10 tablets during the day. Side effects in the form of nausea, dizziness, skin rashes, and severe depression of neutrophil leukocytes occasionally contraindicate the use of the drug. Dilantin, in doses of 100 mg. three times a day, is less effective than carbamazepine.

Surgical measures are necessary if carbamazepine (Tegretol) produces too many side effects or if, as sometimes happens, the patient acquires a tolerance to the drug. The most reliable surgical measures are injections of alcohol into the roots or trigeminal ganglion, and section of the sensory root. These procedures lead to complete sensory loss with relief of the pain, but in some cases the patient is troubled by unpleasant burning paresthesias in the affected area of the face. This discomfort cannot be relieved by further injection or by root section.

It may be mentioned in passing that carbamazepine is also effective in the treatment of the lightning pains of tabes dorsalis.

References

Elliott, F. A.: Clinical Neurology, 2nd Ed., pp. 156–158. Philadelphia, W. B. Saunders Co., 1971.
White, J. C., and Sweet, W. H.: Pain and the Neurosurgeon. Springfield, Charles C Thomas, 1969.

4. Bell's Palsy

Frank Elliott

Cause: An inflammatory condition of the seventh nerve as it lies in its bony canal proximal to the stylomastoid foramen.

Early Manifestations: Rapid onset of facial paralysis, sometimes accompanied by pain over the mastoid.

Treatment: Steroids and physiotherapy.

Possible Dire Consequences without Treatment: Permanent facial paralysis.

Bell's palsy is predominantly a disease of young adults. The incidence is the same for both sexes. Pain behind the ear is sometimes present at the onset, and at this stage there may be deep tenderness behind the angle of the jaw. The affected side of the face feels stiff and numb, and paralysis comes on rapidly, becoming complete within twelve to twenty-four hours. The eye cannot be closed, and retraction of the angle of the mouth is impossible. The unopposed muscles on the sound side pull the mouth over to that side. Despite complaints of a sense of numbness in the face, there is no superficial sensory loss. Sometimes there is loss of taste over the anterior two-thirds of the tongue on the affected side. Occasionally, hyperacusis occurs, probably from involvement of the nerve to the stapedius muscle. The lower lid falls away from the eye, allowing tears to escape onto the cheek.

In about 70% of all cases, fibrillation is found on electromyography, without a reaction of degeneration; in such cases recovery is quick and complete. In the remainder, degeneration of the nerve occurs and recovery may not start for three months or more. The measurement of the conduction time in the facial nerve, between the front of the ear and the angle of the mouth, can be helpful in that full recovery is to be expected if conduction time is less than 4.0 milliseconds. Partial denervation is indicated if conduction time exceeds 4.0 milliseconds. When complete denervation is present, the nerve becomes inexcitable by the end of the first week.

Recovery may be incomplete, and contracture can lead to displacement of the angle of the mouth toward the paralyzed side. Misdirection of regenerating nerve fibers sometimes leads to troublesome synkinesia; for instance, the eye may close when the patient smiles.

Unilateral facial paralysis is seen in poliomyelitis, encephalitis, acute infective polyneuritis, and many forms of meningitis, both acute and chronic, but in such cases the general setting indicates its origin. In geniculate herpes there is a herpetiform rash in the auditory meatus, on the pinna, and on the anterior wall of the fauces. Facial paralysis can occur with affections of the parotid gland, including uveoparotid polyneuritis, a manifestation of sarcoidosis. Chronic otitis media, with or without cholesteatosis, is an occasional cause of facial palsy associated with deafness. Fracture of the petrous temporal bone is an obvious explanation for facial paralysis occurring at the time of an injury, but it may also occur a week to ten days after the injury.

Facial paralysis of slow onset does not enter into the differential diagnosis of Bell's palsy.

High doses of steroids or ACTH should be given as soon as the palsy develops, in order to inhibit the inflammatory process. This applies to both Bell's palsy and facial paralysis from geniculate herpes. Facial massage and electrical stimulation of the facial muscles should be started at once, but electrical stimulation should be stopped if signs of contracture appear. Facial movements can be practiced in front of a mirror as soon as there is some return of movement. Decompression of the facial nerve in its bony canal has not proved effective. Hypoglossal-facial anastomosis can be effective in selected cases of persistent paralysis.

Reference

Traverner, D.: Bell's Palsy. A Clinical and Electromyographic study. Brain, *78*:209, 1955.

5. Neuralgic Amyotrophy (Paralytic Brachial Radiculitis, Brachial Plexus Neuropathy)

Frank Elliott

Cause: An allergic disorder related to serum neuritis.

Early Manifestations: Severe pain followed within days by weakness or paralysis of proximal muscles, usually in the shoulder girdle.

Treatment: Steroids.

Possible Dire Consequences without Treatment: Continued symptoms.

In more than 50% of cases, the condition arises during convalescence from an infection, after a minor operation, or following inoculation.

The pain starts acutely and is severe. Usually it is felt in the region of the scapula or deltoid, but may radiate down the arm as far as the elbow or even further. The pain lasts from a few hours to three weeks and then usually improves, but in some cases intermittent pain continues for several months. Weakness or paralysis of muscles usually appears within the first three days. It is confined to the shoulder girdle in about half the cases. Rarely, the entire arm is paralyzed. Occasionally, the paralysis or weakness is confined to muscles supplied by a single peripheral nerve, such as the long thoracic nerve, the suprascapular nerve, or the radial nerve. The most common combination is paralysis of the spinati and deltoid. The diaphragm may be paralyzed on the affected side. Transient minor sensory impairment may occur within the territory of the affected root or nerve. Occasionally both shoulders are affected, and there may be an interval of several weeks between the involvement of the two sides. The spinal fluid is normal.

The diagnosis is simple provided the existence of this disorder is remembered. It may mimic bursitis since passive movement of the shoulder may increase the pain, but the rapid onset of paralysis and the presence of sensory impairment are diagnostic. The rapid onset and severe degree of paralysis distinguish the condition from root pain due to a prolapsed disc. The sensory impairment, the severe pain, and the restriction of the paralysis to a single group of muscles together exclude the possibility of a localized poliomyelitis.

Prednisone should be given in daily doses of at least 60 mg. for ten days, the dose being reduced thereafter over a period of ten days. The shoulder joint should be put through a complete range of movement three times daily, and electrical stimulation of the weakened muscles should be given when the acute pain has subsided. In untreated cases, full motor recovery may be delayed for one or two years.

Reference

Tsairis, P., Dyck, P. J., and Mulder, D. W.: Natural History of Brachial Plexus Neuropathy. Arch. Neurol. *27*:109, 1972.

6. Temporal Lobe Epilepsy

Frank Elliott

Cause: Glial scars and other structural lesions involving the temporal lobe.

Early Manifestations: Brief, recurrent, abrupt disorders of thinking, emotion, the special senses, or behavior.

Treatment: Anticonvulsant medication. Rarely, temporal lobectomy.

Possible Dire Consequences without Treatment: Continued symptoms.

All forms of epilepsy are treatable, to some extent, but this discussion is limited to the identification and treatment of temporal lobe seizures, which used to be called "epileptic equivalents" because the attacks bear so little resemblance to the conventional epileptic convulsion. However, they fall within the definition of epileptic seizures; namely, a recurrent, abrupt, brief disorder of cerebral function caused by a "sudden, excessive, rapid, and local discharge of grey matter" (Hughlings Jackson 1870). The discharging focus is usually in the temporal lobe, but some attacks have their origin in the orbital area of the frontal lobe. Occasionally, a temporal lobe seizure terminates in a generalized convulsion.

It is thought that the cause of temporal lobe epilepsy is always a structural lesion. Pathologic examination, by serial section, usually discloses some abnormality. The most common is glial scarring. Small vascular malformations or areas of gliosis are not uncommon. Cerebral tumors, and pressure on the medial aspect of the temporal lobe by pituitary and parapituitary tumors can be responsible.

The attack is sometimes ushered in by a sensory experience. Uncinate attacks, which arise from a discharging focus in the region of the uncinate gyrus, are marked by a peculiar dreamy state associated with hallucinations of smell, usually unpleasant, and this may be followed by smacking of the lips, swallowing movements, and chomping of the jaws. Or the hallucination of smell may be followed by Lilliputian hallucinations; the patient sees small highly colored figures, human or animal, during the dreamy state. Visual hallucinations of human figures or faces, or animals, or visual memories from the past, combined with a sense of unreality, may constitute the entire attack. Thus, one patient saw the face of a hideous woman approaching her; this was accompanied by extreme terror. Unformed visual fields or scintillating scotomas are commonly due to disease of the retina or occipital lobe.

Auditory attacks are uncommon, and usually consist of noises such as hissing, booming or ringing. Sometimes there may be a sudden sense that all outside sounds have ceased or that the tempo of ambient noises has suddenly accelerated or slowed down. *Formed* auditory hallucination, such as a voice speaking, may occur in disease of the temporal lobe, but the hearing of voices is more often the result of a psychosis than of structural disease of the brain.

Vertigo of abrupt onset and brief duration may precede a generalized seizure arising in the temporal lobe. Sometimes the patient complains that the entire attack consists of a feeling of turning a somersault. The vertigo is distinguished from aural vertigo by the brevity of the attack and by the absence of other aural symptoms. Occasionally, however, vertigo arising in the internal ear causes either syncope or an evoked epileptic convulsion.

Another form of temporal lobe epilepsy is the psychomotor seizure, which consists of a series of coordinated acts that are out of place, bizarre, and serve no useful purpose. For instance, one patient experienced a sudden sense of fear, which was so intense that she made violent attempts to escape from her surroundings. In "cursive" epilepsy, the patient starts running about in an aimless fashion. Sudden brief spells of laughing may constitute the entire attack (gelastic epilepsy). Some patients may go on an unnecessary journey during which they may behave normally; if driving a car, road signs and traffic lights are obeyed but there is complete amnesia, and when the attack comes to an end, the patient finds himself far from home and unable to explain how he got there. Clearly, such attacks last much longer than the ordinary temporal lobe seizure, and in some cases it has been found that the epileptic discharge from the temporal lobe was almost continuous. This situation corresponds to "status epilepticus."

Rarely, temporal lobe seizures take the form of rage or physical aggression without provocation. It should be noted, however, that criminal assaults are not more common in epileptics than in non-epileptics.

An episode of extreme fear may constitute the entire attack, or the sense of fear may be accompanied by hallucinations or forced thinking. Sensations of pleasure are rare. Uncontrolled crying without provocation and unassociated with a feeling of depression may occur.

Episodes of abdominal discomfort, such as epigastric pain or a "funny feeling" accompanied by a desire to defecate, may precede other manifestations of psycho-motor epilepsy, or they may occur on their own. In yet other cases the visceral sensa-tions are precordial, such as a sense of pressure or a sense of fluttering in the chest with tachycardia. When visceral sensations constitute the entire attack, the possibility of epilepsy is easily overlooked. One patient had more than 20 attacks of constricting pain in the chest, which was always thought to be anginal, but was never associated with any abnormalities in the EKG. The attacks were controlled by Dilantin. Episodic visceral disturbances are also seen in diencephalic autonomic epilepsy, in which the epileptic discharge is thought to arise in the hypothalamus or the anterior part of the thalamus, rather than the temporal lobe. The patient experiences fullness in the abdomen, nausea, rapid breathing, tachycardia, elevation of blood pressure, flushing, salivation, lacrimation, perspiration, and pilo-erection. The pupils are widely dilated and the general picture is one of extreme terror. Such an episode can last from seconds to several minutes. Sometimes it progresses into a generalized seizure, but when this does not occur the attack is apt to suggest an attack of paroxys-mal tachycardia or an anxiety neurosis or a carcinoid tumor.

Diagnosis requires two steps. The first is to prove that the seizure is coming from the temporal lobe, and the second is to try to establish the nature of the under-lying disease. An electroencephalographic abnormality arising in the temporal lobe can usually be recorded during an attack; between attacks the EEG may be normal or abnormal. If it is normal when the patient is awake, a sleep record often discloses spike activity. Special placement of the electrodes, *e.g.*, in the nasopharynx, increases the chance of finding an abnormal discharge. Whatever the outcome of the EEG examination, the patient should be thoroughly studied by x-ray examination, brain scan, arteriography, pneumoencephalography, and spinal tap in an attempt to identify the cause of the attacks.

The treatment of temporal lobe seizures is anticonvulsant drugs. Temporal lobec-tomy is resorted to in rare instances, if medication fails to bring about reasonable control of the attacks.

The most effective drug is Phenytoin sodium (Dilantin), starting with 200 mg. in the morning and 100 mg. in the evening. In most cases, a daily dose of 400 mg. is adequate. Another derivative of the hydantoins, Mesantoin, also can be used, in doses up to 600 mg. a day. Mysoline can be given alone or in combination with Dilantin, the average daily dose for an adult being 1.0 to 1.5 gm. daily. On the whole, phenobarbitone is less effective than the foregoing, but it can be tried either alone or in combination with Dilantin. Carbamazepine (Tegretol) is another alternative that is used in the treatment of both grand mal and temporal lobe seizures; the dose for adults ranges from 400 to 800 mg. a day.

As in all types of epilepsy, seizure may be precipitated by fatigue, excessive fluid intake, and emotional stress; patients should be advised to avoid the first two, but the third is often inescapable.

Reference

Elliott, Frank A.: Clinical Neurology, 2nd Ed. Philadelphia, W. B. Saunders Co., 1971, p. 130.

7. Headaches

Perry MacNeal

Cause: Tension, migraine, cluster.

Early Manifestations: Hostility, headache, unknown.

Treatment: Aspirin, ergotamine, steroids, and others.

Possible Dire Consequences without Treatment: Continued symptoms.

The pain of *tension headache* is presumably produced by muscle contraction about the head and scalp, but it seems quite possible that, as our understanding of the chemistry of emotion increases, other mechanisms—hormonal or enzymatic—may be revealed. The most common psychodynamic factor is repressed hostility. Even the patient who relates his symptoms to "pressure at work" or "long hours" reveals on detailed inquiry, the fact of person-to-person hostility. In severe cases, sometimes leading to almost total disability, the hostility may have been so thoroughly repressed as to defy conventional rational approaches by the therapist.

TABLE V–1.
REGIMEN FOR CLUSTER HEADACHE

	Day	1	2	3	4	5	6	7	8	9	10	11	12	13	14	15	16
Ergotamine* tartrate, 1.0 mg.	Breakfast	1	1	1	1	1	1	1	1	1	1	1	1	1	0	0	0
	Lunch	1	1	1	1	1	1	1	1	1	1	1	1	0	0	0	0
Caffeine	Supper	0	0	0	0	0	0	0	0	0	0	0	0	0	0	0	0
Citrate, 100 mg.	Bedtime	0	0	0	0	0	0	0	0	0	0	0	0	0	0	0	0
Ergotamine* tartrate, 1.0 mg.	Breakfast	0	0	0	0	0	0	0	0	0	0	0	0	0	0	0	0
Caffeine	Lunch	0	0	0	0	0	0	0	0	0	0	0	0	0	0	0	0
Citrate, 100 mg.	Supper	2	2	2	2	2	2	2	1	1	1	1	1	0	0	0	0
Pentobarbital, 30 mg. Bellafoline, 0.125 mg.	Bedtime	2	2	2	2	2	2	2	2	2	2	2	1	1	1	1	0
	Breakfast	1	1	1	1	1	1	1	1	1	0	0	0	0	0	0	0
Triamcinolone, 4.0 mg.	Lunch	1	1	1	1	1	1	1	0	0	0	0	0	0	0	0	0
	Supper	1	1	1	1	1	1	1	1	0	0	0	0	0	0	0	0
	Bedtime	1	1	1	1	1	1	1	1	1	1	0	0	0	0	0	0

* Cafergot (Sandoz)

The perfect prophylaxis for *migraine* has not yet been found. Methysergide is frequently useful, and the dose schedule recommended at present (2 mg. three times daily for not longer than six months, followed by a three months' "break") seems directed toward avoiding the side effects encountered with the larger doses formerly prescribed. During the three month "break," or in cases in which methysergide is either unsuccessful or contraindicated, we have been using ergotamine tartrate by mouth in the form of a 1-mg. tablet, four times a day initially. This is then gradually reduced to the minimum amount necessary to control the symptoms. Thus far, in experience extending as long as six years with some patients, we have seen no untoward effects. Nonetheless, this program must be carefully supervised, with frequent checks on the heart, retinal vessels, and peripheral circulation, and must still be considered to be in the investigational stage. It should be reserved for those patients in whom the degree of their disability warrants acceptance of the theoretical risks involved.

The causes and "cure" of the *cluster headache* (Horton's cephalgia, histamine cephalgia) remain unknown. However, if the diagnosis is carefully established (excruciating, unilateral, sudden pain in the head and eye, accompanied by epiphora and ocular congestion, lasting one-half to two hours, occurring several times daily for a variable period of four to sixteen weeks, followed by months or years of complete freedom), the distress can usually be completely controlled by the program in Table V–1.

The usual precautions in the use of ergot and steroids must be observed, and the medication discontinued from time to time to determine when the "cluster period" has come to its own conclusion. It is quite likely that further exploration of the chemistry of emotion may well lead to final resolution of this peculiar mystery.

Reference

MacNeal, P. S.: The patient with headache. Postgrad. Med., *42*:249, 1967.

8. Parkinsonism

Henry R. Schutta and Victor Robert

Cause: Arteriosclerosis, postencephalitis, manganese and carbon monoxide poisoning.

Early Manifestations: Bradykinesia, tremor and rigidity, loss of facial expression, micrographia.

Treatment: Medical: Levodopa therapy, atropine-like drugs, amantadine, and antihistamines; physiotherapy; surgical: stereotaxic procedures.

Possible Dire Consequences without Treatment: Progressive disability.

The majority of patients with parkinsonism suffer from a degenerative condition of unknown etiology, also known as Parkinson's disease or paralysis agitans. Parkinsonism is a common side effect of phenothiazine medication; it may be the result of a variety of encephalitides; it occasionally follows severe head injuries and can be caused by manganese or carbon monoxide poisoning. Diffuse vascular disease, leading to damage of the basal ganglia, results in arteriosclerotic parkinsonism.

The prevalence rate of paralysis agitans is 157 per 100,000. Males are affected twice as frequently as females, and the disease begins most commonly in the fifties and sixties and is usually sporadic.

Pathologic changes are most evident in the substantia nigra and corpus striatum. There is depigmentation of the substantia nigra and a loss of neurons can be seen. Some neurons contain large eosinophilic inclusions known as Lewy bodies. A certain degree of neuronal loss also occurs in the cerebral cortex.

Recent chemical studies revealed abnormally low concentration of dopamine in the basal ganglia of patients with parkinsonism, and therefore a disturbance of catecholamine metabolism has been postulated as the basis for parkinsonism.

The onset is insidious and the progress is usually slow. Early in the disease the signs may be asymmetrical. The initial complaints are either tremor or progressive stiffness and slowness of movements, and difficulty with gait. Loss of facial expressiveness may be noted by the family, and changes in speech commonly draw attention to the fact that something is wrong. Micrographia is frequently an early symptom.

Of the three major components of parkinsonism (bradykinesia, tremor, and rigidity), bradykinesia is always present, but some patients may suffer only from tremor or only from rigidity; most patients, however, have tremor and rigidity.

Tremor is generally most pronounced in the hands, but also may involve the legs, the lips, the tongue, and the neck muscles. It is intermittent at first, but as time passes it becomes more and more persistent. The tremor is a coarse, rhythmic movement at the rate of about four to six cycles per second, and is frequently of the "pill-rolling" type. It is a static tremor and tends to disappear with movement and during sleep, but is increased by stress.

Rigidity is present in most patients with parkinsonism; it eventually spreads to all extremities, but it may begin in only one. "Cogwheeling" frequently accompanies rigidity. When there is doubt about the presence of rigidity, it can be verified by having the patient perform alternating movements in the extremity opposite to the one being tested.

As the disease advances, a generalized attitude of flexion develops; the arms tend to be adducted, flexed at the elbows, and the knees are slightly flexed.

Bradykinesia, or poverty of movements, is first manifested in the face. The patient tends to blink less than normally and the face is expressionless. Also, voluntary movements are initiated and performed slowly. Patients with parkinsonism do not fidget; they sit still. They require increasingly more time for dressing; initiation of movement becomes more difficult. A combination of bradykinesia and rigidity leads to a decrease in the swinging of the arms when the patient walks, and a slow, shuffling, small-stepped gait.

There are certain minor signs that are helpful in confirming the diagnosis of parkinsonism. When the patient is asked to close his eyes lightly, the eyes will flutter (blepharoclonus). A tapping on the forehead will produce continued blinking even though the patient is asked not to blink (positive glabellar tap test.) Scratching the palm frequently produces a twitch of the mentalis muscle in extrapyramidal disorders (palmo-mentalis reflex). None of these signs is specific for parkinsonism, but when present in association with other suspicious signs of extrapyramidal disease, they help in the diagnosis.

The speech is frequently monotonous and somewhat slurred, and occasionally, patients with parkinsonism display palilalia (they repeat parts of sentences).

Intellectual deterioration is not a consistent accompaniment of Parkinson's disease, but in advanced stages, varying degrees of intellectual deterioration may occur. In other forms of parkinsonism, notably the arteriosclerotic type, dementia is commonly present.

The reflexes may be normal, or they may be submerged in the rigidity; often the reflexes vary, depending at what phase of the tremor the tendon is struck. Plantar responses in Parkinson's disease are flexor, but they may be extensor in arteriosclerotic or postencephalitic types, where corticospinal tract damage is also frequently present. The EEG and spinal fluid examination usually reveal no abnormalities.

The disease progresses at varying rates; generally speaking, within five years 25% of patients are severely disabled; ten to fifteen years from the onset, 70% are completely disabled or dead. Major causes of death are bronchopneumonia and urinary tract infections.

There is no cure for parkinsonism, but the symptoms can be alleviated by various means.

At present the treatment of choice is L-dopa (L-dihydroxyphenylalanine). The drug is given orally in four divided doses, and the doses are gradually increased. It may be started at 250 mg. q.i.d. and increased by 125 mg. daily, or every second day, until the desired effects occur, or side effects prevent further increments. The effective daily dose varies between 3 and 8 gm. Rigidity and akinesia respond best to L-dopa, whereas tremor responds least, and occasionally it is made worse by L-dopa therapy.

The most troublesome side effect of L-dopa is anorexia, nausea, and vomiting. Postural hypotension and drenching sweats are not uncommon. About 50% of patients develop dyskinetic movements, and a considerable proportion develop mental disturbances, confusion, psychosis, and depression. All the side effects are dose-dependent, and disappear when the dose is reduced. Failure or success of L-dopa therapy generally depends on how well the patient can tolerate the drug, although some patients, even on large doses of L-dopa, fail to respond.

Amantadine hydrochloride has also been found helpful in parkinsonism. It reduces rigidity and bradykinesia. It can be used as an adjuvant to the L-dopa therapy.

A large number of atropine-like compounds have been used in the past, and are moderately effective. The more common ones are trihexyphenidyl (Artane), benztropine mesylate (Cogentin) and procyclidine (Kemadrin). When a patient has been treated with these drugs for a while, and then it is decided to put him on L-dopa therapy, it is unwise to discontinue these drugs because, very often, the patient becomes completely rigid before the L-dopa has a chance to act.

Certain antihistamines are also useful. Diphenhydramine hydrochloride (Benadryl) will occasionally influence the tremor favorably.

The importance of physical therapy cannot be overemphasized. All patients with parkinsonism should be encouraged to take regular exercises which, in severe cases, should be initially supervised by a skilled physical therapy staff.

Surgical treatment, which was a common means of relieving the symptoms of parkinsonism in the past, relieved tremor and rigidity, but had no influence on the bradykinesia. With the advent of L-dopa, the indications for surgery have become very uncertain. It is probable that a few patients who do not benefit from L-dopa will be advised to submit to surgery.

Addition of a variety of drugs that inhibit the breakdown of L-dopa is used as an adjuvant in L-dopa therapy. These drugs are still at the stage of clinical investigation in the U.S.A. The advantage of this is that the dose of L-dopa can be much smaller and therefore some of the side effects, such as nausea and vomiting, may not occur. The side effects due to disturbance of the central nervous system, such as the dyskinesias and psychiatric abnormalities, are not reduced. It is too early to say yet whether or not L-dopa therapy eventually will lose its effectiveness as the disease progresses.

References

Brain, L., and Walton, J. N.: Diseases of the Nervous System. 7th Ed. London, Oxford University Press, 1969.

Cotzias, G. C., Papavasiliou, P. S., and Gellene, R.: Modification of Parkinsonism—chronic treatment with L-dopa. New Eng. J. Med., *280*:337, 1969.

McDowell, F. H., and Lee, J. E.: Extrapyramidal diseases. *In* Clinical Neurology. Edited by A. B. Baker. New York, Harper & Row, 1971.

9. Myasthenia Gravis

HENRY SCHUTTA AND VICTOR ROBERT

Cause: Disorder of neuromuscular transmission, which is relieved to varying degrees by cholinesterase inhibitors. The etiology remains unknown.

Early Manifestations: Fatigability, ptosis, diplopia, dysphagia, difficulty in chewing and weakness, generally more pronounced in the face and limb girdle muscles. These symptoms are more pronounced after exercise and toward the end of the day. The onset is usually insidious.

Treatment: Anticholinesterase drugs, steroids or ACTH, thymectomy.

Possible Dire Consequences without Treatment: Respiratory failure and death.

Myasthenia gravis is a disease characterized by fatigability and weakness. Striated muscles supplied by cranial nerves tend to be affected early. The disease varies in severity, and is relieved to varying degrees by anticholinesterase drugs.

Myasthenia gravis affects mostly young adults, but it may occur at any age. Among young adults, women are affected three times as often as men, but after the age of forty years, men and women are affected equally. The prevalence rate in the United States and Britain is about 3 per 100,000. Neonatal myasthenia is seen in approximately 1 in 7 children born of myasthenic mothers. This disorder responds to neostigmine and subsides in two or three weeks, the child being normal thereafter.

The etiology of myasthenia gravis is uncertain, but an autoimmune mechanism is suspected. The symptoms of the disease are related to a disturbance of acetylcholine metabolism at the neuromuscular junction.

The pathologic findings in patients with myasthenia gravis are scant. The affected muscles often appear normal. Small focal collections of interstitial lymphocytes (lymphorrhages) and degenerating or necrotic fibers are occasionally found. More severe inflammatory changes are uncommon and seem to occur more often in patients with thymoma. Myocarditis has been reported in a few cases.

Tumors of the thymus (thymoma) are found in 10% of all cases. In about 70%, germinal center hyperplasia is observed. The glands appear normal in about 20% of the patients with myasthenia gravis. There is no characteristic pathologic condition in other organs.

The onset is usually insidious, and the first symptoms are commonly related to weakness of the ocular muscle, giving rise to ptosis or diplopia. The ocular muscle weakness may be unilateral or bilateral, and may vary from day to day. Symptoms frequently fluctuate, and they typically appear toward the end of the day, and improve or disappear with rest. When the bulbar musculature is affected, difficulty in swallowing and chewing occurs, and this again is more evident toward the end of the meal. Speech may become progressively weak and slurred as the patient speaks. Palatal weakness gives rise to a nasal voice, and a nasal regurgitation of liquids can occur. Other symptoms are due to weakness of trunk and limb muscles, such as difficulty in holding up the head, elevating the arms, and walking or climbing stairs. Dyspnea is always a sinister symptom in patients with myasthenia gravis, as respiratory failure may develop rapidly and can be fatal.

The findings on clinical examination depend on the extent of the muscular involvement, but weakness is the only abnormality. Ptosis is often found and sometimes, when not present initially, can be induced by asking the patient to gaze upward for a few minutes. Weakness of the extraocular muscles is usually asymmetrical and may be confined to one muscle, or there may be complete external ophthalmoplegia of one or both eyes.

Bilateral facial weakness is often present, the face appearing flat and expressionless. The patients have difficulty in closing the eyes tightly and they have a characteristic myopathic smile.

Weakness of bulbar or spinal muscles, when present, can be detected by appropriate tests. The muscle power may initially be reasonably good, but after a particular movement is tested several times, the strength may decline. Muscles of the shoulder and hip girdle tend to be weaker than the more peripheral muscles. The reflexes and sensation are normal. A normal neurologic examination, at a time when the patient is complaining of symptoms suggestive of myasthenia gravis, is virtually incompatible with the diagnosis (Rowland).

The diagnosis of myasthenia gravis can be confirmed or excluded by pharmacologic tests in the majority of cases. The most frequent errors in the diagnosis of myasthenia result from errors in applying and interpreting these tests. The most commonly used test in the diagnosis of myasthenia gravis, and one which often confirms the diagnosis, is the Tensilon test. Tensilon (edrophonium) is a quick-acting cholinesterase inhibitor, and is given intravenously. The initial dose is 2 mg., followed immediately by a further 8 mg., if there is no adverse reaction to the initial smaller dose. There should be an improvement of muscle power within sixty seconds. The improvement lasts only a few minutes.

4

In the small number of patients in whom the Tensilon test is inconclusive, the Curare test can be of great help. It is the most reliable test for excluding myasthenia gravis, but should be performed only by an experienced examiner in the presence of an anesthesiologist. The myasthenic patient is unduly sensitive to Curare, and marked weakness can be produced by one-fifth of the average curarizing dose. When weakness occurs it can be easily reversed by Tensilon or Prostigmin. The absence of weakness upon administration of one-fifth of the average curarizing dose excludes the presence of myasthenia at the time of testing.

Electromyography may supply evidence of a defect in the neuromuscular transmission, and can be of value in confirming the diagnosis.

At the time of onset, it is impossible to predict the outcome of the disease in any case. The disease is chronic, and remissions and exacerbations are common. Myasthenia may remain limited to the external ocular muscles, or it may be generalized from the onset. Symptoms may be very mild, or can become severe rapidly. Partial or complete remissions may occur in approximately 25% of cases, usually within the first five years. Patients with thymoma appear to have a poor prognosis for survival even when thymectomy is performed. Pregnancy has no consistent effect on the disease.

The treatment of myasthenia gravis is medical in the first instance. The standard treatment consists of neostigmine or pyridostigmine (Mestinon); the latter has largely replaced neostigmine because it has a more prolonged action (from three to six hours). The usual initial dosage of Mestinon is one tablet (60 mg.) three or four times daily. The dose is then gradually increased until maximum benefit is obtained. More than 120 mg. every two hours is rarely needed.

Overdosage with anticholinesterases may result in a cholinergic crisis, which consists of increasing weakness and respiratory insufficiency. A myasthenic crisis, which can be precipitated by intercurrent disease or undermedication, manifests itself in the same way.

Patients with either type of crisis must be managed in an intensive care unit, and the question whether one is dealing with a myasthenic or cholinergic crisis can be resolved by the Tensilon test. Weakness is myasthenic if symptoms improve after Tensilon, but when the symptoms are increased by Tensilon, or if no improvement occurs, the patient is suffering from an overdosage of anticholinesterase drugs, *i.e.*, cholinergic crisis.

In either instance the patient is managed by vigorous treatment of intercurrent disease. In myasthenic crisis, the prostigmine is increased; in the cholinergic crisis it is reduced. Respiration is supported as needed.

Corticosteroid therapy may be useful in the management of severe myasthenia gravis. Treatment with ACTH, 1,000 units in divided doses for ten days, should be instituted in an intensive care unit, because a period of deterioration occurs in most cases before improvement takes place. The improvement is transient, lasting from weeks to months, and re-treatment is often necessary. Some patients also respond to large doses of prednisone; 100 mg. on alternate days has been recommended.

Although the relationship of the thymus to myasthenia gravis is not well understood, thymectomy induces a complete remission of the disease in 17 to 25% of all cases, and considerable improvement in a further 29%. There are no absolute rules for the selection of patients for surgery, but thymectomy should be recommended when myasthenia is functionally disabling in spite of adequate medical treatment for at least six months.

References

Mayo Clinic: Clinical Examinations in Neurology. 3rd Ed. Philadelphia, W. B. Saunders Co., 1971.

Osserman, K. E.: Myasthenia Gravis. New York, Grune & Stratton, 1958.

Perlo, V. P., Poskanzer, D. C., Schwab, R. S., Viets, H. R., Osserman, K. E., and Genkins, G.: Myasthenia gravis: evaluation of treatment in 1,355 patients. Neurology, *16*:431, 1966.

Rowland, L. P., and Layzer, R. B.: Muscular dystrophies, atrophies and related diseases. *In* Clinical Neurology. New York, Harper & Row, 1971.

10. Subclavian Steal Syndrome

CAROLYN PARRY

Cause: Stenosis or occlusion of the subclavian or innominate artery proximal to the vertebral artery.

Early Manifestations: Vertigo, ataxia, diplopia, decreased visual acuity, paresthesias and/or coldness in the arm. Systolic blood pressure difference of 20 to 40 mm. Hg between right and left arms.

Treatment: Surgical correction of stenosis or occlusion.

Possible Dire Consequences without Treatment: Stroke.

It has been estimated that 3 out of 4 stroke victims have had warning symptoms of impending stroke in the form of transient cerebral ischemia (Henzel, 1971). It has also been estimated that as many as 50% of patients with symptoms of cerebral insufficiency have extracranial occlusive vascular disease (Mishkin, 1967). This type of occlusive vascular disease is readily amenable to surgery with high percentages of success. It is apparent that prompt and accurate diagnosis of the cause of transient ischemic attacks and surgical correction of the specific abnormality may prevent or postpone the devastating consequences of an irreversible stroke.

A subclavian steal is an example of a localized, correctable, extracranial lesion that produces characteristic signs and symptoms. There is stenosis or occlusion of the subclavian or, less frequently, the innominate artery, proximal to the origin of the vertebral artery. The stenosis or occlusion is almost always caused by atherosclerosis, but tumor, congenital anomaly, or previous surgery (Blalock-Taussig) may also cause the constriction (Piccone et al., 1970). The blood pressure in the distal subclavian artery decreases because of the stenosis proximally, and when it falls 10% of its usual level it becomes lower than the pressure in the vertebral-basilar arterial system. There is "siphoning" of the blood from the contralateral vertebral artery, the basilar artery, and then reversed flow, or caudad flow, in the ipsilateral vertebral artery to supply the distal subclavian. The result is a "stealing" of blood from the brain to supply the subclavian and the arm. The left subclavian artery is affected two to two and one-half times as frequently as the innominate artery. Males are predominantly affected in the ratio of 2 or 3:1. The usual age of presenting symptoms is fifty to fifty-five years. Any intra- or extravascular process capable of stenosing or occluding the proximal subclavian artery can set the stage for the hemodynamics of the retrograde flow in the ipsilateral vertebral artery and possibly basilar insufficiency (Henzel, 1971). The subclavian steal phenomenon is one of many "steal" phenomena that may exist in the body with vascular compromise, but space permits discussion of only this form of "steal." The classic presentation of a subclavian steal is a patient who complains of vertigo, ataxia, diplopia, or decrease in visual acuity. Classically, the symptoms are aggravated by exercise of the affected arm. There is often a bruit over the stenosed portion of the subclavian (Newton and Wylie, 1964).

Claudication symptoms in the affected arm are occasionally the presenting complaint, but more often the patient complains of paresthesias, coldness, or anesthesia. There is almost always a systolic blood pressure difference between the two arms of at least 20 to 30 mm. Hg. Piccone has noted that cerebral symptoms may be relieved by an inflated blood pressure cuff on the affected arm. By occluding the brachial artery, the pressure in the subclavian is raised and returns the vertebral circulation to its normal antegrade flow. Piccone has also stated that amelioration of the CNS symptoms with this simple mechanical device indicates a good prognosis for surgery.

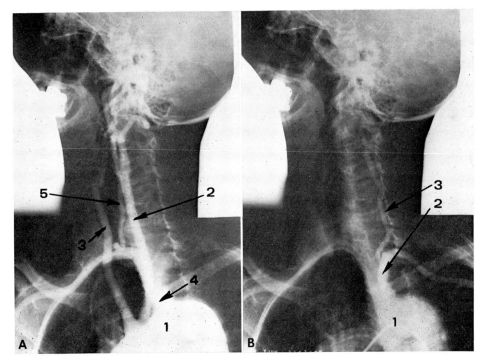

Fig. V–1. A. Injection of contrast material into the aortic arch (1) demonstrates immediate filling of the right common carotid (3), right subclavian (4), right vertebral (5), and left common carotid (2) arteries. The left subclavian artery is occluded at its origin. There is an incidental anomaly of an aberrant right subclavian artery (4) originating from the thoracic aorta distal to the origin of the left subclavian.

   B. Several seconds later when most of the contrast material has disappeared from the carotids and the right subclavian artery there is retrograde flow in the left vertebral artery (3) to fill the subclavian artery (2) distal to its occlusion. (Courtesy of Koson Kuroda, M. D., Thomas Jefferson University Hospital.)

Katsilabros has utilized this principle in more severely affected individuals. He found that when the subclavian steal phenomenon exists, elevating the affected arm and/or suspending the arm from an overhead frame on a bed may improve the mental status of stuporous, semicomatose, or comatose patients.

Reivich first described the reverse blood flow in the vertebral artery associated with a subclavian stenosis in two patients in 1961. He then proceeded with animal experiments to determine cerebral blood flow in various extracranial occlusive states. An editorial in the same year coined the name "subclavian steal," and commended Reivich for the first sound attempt to elucidate patterns of blood flow in cerebrovascular insufficiency.

The occluded or partially occluded subclavian artery usually steals blood from the vertebral artery, but other pathways are also available. The vertebral-basilar-vertebral arterial pathway is the most common and potentially the most dangerous, since it takes blood from the posterior brain, but occasionally may also "steal" from the anterior brain via the posterior communicating arteries. If there is coexistent carotid disease, the entire brain may be deprived of its usual blood supply. Other pathways include collateral supply from the thyrocervical trunks, internal mammary arteries and external carotids via the superior and inferior thyroid arteries (Newton and Wylie, 1964).

Surgical correction in the past has been primarily endarterectomy with good results. This procedure was utilized primarily with a segmental stenosis from an atheromatous plaque. A patch graft was frequently used when the stenosis occurred at the origin of the vertebral artery, and a bypass graft was used when the stenosis occurred at the subclavian artery (Ponsdomenech and Le Pere, 1969). Several of these procedures necessitate an intrathoracic approach from all the morbidity of this extensive procedure. Forestner et al. reported, from a series of dogs and one patient, experience with a subclavian-to-subclavian bypass graft in January, 1972. In the same journal, Finkelstein et al. described the operation and results in 15 patients with a subclavian-to-subclavian Dacron bypass graft. This procedure was entirely extrathoracic, and the rate of success was 100%. The patients remained free of symptoms and had equal blood pressure in both arms in their six-month to four-year follow-up. Since 200,000 people die of strokes in the United States annually and 2,000,000 are living with various sequelae, it is imperative to diagnose accurately and treat surgically the high percentage of extracranial lesions causing cerebral ischemia such as the subclavian steal. Fig. V–1A & B.

References

Editorial: A new vascular syndrome—the subclavian steal. New Eng. J. Med., *265*:912, 1961.

Finkelstein, N. M., Byer, A., and Rush, B. F.: Subclavian-subclavian bypass for the subclavian steal syndrome. Surgery, *71*:142, 1972.

Forestner, J. E., Ghosh, S. K., Bergan, J. J., and Conn, J., Jr.: Subclavian-subclavian bypass for correction of the subclavian steal syndrome. Surgery, *71*:136, 1972.

Heidrich, H., and Bayer, O.: Symptomatology of the subclavian steal syndrome. Angiology, *20*:406, 1969.

Henzel, J. H., Dexter, J., and Doerhoff, A.: Stroke prevention by early recognition of correctable cerebrovascular ischemia. Missouri Med., *68*:321, 1971.

Katsilabros, L., and Katsilabros, N. L.: The arterial steal phenomenon as an explanation of the angina pectoris and the pain of intermittent claudication. Angiology, *22*:575, 1971.

Mishkin, M. M.: Extracranial ischemic lesions which secondarily involve the brain. Radiol. Clin. N. Amer., *5*:395, 1967.

Newton, T. H., and Wylie, E. J.: Collateral circulation associated with occlusion of the proximal subclavian and innominate arteries. Amer. J. Roentgenol., *9*:394, 1964.

Piccone, V. A., Karvounis, P., and Le Veen, H. H.: The subclavian steal syndrome. Angiology, *21*:240, 1970.

Ponsdomenech, E. R., and Le Pere, R. H.: Obstruction of the subclavian artery. Vasc. Surg., *3*:211, 1969.

Reivich, M. H., Holling, H. E., Roberts, B., and Toole, J. F.: Reversal of blood flow through the vertebral artery and its effect on cerebral circulation. New Eng. J. Med., *265*:878, 1961.

11. Intermittent Claudication of the Cauda Equina

ORVILLE HORWITZ

Cause: Space-occupying mass in cauda equina.

Early Manifestations: Intermittent claudication accompanied by paresthesia.

Treatment: Surgical removal of mass.

Possible Dire Consequences without Treatment: Continued symptoms. Possibly paralysis.

The cause of the syndrome is thought to be largely mechanical, insofar as there appears to be a gradual increase in the size of an otherwise symptomless lumbar disc protrusion with each weight-bearing step until a critical point is reached and the patient experiences pain and begins to limp.

There is genuine intermittent claudication. The patient gives a history of being able to walk a certain distance before noticing pain in the extremity or extremities. In other words there is a latent period between the onset of activity and the onset of symptoms.

This is an uncommon condition, as well over 95% of intermittent claudication is due to arterial insufficiency.

The symptom, strongly suggestive, is that of paresthesia of the extremity or part of the extremity or paresthesia of the scrotum, which practically never occurs with intermittent claudication induced by arterial insufficiency.

References

Horwitz, O.: Diseases of the arteries of the extremities. *In* Cardiac and Vascular Diseases. Edited by H. L. Conn and O. Horwitz. Philadelphia, Lea & Febiger, 1971.

Jaffe, R., Appleby, A., and Sejonia, V.: Intermittent ischemia of the cauda equina due to stenosis of the lumbar canal. J. Neurol. Neurosurg. Psychiat., *29*:315, 1966.

12. Space-Occupying Lesions of the Spinal Cord

FREDERICK A. SIMEONE

Cause: Tumors, abscesses, discs, degenerative spine disease.

Early Manifestations: Pain, weakness, numbness, bladder difficulty.

Treatment: Surgical excision or decompression.

Possible Dire Consequences without Treatment: Paralysis, incontinence, impotence.

Since the care of space-occupying lesions within the spinal canal is usually surgical, no specific consideration of new operative techniques will be made except to encourage the reader to consult a neurosurgeon promptly after the condition is suspected.

The spinal canal is bounded anteriorly by the vertebral bodies, laterally by the vertebral pedicles, and posteriorly by the laminae. Masses within the confines of this structure produce symptoms that are rather stereotyped, and are related principally to the speed of progression.

Rapidly Progressing Intraspinal Lesions. These lesions include metastatic (usually epidural) tumors, abscess, collapsed disc or vertebrae, hemorrhage. Here one finds that pain is the first and most consistent symptom. Pain is located in the spine directly over the lesion. If the lesion involves a nerve root, as it must in the lumbar spinal canal where only nerve roots are present, pain radiating into an extremity or other part of the body is present. Pain may precede the development of neurologic signs and symptoms for some time. If the lesion is a progressive one, such as a tumor, abscess, or hemorrhage, neurologic signs follow rapidly. Signs that are of a relatively acute onset, but fairly static after their presentation (such as herniated discs), may produce pain initially with slowly progressive neurologic signs depending on the severity of compression. In the cervical or thoracic region, spinal cord compression is the prime consideration. The patient first experiences difficulty with walking, develops a wide-based gait, and ultimately complains truly of weakness. During this time he may have bladder difficulty consisting of either retention or frequency. In thoracic cord lesions, only the legs are involved. In the cervical region it seems that the legs are involved before the arms, regardless of the cause of compression.

Although acute cervical disc disease frequently affects only a nerve root supplying the arm, in occasional cases spinal cord compression is produced, creating a true surgical emergency. On neurologic examination, one may find depressed or absent reflexes in the lower extremities with no plantar signs. This is true if the patient is examined within the first few days of symptoms, and if the onset of spinal cord compression has been abrupt. After some delay, or in more gradually produced spinal cord compression, the more characteristic hyperreflexia and extensor plantar response occur. If loss of sensation occurs, it frequently involves only sensations of pain and temperature in a segmental distribution beginning several levels below the site of the spinal cord lesion. When nerve root compression is present alone, or combined with spinal cord compression, there may be numbness in the distribution of the affected nerve root, and loss of reflex or strength in the same distribution.

In all cases in which a progressive lesion is suspected, prompt myelography and surgical decompression are indicated. A possible exception in the category of acute, progressive intraspinal lesions would be malignant lymphoma, which can respond adequately to x-ray therapy. However, many believe that x-ray therapy should be combined with surgical decompression.

Chronic or Slowly Progressive Intraspinal Space-taking Lesions. These include meningiomas, neurofibromas, cervical spondylosis, or degenerative disc disease. More slowly progressive intraspinal tumors can produce weakness, numbness, and bladder difficulty in such an indolent fashion that the neurologic deficit often goes unnoticed for several months or years. When situated near a nerve root, these benign intraspinal tumors can produce significant pain. The pain is characteristically felt at night. It is located at the site of the tumor and frequently radiates along the chest or the abdominal wall, or into an extremity. The patient may have to sleep propped up in bed or in a chair in order to obtain relief. Neurologic signs are as mentioned above, except that hyperreflexia and extensor-plantar responses are typical. Myelography confirms the diagnosis and surgical excision produces excellent results in benign intraspinal tumors.

Chronic degenerative disease of the spinal canal, with proliferative changes of the disc spaces and ultimate spinal cord compression, is an extremely common syndrome. Although radicular pain is common, it is not unusual to see progressive spinal cord involvement from chronic cervical disc degeneration in the absence of pain. When pain is present, it is usually low-grade and radiates in a monoradicular distribution. As the syndrome progresses, the patient develops a wide-based gait, with ultimate weakness in the arms and legs.

Treatment of chronic degenerative disc disease, like treatment of herniated cervical and lumbar discs, is somewhat variable. Patients with chronic cervical degenerative disc disease are frequently elderly, and may be unable to withstand the required surgery. Here, long-term use of a collar may be effective, at least in arresting symptoms. This is true of patients with focal cervical disc degeneration who have only radicular pain. For patients with lumbar and cervical disc herniations who are free of neurologic deficit, a trial in a brace or cervical collar is frequently indicated prior to surgery. In the absence of significant neurologic deficit, the main indication for operation in cervical and lumbar disc disease is the presence of intractable and disabling pain. Patients with acute cervical or lumbar herniations may respond to their first attack with rest and be free of subsequent attacks. In patients in whom symptoms recur, surgical excision offers the best chance of permanent relief.

Reference

Guttman, L.: Clinical symptomatology of spinal cord lesions. Handbook of Clinical Neurology. Edited by P. J. Vinken and G. W. Bruyn. Amsterdam, North Holland Publishing Co., 1969.

13. Carpal Tunnel Syndrome

FREDERICK A. SIMEONE

Cause: Thickening of transverse carpal ligament at wrist or compression of median nerve by structures under the carpal ligament; can be associated with myxedema, diabetes, pregnancy, or occupational trauma.

Early Manifestations: Numbness, difficulty in picking up fine objects, weakness of opposition of thumb; later, pain and numbness on volar surface of hand, excluding small finger. Discomfort most likely to occur in early morning hours.

Treatment: Local steroids, wrist splint, or section of carpal ligament and decompression of median nerve.

Possible Dire Consequences without Treatment: Numbness of palmar surface of first four fingers, atrophy of thenar eminence with impaired function.

This condition most often occurs in middle age and seems to affect more women than men. Initially there is no difficulty with the hand, except during the early morning. After a few hours of sleep the patient awakens with an uncomfortable, "woody" feeling on the volar aspect of the hand involving the thumb, and the index, middle, and perhaps ring fingers. She may rub the hand, shake it about, and eventually return to sleep after the symptoms have subsided. In more severe cases, the discomfort may be present during the day, and ultimately persistent numbness follows. The patient notices early that she is unable to pick up needles, pins, or other small objects. Because of the associated proprioceptive difficulty, there is clumsiness in the performance of activities such as the buttoning of a blouse. If weakness follows it involves the thenar eminence, since the median nerve supplies the opponens pollicis muscle. This may be appreciated by the inability to turn a key in a lock, dropping of objects from the hand, and a deterioration in handwriting. Ultimately, atrophy ensues, most noticeably on the radial side of the thumb between the metacarpal-phalangeal joints and the wrist.

During examination one must seek possible causes for the carpal tunnel syndrome, although in more than half the cases none can be found. It is seen in conditions that cause tissue swelling, such as myxedema, pregnancy, and diabetes. It may be related to occupational trauma, particularly in male patients. Activities that require prolonged flexion and extension of the wrist, or forceful hyperextension, may thicken the transverse carpal ligament. An indistinguishable syndrome, though rarer, may be seen with abnormalities of the bones and tissues of the wrist, particularly if they result in synovial thickening or outpouching.

Neurologic examination in early cases may be entirely normal, despite significant symptoms. The first signs may be numbness at the tips of the thumb and the index and middle fingers. When the ring finger is involved, only its radial half is numb. Subsequently the numbness may extend up the fingers toward the palms. Numbness does not involve the dorsal surface of the hand.

Weakness may be detected by having the patient hold a card between the tips of his thumb and small finger. A significant difference between the two hands is suggestive. (Since this condition is commonly bilateral, this test is less valid when both hands are symptomatic.) Atrophy on the thenar eminence, as described above, may be present before significant weakness is detected.

Much has been said about the so-called Tinel's sign in the diagnosis of carpal tunnel syndrome. This is a shock-like sensation in the distribution of the median nerve, effected when the midportion of the volar surface of the wrist is tapped with the examiner's finger. Normal individuals, however, experience a similar sensation on the percussion of a peripheral nerve. Since the response cannot be quantified, this sign should not be used as the basis for selecting treatment. An extremely valuable diagnostic test, however, is the conduction velocity determination. In this test, the electromyographer stimulates the median nerve above the wrist, and records the response in a digital nerve. A significant delay in conduction across the wrist, when compared to the velocity of conduction in another portion of the nerve above the wrist, is strongly suggestive of a carpal tunnel syndrome. Patients with this syndrome who show numbness and weakness invariably have delayed conduction. Patients who are symptomatic, but in whom the conduction velocity is normal, often have a prompt, spontaneous recovery. Surgery is rarely indicated in the presence of a normal conduction velocity determination. In addition, the electromyographer may detect fibrillation in the opponens pollicis muscle, which further confirms this diagnosis.

The form of treatment depends on the duration of the symptoms and the degree of neurologic compromise. In patients with a relatively short history, who have no evidence of persistent numbness or weakness, one may consider a mid-position wrist splint, which can be applied at bedtime and removed in the morning. In many cases, this splinting eliminates the symptoms and can be discontinued when no longer needed. In more severe cases, local injection of steroids into the carpal ligament can produce prompt, long-lasting relief. The injection may have to be repeated, though in occasional cases, the condition responds to a single injection. When persistent numbness, atrophy, or intractable discomfort are present, only surgical section of the carpal ligament is effective. This is a benign procedure, with negligible risk and a high incidence of success. Under regional block anesthesia, the surgeon, by one of a variety of available techniques, can section the carpal ligament throughout its extent, and decompress the median nerve. The relief of discomfort is prompt. Usually numbness and weakness disappear, unless they are far advanced at the time of operation.

Reference

Grossman, L. A., Kaplan, H. J., Ownby, F. D., and Grossman, M.: Carpal tunnel syndrome— initial manifestation of systemic disease. J.A.M.A., *176*:259, 1961.

14. Thoracic Outlet Syndrome

FREDERICK A. SIMEONE

Cause: Abnormal cervical rib; compression by scalenus anticus or medius muscle; compression by clavicle against first rib (costoclavicular syndrome).

Early Manifestations: Usually paresthesias of hand and arm.

Treatment: Exercises, splinting, removal of offending rib or scalene muscle.

Possible Dire Consequences without Treatment: Continued pain, atrophy of muscles of arm and hand, vasomotor symptoms.

To some extent, the symptoms depend on the nature of the compressing force. The thoracic outlet roughly includes the area behind the clavicle extending from the cervical spine to the shoulder musculature, and bounded posteriorly by the upper portion of the rib cage. The patient experiences a constant dull, aching pain, or a sharper, shooting pain, which is aggravated by certain movements of the shoulder girdle. When there is a radiation into the hand, it frequently involves the ring and small fingers. Certain positions, particularly those that alter the dimensions of the thoracic outlet (such as holding the arm higher than horizontal) can aggravate the discomfort. Often the patient can keep his arms in this position for a few minutes, after which he is forced to let them drop by his side to relieve the pressure. Elevation of the hands above the horizontal plane causes the brachial plexus to arch under the abnormal rib and thereby aggravate the compression. In patients with scalenus anticus syndrome, rotation of the neck or even extension of the arm can be uncomfortable. In the costoclavicular syndrome, actions that pull the clavicle closer to the rib cage, such as hyperextension of the neck, or movement of the shoulders backward and downward, can be uncomfortable. Although most of the symptoms in these syndromes are caused by compression of the brachial plexus, vasomotor disturbances such as a feeling of coldness in the hand or a Raynaud's-like syndrome have been described, presumably due to compression of the subclavian artery. Rarely, this artery actually may become thrombosed.

More severe cases may produce actual weakness and atrophy in the upper extremity. The distribution of this motor involvement varies with the point of brachial plexus compression. Cervical rib is most likely to produce atrophy of the small muscles of the hand due to compression in an ulnar distribution. The scalenus and costoclavicular syndromes rarely include weakness.

Diagnosis of the cervical rib syndrome is occasionally simplified by palpation of the enlarged rib in the supraclavicular fossa. Anomalous ribs, however, are not frequently large enough to be palpated with certainty. Occasionally a bruit can be heard in the supraclavicular fossa, particularly with movement of the arm. Test positioning of the neck and shoulders, the so-called "thoracic outlet maneuvers," can sufficiently compress the subclavian artery so that the radial pulse is obliterated. Unfortunately, these maneuvers can lead to pulse obliteration in normal individuals, so their results are not diagnostic. These tests should be considered positive only when the pulse totally disappears, since reduction in the radial pulse is of little significance. In the cervical rib syndrome, the pulse may be obliterated when the arm is elevated and hyperabducted at the shoulder. Rotation of the head toward the affected side, associated with hyperextension of the neck, may be sufficient to occlude the subclavian artery in the scalenus anticus syndrome. More important, if the symptoms are aggravated by these maneuvers, one can then expect with greater confidence a thoracic outlet syndrome. Maneuvers that aid in the diagnosis of the scalenus anticus syndrome are essentially the same as those for cervical rib compression. In the costoclavicular syndrome, extension of the neck and backward placement of the shoulders may be sufficient to obliterate the pulse.

Specific diagnostic tests, such as electromyography, brachial angiography, and oscillometry, can occasionally confirm what is essentially a clinical diagnosis. Roentgenograms of the cervical spine, of course, are essential.

Treatment consists of avoidance of activities that can produce thoracic outlet compression. With cervical rib and scalenus anticus syndromes, activities that require the arms to be kept above the horizontal should be avoided. Exercises in these two syndromes are rarely of help. In patients who are more uncomfortable in the supine position, splinting has occasionally been helpful as a bedtime treatment. Very often, for reasons that remain unclear, the symptoms may spontaneously subside after several weeks or months.

In scalenus anticus syndrome, rotation of the head to either side should be avoided, since this will tighten or stretch the offending muscle. Occasionally direct injection of local anesthetic into the belly of the muscle can produce temporary relief.

Therapy in the costoclavicular syndrome is to be directed to those activities that pull the shoulders downward and the neck backward. Therefore, patients who carry heavy objects on their shoulders, use a wheelbarrow, and the like may be required to change their occupation.

If the pain is intractable, or evidence of weakness evolves, surgery is required. Removal of the offending cervical rib, section of the scalenus anticus muscle, or removal of a portion of the first thoracic rib is indicated, according to the nature of the compressing forces. Although the operation should be tailored to the specific condition, recently more aggressive operation involving decompression of the entire thoracic outlet through an axillary incision has been recommended. This procedure may be employed when the exact cause of the thoracic outlet compression is uncertain.

References

Noffziger, H. C., and Grant, W. T.: Neuritis of the brachial plexus mechanical in origin: the scalenus syndrome. Surg. Gynec. Obstet., *67*:722, 1938.
Rosati, L. M., and Lord, J. W.: Neurovascular Compression of the Shoulder Girdle. Modern Surgical Monograph, New York, Grune & Stratton, 1961.

15. Idiopathic Night Cramps

ORVILLE HORWITZ

Cause: Unknown.

Early Manifestations: Severe and painful cramps usually of gastrocnemius.

Treatment: Quinidine sulfate, 500 mg., Quinimine sulfate, 300 mg., or Benadryl, 50 mg. orally before retiring.

Possible Dire Consequences without Treatment: Continuation of symptoms.

Night cramps also may be due to improper drainage from the calf, as seen in deep varices, as well as to salt depletion from such causes as excess sweating. Respectively, these may be controlled by elevation of the legs or the foot of the bed, and ingestion of salt tablets.

Idiopathic cramps may be controlled by the above-mentioned drugs, which act prophylactically but not therapeutically.

Reference

Geschwind, N.: Skeletal muscle cramps. J. Clin. Pharmacol. Ther., *5*:859, 1964.

16. Treatable Intracranial Space-Occupying Lesions

Frederick A. Simeone

Cause: Brain abscess, benign tumor, aneurysm, subdural hematoma.

Early Manifestations: Signs and symptoms of increased intracranial pressure: Deafness, cranial nerve involvement, change of mood, personality, and behavior, contralateral palsy, ataxia, Jacksonian seizures, contralateral weakness, occasionally involvement of both legs, hemianopsia, oculomotor discrepancies. Many patients with temporal lobe pressure may be admitted to mental wards before proper diagnosis is made and at this point *all* other signs, symptoms, and x-ray and laboratory findings may be normal.

Treatment: Surgery and, in the case of brain abscess, antibiotics.

Possible Dire Consequences without Treatment: Increased intracranial pressure, death.

Depending on its location, the lesion may at first cause any of the aforementioned symptoms, and these may become more severe as more space is occupied. Alternately the symptoms may disappear temporarily only to recur with increased intensity, a pattern presumably attributable to the brain's temporary accommodation to its more cramped quarters.

Sometimes the history and physical examination reveal specific distinguishing symptoms. For instance, in patients who have, in addition to signs of intracranial pressure, leukocytosis, fever and sinusitis or bronchiectasis, brain abscess is the most likely diagnosis, whereas subdural hematoma is suspected in patients who have suffered a recent accident. It is not unusual, however, to find nothing other than one or two of the above symptoms, with no indication of the causes. High index of suspicion is most helpful.

The most dangerous error is to mistake one of the treatable conditions for vascular insufficiency.

In the past, diagnosis was based on signs of increased intracranial pressure. Fortunately, however, owing to an increased index of suspicion among physicians and vastly improved diagnostic facilities, earlier diagnosis is possible. The triad of headache, vomiting, and papilledema is found in toto in only 50% of all cases; these symptoms also can occur in any sequence. Bradycardia and increased blood pressure also may be noted.

Brain scan, electroencephalography, angiography, and pneumoencephalography are the ultimate guides to the size, location, and often the nature of these conditions.

References

Allen, N., and Mustian, V.: Origin and significance of vascular murmurs of the head and neck. Medicine, *41*:227, 1962.

Courville, C. B., and Rosenvold, L. K.: Intracranial complications of infections of nasal cavities and accessory sinuses; a survey of lesions observed in a series of 15,000 autopsies. Arch. Otolaryng., *27*:692, 1938.

Dandy, W. E.: Intracranial arterial aneurysms. New York, Comstock Publishing Co., Inc., 1944.

Elliott, F. A.: Clinical Neurology. 2nd Ed. Philadelphia, W. B. Saunders Co., 1971.

Elliott, F. A., and McKissock, W.: Acoustic neuroma: early diagnosis. Lancet, 2:1189, 1954.

Givre, A., and Olivecrona, H.: Surgical experiences with acoustic tumors. J. Neurosurg., 6:396, 1949.

Hoefer, P. F. A.: The electroencephalogram in cases of head injury. *In* Injuries of the Brain and Spinal Cord and Their Coverings. 4th Ed. Edited by S. Brock. New York, Springer Publishing Co., 1970.

Zulch, K. J.: Brain Tumors: Their Biology and Pathology. New York, Springer Publishing Co., 1965.

Chapter VI

Abdominal and Gastrointestinal Diseases

Introduction

Of the seventeen disorders mentioned, ten are definitely surgical, four potentially surgical, and three definitely medical. Therapeutically, then, the abdominal cavity is fundamentally a surgical area. Other lesions for which operation is surely the treatment of choice are discussed in the vascular and urinary sections of this book.

The cardinal sign of abdominal disease is pain. Regardless of its source, the pain is referred to some cutaneous segment more or less near the area of origin, but with overlap. Painful melena and painful hematuria point to local disorder; bleeding alone is much less significant. Bleeding may be due to primary intestinal disorders, such as ulcers, polyps, diverticula, telangiec-tases, or infections, the latter including such conditions as masquerading tuberculosis, syphilis, typhoid fever, and other bacterial or parasitic condi-tions. It may be due to local (ruptured aneurysm, mesenteric occlusion) or to widespread disorders (polycythemia, purpura, scurvy, anticoagulant dis-orders, hemophilia) and not to intestinal diseases alone.

In its other role this chapter is concerned with the gastrointestinal tract as a structure that happens to traverse the abdomen. Here we are in a less surgical domain, which in theory extends from glossitis to hemorrhoids. Hiatal hernia is included; colitis is not. Symptoms are more nondescript than in abdominal disease broadly. Nausea accompanies acute neurologic syndromes from head injury to hypercalcemia, to heat stroke with fever, to exertion or labyrinthitis without fever or fever with little else. It, of course, may accompany gut disease simply; the first symptom of gut bleeding may be thirst and restlessness, and the principal symptom of dumping may be syncope.

Of all the classically surgical conditions appendicitis is surely the foremost and was once perhaps the only specifically treatable disease with almost assured excellent results. For this reason professors of surgery encourage such conversations as this:

Q: "When encountering an acute abdomen, what's the first thing you think of?"
A.: "Acute appendicitis."
Q: "What's the last thing?"
A: "Acute appendicitis."

Many surgeons state that a medical service is the worst place in the world to develop this disease.

I once had a man's gangrenous appendix removed for the sole reason that he was a friend of my father's from whom I was accustomed to take orders.

Now there are other lesions which we can treat. Some are mentioned under infectious disease under "pus below the diaphragm." Some others are mentioned below.

Neoplasms have not been considered, although certain malignancies of the large bowel are not too rarely completely excised, particularly if the presenting symptoms are localized in the case of obstruction rather than generalized as in the case of weakness and anemia. Even patients suffering from such monstrous conditions as esophageal carcinoma and leiomyosarcoma of the stomach sometimes yield to x-ray treatment upon occasion, but this, unfortunately, is excessively rare.

Other conditions which may present as gastrointestinal disease include: Purpura. Scurvy. Polyps. Anti-coagulant therapy. Hemophilia. Tuberculosis. Syphilis. Typhoid Fever. Interspinal paralysis. Ruptured Aneurysm. Mesenteric Arterial Occlusion. Telangiectasis. Tabes dorsalis.

1. Achalasia

SIDNEY COHEN

Cause: Unknown. Degeneration of neural elements in the brain stem, vagal nerves and Auerbach's plexi.

Early Manifestations: Dysphagia, chest pain, nocturnal regurgitation.

Treatment: Pneumatic dilatation or surgical myotomy of the lower esophageal sphincter.

Possible Dire Consequences without Treatment: Aspiration pneumonia, lung abscess, bronchiectasis.

Achalasia of the esophagus is a disorder that affects both sexes at any age but is seen most commonly in young adults and middle aged persons. The etiology is not clear. It may be viral or degenerative. Neural changes have been shown in the dorsal vagal nucleus in the brain stem, the vagal trunk, and the myenteric ganglia in the body of the esophagus. Patients with achalasia always have dysphagia (a subjective awareness of the passage of a bolus). The dysphagia is for both liquids and solids. Regurgitation (usually nocturnal) occurs in about 70% of patients. Chest pain is present in about 30%. Weight loss, although present, is not a prominent symptom.

The diagnosis of achalasia is best made by history and x-ray examination. X-ray examination shows esophageal dilatation, aperistalsis and a symmetrically tapered (bird beak) distal esophagus corresponding to the lower esophageal sphincter. Esophagoscopy is done to exclude conditions that may mimic achalasia. The instrument should pass easily into the stomach. In carcinoma and stricture, the esophagoscope cannot be passed into the stomach.

Esophageal manometry shows absence of peristalsis with or without simultaneous, non-peristaltic, repetitive contractions (tertiary waves). The lower esophageal sphincter pressure is markedly elevated as compared to normals (50 mm. Hg in achalasia as compared to 20 mm. Hg in normals). During swallowing sphincter pressure relaxes but only partially. In normals, pressure in the sphincter decreases by about 95% during swallowing, whereas in patients with achalasia, the drop in pressure is about 30 to 40%. The partial decrease in pressure leaves a residual pressure which acts as the obstruction at the cardio-esophageal junction.

Therapy of achalasia, pneumatic dilatation and Heller cardiomyotomy, reduces the level of sphincter pressure. Therapy does not restore peristalsis nor does it make the sphincter relax to a greater degree during swallowing. The decrease in sphincter pressure by both forms of therapy allows the esophagus to empty in the upright position and thus diminishes esophageal retention and subsequent regurgitation.

Pneumatic dilatation is successful in 90% of patients but repeat treatments may be required. A small risk of esophageal rupture is present with dilatation. Heller myotomy is also highly successful, and provides more permanent results than pneumatic dilatation. However, surgery produces sphincteric incompetence in about 20% of patients. Most clinicians use pneumatic dilatation initially and surgery in cases requiring multiple treatments.

At present, achalasia is a treatable disease. However, both forms of treatment have serious drawbacks. The future management of achalasia may be modified by the recent demonstration that sphincter pressure is elevated because of a supersensitivity to the gastrointestinal hormone, gastrin.

References

Cohen, S. and Lipshutz, W.: Lower Esophageal Sphincter Dysfunction in Achalasia. Gastroenterology *61*:814, 1971.

Cohen, S., Lipshutz, W., and Hughes, W.: Role of Gastrin Supersensitivity in the Pathogenesis of Lower Esophageal Sphincter Hypertension in Achalasia. J. Clin. Invest. *50*:1241, 1971.

Bernstein, L. M., Fruin, R. C., and Pacini, R.: Differential of esophageal pain from angina pectoris: Role of the esophageal acid perfusion test. Med. *41*:143, 1962.

2. Hiatal Hernia

ORVILLE HORWITZ

Cause: Relaxing of supporting tissue of diaphragm with herniation of abdominal organs into chest. This is a common disorder and is said to occur to a greater or a lesser extent in almost half the individuals over fifty years of age.

Early Manifestations: Generally none. Symptoms probably vary with the size of the hiatus, and are more pronounced in the recumbent position. This is dull, postprandial, retrosternal fullness, disappearing spontaneously, and later possible dyspnea, in large hernias from crowding of the thoracic structures.

Treatment: Early: antacid and position. Late: surgical repair.

Possible Dire Consequences without Treatment: Pain, mimicking angina, acute or chronic hemorrhage, anemia.

This is a common disorder which occasionally gives rise to serious and debilitating symptoms, especially if reflux esophagitis occurs. Usually, however, it is asymptomatic and the problem for the physician is to decide whether or not the hernia is responsible for the symptoms. Certainly a very small percentage of patients require surgical intervention which is fortunate as the necessary procedure is still far from satisfactory in many instances.

Reference

Fleischner, F. G.: Hiatal hernia complex. J.A.M.A., *162*:183, 1956.

3. Hypertrophic Pyloric Stenosis

DAVID MORRIS

Cause: Primary pyloric muscle hypertrophy; secondary scarring

Early Manifestations: Slowly progressive obstruction and gastric retention

Treatment: Limited gastric resection with a drainage procedure

Possible Dire Consequences without Treatment: Prolonged gastric retention

---

Two varieties of hypertrophic pyloric stenosis can be differentiated. The more common is a secondary hypertrophy usually in association with chronic gastritis or duodenal ulcer disease, occasionally from carcinoma (both gastric and pancreatic) and rarely from a foreign body or gastric polyp with a long pedicle creating a ball-valve obstruction. The primary or idiopathic form in adults (usually males) shows only pyloric hypertrophy. Though not seen as frequently as in infants, primary hypertrophic pyloric stenosis is probably more common than believed.

Symptoms are quite variable. Ulcer-like pain is most common. Vomiting is frequent. Proportional to the severity of emesis, one sees dehydration, hypochloremia and alkalosis. Weight loss is common, but is not necessarily associated with vomiting. Minimal symptoms such as "bloating" after eating may be the only complaint.

For diagnosis the presence of gastric retention should be verified. When previous ulcer disease is known, the diagnosis is immediately suggested. The primary form should be considered when the upper gastrointestinal series shows a long narrow smooth pyloric channel. Total obstruction is rare as contrasted to that from malignancies in this area. Gastroscopy is not usually diagnostic but the presence of the "cervix sign" is described as being characteristic in the primary form. Gastroscopy and cytologic studies can definitely help rule in a malignant lesion.

Surgery is indicated for a high-grade obstruction or when carcinoma is suspected. The Fredet-Ramstedt pyloromyotomy although highly successful in infants allows no inspection of the gastric mucosa and does not give optimal results in adults. Gastric complications of hypertrophic pyloric stenosis in adults are relatively frequent and will not necessarily be seen on roentgenography. Gastritis, gastric ulcers or carcinoma may remain undetected. Pylorectomy and mucosal inspection with a drainage procedure are recommended. Prognosis is good.

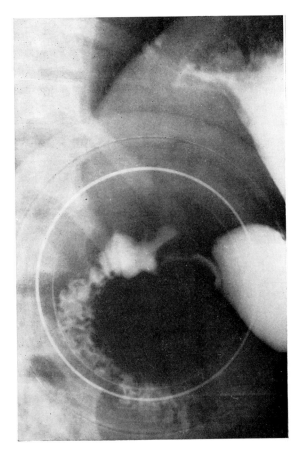

Fig. VI–1. Forty-five-year-old male presenting with low sternal chest pain and post-cibal bloating for the preceding several years. The symptoms were relieved by induced vomiting. An upper gastrointestinal series showed a hiatal hernia and a relatively fixed zone of narrowing in the antrum and pylorus. Carcinoma could not be excluded. Cytologic studies were negative. Gastroscopy showed a cobblestoned, deformed antrum with a "pseudo-pylorus." Surgery revealed only hypertrophic pyloric stenosis.

References

Boyle, J. D. and Goldstein, H.: Management of pyloric obstruction: Med. Clin. N.A. *52*:1329, 1968.

DeMuth, W. E., Jr., et al.: Gastric complications of hypertrophic pyloric stenosis in adults. Amer. Surg., *36*:428, 1970.

Hakhamini, H. and Cogbill, C. L.: Primary adult hypertrophic pyloric stenosis. Case report and review of literature. Amer. Surg. *34*:446, 1968.

Ittzes, E.: Pyloric obstruction in adults caused by congenital stenosis. Amer. J. Surg. *116*:97, 1968.

Milano, A. M., Lindner, A. E. and Marshak, R. H.: The Radiology Corner. Primary hypertrophic pyloric stenosis in the adult. Amer. J. Gastroenterol. *55*:174, 1971.

Shuster, M. M. and Smith, V. M.: The pyloric "cervix sign" in adult hypertrophic pyloric stenosis. Gastroint. Endosc. *16*:210, 1970.

4. Zollinger-Ellison Syndrome— Hypergastrinemia

ALEXANDER RUSH

Cause: Non-insulin secreting tumor of the pancreas.

Early Manifestations: The presenting symptoms and signs may be quite variable. In addition to the above, some patients describe bouts of abdominal cramps and diarrhea; others, nausea and vomiting of sour, scalding material upon awakening. If they are able to vomit this material, they manage to get through the remainder of the day without too much discomfort.

Treatment: Presently limited to surgery—(a) removal of the secreting tumor, or (b) total gastrectomy. The localization of the tumor(s) may be difficult.

Possible Dire Consequences without Treatment: Pain, discomfort, death.

In 1955 Zollinger and Ellison presented a syndrome characterized by (1) fulminating ulcer diathesis; (2) gastric hypersecretion; (3) presence of a non-beta islet cell tumor of the pancreas. They speculated that these symptoms were related to the release by the tumor of a potent gastric secretogogue. Gregory subsequently demonstrated that the potent secretogogue was indeed gastrin. Zollinger subsequently analyzed some 700 reported cases. In 46% intractable ulcerlike pain was described. The usual complications of ulcer were encountered as follows: perforation 24%; hemorrhage 15%; obstruction 2%. Of particular significance is the fact that in 17% of the reported cases peptic ulceration was not a prominent feature in the clinical picture.

The diagnosis is based on the clinical history as noted. Upper gastrointestinal x-ray examination may reveal evidence of gastric hypersecretion with giant folds of the mucosa, ulcerative lesions in the duodenum that are particularly prone to involve the post-bulbar area and even beyond the ligament of Treitz. Laboratory aids to the diagnosis include the demonstration of a twelve-hour gastric secretory volume of 1 liter or more; and a ratio of Peak Acid Output Basal-HCL mEq./L/hr. (add 4 successive 15-minute samples) to Peak Acid Output Histalog HCL mEq./L/ (highest output for any two successive 15-minute periods $\times$ 2) greater than 0.6 (Z-E: $\dfrac{\text{PAO Basal}}{\text{PAO Histalog}} = 0.6$). This is interpreted as indicating that the stomach of the patient with Z-E is being maximally stimulated at all times and thus additional stimulation by Histalog does not produce the increase such as occurs in patients with the ordinary duodenal ulcer. Radio-immunoassay now provides the most reliable method of diagnosis since it has been demonstrated by McGuigan that, in contrast to normal individuals and to patients with common peptic ulcer, serum gastrin concentrations are found to be above 600 $\mu\mu$g./ml. even as high as 300,000 $\mu\mu$g./ml.

Pancreatic scanning and selective angiography may in some cases be most helpful. If localization of the tumor cannot be made, then total removal of the target organ-gastrectomy is advocated by Zollinger on the grounds of a high degree (50%) of malignancy, the frequency of adenomatosis throughout the pancreas, and aberrant locations of functioning islet tissue *e.g.*, the walls of the duodenum. The results of total gastrectomy in young individuals appear to be far better than might be anticipated from the results of a similar procedure for gastric malignancy in older individuals.

References

Zollinger, R. M.: The GI effects of pancreatic tumors. Phila. Med. *66*:219, 1970.
————: Pancreatic problems. Chronic pancreatitis and pancreatic tumors. Postgrad. Med. *49*:145, 1971.

5. Peptic Ulcer

ALEXANDER RUSH

Cause: Unknown. Development of ulceration believed to be acid-pepsin secretion acting on area of lowered mucosal resistance for whatever reason—vascular, neural, humoral, etc.

Early Manifestations: Epigastric pain-food-ease syndrome. Pain may be absent. It has been estimated that about 25% of patients presenting with massive gastrointestinal hemorrhage from active ulcer provide no other symptom suggestive of the disease.

Treatment: Principles are rest, feedings, sedation, antacids and anticholinergenics.

Possible Dire Consequences without Treatment: Perforation, bleeding, obstruction, death.

Pain, when present, may be centered anywhere in the abdomen other than the usual epigastrium and may mimic that of acute appendicitis or sigmoid diverticulitis. The pain may be described as low substernal resembling the "heartburn" of lower esophageal reflux. Particularly deceiving is the location of pain in the lower thoracic or lumbar area. This type of pain is usually associated with penetration of the ulcer deep into the posterior wall and into the pancreas. The correct interpretation of the pain is further complicated by the loss of the usual rhythm and periodicity and by an inconclusive or lack of response to food and antacids. When the pancreas is penetrated, there may even be a misleading elevation of the serum amylase but seldom does this elevation reach the proportions expected in acute pancreatitis. Non-specific symptoms to be looked for are "emotional ulcer equivalents"—unusual fatigue, depression, or irritability. The classical positive physical sign of acute tenderness localized in the epigastrium in the midline or a little to the right may be entirely absent. On the other hand spot tenderness over a lower thoracic vertebra may be striking if looked for and found.

Diagnosis. The clinical diagnosis of peptic ulcer should be confirmed by appropriate radiologic examination. The demonstration of a persistent crater is considered direct and conclusive evidence of ulcer. Indirect evidence consists of irritable deformity in the absence of demonstrable crater. A positive radiologic diagnosis is possible in better than 85% of patients. When the x-ray evidence is absent or equivocal and yet the clinical evidence is strong, a useful diagnostic aid is the Palmer Acid Test; 200 ml. 0.1 N HCL are instilled through a catheter with the tip within the fasting stomach that has previously been emptied. The prompt development of typical distress which is relieved on aspiration of the acid and replacement with 200 ml. 2% NaNCO₃ constitutes strong evidence of active ulcerative disease. Additional laboratory studies such as determinations of basal acid output, peak acid output following maximal stimulation with Histalog serum gastrin levels are not useful as routine procedures. They do have an important role in differential diagnosis of certain gastric lesions, Zollinger-Ellison syndrome and perhaps in decisions as to prognosis and the need for possible surgical interventions.

Reference

Palmer, W. L.: Portis' Diseases of the Digestive System. Philadelphia, Lea & Febiger, 1941.

6. Chronic Active Liver Disease

R. D. SOLOWAY, W. H. J. SUMMERSKILL, A. H. BAGGENSTOSS AND L. J. SCHOENFIELD

Cause: Australia antigen, other viruses, drugs (oxyphenisatin), alcohol.

Early Manifestations: Jaundice 56% fatigue 67%, anorexia 27%, arthralgias 25%, acute onset 56%, amenorrhea 48%.

Treatment: For disease with 10-fold increase in SGOT or 5-fold increase in SGOT with 2-fold rise in gamma globulin: prednisone 60 mg. initially, 20 mg. maintenance or prednisone 30 mg. initially, 10 mg. maintenance coupled with 50 mg. azathioprine daily.

Possible Dire Consequences without Treatment: Continued liver disease, possibly death.

Criteria for the selection of patients include chronicity, documented by liver function tests, of at least ten weeks' duration without improvement; activity, biochemically characterized by a persistent 10-fold rise in SGOT, or a 5-fold rise in SGOT coupled with a 2-fold rise in gamma globulin; and the demonstration on liver biopsy of moderate to severe piecemeal necrosis, portal round cell infiltration and Kupffer cell proliferation with or without subacute hepatitis or cirrhosis.

The differential diagnosis of CALD includes Wilson's disease, chronic persistent hepatitis, primary biliary cirrhosis, hemochromatosis and the pericholangitis associated with ulcerative colitis and regional enteritis. These conditions are almost

TABLE VI–1. TREATMENT PROGRAMS FOUND EFFECTIVE
FOR CHRONIC ACTIVE LIVER DISEASE

Date	*Prednisone (Pred)*	*Prednisone and Azathioprine (Comb)*	
1st week	60 mg. daily*	30 mg daily*	50 mg. daily*
2nd week	40	20	50
3rd & 4th wks	30	15	50
Maintenance	20	10	50

* Medications given as one dose daily at 8 A.M.

always separable on clinical, biochemical and histologic grounds or by the use of specific laboratory tests. The two conditions presenting the most frequent problems in differential diagnosis are acute and chronic persistent hepatitis. Chronic persistent hepatitis usually follows a benign course and does not eventuate in either cirrhosis or death if untreated. It is arbitrarily distinguished from CALD on histologic grounds by the presence of minimal or absent piecemeal necrosis. From a review of the literature, only 5 of 306 United States patients with acute hepatitis fulfilled the criteria and had a 10-fold elevation of SGOT at ten weeks after the onset of their illness. Five of 37 patients with persistent hepatitis had a persistent elevation of SGOT of this magnitude.

Table VI–1 indicates the Pred and Comb regimens we are presently using to treat CALD. During this study, 2 other groups received placebo or azathioprine 100 mg. daily.

The first 63 patients studied ranged from twelve years (the lower limit for entrance into study) to seventy-five years of age. Females comprised 71% of the series.

Prednisone or a combination of prednisone and azathioprine have been found to be superior to azathioprine alone or placebo for the treatment of severe chronic active liver disease. On the successful regimens outlined, fewer patients developed encephalopathy, ascites and increasing jaundice, or died, while more patients developed clinical, biochemical and histologic resolution.

Chronic Active Liver Disease (CALD) is a condition characterized by biochemical and histologic signs of continuing hepatic inflammation and necrosis. From a review of the literature, up to 50% of patients with severe CALD will die within three years of initial diagnosis if untreated.

Until the past few years, the management of this condition has not been subjected to controlled trials of drug therapy. Guidelines for management had been suggested from the results of nonuniform treatment but decisions had not been made concerning whether or not the benefits of the drugs used exceeded their toxicity. Results from the Copenhagen study group for liver disease suggested that prednisone prolonged survival in females with cirrhosis and without ascites. Immunosuppressives, such as 6-mercaptopurine and azathioprine, had been used alone and in combination with steroids in such a variety of schedules that conclusions concerning efficacy could not be drawn.

The aim of our study was to assess the effect of Prednisone (Pred), Azathioprine (Azp), a combination of prednisone and azathioprine (Comb) and placebo (Plac) on chronic active liver disease (CALD) in a randomized double-blind trial with predefined criteria for improvement or deterioration.

The onset was acute and clinically biochemically indistinguishable from acute hepatitis in 51%. The clinical duration of disease had been greater than eighteen months in 16%, between six and eighteen months in 35% and between 2.5 and six months in 49%. Fifty-eight percent of patients described a decrease in their ability to carry on normal daily activities and 24% complained of a decreased appetite. Prior variceal bleeding had occurred in 5% and prior encephalopathy in 8%. Ascites and/or peripheral edema were present in 17%.

Prior to treatment, the range of SGOT in these patients was between 125 to greater than 3000 (our normal was less than 25 IU/L). The serum bilirubin was greater than 1.0 mgm% in more than 90%. An elevated gamma globulin was present in 92% and 95% had a depressed albumin. The prothrombin time was significantly elevated in 50%. In contrast, only 19% had a marked elevation of alkaline phosphatase (greater than 200 IU/L, normal less than 70). IgG was increased in 88%, IgA in 30% and IgM in 71%. The Australia antigen was positive in 7% and the LE clot test in 36%.

Liver biopsies uniformly showed piecemeal necrosis, round cell infiltration and Kupffer cell proliferation.

In order to evaluate the response of CALD to treatment, we defined the therapeutic end points of remission and treatment failure. Remission indicated achievement of clinical and biochemical normality, and loss of features characteristic of CALD on biopsy. Treatment failure indicated the development of encephalopathy or increasing ascites with a two-fold increase in serum bilirubin to greater than 12 mg.%.

In terms of overall response to treatment, Pred or Comb were superior to Azp or Plac. Forty-seven percent of patients receiving Pred or Comb and 19% of patients receiving Azp or Plac remitted (P<0.05%) while 6% of patients receiving Pred or Comb and 45% patients receiving Azp or Plac failed treatment (P <0.02%). Subsequent follow-up of these and additional patients has demonstrated that 80% of patients receiving Pred or Comb remit within two years of beginning therapy. The efficacy of prednisone in enhancing survival in CALD has been demonstrated in a concurrent study by Cook et al. Little histologic resolution occurred, perhaps due to the lower dose of prednisone used.

No one in the Pred or Comb groups developed a loss of appetite and only the two patients who failed developed encephalopathy. Ascites developed in only one patient during the course of treatment and cleared in 90% of those patients on Pred and Comb in whom it had been initially present. In contrast, among patients receiving Azp or Plac, a decrease in appetite was noted in 25%, and encephalopathy and ascites each developed in 33%. In addition, only 33% of patients in these groups experienced clearing of ascites, if it was present initially. Elevated levels of SGOT, gamma globulin, serum bilirubin, albumin and alkaline phosphatase returned to normal significantly more frequently among patients receiving Pred or Comb. With the use of serial liver biopsies, there was a significantly increased incidence of resolution of features characteristic of CALD among patients receiving Pred or Comb. This resolution followed clinical and biochemical resolution by six to eighteen months and was the determining feature in assessing when to discontinue maintenance therapy.

Severe toxic reactions to prednisone included vertebral collapse, aseptic necrosis of the hip and cataracts and occurred on 10% of patients receiving prednisone for one year or more. These complications were not significantly more frequent than among patients on regimens not containing prednisone. A cushingoid appearance developed in most patients receiving regimens containing prednisone, even when the maintenance dose was 10 mg. per day. These features generally regressed when the medication was discontinued. Features ascribed to azathioprine toxicity, thrombocytopenia and leukopenia, or ascites coupled with deteriorating liver function developed more frequently in patients receiving Azp or Plac. Each of these toxic features developed in patients receiving placebo, making difficult the separation of drug toxicity from the natural course of the disease.

References

Treatment

Ammon, H. V., Baggenstoss, A. H., and Summerskill, W. H. J.: Characterization and incidence of remission and relapse in chronic active liver disease (CALD). Abstract: Gastroenterology *62*:173, 1972.

Boyer, J. L., and Klatskin, G.: Pattern of necrosis in acute viral hepatitis prognostic value of bridging (subacute hepatic necrosis). New Eng. J. Med., *283*:1063, 1071, 1970.

Cook, G. C., Mulligan, R., and Sherlock, S.: Controlled, prospective trial of corticosteroid therapy in active chronic hepatitis. Quart. J. Med. *40*:159, 1971.

Copenhagen Study Group for Liver Diseases. Effect of Prednisone on the survival of patients with cirrhosis of the Liver. Lancet, *1*:119, 1969.

Geall, M. G., Schoenfield, L. J., and Summerskill, W. H. J.: Classification and treatment of chronic active liver disease, Gastroenterology, *55*:724, 1968.

Soloway, R. D., Summerskill, W. H. J., Baggenstoss, A. H., Geall, M. G., Gitnick, G. L., Elveback, L. R., and Schoenfield, L. J.: Clinical, biochemical and histologic remission of severe chronic active liver disease: A controlled study of treatments and early prognosis. Gastroenterology, *63*:820, 1972.

Supplemental

Mackay, I. R.: Chronic hepatitis: effect of prolonged suppressive treatment and comparison of azathioprine with prednisone. Quart. J. Med., *37*:379, 1968.

Mistilis, S. P. and Blackburn, C. R. B.: Active chronic hepatitis. Am. J. Medicine, *48*:484, 1970.

Page, A. R., Good, R. A. and Pollara, B.: Long-term results of therapy in patients with chronic liver disease associated with hypergammaglobulinemia. Am. J. Med., *47*:765, 1969.

Sherlock, S.: The immunology of liver disease. Am. J. Med., *49*:693, 1970.

7. Pseudocyst of Pancreas

Peter Moulder

Cause: Often trauma or pancreatitis.

Early Manifestations: Often presents as persistent epigastric pain without fever and without weight loss. Pain is not necessarily either continuous or severe. It is sometimes accompanied by fever, nausea and vomiting. Negative x-ray studies are not unusual.

Treatment: Decompression into stomach commonest present surgical procedure.

Possible Dire Consequences without Treatment: Continuing symptoms. Sometimes death.

Clinical suspicion is a vague upper abdominal symptom-set. Careful palpation of the abdomen will find a mass or fullness in many patients, and upper gastro-intestinal x-ray examination will show displacement of the stomach or change in duodenal configuration in three-quarters of those that are of clinical significance. Additional Studies: Radionuclide studies are useful when deciding between normal and abnormal, but not for distinguishing a lesion such as pseudocyst; this holds true for subtraction analysis [liver (Tc^{99m}) + pancreas (Se^{135})]—liver (Tc^{99m}). Celiac and superior mesenteric arteriography will indicate a space-occupying lesion which can be a cyst of any type, a tumor (since many in the pancreas are not hypervascularized) or just pancreatitis. A "blush" in the arteriogram which usually indicates tumor can occur when there is hemorrhage or bleeding into a pseudocyst; and, since this is common in the symptomatic phase of these cysts, care must be taken in judgment until there are enough data to indicate the importance of this.

TREATMENT

Treatment is temporarily medical when in the acute phase to allow the wall to thicken. Rarely will the pseudocyst disappear and generally the patient should be planned for surgical treatment. When the pseudocyst has been present for some time, or if threatening to rupture (rapid enlargement, peritoneal irritation, diaphragmatic irritation), pleural fluid will usually form. Then surgical exploration should be prompt. Medical therapy is the same as for acute pancreatitis, *i.e.* those modalities, such as gastric decompression that depress the exocrine pancreatic function since the pseudocyst is filled from the ductal system of the pancreas. There is a variety of surgical maneuvers: decompression into the stomach is the most common procedure, but decompression into an isolated small-bowel segment—Roux-en-Y is preferred by many. External decompression was common in the early days of surgical therapy, and on occasion can be used in extreme situations; however it is not "better" for the friable wall, since it is more dependent on a firm suture connection for its integrity than internal decompression, because of the distance between skin and cyst, their different directional mobilities.

References

Hess, W.: Surgery of the Biliary Passages and the Pancreas. Princeton, D. Van Nostrand Co., 1965.

Jordan, G. L.: Pancreatic Cysts, in Surgical Diseases of the Pancreas. Howard, J. M. and Jordan, G. L., Eds. Philadelphia, J. B. Lippincott Co., 1960, pp. 283–320.

Landman, S., Polcyn, R. E., and Gottschalk, A.: Pancreas imagery—Is it worth it? Radiology, *100*:631, 1971.

Rhoads, E.: Pancreas Chap. 33, p. 916. *In* Surgery, Principles and Practice, E. Rhoads, J. G. Allen, H. N. Harkins, and C. A. Moyers (Eds.) 4th Ed. Philadelphia, J. B. Lippincott Co., 1970.

8. Acute Cholecystitis

PETER MOULDER

Cause: (a) Primary   —Undetermined
        (b) Proximal   —Gallstones
                             Previous inflammation of gallbladder
        (c) Local   —Vascular deficiency (edema, tumor, etc.)
                             Infective bacterial organism
        (d) Systemic   —Diabetes
                             Homo Sapiens
                             Female in central age range   Estrogenics

Vaguely— Multiparity / Vagal hyper- or mal-function

        (e) Unique   —Hemolytic disorder
                             Hypercholesterolemia
        (f) Inter-related —Pancreatitis
                             Myocardial coronary disease

Early Manifestations:

1. "Fecund, fat female of forty" with right upper quadrant abdominal pain occasionally referred to scapula

     Examination   (a) Tender to finger-tip pressure over the gallbladder. The gallbladder nestles into the palm of the hand as a rounded mass.
                              (b) Hyperesthesia over a localized area of the abdomen anterior to the gallbladder.
                              (c) Often right upper quadrant referred pain with *vigorous* jostling of the abdomen elsewhere.

     Variations   Left upper quadrant pain or only the scapular pain.

2. "Just not well." Loss of appetite, weak, sweaty and no desire to move. Occasionally nausea and vomiting.

     Examination   (a) Fever—102°
                              (b) Tachycardia—120
                              (c) Patient is irritable during the query and abdominal examination
                              (d) Leukocytosis and/or polymorphonuclear leukocytes 90%
                              (e) Diabetes present, newly found, or worsened

3. Occasionally Early:
                              (a) Jaundice from biliary obstruction or possibly from hemolytic disease
                              (b) Signs of accompanying pancreatitis
                              (c) Signs of bile peritonitis—disastrous

Treatment

This should be a systems approach and preferably one developed in a collaborative way by the practitioner-internist and the surgeon to suit the local dynamics and the skills of each. There are many courses to follow, and most work quite well. The greatest variations relate: (1) to early versus delayed operation in the non-perforative variety, (2) to the extent of delay if not done in the acute situation and (3) to the election of surgery after the first attack. Under any circumstance *cholecystectomy* is the curative treatment and for practical purposes non-resective therapy is delaying (even though for many years—and this can be the correct treatment in certain situations).

The following schema is a reasonable indicator of the various plans in use today.

SCHEMA

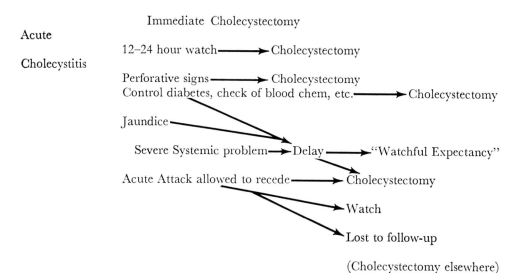

(Cholecystectomy elsewhere)

According to Hofmann and Thistle, "When clinical studies of potential gallstone-dissolving agents began, it was thought that all the natural bile components might be suitable and that the goal of pharmacologic dissolution might be achieved through expansion of the bile acid pool. But the experience described here showed that only chenodeoxycholic acid dissolved stones, that it dissolved only cholesterol gallstones, and that it acts by rendering bile unsaturated in cholesterol."

POSSIBLE DIRE CONSEQUENCES WITHOUT TREATMENT

1. Perforation with bile peritonitis and death.
2. Localized perforation with severe chronic inflammation
3. Prolonged near total disability
4. Uncontrollable diabetes
5. Myocardial infarction
6. Pancreatitis
7. Cholecystectomy elsewhere

References

Danzinger, R. G. et al.: Effect of oral chenodeoxycholic acid on bile acid kinetics and biliary lipid composition in women with cholelithiasis. J. Clin. Invest., *52*:2908, 1973.
Hofmann, A. F. and Thistle, J. L.: Chenodeoxycholic acid: The Mayo Clinic experience. Hosp. Pract. *9*:41, 1974.
Standard Medical Surgical Texts.
Schein, C. J.: Acute Cholecystitis. New York, Harper & Row, 1972.

9. Intussusception

ORVILLE HORWITZ

Cause: Usually protrusion of wall of the ileum near the ileocecal valve in the lumen.

Early Manifestations: Pain and signs of obstruction near the ileocecal valve.

Treatment: Surgery

Possible Dire Consequences without Treatment: Continued intestinal obstruction and death

This is usually a disease of children in the first two years of life. However, it may also occur in adults. In the latter case, there is frequently a tumor, benign or malignant, associated with the disease. In a few cases the intussusception reduces without treatment leaving an intact intestinal tract. However, operation, particularly in older patients, is almost always necessary.

References

Rhoads, J. E., Allen, J. G., Harkin, H. N., and Moyer, C. A.: Surgical management of dead and distended bowel. *In* Surgery—Principles and Practice, 4th ed. Philadelphia, J. B. Lippincott Co., 1970, p. 1098.
Ibid. p. 1521.

10. Non-Tropical Sprue

JULIUS J. DEREN

Cause: Sensitivity to or toxicity of gluten.

Early Manifestations: Weight loss, diarrhea, bulky stool, specific nutritional deficiencies, *i.e.* vitamin B_{12} (megaloblastic anemia), vitamin K (hemorrhage), calcium and vitamin D (tetany and bone lesions).

Treatment: Avoidance of gluten-containing foods.

Possible Dire Consequences without Treatment: Continued symptoms and death.

Classic presentation—bulky stools, weight loss, malnutrition.
Subtle presentation—one or more of the following may be the predominating presenting feature:
Weight loss
Steatorrheic stool (diarrhea may or may not be present)
Generalized malnutrition

Vitamin or mineral deficiency
  1. Vitamin B_{12}—megaloblastic anemia
  2. Iron deficiency unrelated to blood loss and nonresponse to oral iron supplement
  3. Vitamin C and Ca^{++} tetany and bone disease
  4. Folic acid deficiency
  5. Vitamin K—Hypoprothrombinemia
Past history of celiac disease
Family history of non-tropical sprue
Abdominal distension
Abdominal pain.

Pathology. Virtual complete atrophy of the villi of the small bowel, lesion is more severe in proximal than distal small bowel.

Severe distortion of the epithelial cell.

Decrease in the microvilli.

Variable cellular infiltrate in lamina propria.

Diagnosis. The essential diagnostic features are the demonstration of a "flat" small bowel biopsy and improvement of biopsy and malabsorption upon gluten withdrawal.

Other laboratory studies are helpful in documenting malabsorption and in its differential diagnosis and include:
  1. Steatorrhea—fecal fat excretion of greater than 6 gm/day is present in 90% of patients with non-tropical sprue.
  2. Serum carotene of less than 50 μg./100 ml. is frequently present. Usefulness limited by rapid decrease in serum level when dietary intake is curtailed and not helpful in differential diagnosis of malabsorption.
  3. Xylose tolerance test. A majority of patients with non-tropical sprue will excrete in the urine less than 4 gm./24 hours following a 25-gm. oral loading dose of xylose. Most helpful in differentiating non-tropical sprue from pancreatic insufficiency.
  4. Schilling Test—Vitamin B_{12} malabsorption is present in patients with severe disease in whom the small bowel lesion extends to ileum.
  5. Small bowel roentgenograms reveal dilatation, coarsening of the folds, segmentation, and flocculation. Small bowel pattern is generally normal in pancreatic insufficiency.

Pathophysiology. Epithelial cells are injured as a result of exposure to gluten fraction of wheat, oats, barley. The injury may be an "allergic" response or may be a consequence of the failure of the epithelial cell from patients with non-tropical sprue to completely degrade a toxic polypeptide in gluten.

  Therapy. 1. Gluten-free diet—eliminates wheat, barley, rye and oats. Gluten is used as a "filler" in a number of prepared foods. Therefore patients must be carefully instructed in the principles of the diet (a detailed review including sample diets may be found in J. Amer. Diet. Assoc. *33*:137, 1957, and in several cookbooks specifically written for gluten-sensitive individual).
  2. Usually clinical improvement results in a week to ten days.
  3. Epithelial cell structure improves within a week but restoration of villous structure may take a longer period.
  4. An occasional patient may require a longer period of gluten avoidance before improvement is noted.

5. In general patients should remain on a gluten-free diet for life. Dietary discretions in some are associated with an acute exacerbation of symptoms (gluten shock), whereas in others dietary discretion merely leads to clinically silent morphological changes and malabsorption.

References

Bayless, T. M., Yardley, J. H., and Hendrix, T. R.: Adult celiac disease: Treatment with a gluten-free diet. Arch. Intern. Med., *111*:83, 1963.
Benson, G. D., Knowlessar, O. D., and Sleisenger, M. H.: Adult celiac disease with emphasis upon response to gluten-free diet. Med. *43*:1, 1964.
Mann, J. G., Brown, W. R. and Kern, F., Jr.: The subtle and variable clinical expressions of gluten-induced enteropathy (Adult Celiac Disease, Nontropical Sprue). Amer. J. Med., *48*:357, 366, 1970.

11. Properitoneal Hernia, Epigastric Hernia

F. Tremaine Billings, Jr.

Cause: Minute openings exist in the aponeurosis of the linea alba for the passage of small blood vessels, which in some individuals are large enough to permit little masses of properitoneal fat to be extruded. If the opening enlarges, the parietal peritoneum may be pushed out and a sac formed.

Early Manifestations: A pea sized mass, the protruding fat, may be accidentally discovered on physical examination without symptoms. If omentum is irreducibly present in a sac, abdominal pain and gastrointestinal symptoms may be so severe as to lead to suspicion of presence of some other upper abdominal disorder.

Treatment: If symptomatic, operative repair is indicated.

Possible Dire Consequences without Treatment: Rarely strangulation of hernial sac and gastric or intestinal contents may occur. Chief adverse result of the presence of a properitoneal hernia is that when undiagnosed it may lead to exploratory laparotomy. If not suspected and reduced, it may remain undiagnosed even postoperatively.

The presence of this herniation may long be unsuspected. The discomfort and pain it causes seem unrelated to usual upper gastric disorders and often lead to a diagnosis of neurosis. Symptoms can usually be elicited by straining or by sitting up from supine position. If irreducible, a nagging discomfort and pain may be present intermittently with any activity. Characteristically symptoms may first follow flexion exercises in treatment of mechanical low back pain.

References

Homans, John: Textbook of Surgery, 5th Ed., Springfield, Charles C Thomas, 1940, page 1008.
Rhoads, J. E., Allen, J. G., Harkin, H. N., and Moyer, C. A.: Epigastric Hernia. *In* Surgery—Principles and Practice. 4th ed. Philadelphia. J. B. Lippincott Co., 1970, p. 1098.

12. Acute Appendicitis

WILLIAM C. STAINBACK

Cause: Bacterial infection.

Early Manifestations: The classical early manifestations of this disease are sudden onset of central abdominal pain, nausea, vomiting and localized tenderness. Under these circumstances the diagnosis is simple. Fever and leukocytosis may also be present. However, none of these may be in evidence. Under certain circumstances a "stitch" in the side may be the only symptom. Signs may be completely absent or limited to right sided tenderness on rectal examination. Diarrhea is rare. A high index of suspicion should accompany the examiner at all times. A medical ward may be the most perilous place to develop an atypical appendicitis.

Treatment: Surgical removal.

Possible Dire Consequences without Treatment: Peritonitis and death.

Acute appendicitis is the most common cause of an acute abdominal emergency. Although it occurs most frequently in patients between the ages of fifteen and thirty years, it can occur in individuals of any age and affects both sexes equally.

The cause of acute appendicitis is bacterial infection. The mechanism involved may be: (1) the result of obstruction with subsequent distention with bacteria and mucus, occlusion of venous and arterial blood supply, and eventually necrosis and perforation, or (2) primary infection which may be transmitted through the gastrointestinal tract, the blood supply or the lymphatics. This latter type of appendicitis is often epidemic and may accompany epidemics of gastroenteritis or other infectious diseases.

The history and physical findings in acute appendicitis may be extremely variable, but the typical ones are: (1) central cramp-like pain eventually localizing in the right lower quadrant of the abdomen, (2) anorexia, nausea and vomiting, (3) tenderness and muscle guarding on palpation of the right lower quadrant, (4) leukocytosis, (5) obstipation, and (6) a low-grade fever.

In my experience the two most reliable findings are the history of sudden onset of mid-abdominal pain followed by anorexia and nausea for several hours and localized tenderness and guarding. If presented with these two findings, the surgeon is obligated to explore the patient unless he can rule out appendicitis with certainty. The diagnosis of appendicitis is much more difficult and the disease more atypical in the very young and the aged. Extreme caution is needed to avoid catastrophic errors in these patients.

The differential diagnosis of acute appendicitis includes almost every other acute abdominal condition. The primary ones, however, are ovulation with bleeding, ruptured ovarian cyst, pelvic inflammation and other pelvic diseases in women; acute mesenteric adenitis in children and young adults; acute diverticulitis, vascular accidents in the elderly; and acute cholecystitis, perforated ulcer and pancreatitis in adults.

It is universally agreed that the most satisfactory treatment of appendicitis consists in removal of the appendix before it has ruptured or before other complications develop. However, a difference of opinion exists concerning the treatment of perforated appendicitis with generalized peritonitis. One group of surgeons advocates the delayed (Ochsner) treatment. In this method therapy is primarily directed toward the peritonitis and consists of putting the intestine absolutely at rest by intestinal intubation, I.V. fluids, electrolytes and antibiotics. Surgery is confined to delayed drainage of abscesses and treatment of other complications. Another group of surgeons, which includes this author, advocates that a patient with appendicitis be operated upon as soon as the diagnosis is made regardless of the stage of the disease. The appendix should be removed if possible and drainage established. In addition, the measures for treating peritonitis are utilized including intestinal intubation, fluids, electrolytes and massive appropriate antibiotics (at least two). There is general agreement that the same affection in children should be treated by immediate operation.

Reference

Allen, J. G.: Appendicitis, Peritonitis, and Intra-abdominal abscesses. *In* Surgery , Principles and Practice, E. Rhoads, J. G. Allen, H. N. Harkins, and C. A. Moyer (Eds.) 4th Ed. Philadelphia, J. B. Lippincott Co., 1970, Chapter 37, p. 1039.

13. Volvulus of Colon

PETER MOULDER

Cause: Twisted colon.

Early Manifestations: Severe abdominal pain with signs of ileus.

Treatment: Decompression. Resection.

Possible Dire Consequences without Treatment: Intestinal obstruction, death.

There is distention of the abdomen and low intestinal obstruction—partial or complete—often recurrent. Added signs of gangrenous bowel occur in the later stages.

Suspect the problem and the diagnosis is often easy, especially for sigmoid volvulus.

Physical Examination: Abdomen distended with large, gas-filled bowel, and the gas will be *contiguous* as determined by scratch-auscultation. It is one huge bubble high in abdomen and under rib cage when the cecum is involved, and it is a folded loop (a pattern which may be visible on abdominal wall) in sigmoid volvulus. The auscultatory signs of obstruction will reflect the stage of the obstruction; evidence of peritoneal irritation is ominous and should be diligently elicited especially in the elderly and in the psychotic patients who are prone to the problem and not easy to examine.

Volvulus of cecum will produce a huge dilated viscus (with fluid level sign if sought) in most of the upper abdomen on regular abdominal film. This can be confused with

5

stomach—check for appropriate gas bubble, or empty the stomach with a Levin tube; barium enema will indicate site of obstruction at beginning of transverse colon or upper ascending colon.

Volvulus of sigmoid will show the huge folded loop ("horseshoe") of the sigmoid loop filling all of the abdomen on the regular film. Barium enema will show complete obstruction with a characteristic "bird's beak" deformity at the junction; sometimes spill will occur into a convoluted segment of sigmoid.

Excision is a necessity even when decompression is accomplished, because the causative factors when present will lead to a recurrence.

Cecum: Decompression should be attempted gently and over only a short period of time in cecal volvulus before surgery is elected. Use of the usual long tube is too time consuming and has such a low yield that it should not be attempted. A gentle barium enema may open it. Resectional therapy with anastomosis can be done with low risk if the patient is in even fair shape. An exteriorization resection can be performed if the patient is moribund.

Sigmoid: Decompression should be attempted by passing an oiled tube through the distal wedge via a proctoscope. This is worth the obvious risk, as decompression can afford time to prepare the bowel for low risk resectional therapy. Needless to say peritoneal irritation, bloody mucus, shock etc., must lead to prompt surgical exploration.

Reference

Gerwig, W. H. Jr.: Volvulus of the Colon. *In* Diseases of the Colon and Anorectum. Turell, R. (Ed.) Philadelphia, W. B. Saunders Co., 1969, pp. 684–691.

14. Barium Enema Complications

John McClenahan

Cause: Impaction, perforation with peritonitis, embolization of barium, cardiac response to bowel distention.

Early Manifestations: Signs of obstruction. Dizziness, nausea, precordial pain, collapse and shock. ECG abnormalities: ventricular bigeminy, coupled PVCs, transient AV and bundle-branch block, RS-T segment depression.

Treatment: Adequate fluids and mineral oil by mouth to prevent impaction. Gentleness during examination: avoidance of balloon catheter, low hydrostatic pressure of barium column. Extraperitoneal perforation will usually reduce itself spontaneously. Intraperitoneal perforation must be surgically drained and the rent repaired.

Possible Dire Consequences without Treatment: Obstruction. Barium peritonitis with adhesions. Death (mortality 47% after intraperitoneal rupture).

Frightened, uncomprehending old people are subject to barium enema complications, especially when they suffer from heart disease, diverticulitis or have had a fresh endoscopic biopsy of the rectum or sigmoid. ECG abnormalities occur in about 46% of these people particularly during evacuation of the enema. Since it is not unusual for them to faint in the toilet and injure themselves they should not be left unattended.

References

Berman, C. Z., Jacobs, M. G., and Bernstein, A.: Hazards of the Barium Enema As Studied by Electrocardiographic Telemetry, J. Amer. Geriatric Soc., *13*:672, 1965.
Eastwood, G. L.: ECG Abnormalities Associated with the Barium Enema, J.A.M.A., *219*:719, 1972.
Gordon, B. S. and Clyman, D.: Barium Granuloma Of the Rectum, Gastroenterology, *32*:943, 1957.
Seaman, W. B. and Wells, J.: Complications Of the Barium Enema, Gastroenterology, *48*:728, 1965.

15. Complications of Diverticulosis of the Colon

DAVID PASKIN

Cause: Probably on the basis of degenerative disease secondary to obstruction of the base of the diverticula with inflammation ensuing.

Early Manifestations: Possibly fever of unknown origin, occult or massive hemorrhage, pain, tympanites, obstipation.

Treatment: Surgery.

Possible Dire Consequences without Treatment: Intestinal obstruction, hemorrhage, peritonitis, and death.

Diverticula are present in the large intestine of many people over the age of fifty. The incidence becomes even greater as the seventh and eighth decades are approached. In most people, these remain asymptomatic and therefore require no treatment. However, in about 30% of cases, complications of diverticular disease occur and require vigorous treatment.

The etiology of diverticula is not known; however, it is felt that this is a degenerative process occurring in the colon. They are present commonly on the mesenteric border at the area where the small blood vessels supplying the wall of the large bowel enter from the mesentery through the seromuscular layers. This is an area of potential weakness. Diverticula of the colon are usually false in that they do not contain all four coats of colonic wall but usually only contain mucosa and submucosa. On the right side of the colon, however, true diverticula do exist though even here the great majority are false.

Left-sided diverticula are commonest. However, if diverticula are present on the right side, a greater proportion will cause symptoms.

The complications of diverticular disease of the colon are hemorrhage, obstruction, perforation with abscess formation, or free perforation, acute diverticulitis and fistula formation.

Hemorrhage. Diverticular disease of the colon is the most common cause of massive gastrointestinal hemorrhage and the second most common cause of moderate hemorrhage in elderly patients (second only to bleeding from an upper gastrointestinal lesion). Occult bleeding from the large bowel is usually not diverticular disease but represents carcinoma. The diagnosis of bleeding from diverticula is not a difficult one. This usually occurs in an elderly patient with massive lower gastrointestinal hemorrhage. Bright red or maroon blood is passed per rectum. Initial sigmoidoscopic examination reveals the presence of blood in the rectum and lower sigmoid. Identity of the bleeding site is rare. Barium enema will demonstrate diverticula but usually no evidence of diffuse inflammation. To locate the bleeding area on the barium enema, especially in a patient with diffuse disease throughout the colon, is impossible. The introduction of selective arteriography through the inferior mesenteric artery has helped in diagnosing the particular area of the colon which is bleeding. However, the patient has to be bleeding at the time of study and at a rate of at least 2 ml. per minute. If this latter set of circumstances exists, this is the procedure of choice for diagnosing lower gastrointestinal bleeding from diverticular disease or other colonic causes. Through this procedure it has been found that the right-sided lesions are indeed the ones that bleed more commonly. Other lesions such as small A-V malformations in the cecum are the bleeding sites in an increasing number of cases, the diverticula being incidental.

The treatment after the diagnosis is established is that of fluid and blood replacement and other general support for the patient. Usually the bleeding will stop without emergency operation being necessary. This may require between 5 and 8 units of blood in the first twenty-four to forty-eight hours. Recurring bleeding is an absolute indication for surgical intervention.

The procedure of choice for diverticular disease with hemorrhage is subtotal colectomy. The results of doing a lesser procedure, such as colostomy, right colectomy, left colectomy or a lesser subtotal colectomy, have been fraught with complications and deaths from recurrent hemorrhage. Patients having total abdominal colectomies with end-to-end ileo-proctostomies have fared much better. Recurrence of bleeding in these patients is extremely rare.

Emergency colectomies in patients with hemorrhage can be done as one stage procedures because the blood acts as a fine cleansing cathartic, therefore allowing anastomosis to be performed without the use of standard bowel preparation.

Obstruction. Chronic recurring diverticular disease or acute diverticulitis can and will frequently cause obstruction of the large intestine. The diagnosis is made by the history of constipation, at times vomiting, and increasing abdominal girth. Physical examination usually reveals a distended hypertympanitic abdomen with mild to moderate tenderness in the left lower quadrant. Sigmoidoscopy may demonstrate spasm in the lower sigmoid colon. X-ray films of the abdomen with the patient in a supine and an erect position are helpful because a cut-off on the left side of the colon can usually be seen and this is indeed the obstructing point. Barium enema will usually show a complete obstruction of the colon. The differential between diverticular disease and carcinoma when it presents with obstruction is at times impossible. The treatment is immediate laparotomy if the cecum is 12 cm. in diameter or greater as determined by x-ray examination. If the cecum is not this large due to the obstruction in the more distal colon, treatment with a nasogastric tube and intravenous fluids may be used until the edema resolves in the involved area. Then elective resection is performed. The reasons for operating electively rather than under emergency condition are as follows: the general condition of the patient is better; and under emergency conditions, in an unprepared obstructed colon, one submits a patient to at least a two-stage and probably a three-stage operative procedure. (The first stage is a colostomy; four to six weeks later the second stage is resection of the involved lesion with an end-to-end colo-colostomy; and the third stage is closure of the proximal protecting colostomy which was done as the first stage. Some have combined two of these stages into one and have therefore created the two-stage procedure by either doing the colostomy and resection at the same time, or the resection and anastomosis and closure of a previously made colostomy at the same time.)

The treatment of any obstructing diverticular disease of the large bowel is usually a surgical procedure. If cecal perforation is not imminent, the best treatment is a trial of non-operative management with nasogastric tube, parenteral fluids, and systemic antibiotics. If in twenty-four to forty-eight hours the patient begins to improve, this course should be continued. If in twenty-four to forty-eight hours the patient's condition is not improving, a decompressing colostomy should be performed.

Perforation Without Abscess Formation A frequent complication of diverticular disease is perforation or perforation with abscess formation. This is a most serious problem and if not treated aggressively and rapidly, diffuse peritonitis and death are the result.

Diagnosis of free perforation is made once again by history, careful physical examination, and radiographic findings. A history of the acute onset of severe abdominal pain frequently radiating to both shoulder areas is common due to the free air collecting under the diaphragm. A pleural effusion due to drainage in the right or left subdiaphragmatic spaces can occur. Signs of peritonitis which include rebound tenderness, decreased bowel sounds and guarding over the area of perforation are present. This is most commonly found on the left side but is certainly not uncommon on the right side. It is rare in the transverse colon. Laboratory studies usually reveal a leukocytosis with a shift to the left and mild to moderate dehydration as evidenced by an increasing hematocrit. X-ray evidence of free air under the diaphragm is present. The treatment is obviously surgical. However, before surgery can be performed, careful and aggressive fluid and electrolyte replacement is mandatory and then operation is of next importance. The procedure of choice is at least a divided colostomy and drainage of the area of perforation. However, resection of the perforated area bringing both the proximal and distal ends of the remaining colon out as an end colostomy and a mucous fistula respectively is preferred. After four to six weeks, the second or third stage of the procedure may then be performed re-establishing continuity of the colon and rectum. A loop decompressing but not totally diverting colostomy is contraindicated and will be of little to no help.

Perforation with Abscess Formation. Perforation with abscess formation will usually present the same as a free perforation except the signs and symptoms of free air in the peritoneal cavity will be absent. Localized evidence of peritonitis is present. One key point to be remembered: In an elderly patient there are times when neither a leukocytic reaction nor a fever is evolved in the presence of an acute abdomen.

However, tachycardia is a good clue to its presence and may be the only positive physical sign of an intra-abdominal catastrophe in the elderly. Tenderness and signs of peritonitis may not be as severe and as obvious as they are in younger patients. The treatment of perforation with abscess formation is drainage of the abscess area and a proximal divided completing diverting colostomy. Four to six weeks later, the area of involved disease may be resected and an end-to-end coloproctostomy performed.

Perforations and perforation with abscess on the right side of the colon may usually be treated primarily by immediate right hemicolectomy with creation of an ileo-transverse colostomy. This is possible on the right side because the blood supply is invariably better and the bowel contents are in a more liquid form.

Acute Diverticulitis. The clinical syndrome of acute diverticulitis is a most common cause of severe abdominal pain in the elderly patient. Usually the history is one of diffuse abdominal pain which localizes to either the right or left lower quadrants. This syndrome is rare in the transverse colon. The pain is usually constant and quite similar to that of appendicitis in younger patients. Physical findings are those of peritonitis which includes rebound tenderness, decreasing bowel sounds and guarding. Fever, tachycardia and leukocytosis with a shift to the left are present. Sigmoidoscopy will usually reveal spasm as the scope is passed beyond 12 to 14 cm. and barium enema will show a typical pattern of acute diverticular disease with spasm in the area of colon involved. The radiographic differential between this and carcinoma of the colon especially on the left side but even on the right side as well is at times a perplexing one and may make operative intervention necessary just for this particular reason. The treatment of acute diverticulitis without complications of perforation, hemorrhage, or obstruction has become more surgically oriented in recent years and many series are now reporting operative intervention on a semi-elective basis in patients who have had just one severe attack of acute diverticulitis. These patients may develop small intramesenteric abscesses which can be demonstrated radiographically and this is certainly indication for semi-elective operation after bowel preparation is undertaken. Non-operative therapy consists of gastrointestinal decompression via nasogastric tube, IV fluids and parenteral antibiotics. Nonabsorbable oral antibiotics should also be used.

Fistula Formation. Diverticular disease is the most common cause of pneumaturia. It is also the most common cause of fistulas between the colon and the uterus in the female. The treatment of this particular complication is surgical. Diagnosis of the acute attack is similar to that of diverticulitis with abscess. The treatment is similar also, except that the fistula must be resected. Fistulization occurs because of inflammation and abscess in close proximity to another viscus.

The entire spectrum of the complications of diverticular disease is a complex and interesting one. It requires aggressive surgical treatment and excellent judgment on the part of the surgeon as to when to operate and which procedure is best suited for the patient.

The results of surgical treatment of diverticular disease are good to excellent. Permanent colostomies in these patients should almost never be necessary.

References

Byrne, R. V.: Primary Resection of the Colon for Perforated Diverticulum, Amer. J. Surg. *112*:273, 1966.
Colcock, B. P.: Surgical Treatment of Diverticulitis, Amer. J. Surg., *115*:265, 1968.

Giffin, J. M., Butcher, H. R., and Ackerman, L. V.: Surgical Management of Colonic Diverticulitis, Arch. Surg., *94*:619, 1967.

Levy, S. B., Fitts, W. T. Jr., Lench, J. B.:   Surgical Treatment of Diverticular Disease of the Colon, Ann. Surg., *166*:947, 1967.

Olsen, W. R.: Hemorrhage from Diverticular Disease of the Colon, Amer. J. Surg., *115*:247, 1968.

Rigg, B. M., Ewing, M. R.: Current Attitudes on Diverticulitis with Particular Reference to Colonic Bleeding, Arch. Surg., *92*:321, 1966.

16. Torsion of Ovarian Cyst

ORVILLE HORWITZ

Cause: Pedunculated ovarian cyst.

Early Manifestations: Sudden or gradual onset of pain.   Tenderness of a cystic mass, later severe.   Frequently leukocytosis.

Treatment: Surgery.

Possible Dire Consequences without Treatment: Necrosis of cyst and gangrene.

This type of lesion may be confused with a twisted pedicle of the uterus, tubo-ovarian abscess, ectopic pregnancy or appendicitis.   It is mentioned here as one of the causes of severe lower abdominal pain.   It can occur at any age and the pain may be periodic as the torsion may be secondary to the position of the patient.   It is usually unilateral and rarely bilateral.   It is usually palpated as a tender cystic mass on pelvic examination.

Reference

Greenhill, J. P.: Office Gynecology, 8th Ed., Chicago, Year Book Medical Publisher, 1965.

17. Telangiectasia of Mucosa of Colon

ORVILLE HORWITZ

Cause: Congenital telangiectasis.   Dilated thinned-out capillaries.

Early Manifestations: Melena, severe or perfunctory.   May, however, be asymptomatic for many years or forever.   May also be preceded or accompanied by hemoptysis from pulmonary lesion or epistaxis, or by an innocuous looking "birth mark."

Treatment: Surgical resection of area if hemorrhage is not controlled otherwise.

Possible Dire Consequences without Treatment: Continued bleeding, severe blood loss, death.

This condition should be suspected in patients who bleed persistently from the colon but have normal barium studies of the upper and lower gastrointestinal tract, particularly if accompanied by a past or family history of telangiectasia. Arteriography may be helpful in making the diagnosis (Fig. VI–2), *if hemorrhage is rapid.*

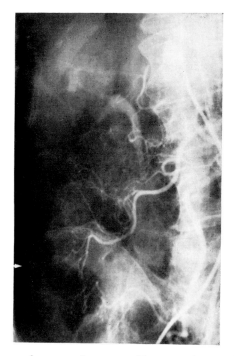

Fig. VI–2. Aortogram of seventy-three-year-old man, who required 17 transfusions in fourteen days in the hospital, showing site of bleeding (arrow) from congenital familial telangiectasis of the lower portion of the ascending colon.

Reference

Allen, E. V., Barker, N. W., and Hines, E. A.: Peripheral Vascular Diseases, 3rd Ed. Philadelphia, W. B. Saunders Co., 1962.

Chapter VII

Fever and Infections

Introduction

Fever must be considered the hallmark of infections. Certainly the large majority of infections present with fever either as the chief complaint or as an accompanying sign or symptom. If a patient presents with fever, the odds are overwhelming that the cause is infection. Conversely if the fever has persisted for more than three weeks and is undiagnosed, the chances are that it is *not* an infection (See Table VII–1). Occasionally patients may be afebrile throughout their infection, thereby rendering the diagnosis most difficult.

My own obviously biased series of patients presenting with fevers of temporarily unknown origin (>ten days >100°F.) includes the following: 8 cranial arteritides, 1 tularemia, 1 brucellosis, 1 bacterial endocarditis, 2 abscessed teeth, and 2 undiagnosed.

We have concentrated on the infections which are the most troublesome. These seem to be tuberculosis, hidden abscesses, and bacterial endocarditis. A large part of the discussion of infections is, therefore, devoted to these three items.

Certain infections, we believed, were best handled in chapters other than this one. For instance, brain abscess is included as a neurological entity, and pyelonephritis is treated as a nephrological lesion.

We have also included diseases which are not prevalent in the United States but have been imported recently at an increased rate because of air travel. Included in these are hookworm, malaria and schistosomiasis.

TABLE VII-1.
FEVER OF OBSCURE ORIGIN

Author	Dates of Collection	Established Causes (no. cases)					Not Diagnosed (no. cases)	Total No. Cases	Criteria for Selection
		Infection	Collagen Disease	Hemic	Cancer	Miscellaneous			
Alt, Barker	1913–1930	10	6	3	3	1	78	101	Fever >99°F., any age after complete study with hospitalization
Kintner, Rountree	1919–1930	2	—	—	1	—	97	100	Fever >100.5°F., excluded patient with chills
Hammon, Wainwright	to 1936	38	—	5	10	1	36	90	Any age, grouped on basis of high fever or low fever
Keefer	1930–1939	43	8	9	10	10	—	80	Excluded cases diagnosed on initial study
Wolf, Jacobs	1940–1944	2	—	1	—	1	32	36	Fever 99.8°F., age 13 yr., duration 10 days after hospital study
Bottiger	1940–1949	16	4	2	9	4	123	158	Duration >10 days
Oppel, Berntsen	1951–1952	62	2	—	1	23	22	110	Not known
Reid	1953–1955	39	2	6	3	22	41	113	Age >14 yr., fever 99.5°F., any duration
Geraci et al.	to 1959	15	1	10	11	5	28	70	Included only patients subjected to laparotomy
Petersdorf, Beeson	1952–1957	36	15	9	11	22	7	100	Fever >101°F., duration >3 wks., after 1 week of study
Sheon, Van Ommen	1959–1960	13	8	6	4	6	—	37	Fever >100.5°F., duration >3 wks., patients older than 16 years

Prominent among the miscellaneous conditions are temporal arteritis and the venous thrombosis pulmonary embolus complex

References

Alt, H. L. and Barker, M. H.: Fever of unknown origin. J.A.M.A., *94*:1457, 1930.

Bottiger, L. E.: Fever of unknown origin. With some remarks on the normal temperature in man. Acta Med. Scandinav., *147*:133, 1953.

Geraci, J. E., Weed, L. A. and Nichols, D. R.: Fever of obscure origin—the value of abdominal exploration in diagnosis; report of seventy cases. J.A.M.A. *169*:1306, 1959.

Hamman, L. and Wainwright, C. W.: The diagnosis of obscure fever; I. The diagnosis of unexplained long-continued, low-grade fever. Bull. Johns Hopkins Hosp., *58*:109, 1936.

Hamman, L. and Wainwright, C. W.: The diagnosis of obscure fever; II. The diagnosis of unexplained high fever. Bull. Johns Hopkins Hosp., *58*:307, 1936.

Keefer, C. S.: The diagnosis of the causes of obscure fever. Texas J. Med., *35*:203, 1939.

Kintner, A. R. and Rowntree, L. G.: Long continued, low grade, idiopathic fever; analysis of 100 cases. J.A.M.A., *102*:889, 1934.

Oppel, T. W. and Berntsen, C. A., Jr.: Symposium on differential diagnosis of internal disease; the differential diagnosis of fevers: the present status of the problem of fever of unknown origin. M. Clin. North America, *38*:891, 1954.

Petersdorf, R. G. and Beeson, P. B.: Fever of unexplained origin: report of 100 cases. Medicine, *40*:1, 1961.

Reid, J. V. O.: Pyrexia of unknown origin; study of a series of cases. Brit. Med. J., *2*:23, 1956.

Sheon, R. P. and Van Ommen, R. A.: Fever of obscure origin: diagnosis and treatment based on a series of sixty cases. Amer. J. Med., *34*:486, 1963.

Wolf, H. L. and Jacobs, S.: Fever of undetermined origin. New Orleans M. and S. J., *99*:441, 1947.

1. Bacterial Endocarditis

Donald L. Bornstein

Cause: Various gram-positive cocci and others.

Early Manifestations: Unexplained fever and heart murmur for one week or more.

Treatment: Large doses of appropriate antibiotic.

Possible Dire Consequences without Treatment: Death.

Bacterial endocarditis, or more properly, infective endocarditis, is a term encompassing infections seated on the heart valves or endocardium, or on the walls of the adjacent great vessels, caused by a variety of microorganisms. The symptoms in all cases reflect an interplay of four factors: local cardiac damage, peripheral arterial embolization, immunologic responses of the infected host, and stigmata of systemic infection.

There are several major varieties of infective endocarditis which differ widely in their etiology, pathogenesis, clinical presentation, prognosis, and therapeutic requirements. These include:

1. Subacute bacterial endocarditis (SBE), the classic illness involving organisms of low grade virulence engrafted onto an abnormal heart as a "susceptible" cardiac site;

2. Acute bacterial endocarditis (ABE), caused by virulent microorganisms such as staphylococcus, pneumococcus, and gram-negative enteric bacilli and capable of attacking normal heart valves;
3. Enterococcal endocarditis, caused by the group D streptococcus, which falls between classical SBE and ABE in its clinical presentation;
4. Endocarditis due to fungi or rickettsiae, and other "abacterial" cases and
5. Endocarditis developing after cardiac surgery.

Subacute Bacterial Endocarditis

The pathogenesis of SBE involves an inciting bacteremia with relatively avirulent normal flora and a particularly susceptible cardiac site. The classical organism responsible for this type of infection is the heterogeneous group of common oral commensal alpha hemolytic streptococci referred to generically as Streptococcus viridans. Other streptococci (non-hemolytic, microaerophilic, anerobic, and rarely non-group A beta hemolytic strains) of the skin or oropharyngeal, gastrointestinal, or genitourinary tracts and other relatively avirulent normal flora (Neisseriae, diphtheroids, Staphylococcus epidermidis) are also capable of producing this disease (Table VII–2). The particularly susceptible cardiac sites are found in patients with known rheumatic heart disease, primarily those with mitral or aortic insufficiency, and in patients with certain types of congenital heart disease (small ventricular septal defects, patent ductus arteriosus, bicuspid aortic valves, coarctation of the aorta, complicated [ostium primum] but not the common [ostium secundum] intra-atrial septal defects, tetralogy of Fallot, and pulmonic stenosis). Pure valvular stenosis is an uncommon setting for this disease, but aortic stenosis of the elderly, which can be a more complex lesion with some associated regurgitation, may also be involved. SBE rarely develops in the presence of long standing atrial fibrillation, chronic congestive failure or myxedema. An attractive theory to account for the localization of endocardial vegetations and the hemodynamic features of the susceptible cardiac sites has been presented by Rodbard.

The bacteremia required to seed a susceptible cardiac site has also been studied in great detail. Any manipulation, disease or trauma of a mucosal surface which has its own microflora can give rise to transient bacteremia with these organisms. Dental extraction or other dental manipulation, gingival disease, tonsillectomy, bronchos-

TABLE VII–2.
CHANGES IN ETIOLOGIC AGENTS RESPONSIBLE FOR CASES OF SUBACUTE BACTERIAL ENDOCARDITIS SINCE THE ADVENT OF ANTIMICROBIAL AGENTS

	Pre-Antibiotic	Recent
Number of Cases of Proved Etiology	*1005*	*284*
Organisms	% of Cases	
Alpha streptococcus	82.4	64
Nonhemolytic streptococcus	5.4	8.8
Microaerophilic streptococcus	1.1	8.1
Enterococcus	3.3	9.5
All staphylococci	5.2	3.9
Hemophilus species	0.6	1.4
Fungus	0	1.4
Others	1.7	2.9

copy, and ulcerative oral lesions are all associated with a high incidence of short-lived bacteremia with oral and gingival flora, primarily alpha hemolytic streptococci. Cystoscopy, indwelling catheters, transurethral resection of the prostate, dilation and curettage, sigmoidoscopy, the third stage of labor, and disease of the bowel or genitourinary tract can cause bacteremia with gram-negative rods, enterococcus, and other normal flora. Patients with known susceptible cardiac sites should be protected with appropriate antibiotic coverage when instrumentation or surgery of such contaminated mucosal surfaces is anticipated. A history of recent dental surgery or gingival disease is frequently found in new cases of SBE with Streptococcus viridans; conversely completely edentulous patients with other oral lesions rarely develop SBE with this organism.

Since the organisms which produce this syndrome tend to possess minimal virulence, the clinical course tends to be insidious. Common early complaints are malaise, lassitude, anorexia, myalgia, sweating, and low grade fever. When first seen by a physician, the patient is frequently considered to have a mild viral illness. Frequently, the patient receives a course of antimicrobial agent which may give symptomatic relief, but shortly after treatment is discontinued, symptoms return as before. A physician should always be suspicious of fevers in any patient with a heart murmur. Recurrence of fever after initial therapy should always alert the physician to the possibility of a more significant cause for the symptoms and to the need for an appropriate diagnostic effort, which includes properly obtained blood cultures.

In about one-third of cases, the symptoms of systemic infection are not prominent and the initial symptoms relate to embolic complications and present as localized back or abdominal pain, hematuria, sudden visual loss, subarachnoid hemorrhage, transient ischemic attacks, mononeuritis, headache and confusion, or rarely as a mycotic aneurysm. Immunologic responses, including circulating antibody-antigen complexes, play a role in the splenomegaly, the nephritis, and the cutaneous vascular stigmata seen in long standing disease. On occasion, a patient may not seek medical assistance until local valve injury has caused cardiac decompensation.

Early in the antibiotic era, it became clear that better acumen was required in the diagnosis of SBE. Although bacteriologic cures could be achieved in 90% of cases, less than 75% of cases survived and many of the survivors were partially disabled. High complication rates were found related to protracted delays in diagnosis and treatment. Classical findings in SBE such as a splenomegaly, clubbing, Osler's nodes, anemia, azotemia, or other embolic episodes were shown to be relatively late developments. If therapy is withheld until events of this sort are apparent, potentially crippling or lethal complications can ensue, which are no longer reversible by antimicrobial therapy. In 1950, Friedberg presented new diagnostic criteria for earlier detection and more effective therapy of SBE: An otherwise unexplained fever (101 °F.) lasting for over one week in a patient with a heart murmur should be considered as a possible case of SBE, and blood cultures should be obtained before embarking on or continuing empiric therapy.

The difficulties in diagnosis have increased in the last two decades as major changes have occurred in the clinical presentation of all endocarditis. The major changes in SBE include: increasing age of patients from a mean of thirty-two in the pre-antibiotic era to over fifty-five today, reflecting control of acute rheumatic fever and its recurrences with a residual aging cadre of persons with rheumatic heart disease; the increased and often careless use of antimicrobial drugs which can obscure this diagnosis; and new modalities of therapy which have introduced new susceptible cardiac sites.

In recent series, over 60% of cases have occurred in patients over fifty years of age. Cases in sixty- to eighty-year-olds are not uncommon. These patients often have murmurs which are ascribed to cardiac dilatation or to other complications of aging and are considered functional; nevertheless, some of these represent compensated rheumatic heart disease or other susceptible cardiac sites and make the patients good candidates for acquiring SBE. Some elderly patients with active renal disease or with congestive heart failure may have SBE without manifesting fever.

Other cardiac lesions found to be involved in SBE in recent years include: perforated or otherwise injured valve cusps from a previous, cured case of acute bacterial endocarditis; mitral insufficiency secondary to post-infarction papillary muscle injury; dilated and calcified mitral or aortic valve annuli; and prosthetic valves and patches.

Rare patients with SBE have lesions seated on the pulmonic or tricuspid valves in the right ventricle or in the pulmonary artery. These are almost without exception patients with congenital heart disease such as VSD, PDA, pulmonic stenosis, or tetralogy of Fallot. Patients with rheumatic heart disease today rarely have significant disease of the tricuspid or pulmonic valves without more serious disease of the mitral or aortic valves and rarely have right-sided SBE. Acute bacterial endocarditis is a much more common cause of such localization as is discussed below. Right-sided SBE should be strongly suspected when recurring pulmonary infiltrates or infarcts are detected by x-ray examination or clinically in a febrile patient with cardiac findings compatible with congenital heart disease. It is not significantly more difficult to isolate the responsible organism by blood cultures in right-sided SBE. Table VII-3 lists some clinical presentations which should raise the possibility of SBE and lead to obtaining blood cultures.

The leukocyte count is generally normal or minimally elevated in SBE, with counts less than 14,000 on admission in over 80% of cases, and less than 10,000 in about 60% of cases. A mild to moderate normocytic "anemia of infection" is commonly found, with hemoglobin concentrations below 12 gm.% in 60 to 70% of

TABLE VII–3.
CLINICAL PRESENTATIONS THAT SUGGEST
SUBACUTE BACTERIAL ENDOCARDITIS AND REQUIRE
OBTAINING BLOOD CULTURES

Patients with any murmur, some fever and:

Recent dental manipulation.
Cerebral embolus or transient ischemic attacks.
Atypical "aseptic" meningitis or focal neurologic signs.
Toxic psychosis or confusion.
Subarachnoid hemorrhage.
Normocytic anemia, high sed rate or positive rheumatoid factor.
Anorexia, weight loss, or persistent lassitude.
Recent arthralgias or clubbing.
Active renal disease or azotemia.
Sporadic hematuria or pyuria.
Splenic infarct or splenomegaly.
Peripheral arterial embolus.
Palpable tender arterial swelling or ruptured mycotic aneurysm.
Instrumentation or surgery of GU, GYN, GI tracts.
Progressive cardiac decompensation.
Recurrent pulmonary infiltrates (Right-sided SBE).

cases. Other laboratory data which may be found are: increased sedimentation rate; significant titers of rheumatoid factor in about 50 to 60% of patients, which fall with appropriate antimicrobial therapy; the presence of cryoglobulin or cryofibrinogens; abnormal phagocytic reticuloendothelial cells in the first drop of ear lobe blood in 15 to 25% of cases; a positive nitroblue tetrazolium (NBT) dye reduction test in most untreated cases, which suggests an ongoing bacterial or fungal infection; periodic microhematuria or pyuria; and, most importantly, positive blood cultures.

The key to diagnosis and to optimal therapy, however, is the isolation of the responsible organism. Mortality and morbidity in series of cases in which the organism has not been identified are significantly greater and the problems of management are greatly increased. Bacteremia is more or less continuous in SBE, and often, rather low grade. In one study, over 50% of patients had less than 30 bacteria per ml. and 24% had 10 bacteria per ml. or less. Some have suggested that 4 or 5 blood cultures are sufficient to recover the etiologic agent in 94 to 98% of cases of SBE. These suggestions are based only on cases in which the causal agent was isolated. Presumably, the number of cultures required to recover the organism responsible in *all* cases would be somewhat larger.

The greatest factor responsible for negative blood cultures in SBE is recent or ongoing antimicrobial therapy. An antibiotic regimen inadequate to cure the disease can render the blood sterile for up to seven to fourteen days or longer and can suppress the bacteria in such a manner that longer periods of incubation are required before growth is apparent in the blood culture bottles.

When therapy is begun in suspected SBE after several blood cultures are drawn but before any have revealed bacterial growth, a significant proportion of such cases (20 to 30% or more) will remain culture negative. This can pose serious problems in diagnosis and management. Of this number, some cases are truly infective endocarditis due to typical bacteria, a few may represent cases due to unusually fastidious organisms, bacterial or non-bacterial, and others are misdiagnosed and are not cases of infective endocarditis.

In this predicament, if no better diagnosis is forthcoming to explain the clinical findings, it is generally wisest to continue with empiric antimicrobial therapy, which should be raised to levels adequate to deal with the enterococcus (see below), since it cannot safely be assumed that the unrecovered organism is highly drug sensitive. The alternative plan of discontinuing antibiotics and re-culturing the blood may be dangerous because after seven to fourteen days of large parenteral doses of antibiotic, which have presumably ensued between drawing the blood for cultures and receiving the official negative report, bacteremia may be suppressed for one to two weeks or more. If it is finally established that SBE is present, weeks of valuable time will have been lost before treatment is instituted.

For these reasons, just as one should be quick to consider SBE and to begin diagnostic studies, one should be circumspect and deliberate about the moment for instituting therapy. In the absence of significant toxemia, embolic events or congestive heart failure, one can safely observe a patient with suspected SBE during a short diagnostic period. The author obtains 4 blood cultures during the first twenty-four hours and 1 or 2 daily thereafter for the first week, maintaining close contact with the bacteriology laboratory. When an organism is first detected, empiric therapy is begun, which is modified, as required, when further laboratory information becomes available. If after seven days, the cultures are still sterile, the case is re-evaluated and empiric therapy is begun or is withheld pending further studies as indicated clinically. Therapy is begun only in patients who would be treated even if cultures remain negative. Cases that are not treated are observed for another few days and again re-evaluated. Patients who have recently received antimicrobial drugs would be expected to require a longer period before yielding positive blood cultures. Before beginning therapy in patients whose initial blood cultures are sterile, several blood cultures may be drawn for special laboratory study for fastidious organisms or for partially cell wall deficient bacteria (see below).

Although one positive blood culture for Streptococcus viridans may be adequate in a suspected case of SBE, a second positive isolation is desirable, as it confirms the etiologic agent and the persistence of the bacteremia. The above considerations are not applicable to the acutely ill and toxemic patient thought to have ABE, in which case one must often complete blood cultures within one to two hours and begin therapy.

Acute Bacterial Endocarditis

The organisms responsible for acute bacterial endocarditis in the pre-antibiotic era were primarily D. pneumoniae, Streptococcus pyogenes (group A), Staphylococcus aureus, N. gonorrheae, N. meningitidis, and rarely gram-negative enteric bacilli or other streptococci. Today, the vast majority of cases are due to Staphylococcus aureus, the balance to gram-negative bacilli, enterococcus, occasionally pneumococcus, and rarely Streptococcus pyogenes or other organisms. Although the incidence of gram-negative bacteremia has risen dramatically in the past two decades, endocarditis due to gram-negative bacilli still is relatively rare. Bacteremia with gram-positive organisms poses a much greater threat of endocarditis than a comparable bacteremia with gram-negative rods. This difference is not fully explained solely by the known complement-dependent bactericidal action of serum against gram-negative bacilli and remains an interesting biological mystery.

The pathogens involved in this disease are not limited by the hemodynamic constraints imposed on relatively avirulent organisms and can attack normal heart valves including the tricuspid valve or, very rarely, the pulmonic valve in 15 to 25% of cases. The left side is still the preferred site of localization, with the aortic valve slightly more commonly involved than the mitral, in contrast to the clear preferential involvement of the mitral valve in SBE. When a susceptible cardiac site is available, however, there is usually preferential localization to that site.

In the pre-antibiotic era and again during the late 1950s when nosocomial drug resistant Staphylococcus aureus was an endemic problem in our hospitals, most cases of ABE developed as a relatively late complication of an uncontrolled local infection such as pneumonia, meningitis, wound infection or the like. Often the endocarditis was first detected at autopsy as its presence in life was masked by the uncontrolled sepsis of the primary infection. In other cases, an exacerbation of fevers and chills, an embolic event, or the sudden appearance of a murmur of valvular insufficiency and the rapid onset of cardiac decompensation allowed the diagnosis to made in life. Today we seldom see endocarditis originating in this manner because we have potent antimicrobial drugs for most bacterial pathogens and we should be able to relieve sepsis and eradicate the bacteremia arising from a focal infection promptly. Some cases will still develop from the early bacteremic phase of local infections before antimicrobial therapy is begun, however. The majority of cases of

ABE today are "primary," originating from blood stream contamination or from superficial or apparently trivial infections. A major source of such blood stream contamination today is iatrogenic and due to complications of the use of indwelling intravenous catheters and intravenous fluid therapy. Infection develops when such catheters are inserted without strict asepsis, when they are left in place for over forty-eight hours or without scrupulous local care, and when sterility of the fluids to be administered is lost due to careless technique during handling, especially with enriched fluids, or due to faulty infusion sets. Sterile phlebitis can develop in reaction to many medications, and if secondarily infected, can develop into septic endophlebitis, a dangerous local situation. A variety of other catheters which are now placed intravenously and left for varying periods of time such as central venous pressure, pacing, or balloon-assist catheters, present similar problems of contamination. Self inoculation by narcotic addicts has been responsible for up to 5% of cases of endocarditis. These cases have been primarily due to Staphylococcus aureus, but a variety of virulent and "avirulent" organisms have been implicated (Table VII–4). The other major group of cases originate from minor or early focal infections including pneumonia, meningitis, skin ulcers, wound infections, infected burns, chronic urinary tract infection or from transient bacteremias from the skin, GI, GU, or female genital tracts, either spontaneous or secondary to local disease, trauma, or surgical procedures.

The clinical manifestations and course of acute bacterial endocarditis tend to be more hectic and fulminant than those of SBE. Untreated cases will die within two weeks in most cases, and within six weeks in virtually all cases. Cardiac valve damage fenestration, perforation, or ulceration may occur within forty-eight to seventy-two hours of the initial fevers. This type of injury is associated with a new or "changing" murmur or valvular injury, usually insufficiency, and is usually followed by rapid and often irreversible cardiac decompensation. Even the most prompt recognition and treatment of this disease may be too late to prevent valvular damage; but in these cases prompt recognition and handling, including acute surgical intervention, may mean the difference between life and death.

Because the clinical course is much more rapid, the late embolic events of SBE are rarely seen in acute bacterial endocarditis unless this disease has been partially treated. Anemia, splenomegaly, azotemia, Janeway spots, Roth spots, embolic

TABLE VII–4.
ENDOCARDITIS IN NARCOTIC ADDICTS
(Three series; 112 cases)

Staphylococcus aureus	46
Staphylococcus epidermidis	3
Candida species	16
Enterococcus	13
Streptococcus viridans	8
Other streptococci	4
Pseudomonas	6
Other gram-negative rods	7
Unknown	9
Left-Sided	79%
Right-Sided	27%
Bilateral	4%

events and, of course, a new murmur of valvular insufficiency should not be anticipated as parts of early recognition of this disease. The endocardial vegetations tend to be larger and more friable and produce larger and more serious vascular occlusions—often of cerebral, coronary, or peripheral arteries. Emboli may go on to suppurate, a complication rarely, if ever, seen in SBE.

Most patients with acute bacterial endocarditis will present with high fever, with or without chills, and with moderate leukocytosis. This combination suggesting bacteremia should prompt immediate blood cultures before beginning empiric antimicrobial therapy. High fever is all one needs to consider seriously the diagnosis of ABE. If, in such a patient, x-ray films reveal a pulmonary infiltrate or density, as would be expected with acute bacterial endocarditis localized on the tricuspid or pulmonic valves, many physicians might erroneously assume the process to be a primary pulmonary infection and treat without obtaining blood cultures. Such therapy might not be adequate for ABE and the outcome, therefore, might be tragic.

From the considerations raised above, we can draw the following guidelines for early recognition of ABE:

1. There need be no specific clues to acute bacterial endocarditis except for high fever and toxemia. Do not require the presence of a significant heart murmur to consider this diagnosis; most cases lack them. Obtain blood cultures, 2 to 4 at thirty- to one hundred and twenty-minute intervals before beginning broadly bactericidal empiric therapy.

2. Be alert for possible ABE in febrile patients who also have:
   —Historical or physical evidence of self-injection (narcotics).
   —Recent hospitalizations which included intravenous therapy, surgery, or surgical instrumentation.
   —Skin infections—decubitus ulcer, wound infection, burn, furuncles.
   —Recent septic abortion.
   —Recrudescent fever and toxemia after apparently successful treatment of a local infection.
   —Recurrent pulmonary infiltrates, cavities, or effusion especially with jaundice, suggesting right sided endocarditis.
   —Any evidence of peripheral arterial embolization.
   —A new murmur compatible with valvular insufficiency or perforation which confirms the diagnosis and may require prompt surgical repair.

3. Positive blood cultures which persist over several hours or more suggest endocarditis or some other intravascular infection. All bacteremias due to Staphylococcus aureus, pneumococcus, beta hemolytic streptococci, or enterococcus merit close scrutiny as potential cases of endocarditis.

Enterococcal Endocarditis

Enterococci (Streptococcus faecalis, Streptococcus faecium, Streptococcus durans) are normal inhabitants of the intestinal and female genital tracts and the oropharynx. The majority of isolates (75%) are non-hemolytic on blood agar, but others are alpha- or beta-hemolytic. Enterococci are distinguished from other streptococci by their resistance to killing by penicillin and by their hardiness, as they will grow at 45° C, at elevated pH, in the presence of sodium azide, and in 6.5% NaCl broth. They belong to the group D streptococci. This group also includes the non-enterococcal species Streptococcus bovis and Streptococcus equinus which do not grow in 6.5% NaCl broth, are penicillin sensitive, and resemble Streptococcus viridans more than enterococci in their pathogenicity.

Enterococcal endocarditis falls between classical SBE and ABE in its pathogenesis, clinical manifestations and course. Some cases can be distinguished from classical SBE only by the isolation of an enterococcus from blood cultures and by the concomitant need for more vigorous antimicrobial therapy, while others present with hectic fevers and follow a septic rapid downhill course. Most cases however are intermediate in their clinical course, and involve older men with prostatic hypertrophy or other genitourinary disease and women of all ages with gynecological or genitourinary problems. Overall, compared with SBE, fevers are higher, chills and leukocytosis are more common, embolic events more destructive, emboli are larger and may suppurate to produce splenic or brain abscesses, valvular injury is more rapid and normal heart valves are frequently attacked, 60% in a series of autopsied cases seen at Mayo Clinic.

In recent years the relative incidence of enterococcal endocarditis has increased, due primarily to increased awareness of the importance of identifying this organism from other streptococci but also due to increased instrumentation and surgery of the GU and GI tracts in an increasingly older population. Clues to this diagnosis are those cited above for SBE and for ABE, especially in patients with recent gynecologic, genitourinary, or gastrointestinal disease, surgery, or instrumentation or in patients on long term penicillin prophylaxis. The presence of a murmur suggestive of valvular disease or of congenital heart disease should not be required in making this diagnosis, since something like 60% of cases will not have a pre-existing susceptible site. Again, diagnosis rests on obtaining blood cultures from febrile patients before embarking on empiric drug therapy or before changing to new therapy.

Fungal, Rickettsial, and Other "Abacterial" Endocarditis

Fungal endocarditis is a rare disease seen as a late complication of a generalized fungal illness or more frequently as a consequence of contamination of the blood stream (as in narcotic addicts or hospitalized patients with infected indwelling venous catheters) or contamination of the heart or great vessels (at cardiac surgery or by penetrating wounds). The majority of cases today occur in patients after cardiac surgery, especially when prosthetic valves or patches are employed. This form of endocarditis is discussed below.

Patients with fungal endocarditis sometimes resemble textbook cases of SBE, with fever, murmurs (70 to 100%), splenomegaly, petechiae, peripheral emboli, and Osler's nodes (25%), but the anticipated streptococcus is not recovered from the blood. Almost all cases involve the mitral or aortic valves, and over 70% or more are superimposed on a "susceptible" cardiac site. Some fungi grow well in routine blood culture media, while other isolates of the same species may not, and special culture media including some hypertonic media should be inoculated when fungal infection is suspected. Organisms which persist in the yeast phase in the body (cryptococcus, histoplasms) tend to form more friable vegetations than fungi which prefer the mycelial form (aspergillus). The latter may shed organisms into the blood stream only on occasion, in contrast to the more or less continuous bacteremia in SBE and ABE.

In earlier series, up to 40% of cases were first diagnosed when a major embolus to the arteries of the extremities or the bowel was removed surgically and found on histological examination to be a tangled mat of hyphae. Emboli this large are rarely seen in SBE and are rare in ABE. These large emboli reflect the large vegetations seated on the heart valves, a consequence of mycelial growth patterns and of the low grade inflammatory response which fungi evoke, allowing this disease to progress for months before being recognized.

Many cases of candidal, cryptococcal, and aspergillal endocarditis are iatrogenic in origin and/or occur in patients with defective host defenses as a result of diabetes, corticosteroid therapy, immunosuppression by drugs or disease, malignancy, or previous antimicrobial therapy, especially when combined with the use and poor care of indwelling intravenous catheters.

Fungal endocarditis can be distinguished from other sources of fungemia by the persistence of fungemia and by peripheral and cardiac manifestations. Cultures of bone marrow, lymph node, and liver biopsy specimens and serologic testing, where applicable, are worthwhile to establish systemic presence of a fungus when endocarditis seems apparent but blood cultures are sterile.

A rickettsia (C. burnettii), the agent of Q fever, was first shown to cause endocarditis in 1959. By 1967, 21 cases had already been reported in the United Kingdom. The disease presents as SBE of great chronicity affecting primarily middle-aged men and involving normal or diseased valves, usually the aortic valve. The source of infection of these cases is often obscure, as has been noted for Q fever pneumonia, in that there is often no obvious exposure to cattle or sheep. Frequently the patient has had a protracted pulmonary infection in the preceding months. Clinical manifestations include low grade or absent fever, increasing murmur or aortic valve injury, a high incidence of congestive heart failure (63%), clubbing (86%), splenomegaly (36%), and emboli (36%). Diagnosis is established by demonstrating high titers of complement fixing antibody to Q fever antigens, especially to the so-called phase I antigen to which antibody is not formed in uncomplicated Q fever, and by isolation of the organism by inoculation of laboratory animals or embryonated eggs.

Although there has been no reported Q fever endocarditis in the United States as yet, these cases are of importance beyond their number as a prototype of a true infective endocarditis from which routine blood cultures would be sterile—*i.e.*, true abacteremic endocarditis. There have been isolated cases of mycobacterial, spirillary, anaerobic bacterial, and even chlamydial endocarditis, but as yet, no bona fide mycoplasmal, viral, or parasitic infective endocarditis in man.

Most cases of suspected endocarditis with sterile blood cultures reflect a misdiagnosis, an inadequate number of cultures or an inadequate culturing period, or recent antimicrobial therapy. Only rare cases are due to uniquely fastidious organisms. Recent antimicrobial therapy can render common organisms partially cell-wall deficient (PCWD) or otherwise suppress the organism so that it will not grow in routine blood culture media for days or weeks after discontinuing therapy. For such cases the use of cultures supplemented with hypertonic sucrose may allow the altered organism to survive, revert to original bacterial form and grow. Supplementary hypertonic media should probably be employed routinely for blood cultures from patients who have received antimicrobial therapy and should certainly be used when rapid recovery of an organism is not forthcoming. Other approaches for special cases include the use of stringently anaerobic media, highly enriched and supplemented media, fungal media, and on rare occasions—mycobacterial media and animal inoculation.

Endocarditis Following Cardiac Surgery

From its inception, cardiac surgery has been associated with new forms of bacterial endocarditis. With the advent of open heart surgery, the incidence of cases rose dramatically from less than 1% of operated patients to as many as 10% in early series of aortic valve replacement operations. With improved surgical techniques and technology, the overall rate of early postoperative endocarditis fell to 3% and then to the current 1.0 to 1.5% of cases. In addition to the early postoperative cases (occurring before the sixtieth day post-surgery), prosthetic valves or patches represent susceptible cardiac sites which can become infected spontaneously at some later date, similar to patients with rheumatic valvular heart disease. Between 2 and 4% of cases in current series have developed endocarditis months to years after the operation.

The organisms responsible for prosthetic valve endocarditis from twelve recent series are recorded in Table VII–5. In the more recent cases, Staphylococcus aureus has been less commonly seen and fungi and nosocomial gram-negative rods have become relatively more frequent. A wide variety of ordinarily effete bacterial (diphtheroids) and fungal (mucor, coprinus, hormodendrum) saprophytes have caused infections on these acquired "susceptible" sites.

TABLE VII–5.
ENDOCARDITIS FOLLOWING OPEN HEART SURGERY
(12 series: 166 patients: 178 organisms)

	Number	*%*
Gram-positive bacteria	141	79
Staphylococcus epidermidis	69	
Staphylococcus aureus	43	
Enterococcus	5	
Streptococcus viridans	8	
Beta hemolytic streptococci	5	
Other streptococci	4	
Diphtheroids	3	
Pneumococcus	2	
Others (Micrococcus, Bacillus sp.)	2	
Gram-negative rods	33	19
Pseudomonas	14	
Coliforms	12	
Mima-herellea	4	
Others (Salmonella, Serratia, Alkaligenes)	3	
Fungi	15	8.5
Aspergillus	9	
Candida	5	
Histoplasma	1	

Prosthetic materials in the body are notoriously difficult to defend from infection. Infection on a prosthetic valve can begin around the sutures at the base of the valve, on thrombus which has accumulated on the struts or body of the valve, or in some cases at the aortotomy site. Once established it is almost impossible to rid a prosthesis of infection and the process can go on to burrow into the wall of the valvular annulus to loosen sutures and unseat the prosthesis to a greater or lesser extent or alternatively to form a large infected thrombus which interferes with valve function. This can cause rapid cardiac decompensation and death unless valve replacement can be carried out in time. The other major complications of prosthetic valve endocarditis are sepsis and arterial embolization to the brain, coronary vessels or other sites, often with large emboli. When endocarditis involves a prosthetic patch as in VSD repair, the infection usually involves the sites of suture and extends onto the patch. This is sometimes first diagnosed when the prosthesis fails and the pre-existing cardiac problem, such as left to right shunt in VSD, recurs. Although sutures may give way for reasons other than infection, endocarditis must always be considered present until ruled out by appropriate studies.

Early infections are generally more serious, more acute, and more difficult to diagnose. The origin of infection is only occasionally intraoperative contamination. More often a septic complication in the early postoperative period such as wound infection, pneumonia, intravenous contamination, urinary tract infection, or transient bacteremias is responsible for seeding the cardiac site. Most surgical services employ prophylactic antibiotics (usually antistaphylococcal agents) from shortly before the procedure until seven to fourteen days postoperative or longer. Many cases of prosthetic valve endocarditis are first detected when fever develops at home, because the fever had been suppressed in the hospital by the continued use of "prophylactic" drugs until discharge. Earlier diagnosis and better prognosis would be aided if prophylactic antibiotics were discontinued by ninety-six hours postoperatively (if appropriate for a given case), when chest tubes have been removed and arterial and venous cannula sites are healing. Blood cultures taken two or three times a week until discharge would help detect bacteremia at the earliest opportunity and allow for the most effective antimicrobial regimen. This information could be used to detect and correct an otherwise unrecognized septic focus which could lead to endocardial infection. Or, if the heart valve is already infected, the data from blood cultures might allow an earlier and more successful surgical removal and replacement of the infected prosthetic valve, or even cure a very early valve infection.

The late infections tend to be easier to diagnose, are frequently due to organisms of low virulence and resemble spontaneous cases of infective endocarditis more closely than do the early postoperative infection. Detection depends on awareness by the physician of the susceptibility of these patients and a high index of suspicion when they develop febrile illness. A corollary here is the need for good prophylaxis before dental extractions and minor surgery just as in patients with other "susceptible" heart lesions. Other late cases are due to pathogenic organisms and carry a worse prognosis.

Early recognition of prosthetic valve endocarditis requires an alertness to the possibility, the earliest discontinuance of prophylactic coverage and frequent blood cultures in the postoperative period, and early blood cultures for any fevers after discharge. Antibiotics should never be given casually to such patients, and never without prior blood cultures. If routine blood cultures are sterile and fever persists without another well-documented cause, one must consider the possibility of fungal endocarditis and obtain special studies (see above). Typical peripheral stigmata are not common in this form of endocarditis. Embolic events can also be a complication of non-infected thrombus on the heart valve and do not prove endocarditis.

Treatment

The basic aims of therapy in infective endocarditis are to kill the offending organism rapidly and completely, so that bacteriologic relapse, with its attendant increased mortality and morbidity, will not occur. To achieve these aims, it is necessary to use bactericidal drugs for a long enough period to allow healing to proceed. For optimal results, it is necessary to have appropriate laboratory assistance in planning therapy and in monitoring its effectiveness.

Bacteriostatic antibiotics cannot cure endocarditis. Sulfonamides which were able to cure acute life-threatening sepsis, meningitis, or pneumonia could cure no more than 4% of cases of SBE. Results with tetracyclines and chloramphenicol were only slightly better, and many patients who had appeared to be cured, relapsed shortly after therapy was discontinued. Penicillin and other related bactericidal agents can, with proper use, approach 100% bacteriologic cure rates in SBE today.

Studies of the healing in SBE indicate that fibrin deposition and phagocytosis of debris cannot begin until organisms in the vegetations have been killed. Major repairs require at least three to four weeks and healing is not completed for two months or more. This may explain in part why the several fourteen-day treatment regimens that have been proposed in SBE have been associated with an unacceptably high bacteriologic relapse rate of 6 to 23% or more. Similarly, oral regimens of penicillin treatment have been generally found to be unacceptable in this disease because of a significant bacteriologic relapse rate. In any relapse, there is an important period of time before the recurrence of fever and bacteremia in which the infection is active on the valve, causing further valve injury and continued threat of serious embolic events.

Even when complete bacterial cures are accomplished, there are still deaths and considerable morbidity due to irreversible cardiac injury or embolic complication. Regimens which allow bacteriologic relapse in even a few cases are therefore not acceptable where more effective alternatives exist. A four-week course of parenteral penicillin or an equivalent bactericidal agent adjusted with laboratory guidance represents the minimum acceptable regimen for the treatment of SBE.

It is not possible to ensure that an adequate bactericidal regimen is being provided unless the responsible organism has been isolated and is maintained and studied in laboratory. Routine disk sensitivity tests are of limited value as they give data only about bacteriostatic activity. Bactericidal drugs deemed sensitive by the disk method may be inadequate in conventional doses to kill the organism in question within the vegetations. Quantitative tube dilution sensitivity testing of the organism to penicillin or another appropriate agent can be most useful in establishing the minimal bactericidal concentration (MBC) of drug required for this isolate. This information can be used to predict the required amount of drug to be administered.

An even more useful determination once the patient is begun on empiric therapy (see below) is determination of the bactericidal potency of the patient's serum against his isolate. Sterile samples of serum are obtained at high or mid and at low points in therapy. The highest dilution of serum samples which can kill a standard inoculum of the organism (5×10^4 ml.) is determined to ensure that effective bactericidal therapy is in fact being delivered. One aims at achieving minimal serum killing

TABLE VII–6.
PRINCIPLES OF MANAGEMENT

1. Isolate the etiologic agent by adequate blood cultures before beginning therapy.
2. Maintain the organism in the laboratory for the duration of the illness.
3. Determine the minimal bactericidal concentration of appropriate drugs for this isolate (if possible).
4. Monitor therapy by measuring serum bactericidal titers and keeping these above 1/8 at all times, if possible, by adjusting antibiotics.
5. Treat parenterally for four weeks for sensitive organisms and six to eight weeks for enterococcus, Staphylococcus aureus or gram-negative rods.
6. Repeat serum bactericidal titers if drug has to be changed during treatment.
7. Maintain scrupulous care of I.V. infusion sites, using scalp vein needles rather than indwelling plastic catheters where possible.
8. Attend to infected teeth or undrained wounds promptly and with appropriate additional antibiotic coverage if needed.
9. Instruct fully about prophylactic antibiotics for dental surgery and other minor surgery.
10. Re-evaluate the patient thoroughly after therapy is completed. Newly acquired valvular injury or possible mycotic aneurysms require further study.
11. Have patient record temperature daily for one to two weeks and obtain a blood culture at one- to two-week and four-week check ups.

TABLE VII–7.
SPECIFIC THERAPEUTIC RECOMMENDATIONS
(To be modified by *in vitro* sensitivity testing, patient's age, renal function, and history of hypersensitivity)

Etiologic Agent	Antimicrobial Drugs and Dose[1]
Streptococcus viridans[2]	Penicillin 6–24 million units/day I.V. for 4 weeks
Enterococcus[3]	Penicillin 30–60 million units/day I.V. or Ampicillin 12–24 gm./day I.V. and Aminoglycoside (SM, K, G) } for 6 weeks
Staphylococcus aureus[4]	Oxacillin 8–12 gm./day I.V. or Methicillin 12–24 gm./day I.V. } for 6–8 weeks
Gram-negative rods[5]	Ampicillin (if S) 12–24 gm./day I.V. or Cephalothin (if S) 12–18 gm./day I.V. or Carbenicillin (if S) 30–40 gm./day I.V. and Aminoglycoside (SM, K, G) } for 6 weeks
Fungi	Surgical approach is required for cure, plus amphotericin B—build to 50 mg./day I.V. to a dose of 2.0 gm. and 5-Fluorocytosine (if S) 150–200 mg./kg./day p.o.
Rickettsia	Surgical approach is required for cure, plus tetracycline 2.0 gm./day p.o. for 8 weeks
Prosthetic Valve Endocarditis	If organism is highly susceptible, appropriate antibiotics as above, with eventual replacement. Surgical removal and replacement if therapy is not rapidly successful. Continue antibiotic regimen for agent isolated for 4 weeks postoperatively

TABLE VII–7 (*Continued*)

Etiologic Agent	Antimicrobial Drugs and Dose[1]
In penicillin hypersensitivity	
Strep. viridans	Cephalothin[4] 12–18 gm./day I.V. or Vancomycin 2 gm./day I.V. or Erythromycin[4] 4 gm./day I.V. or Clindamycin[4] 2.4–3 gm./day I.V. } for 4 weeks
Enterococcus	Generally no good alternative agents. Consider desensitization to penicillin
Staphylococcus	Cephalothin[4] 12–18 gm./day I.V. or Vancomycin[6] 2 gm./day I.V. } for 6–8 weeks

[1] Penicillin, ampicillin, cephalothin in divided doses at three- or four-hour intervals
Carbenicillin in divided doses at two- or three-hour intervals
Vancomycin, clindamycin, and erythromycin in divided doses at six-hour intervals
Aminoglycosides: Gentamicin 1 mg./kg. q 8 hrs. I.M.
           Streptomycin 0.5 gm. q 8 or q 12 hrs. I.M.
           Kanamycin 0.5 gm. q 12 hrs. I.M. (15 day limit)
    Doses require reduction when renal function is decreased
[2] Some strains (10 to 15%) are highly PCN resistant and should be treated as enterococcus. These will be detected on *in vitro* tests.
[3] Enterococcus requires careful laboratory monitoring to ensure that adequate serum bactericidal levels are obtained.
[4] Occasionally, aminoglycosides are required in addition to maintain good serum bactericidal activity.
[5] Any other regimen (chloramphenicol and aminoglycoside, or aminoglycoside alone) may not reach adequate serum bactericidal concentrations. In this case, clinical results will be poor and surgical attack with valve replacement may be required.
[6] Use for more than three weeks is not recommended. Complete course with alternative therapy.

titers at 1/8 or higher at all times, where this is achievable. Serum killing titers of 1/128 or more are usually achieved at high points in therapy (one hour after I.V. administration completed) when the organism is a sensitive Strep. viridans and the suggested regimen (see below) is followed.

The use of oral probenecid to raise the concentration of a penicillin or cephalosporin drug in the blood is generally not indicated. It is simpler and more clear cut and not much more expensive simply to increase appropriately the amount of drug administered, and so to avoid the gastrointestinal disturbances of probenecid as well as the occasional allergic reactions to this drug which can be mistakenly diagnosed as penicillin allergy, to the patient's detriment.

For some organisms (most enterococci, some Staphylococcus aureus, most pseudomonas, many gram-negative rods), no single drug provides adequate bactericidal effect and a combination of bactericidal agents may provide synergistic or at least additive effect. The classic example of synergistic effect has been that of penicillin and streptomycin (or other aminoglycoside) on the enterococcus. This organism is usually inhibited by concentratons of penicillin of 1 to 12 μgm./ml. (mean of 6 μgm./ml.) but is usually not killed at concentrations of 50 or 100 μgm./ml. This explains why less than 25% of enterococcal endocarditis can be cured by penicillin alone.   This is in contrast to the majority of Streptococcus viridans (over 70%) which are inhibited and killed by penicillin at less than 0.1 μgm./ml.   Recently, the long-known fact that streptomycin (SM) or kanamycin (KM) can act synergistically with penicillin despite resistance of the organism to the SM or KM alone at concentrations achievable *in vivo* has been explained by Standiford and co-workers.   They showed that in many enterococci resistance to SM or KM can be removed by the action of the penicillin which allows SM or KM to enter the cell and attack the organism at a ribosomal site.   Organisms not susceptible to SM or KM synergism were found to be resistant to that drug at the ribosomal level.   The non-synergistic ribosomal resistant strains could be distinguished by the ability to resist very high concentrations of SM (6,000 μgm./ml.)—whereas the SM-synergistic strains were sensitive to less than 1000 μgm./ml.   In their study of selected enterococci, 63% showed synergism of SM and penicillin while 91% of their strains showed synergism to KM and penicillin.

Some forms of endocarditis are not amenable to cure with antimicrobials alone, including all rickettsial and fungal endocarditis, and some cases due to gram-negative rods which are not sensitive to any penicillin or cephalosporin.   It is often not possible to cure endocarditis with an aminoglycoside alone or combined with a bacteriostatic agent, and the best approach may be to consider early surgical removal of the valve if the blood is not rapidly rendered sterile.   Prosthetic endocarditis requires re-exploration, sooner or later, depending on the case.   Other specific details of therapy are described in the references.   Guidelines to management and specific therapeutic recommendations are cited in Tables VII–6 and VII–7.

References

Bain, R. C., et al.:   Right-sided bacterial endocarditis and endarteritis: A clinical and pathologic study.   Amer. J. Med. *24*:98, 1958.

Block, P. C., De Sanctis, R. W., Weinberg, A. N., and Austen, W. G.:   Prosthetic valve endocarditis.   J. Thor. Cardiovas. Surg. *60*:540, 1970.

Bornstein, D. L.:   Bacterial endocarditis Chapter 31.   *In* Cardiac and Vascular Diseases. Conn, H. L., Jr. and Horwitz, O. (eds.).   Philadelphia, Lea & Febiger, 1971.

Friedberg, C. K.:   Subacute bacterial endocarditis: Revision of diagnostic critera and therapy. J.A.M.A. *144*:527, 1950.

Geraci, J. E., Frye, R. L., and Titus, J. L.:   Methicillin and other semisynthetic penicillins in the management of staphylococcal endocarditis.   Circulation *32*:95, Suppl. II, 1965.

Geraci, J. E., and Martin, W. J.:   Antibiotic therapy of bacterial endocarditis. VI. Subacute enterococcal endocarditis: clinical, pathologic, and therapeutic consideration of 33 cases. Circulation *10*:173, 1954.

Hairston, P. and Lee, W. H., Jr.:   Management of infected prosthetic heart valves.   Ann. Thorac. Surg. *9*:229, 1970.

Hook, E. W., and Kaye, D.:   Prophylaxis of bacterial endocarditis.   J. Chron. Dis. *15*:635, 1962.

Kristinsson, A., and Bentall, H. H.:   Medical and surgical treatment of Q-fever endocarditis. Lancet *2*:693, 1967.

Lerner, P. I. and Weinstein, L.:   Infective endocarditis in the antibiotic era.   New Eng. J. Med. *274*:199, 259, 323, 388, 1966.

Mandell, G. L., et al.:   Enterococcal endocarditis.   Arch. Intern. Med. *125*:258, 1970.

Morgan, W. L., and Bland, E. F.:   Bacterial endocarditis in the antibiotic era with special reference to the later complications.   Circulation *19*:753, 1959.

Neu, H. C., and Goldreyer, B.:   Isolation of protoplasts in a case of enterococcal endocarditis. Amer. J. Med. *45*:784, 1968.

Okies, J. E., Viroslav, J., and Williams, T. W., Jr.:   Endocarditis after cardiac valvular replacement.   Chest *59*:198, 1971.

Pankey, G. A.: Acute bacterial endocarditis at the University of Minnesota Hospitals. 1939–1959. Amer. Heart J. *64*:583, 1962.

Roberts, W. C., and Morrow, A. G.: Bacterial endocarditis after cardiac valvular replacement. Chest, *59*:198, 1970.

Rodbard, S., and Yamamoto, C.: Effect of stream velocity on bacterial deposition and growth. Cardiovas. Res. *3*:68, 1969.

Soler-Bechara, J., et al.: Candida endocarditis. Amer. J. Cardiol. *13*:820, 1964.

Standiford, H. C., de Maine, J. B., and Kirby, W. M. M.: Antibiotic synergism of enterococci: Relation to inhibitory concentrations. Arch. Intern. Med. *126*:255, 1970.

Williams, T. W., Jr., Viroslav, J., and Knight, V.: Management of bacterial endocarditis— 1970. Amer. J. Cardiol. *26*:186, 1970.

Wilson, L. C., et al.: Valvular regurgitation in acute infective endocarditis: Early replacement. Arch. Surg. *101*:756, 1970.

2. Collection of Pus

C. W. HANSON

Cause: Direct, hematogenous or lymphogenous extension of various organisms.

Early Manifestations: Often cryptic fever. Sometimes local symptoms. Unusually diverse presentation.

Treatment: Surgical drainage, identification of the organism and its sensitivity, and proper antibiotic therapy.

Possible Dire Consequences without Treatment: Death, peritonitis, septicemia, other abscess, and local suffering.

Purulent Complications of Upper Respiratory Infection

PHARYNGITIS

Cause. Inoculation by air droplets of a susceptible individual, giving rise to an inflammatory and often suppurative process in the upper respiratory tract. The agent may be viral, bacterial (streptococcus, gonococcus, diphtheria bacillus), or on rare occasions fungal or spirochetal.

Early Signs and Symptoms. These are fever, pain in the throat especially upon swallowing, and cervical lymphadenopathy. Further differential information, favoring a bacterial etiology, comes when an adherent membrane is identified, when the lymphadenopathy is unusually large or painful, or when the degree of toxemia is great. A specific diagnosis is approached by the clinical picture, by blood count, by bacteriologic study (here gram stain generally has little usefulness), and with serologic aids. Knowledge of the organisms which are epidemiologically prevalent in the community is of great importance. It is to be emphasized that the clinician's assessment of the throat has, upon critical analysis, been credited with just slightly greater than coin-flipping accuracy in differentiating viral from bacterial infection; the custom of obtaining throat cultures should be an invariable routine. Infectious mononucleosis must also be kept in mind in the appropriate clinical settings.

Treatment is initially symptomatic, as culture results can often be returned within twenty-four hours, and then directed at the primary condition when it is identified, as with penicillin, other antimicrobials, antitoxins, steroids, etc.

In the following discussion, many of the entities begin with a pharyngitis, and it is spread of that infection to adjacent structures which brings about many of the serious complications of pharyngeal infection.

1. Peritonsillar, tonsillar, pharyngeal, and retropharyngeal abscesses may follow by several days the primary episode. There is a partial subsidence of the inflammatory manifestation, but the temperature does not return entirely to normal. Within a few days, it rises again and is joined by other complaints. These may include dysphagia, unilateral or diffuse throat pain, trismus, torticollis, pain upon head movement, neck stiffness, or obstruction of the airway or upper digestive tract. Physical examination may show a mass, displacing posterior pharyngeal structures, or if the lesion is in the more inferior portions, radiographic techniques may have to be employed. Treatment is with general supportive measures, appropriate antimicrobials, incision and drainage when a fluctuant mass is identified, and occasionally anticoagulants for associated cervical thrombophlebitis. Because the responsible microbes are generally penicillin-sensitive, as represented by Streptococci and indigenous mouth flora, this drug is almost invariably selected first. Circumstances likely to have given rise to staphylococcal infections should dictate consideration of penicillinase resistant penicillins, and the occasional recovery of mycobacteria, when appropriate efforts are made, will occasionally necessitate antituberculous therapy.

Dire consequences if untreated include obstruction of airway or upper digestive tract, metastatic infection (with a particularly ominous association with brain abscess), hemorrhage, and aspiration of pus into the respiratory tree.

2. Otitis media

Early Manifestations. Difficulty in hearing, earache, fever, and toxemia.

Cause. Accumulation of fluid and proliferation of microorganisms in the closed space bounded by the tympanic membrane on the one side and the eustachian tube orifice on the other, particularly when the latter is blocked by an inflammatory process.

Diagnosis. Made by otoscopic visualization, and under special circumstances with radiographic techniques. A specific etiologic diagnosis, made by culture of the pharynx or of directly obtained pus through the tympanic membrane, will enable better therapy directed at whatever organism may be recovered.

Treatment. Decongestants; analgesics; antimicrobials (particularly ampicillin until culture results are known, as it is expected to work against 95% of the anticipated organisms in both adults and children); myringotomy, when pain is severe and rupture threatens.

Dire Consequences. Possible spread to the mastoid, to the venous sinuses and meninges, to the labyrinth, and to the brain substance.

3. Sinusitis

Cause. Upper respiratory infection progressing to obstruction of drainage of the sinus orifices, contributed to by such factors as septal deviation, swollen or hypertrophied turbinates, or allergic polyps. Only in the maxillary sinus, apical tooth infection may spread into the antrum without prior respiratory infection.

Early signs and/or symptoms include pain in the sinus regions; tenderness; headache; odontalgia; disturbances of the sense of smell; swelling and edema of the eyes or lids; and nasal discharge, particularly if purulent. With the otoscope, pus may be seen discharging below the middle turbinate in frontal and ethmoid sinusitis, and/or above the middle turbinate in the ethmoid and sphenoid sinusitis. Further diagnostic information may be gained by transillumination, radiographic techniques, and diagnostic puncture. When the structures are close to the surface, tenderness may be felt: supra-orbitally in frontal sinusitis; near the inner angle of the orbit in ethmoid sinusitis; and over the canine fossa in maxillary sinusitis.

Treatment is with humidification, decongestants, and analgesics. Antimicrobials are generally employed; penicillin and other drugs (erythromycin, cephalothins) effective versus endogenous flora appear to be most useful. Initially, drainage is performed by suction irrigation. More drastic surgical techniques are limited to such indications as threatened intracranial extension of infection, when there is a persistent pain or discharge, when there is evidence of bone involvement, or when there is the development of a mucocele or pyocele.

Dire consequences if untreated include extension into contiguous structures, such as the orbit or intracranial contents, and metastatic spread by septicemia.

Reference

Ballenger, J. J.: Diseases of the Nose, Throat, and Ear, 11th Ed. Philadelphia, Lea & Febiger, 1969.

Purulent Complications in the Lower Respiratory Tract

LUNG ABSCESS

Cause. Most commonly seen as a result of aspiration of mouth contents, gastric juice, or foreign body. This typically occurs during a period of depressed consciousness with inadequate cough reflex, such as alcoholic or drug-induced stupor, during the conduct of general anesthesia, or as a consequence of a generalized seizure. Also to be incriminated are poor oral hygiene, esophageal disease such as achalasia or tracheo-esophageal fistula, and lung tumor. In the absence of the latter two factors, the condition rarely occurs in the edentulous individual.

Early Manifestations. Cough, putrid sputum, chest pain which is often pleuritic, fever, the demonstration of lung consolidation and/or cavity formation by appropriate clinical and radiographic techniques, and rapidly developing finger clubbing. The typical position of the dependent segments at the time of aspiration, combined with basic bronchial anatomy, gives rise to a striking predisposition for involvement of the right lung and its posterior segments.

Treatment. Prolonged antimicrobial therapy combined with postural drainage. I.V. penicillin has greatest usefulness in those lesions associated with mouth organisms which, because of their difficulty of culture, are generally reported as having non-specific bacteriologic results. Appropriate studies should be done, however, to indicate other treatments as appropriate for Staphylococcus, Klebsiella-Aerobacter, tuberculosis, carcinoma, etc. Surgical excision of large (greater than 4 cm.) or prolonged (greater than one month) cavities is generally necessary, because their walls fail to collapse, a necessary step in the process of healing, despite well-designed chemotherapy and drainage.

Dire Consequences. Toxemia, metastatic abscesses both through the bronchi to other parts of the lung and via the blood stream (notably brain abscess); suffocation, due to aspiration of large amounts of pus; hemorrhage; and death by a variety of means.

THORACIC EMPYEMA

Cause. Extension of infection into the pleural space from a contiguous area, such as the lung; mediastinal structures especially the esophagus; transdiaphragmatically from gut lesions; from penetrating trauma; or as a complication of thoracic surgical procedures.

Early Manifestations

1. Toxemia
2. Cough
3. Pleural pain
4. Fluid accumulation as demonstrated by a variety of clinical and radiographic techniques
5. Pericardial involvement

Demonstration of pus in the pleural space by needle or trocar aspiration is the master stroke, confirming the diagnosis, relieving the pressure and toxemia, and procuring material which should enable one to make a bacteriologic diagnosis.

Treatment. Drainage by needle, tube, or thoracostomy; to be combined with appropriate chemotherapy, systemically and by the intracavitary route. For the late fibrotic stage, decortication may be necessary.

Dire Consequences. Bronchopleural fistula, pericardial involvement, abscess in the mediastinum, chest wall, or bone; and later, restrictive lung disease.

Notable microorganisms here have been the Pneumococcus (or any other organism giving rise to pneumonia but especially Streptococcus or Klebsiella), the anaerobes of the mouth if the condition follows aspiration, Mycobacteria, Entamoeba histolytica, and actinomycosis.

Reference

Gibbon, John H., Jr.: Surgery of the Chest. Philadelphia, W. B. Saunders Co., 1962.

ABSCESSES IN THE ABDOMINAL CAVITY

Purulent collections in the abdomen arise from a variety of etiologic developments, they occur in all quadrants, exhibit a wide variety of clinical pictures, may only be diagnosed by maintaining a high degree of clinical suspicion, and occasionally with the aid of several increasingly sophisticated diagnostic techniques. They almost invariably require surgical drainage for a long-term cure. Those which occur close in time to a surgical procedure lend themselves relatively readily to diagnosis and therapy; those which do not may present in quite variable and difficult categories of differential diagnosis, such as fever, abdominal mass or pain, weight loss, leukemoid reaction, specific organ dysfunction, and even psychiatric illness, as well as combinations thereof. In Petersdorf and Beeson's Classical Series of 100 Fevers of Unknown Origin, 4 were eventually shown to have deep abdominal abscesses. One each was of tubo-ovarian and appendiceal origin, one was found in the lesser sac after a perforated gastric ulcer (and containing Salmonella), and the last was a cryptogenic collection in the left subphrenic region, also Salmonella, presumably from an earlier unrecognized bacteremia.

In the following discussion, subphrenic abscess is taken as the exemplar; it has been most widely encountered and written about, and many of its lessons are common to other purulent abdominal collections.

References

Petersdorf, R. G. and Beeson, P. B.: Fever of unexplained origin: report of 100 cases. Medicine, *40*:1, 1961.

Rhoads, Allen, Harkins, and Moyer: Surgery: Principles and Practice, 4th Ed. Philadelphia, J. B. Lippincott Co., 1970.

SUBPHRENIC ABSCESS

Cause. Inoculation of this potentially susceptible area with bacteria from a septic focus elsewhere in the body, which is commonly, but not invariably, intra-abdominal.

Early signs and/or symptoms are upper abdominal pain, intensified by respiration, probably referred to shoulder; mass in the upper abdomen; fever and tachycardia; leukocytosis and increased sedimentation rate; altered gastrointestinal tract function; icterus (only as a late and dire manifestation); reaction in or displacement of adjacent bodily structures, *i.e.* transdiaphragmatically. The responsible organisms are often mixed, but under varying circumstances, Staphylococcus, fecal organisms including Bacteroides and anaerobic streptococci, tuberculosis, Entamoeba histolytica, and actinomycosis have been found. Associated conditions may include: especially now, recent hepatobiliary surgery; any other surgery of the upper abdomen, particularly gastroduodenal; recent pancreatitis (with a particular likelihood of spread to the lesser peritoneal sac, see below); appendicitis, diverticulitis; liver abscess either pyogenic or amebic; trauma; cancer; or septicemia elsewhere in the body. In a recent large series, 40% were *not* associated temporally with surgery. The time relationship requires definition. A range of five to one hundred and thirty-one days from surgery to discovery of abscess has been cited, with an average of just over thirty days. However, cases have been described up to twelve years following a surgical procedure in which contamination of the subphrenic space was demonstrated or suspected. The longer incubation periods are often associated with partially suppressive antimicrobial therapy and/or inadequate surgical drainage, with early masking of the more typical features. In the pre-antimicrobial days, 60% of these lesions occurred following perforated peptic ulcer or ruptured appendicitis, each accounting for half of this figure. Now, a more varied pathogenesis is seen in the lesser number of cases we see today, since surgical technique has circumvented many of these problems.

Diagnosis is initiated by clinical suspicion, but radiographic techniques are particularly useful and appropriate here. They consist of the following:

1. Reactive changes in the lungs, pleura, or diaphragm, such as decreased mobility or fixation, elevation, effusion, atelectasis, or real or apparent pneumonia.
2. When seen (3% or less), air in the abscess cavity is virtually diagnostic.
3. Displacement of adjacent abdominal viscera, as seen by plain or contrast roentgenograms of upper or lower gastrointestinal tract, kidneys, spleen, etc. Except following gastric surgery, occurrence on the right is far more common than on the left.
4. Other techniques to be considered are the injection of a fistula tract when present, pneumoperitoneum, celiac angiography, and combined liver and/or lung scans, etc.

Needling the abscess for pus is confirmatory, when its location makes this feasible.

Treatment is by surgical drainage, so designed as not to contaminate uninvolved structures, and by chemotherapy. Prevention (when possible), high suspicion of the possibility, and therefore early diagnosis should characterize our efforts to lessen the discouraging morbidity and mortality figures still associated with this condition. Even when established during life, the mortality rate from subphrenic abscess is still considerably in excess of 30%.

Dire Consequences If Not Treated.   Septicemia and metastatic abscesses, internal and external fistulae, empyema thoracis, spreading peritonitis, vascular occlusion or hemorrhage, and death.

Reference

Konvolinka, C. W., and Olearczyk, A.:   Current Problems in Surgery, Chicago, Year Book Medical Publishers, Inc., 1972.

PYOGENIC LIVER ABSCESS

Cause.   Pyogenic liver abscess arises when a suppurative lesion, especially in the portal bed, or occasionally elsewhere, produces a liver cellulitis or phlegmon, one day to four months after the primary event, averaging about thirty days.   This may then proceed to the development of pus in the liver, resulting in a clinical picture which may be (if removed in time from the initiating event) among the most perplexing of fevers of unknown origin and problems in abdominal differential diagnosis.   Most commonly occurring in the past after appendicitis or diverticulitis, the major associations now seen are with sepsis in the biliary tree or with no event at all (cryptogenic) from some totally unrecognized general or portal bacteremia.

The major signs and symptoms are fever, chills, weight loss, a variety of alimentary dysfunctions, tender hepatomegaly, supradiaphragmatic reaction, and late and ominously, jaundice.   Laboratory findings include anemia, leukocytosis, active sedimentation rate, and until late or unless multiple, surprisingly normal liver function studies.   The aspiration of foul pus favors a bacterial over an amebic origin; amebic liver abscess is discussed elsewhere in this volume (p. 155).   For differential purposes, let it be said here that amebic abscess is more likely when there is a history of travel in areas endemic for amebic dysentery, or when there is a history of prior or concurrent diarrhea, or certainly when there is recovery of cysts or trophozoites from the stool or cavity contents.   Recently, amebic serology has become available for further differential usefulness.   For either kind of liver abscess, radioisotopic liver scanning has come to be the premier diagnostic technique.

Fundamental steps in therapy are drainage and antimicrobial therapy.   Drainage may be accomplished by needle once or repeatedly, and this alone often suffices for the amebic variety, or by the bigger procedure of open surgery for mixed or bacterial abscesses.   Emetine, and more recently, Flagyl are the preferred drugs for treatment of amebic involvement of the liver, while antibiotics should be selected for the pyogenic variety on the basis of cultural diagnosis and sensitivity determinations.

Dire consequences of this condition untreated include a mortality rate variously reported as 40 to 90% for bacterial liver abscess, averaging about 70%, almost invariably fatal if the abscesses be multiple.   This is to be contrasted with amebic liver abscess, where good diagnostic and therapeutic efforts will result in a mortality rate ranging between 10 and 20%.

Reference

Barbour, G. L., and Juniper, K., Jr.:   A Clinical Comparison of Amebic and Pyogenic Abscess of the Liver in Sixty-Six Patients.   Amer. J. Med., 53:323, 1972.

TUBO-OVARIAN ABSCESS

Cause. Bacterial infection of the pelvic adnexal structures, commonly but by no means invariably associated with recent or remote gonorrheal infection and scarring. While we tend to think of this as a disease of the young, a recent survey indicated that 40% occurred in women over the age of forty, that only a third had a prior history of PID, and only a half had a prior history of any form of gynecologic disease.

Early Signs and/or Symptoms. Pelvic pain, often lateralized, accompanied by a mass and (if ruptured, a common development) signs of spreading peritonitis, an extremely septic course, and paralytic ileus. Characteristically, there is but little help to be had from the laboratory, beyond abnormalities in the indices of inflammation. The recently developed technique of culdocentesis has led to a much better diagnostic record, with the procurement of pus or seropurulent fluid enabling an immediate anatomic diagnosis, hastening the recovery of the responsible organism, and leading to treatment with appropriate antibiotics.

Treatment. With general support, a surgical procedure accomplishing drainage, and antimicrobials guided by sensitivity testing. The drainage concept was formerly limited to local efforts, and with no more than limited resection; recent experience may now indicate the preferability of removal of the uterus and both adnexal structures at the initial procedure.

Dire Consequences if Untreated. Continued symptoms, a variety of metastatic infections, spreading peritonitis, and cardiopulmonary complications.

Reference

Nebel, W. A., and Lucas, W. E.: Management of Tubo-ovarian abscess. Obstet. & Gynec. *32*:382, 1968.

PANCREATIC ABSCESSES AND LESSER SAC COLLECTIONS

Pancreatic abscesses and lesser sac collections predominantly follow acute pancreatitis, pancreatic surgery, peptic ulcer disease and its surgery, and trauma. The precipitating event is generally quite dramatic, and should have the clinician alert to purulent complications. Unique features here include elevation of the serum amylase, left pleural effusion, pressure effects displacing the stomach or duodenum, and/or gas in the retro-colic region. The overall mortality may exceed 50%.

Reference

Bolloki, H., Jaffe, B., and Gliedman, M. L.: Pancreatic Abscesses and Lesser Omental Sac Collections. Surg. Gynecol. Obstet., *126*:1301, 1968.

RETROPERITONEAL ABSCESS

Retroperitoneal abscesses arise in a setting of infection, injury, or carcinoma in retroperitoneal organs or structures, or those just adjacent. Common source examples are to be found in the retroperitoneal portions of the colon, either kidney, osteomyelitis in the vertebral column or in the 12th rib, suppurative regional lymphadenitis (often initiated by intra-abdominal sepsis), or generalized bacteremia. Outstanding features of collections in this area are an occasional presentation with lower extremity pain, referred to the hip or knee region or even lower, and spasm of the lumbar musculature, with resultant spinal rigidity and deformity. Tuberculosis and actinomycosis are found retroperitoneally out of proportion to their representation in collections of pus in other abdominal locations.

Diagnostic aids may be found when there is gas in the retroperitoneal tissues (unfortunately rare), from the demonstration of bone destruction when this is the point of origin, and from hints to be obtained fairly frequently during the performance of intravenous urography, including the demonstration of mass, distortion, obstruction, etc.

Reference

Altemeier, W. A., and Alexander, J. W.: Retroperitoneal Abscess. Arch. Surg. *83*:512, 1961.

ABSCESSES IN THE LUMBAR GUTTERS

Cause. These are particularly associated with perforations of the large intestine or its appendix, thereby giving rise to a general numerical association with appendicitis on the right side of the abdomen, and with diverticulitis on the left. However, the various possible anatomic locations of the appendix give rise to a corresponding variability in the clinical presentation of appendicitis and its subsequent appendiceal abscess, *i.e.* intraperitoneally, retroperitoneally, occasionally on the left because of unusual appendiceal length or mobility, and rarely in the other quadrants because of intestinal malrotation. Colonic diverticula, while predominantly a left lower quadrant phenomenon, also may be found in any abdominal sector.

In addition to the usual characteristics of a purulent collection in the abdomen, the notable features here may include a particular applicability of the rectal examination, which may be the best way to find a tender bulging mass; also, when the abscess lies upon the lumbar musculature, there is reference of pain to the lower extremity, and pain upon extension of the leg (psoas sign).

Reference

Rhoads, Allen, Harkins, and Moyer: Surgery: Principles and Practice, 4th Ed. Philadelphia, J. B. Lippincott Co., 1970.

SPLENIC ABSCESS

Cause. Prior septicemia, with lodgement of bacteria in the splenic pulp. There is now a particular association with splenic trauma or infarction, as in sickle cell anemia, while in the past the association had been with endocarditis due to organisms of fecal origin, *i.e.* Enterococcus. The outstanding physical finding here should be a tender, left upper quadrant mass with movement upon respiration.

Reference

Rhoads, Allen, Harkins, and Moyer: Surgery: Principles and Practice, 4th Ed. Philadelphia, J. B. Lippincott Co., 1970.

3. Tuberculosis

Frank McBrearty

Cause: Mycobacterium tuberculosis

Early Manifestations:

Pulmonary	Positive PPD skin test, changes in roentgenogram, fever
Miliary	Fever, malaise, weight loss
Skeletal	Fever, persistent bone pain, positive PPD skin test
Genitourinary	Painless hematuria, pyuria, ureteral colic, fever
Neurological	Symptoms of encephalitis, meningitis, intervertebral disc, space consuming lesion, fever
Pericardial	Fever, friction rub, ascites, hepatomegaly, congestive failure
Peritoneal	Ascites, pain, fever, night sweats, anorexia, malaise

Treatment: Isoniazid, para-aminosalicylic acid. Streptomycin and others. (Table VII–8)

Possible Dire Consequences without Treatment: Continued morbidity and death.

Introduction

The mortality and morbidity from tuberculosis have decreased markedly during the first half of this century. In 1900, the mortality from tuberculosis in the United States was roughly 200 per 100,000 population. In 1968, the rate had plummeted to 3.2 per 100,000. Because of this fall, we as clinicians tend to neglect an equally impressive fact: In 1973, despite the obvious radical decline in mortality, tuberculosis is still the major "infectious" cause of death on a world-wide basis. The World Health Organization estimates that as many as 1.5 billion persons are infected with Mycobacterium tuberculosis. Of these, perhaps 10 to 12 million cases are infectious. Each year, 50 to 100 million "new" infections occur, and each year 2 to 3 million persons die of their infections. If one considers only the United States, one finds an estimated 25 million persons with positive tuberculin reactions. That is, one finds 25 million potentially active cases of tuberculosis. Indeed, at the end of 1967 the incidence of active tuberculosis in the United States was reported as 23.1 per 100,000 population. In other words, during 1967, 45,600 new cases of active tuberculosis were reported in the United States alone. Obviously not included in that figure are the estimated 30 to 40 thousand active cases which were never detected and which, therefore, were never reported. All of this leads to the point of the present discussion: Tuberculosis is a prevalent and eminently treatable disease.

Bacteriology

In current terminology the expression "tuberculosis" refers specifically to granulomatous and fibrocaseating infections caused by the strictly aerobic, non-motile, non-encapsulated, non-sporogenic and acid-fast bacillus, Mycobacterium tuberculosis. Clinically and pathologically, however, a disease complex indistinguishable from "tuberculosis" can be caused by a variety of other, related mycobacteria. The latter include Myco. bovis, Myco. avium, Myco. ulcerans, Myco. marinum (Myco.

TABLE VII-8. (ADAPTED FROM MITCHELL)

Drug (Abbreviation)	Usual Dosage/Diem (mg./kg., where indicated)	Route and Frequency of Administration	Major Toxicities and Miscellaneous Comments
First-line Drugs: Isoniazid (INH)	300 mg. [Range: 0.2–1.8 gm./diem] (10–20 mg./kg./day in children) given with 50–100 mg. pyridoxine per diem	p.o., given in one dose or in three divided doses	Most common: virus-like syndrome comprising anorexia, nausea, myalgia, fever, rash, vomiting. Peripheral neuropathy especially in patients with renal failure or vitamin deficiency. Elevated SGOT. Sideroachrestic anemia
Para-aminosalicylic Acid (PAS)	12 gm. [Range: 6.0–15 gm./diem] (200 mg./kg./diem as Na or Ca salt) (100–150 mg./kg./diem as Ascorbic Acid Salt, PAS-C)	p.o., given in one, two, or three divided doses *Note:* only fresh preparations must be used, as toxicity increases with the age of the drug	Hypersensitivity reactions common. Nausea, vomiting, anorexia, abd. cramps and diarrhea frequent. Interferes with SGOT colorimetric methods. SLE syndrome, blood dyscrasias and hepatotoxicity also occur. Ascorbic Acid Salt preferred in cardiac and hypertensive patients.
Streptomycin (SM)	1 gm. [Range: 0.25–1.0 gm./diem] 0.75 gm. in patients over 45 and in patients with renal impairment	I.M., o.d.	Vertigo and nystagmus are more common than hearing loss and tinnitus. Renal, cutaneous, and blood involvement occur but are rare. Circumoral paresthesia common.
Ethambutol (EMB)	1.2 gm. [Range: 0.8–2.0 gm./diem] (Given as 20–25 mg./kg./diem × 30 days, then 15–20 mg./kg./diem)	p.o., o.d.; or in two to three divided doses	Optic toxicity dose-related. At 25 mg./kg. dose, 3–6% develop loss of blue-green discrimination, blurred vision or scotomas. Permanent retrobulbar optic neuritis develops in smaller %.
Rifampicin (RF, RM)	400–600 mg./diem	p.o., once daily	Hepatotoxicty, nephrotoxicity, thrombocytopenia, hypersensitivity reactions [rash, fever, arthralgia, etc.] and positive Coombs' test are reported but are rare.

Second-line Drugs:

Drug	Dose	Route	Toxicity
Ethionamide (ETA) Prothionamide (PTA)	0.5–1.0 gm./diem	p.o., o.d. before bed, or in two to three divided doses	Causes frequent gastrointestinal upset and hepatotoxicity. Also teratogenic and has been reported to cause gynecomastia, as well as seizures, neuritis and impotence.
Pyrizinamide (PZA)	2.0–3.0 gm./diem (40 mg./kg./diem)	p.o., once daily or in two to three divided doses	Hepatotoxic in approx. 10% of cases. Reported to cause flare-up of clinical gout. Hyperuricemia common.
Capreomycin (CPM) *	0.5–1.5 gm./diem (15 mg./kg./diem)	I.M., o.d.	Nephrotoxicity common, and includes proteinuria, cylinduria and elevated BUN (especially in elderly). Hypokalemia, hypocalcemia, lethargy, stupor, and muscle weakness occur rarely. Ototoxicity in 10–12%, and is mostly vestibular.
Kanamycin (KM) *	0.5–1.0 gm./diem	I.M., o.d. to b.i.d.	Nephrotoxic and ototoxic (both cochlear and vestibular divisions of eighth cranial nerve are affected). Also occasionally hepatotoxic.
Cycloserine (CS)	0.5–1.0 gm./diem	p.o., t.i.d.	CNS symptoms predominate with depression, confusion, and seizures. The latter may be reduced by prophylactic use of anticonvulsants.
Viomycin (VM) *	0.5–1.0 gm./diem	I.M., o.d. for 2 to 7 weeks	Balance and gait disturbances are common. Renal damage, and blood dyscrasias seldom occur.
Thiacetazone (TB-1)	0.1–0.15 gm./diem	p.o., t.i.d.	Allergic reactions are severe. Toxicity substantially increased when dose is greater than 150 mg. per day. Should not be given to any patient allergic to other TB drugs.

* Cross-resistance shared by these drugs.

balnei), Myco. kansasii (Runyon Group I), Myco. scrofulaceum (Runyon Group II), Myco. xenope (Runyon Group III), Myco. intracellulare (Myco. battey, Runyon Group III), and Myco. fortuitum (Runyon Group IV). Traditionally, and perhaps somewhat ironically, the last five organisms mentioned are grouped together as the "unclassified," "anonymous" or "atypical" mycobacteria. Taken as a unit, they account for 2 to 3% of all infections clinically labeled as "tuberculosis," and are differentiated from Myco. tuberculosis by their negative niacin reduction test, their strongly positive catalase reaction, their relatively low guinea pig virulences, and their variable ability to form pigments when grown in the light or in the dark. The photochromogenic mycobacteria (Runyon Group I) are those which roughly double their pigment production after exposure to a source of bright light for one hour. On the other hand, the "scotochromogenic" mycobacteria (Runyon Group II) produce pigment regardless of whether they are cultured in the light or in the dark. A third group, the so-called "nonchromogenic" (Runyon Group III) mycobacteria, produces little or no pigment under most growth conditions. Runyon Group IV includes a number of brilliantly-colored saprophytes (with the exclusion of the non-pigmented Myco. fortuitum) which grow on standard media within seven to fourteen days when cultured at 37 °C.

In general, the atypical mycobacteria tend to be somewhat more drug-resistant and somewhat less prone to miliary spread than Myco. tuberculosis. Furthermore, persons with underlying chronic lung disease (*e.g.* silicosis, emphysema, idiopathic pulmonary fibrosis, etc.) are usually more prone than others to infection by "atypical" organisms. Another characteristic of atypical infections is their geo-demographic distribution. The photochromogen Myco. kansasii, for example, appears to be somewhat more prevalent in urban areas of the Western and Mid-Western United States, and most often causes pulmonary infection. Likewise, the non-chromogenic Myco. battey causes mostly pulmonary disease, but by contrast, is more commonly found in rural areas of the American South. Scotochromogenic bacteria are known to cause both local cutaneous infections and cervical lymphadenitis (especially in children). Myco. balnei is a photochromogen resembling Myco. kansasii, and is the purported cause of "fish-tank" or "swimmer's" granuloma, a local, self-limited granulomatous skin infection.

With control of tuberculosis in cattle, Myco. bovis is becoming an increasingly rare cause of human disease in the Western Hemisphere. In the past bovine tuberculosis was typically "primary" and consisted mainly of gastrointestinal, lymphoreticular or skeletal disease. At present the majority of cases are of the "secondary" or "reactivation" variety (see below) and involve the lungs. Myco. avium is a distinctly uncommon cause of human disease.

Other reasons notwithstanding, because of the possibility of infection with atypical organisms, and because the atypical mycobacteria show such a wide spectrum of response to chemotherapy, every effort should be made to determine both the species and the drug sensitivities of any organism isolated from a case of clinical "tuberculosis."

Pathology, Pathogenesis and Classification

Although various authors divide the clinical course of tuberculosis into various stages, for simplicity's sake one can usefully recognize three phases of tuberculosis infection: Primary, Latent and Post-primary.

Primary tuberculosis refers to infection occurring in a previously uninfected, unsensitized, susceptible individual. Despite the fact that the initial inoculum may enter its host via several routes, by far the most frequent route of infection is via the lung. Once primary infection occurs, the disease spreads according to the immune state, age, sex, race and state of health of the host. At the site of entry, the organism multiplies slowly and excites a variable degree of tissue reaction. The infection may then be contained locally or it may continue to proliferate and spread. Within hours of the latter event, the invading bacilli may pass in sequence to the local lymphatics, to the surrounding lymph nodes, and thence, into the blood stream. Once in the systemic circulation, the tubercle bacillus may settle in any organ system. As previously mentioned, since Mycobacterium tuberculosis is a strict aerobe, the organs most frequently involved in clinical disease are those with the highest tissue oxygen tension. These are, in order of frequency: lung apex, bone, kidney, brain, and serous membranes. Whereas the liver and spleen are common sites of histologic involvement, they are comparatively infrequent sites of gross clinical disease because of their relatively meager tissue oxygenation. It should be noted that once it has reached its end organ, the bacillus may be killed, become dormant, or proliferate. In the last case, clinical disease will appear in a manner consistent with the organ system involved. Dissemination of the disease to organ systems other than the lung is most likely to occur in the young, the elderly, the immunosuppressed, and the debilitated. It is somewhat more common in males and in nonwhites. If miliary spread occurs after primary infection, it most often occurs within twelve months of contact with the disease, and rarely occurs after two years. One must bear in mind however, that dissemination may also complicate chronic post-primary tuberculosis at any time.

The term latent tuberculosis is applied to the stage of the disease during which tubercle bacilli are present in the body, but are not multiplying and are not producing symptoms. This situation follows primary or post-primary infection and may last days, months or years.

Post-primary or "re-activation" tuberculosis usually follows the latent phase and represents recrudescences of disease possibly acquired years previously. During this stage massive caseation necrosis and cavitation are most likely to take place, possibly as a result of the body's protective, cell-based immune reaction against the invading tubercle bacillus. Currently the overwhelming majority of cases of classical chronic cavitating pulmonary tuberculosis are thought to be of the post-primary type. Reinfection is rarely, if ever, a cause of chronic cavitary tuberculosis.

DIAGNOSIS OF PRIMARY TUBERCULOSIS—*with a word or two about PPD and sputum*

In 1955, the World Health Organization published results of an international study which compared tuberculin reactor rates among 34,000 schoolchildren and 3,600 patients with known active tuberculosis. All subjects were given intradermal injections containing 5 tuberculin units (TU) of a standard purified protein derivative (intermediate-strength PPD-S, Mantoux). None of the subjects had previously received BCG vaccination. Among other things, it seemed clear from the data gathered that roughly 91% of American children under the age of thirteen had a negative Mantoux test. Likewise, it seemed apparent that almost 96% of patients with active tuberculosis gave a positive reaction to the same test. It was, therefore, generally concluded that infection with tubercle bacilli was becoming quite uncommon in American children, and that in the absence of anergy* a negative PPD was strong evidence against a diagnosis of tuberculosis. In the light of more recent investigations, both of these assumptions—especially the latter—must be called into serious question.

Holden and colleagues tested 115 consecutive hospitalized patients with bacteriologically-proved tuberculosis. Of these, 34% gave a negative reaction to 5 units of PPD-S, 49% had no reacion to 5 units of commercially-prepared PPD, and 17% did not react to 5 units of Tween-80-stabilized PPD. All tests were performed by the Mantoux method.

The authors speculated that reduced tuberculin skin sensitivity was related to adsorption of the test antigen by the glass walls of the container in which it had been stored. Tween-80 seemed to reduce this effect, but did not completely ablate it. PPD is similarly adsorbed by plastic surfaces.

A further study by Wijsmuller and Termini demonstrates that storage of PPD in glass containers for as little as two weeks after reconstitution leads to a 50% decrease in the tuberculin reactor rate if no Tween is added. The greatest part of this decrease occurs within the first day—and perhaps within the first hour—after dilution of the antigen. In addition, even when used immediately after reconstitution, commercially available PPD and PPD-S seemed somewhat inferior to Tween PPD in eliciting a positive tuberculin reaction.

Regardless of the technical reservations imposed by the preceding statements a freshly prepared intermediate-strength PPD should be applied, nevertheless, to all children or young adults with any of the signs and symptoms to be outlined. If this is positive (*i.e.* shows greater than 10 mm. induration in largest diameter forty-eight to seventy-two hours after the test is applied), the diagnosis of tuberculosis should be assumed until proved otherwise. Accordingly, a vigorous attempt should be made thereafter to culture all pertinent body fluids—especially sputum and urine—for acid-fast bacilli (AFB). For the most part, at least three specimens of sputum and urine are needed for adequate diagnosis. Ideally, these should be collected in the morning from a fasted patient. When the patient is unable to produce sputum spontaneously, fasting gastric washings and/or sputum induction may be performed. It should be noted, however, that repeated sputum collection will confirm the diagnosis in only 25 to 30% of cases of primary pulmonary tuberculosis. In the same vein, it should be recognized that negative sputum *smears* do not necessarily imply negative sputum *cultures*. In fact, to quote Gruft, Gaefer and Kaufmann: "Almost 50% of active open cases may be negative on microscopic examination regardless of the staining procedure used, such as Ziehl-Neelsen, Auramine-Rhodamine Fluorescent staining or any of the modifications. The positive smear is a function of the concentration of organisms in the sputum, approximately 10,000 organisms per ml. being required for a positive direct smear."† A diagnosis of tuberculosis cannot be discarded, therefore, on the basis of normal AFB smears alone. Conversely, a positive AFB smear does not *necessarily* imply a definite diagnosis of tuberculosis. Ambient, non-pathogenic, acid-fast saprophytes such as Myco. butyricum and Myco. smegmatis may be present as sputum or gastric fluid contaminants. These organisms are gener-

---

* Which might be expected to occur in patients with overwhelming illness, Hodgkin's disease, viral illness such as measles, and in patients receiving corticosteroids.

† This figure falls into the neighborhood of 1,000 organisms per ml. using fluorescent staining techniques.

ally indistinguishable from Myco. tuberculosis on microscopic examination alone. Consequently, the diagnosis can only be provisional in the absence of culture confirmation.

Pleural fluid should also be examined when present. This is usually a clear yellow exudate which may rarely be blood-tinged and which will frequently show the classic lymphocytic pleomorphism on cell count. Unfortunately, culture and smear of the pleural fluid will be diagnostic in considerably less than one-half of cases. A more predictable result can be obtained via percutaneous Adams or Cope needle biopsy of the pleura, which yields positive information in 80 to 90% of patients presenting with tuberculous pleural effusion. As with all other specimens, the biopsy should be cultured as well as examined microscopically. Given a pleural effusion of undetermined etiology and a positive PPD, open pleural biopsy should be seriously entertained in the remaining patients whose cultures and percutaneous pleural biopsy are negative.

Hematologic abnormalities seen with tuberculosis will be discussed under a separate heading. Suffice it to say here that the white blood cell count may be high, low, or normal. There may be mild anemia and/or thrombocytopenia, and the erythrocyte sedimentation rate may be normal or accelerated.

In summary, any of the following should particularly inspire the diagnosis of primary pulmonary tuberculosis.*

1. Middle or lower lobe pulmonary infiltrate associated with hilar adenopathy.
2. Pleurisy with effusion in the absence of demonstrable parenchymal lung disease (30% of cases will eventually develop a parenchymal lesion if untreated).
3. Lower lobe or anterior segment upper lobe pulmonary parenchymal lesion which clears with anti-tuberculous chemotherapy.
4. Flu-like symptoms associated with a persistent lung lesion in a child or young adult.
5. Recent, documented PPD conversion in a person of any age.
6. A positive PPD in any child or young adult.

It takes three to eight weeks after primary infection for tuberculin skin reaction to become positive. For this and other reasons, therefore, the intermediate-strength PPD should be repeated in any patient who is suspected of having tuberculosis but whose initial PPD is negative. Contrary to previous theory, repeated tuberculin skin testing does not "convert" a reaction from negative to positive, but only enhances preexisting skin sensitivity. Secondly, if the intermediate PPD is equivocal (*i.e.* 5 to 9 mm. induration) and yet the clinical suspicion of tuberculosis remains high, a repeat 5-TU Mantoux and specific skin tests for atypical mycobacteria (PPD-B, PPD-G and PPD-Y) should be performed. Lastly, when the diagnosis remains elusive in the face of a strongly suggestive clinical setting and negative routine AFB culture results, guinea pig inoculation cultures of the appropriate body fluids might reasonably be obtained. The latter may be positive in as many as 15% of culture negative cases caused by Myco. tuberculosis.

Once the diagnosis of primary tuberculosis is established, a careful epidemiologic search for the source of infection must be made, and therapy should be instituted immediately (as outlined below under therapy of pulmonary tuberculosis). If undiagnosed and untreated, some 10% of patients with primary disease will progress to a post-primary phase. As the latter is the infectious stage of the disease, the cycle for the propagation of new cases will again be set in motion.

---

* The first three of these are quite uncommon in post-primary tuberculosis.

POST-PRIMARY PULMONARY TUBERCULOSIS

As mentioned earlier, most cases of classical, chronic, cavitary, caseofibrotic pulmonary tuberculosis are of the "post-primary" type. That is, most cases arise not from re-infection of an already sensitized host, but rather from "reactivation" of tubercle bacilli acquired during previous primary infection. Reactivation may occur weeks, months, years, or decades after the primary phase. Although reasons for reactivation are not precisely understood, recrudescent tuberculosis is most likely to take place in patients with diminished immunoresponsiveness; for example, in patients with severe intercurrent disease (silicosis, diabetes, cirrhosis, lymphoma) or in patients receiving corticosteroid or immunosuppressive chemotherapy. All patients with a positive tuberculin skin reaction who have not received prior BCG inoculation are, however, candidates for reactivation of disease.

In contrast to primary tuberculosis, the lesions of reactivation tuberculosis tend more toward parenchymal caseating necrosis, cavitation, abscess formation, and bronchopneumonic propagation. In addition, post-primary disease most often affects the apical segments of the lower lobes and the apicoposterior segments of the upper lobes. Involvement may be unilateral or bilateral. The pathologic spectrum produced is vast, and includes asymptomatic apical scarring, overwhelming tuberculous bronchopneumonia with basilar spread, diffuse or localized cavitation, tuberculous pleurisy with or without effusion, solitary pulmonary nodules, tuberculous empyema, and local to diffuse interstitial, pleural and/or mediastinal fibrosis. The disease varies from indolent to fulminant in onset and course.

Presentation. As with primary disease, some patients are totally asymptomatic and are discovered by routine chest roentgenogram, or as part of investigation of another illness, to have an abnormal chest roentgenogram suggestive of pulmonary tuberculosis. Other patients may offer any combination of the following complaints: "smoker's cough," morning cough productive of yellow, green or blood-streaked sputum, pleuritic or other chest pain, breathlessness, nocturnal or post-exertional fever, drenching or non-drenching sweats, weight loss, anorexia, abdominal pain, lassitude, fatigue, or laryngitis (in advanced cavitary disease). Symptoms produced parallel systems involved, and may, therefore be extrapulmonary in origin (skeletal, renal, neurologic for example.) Likewise, symptoms may largely reflect the underlying disease states which predispose toward reactivation of the tubercle bacillus; for example, chronic obstructive lung disease, silicosis, diabetes, cirrhosis, alcoholism, and lymphoma as mentioned above. According to Robson and Emerson, symptoms tend to appear prior to the development of physical signs and in the following order of decreasing frequency: cough, dyspnea on exertion, lassitude, loss of weight, chest pain, dyspepsia, night sweats, and hoarseness. Unlike primary tuberculosis, most patients with post-primary infection give no history of recent tuberculosis exposure.

Physical signs, like symptoms, vary from minimal to marked. One may detect any or all of the classical features such as apical dullness to percussion, decreased apical breath sounds, apical rales or sub-clavicular chest-wall flattening.

The Chest Roentgenogram

Radiologic presentations of chronic tuberculosis are myriad and non-specific. The most common picture is that of mottled, hazy, often bilateral, apicoposterior segment opacification. Frequently, thin- or thick-walled cavities, with or without air-fluid levels may be seen. After adequate anti-tuberculous chemotherapy, aspergilloma will eventually develop in 11 to 17% of cavities greater than 2.5 cm. in diameter. The first signs of the latter event are usually thickening of the cavity wall and increase in the surrounding pleural shadow. Subsequently, the radiographically typical, air-ringed central opacity may become apparent. Alternatively, a solitary nodule indistinguishable from pulmonary carcinoma may be seen on the x-ray film. Particularly in childhood and in adolescence, marked mediastinal or hilar lymphadenopathy may be seen, sometimes in conjunction with segmental consolidation, collapse or cavitation. A reticulo-nodular interstitial pattern or a more gross miliary pattern may also become manifest, as may shift of the trachea, mediastinum and/or interlobar fissures. Stead claims that fibronodular or apical scarring may be detected on chest roentgenogram in 80% of those over the age of fifty who will eventually develop active tuberculosis.

To recapitulate, the chest x-ray findings of post-primary pulmonary tuberculosis are not absolutely diagnostic of either the disease or its activity. Some 25% of sputum-positive cases will have chest roentgenograms which are interpreted as being "normal" or as showing "no active disease." Furthermore, presence of calcium or scarring in the lesion indicates only that the process was established at least nine to twelve months prior to the taking of the x-ray film, and in no way correlates with activity or healing. Sputum or tissue culture of AFB is the only definitive diagnostic procedure. All other methods merely *suggest* the diagnosis, but do not *prove* it.

Laboratory

Comments already made regarding the PPD and the examination of sputum and peripheral blood also obtain in a discussion of chronic tuberculosis. A few additional comments are in order, however. First, the tubercle bacillus is rather fastidious. It is inactivated by ultraviolet light, sunshine, heat, drying, and prolonged exposure to air. Accordingly, if one waits for twenty-four hours after obtaining a sputum sample before culturing that sample, the probability of recovering Myco. tuberculosis on culture is reduced by almost 50% (Robson and Emerson). Second, finding of AFB on the direct sputum smear correlates directly with the infectiousness of the patient from whom the sputum is obtained. Furthermore, patients with reactivation tuberculosis are much more likely than primary tuberculosis patients to have positive sputum smears for AFB. Therefore, even though acid-fast organisms seen on smear may represent non-infective contaminants (especially in patients with chronic lung disease or in those already treated for tuberculosis), one should assume the diagnosis of tuberculosis, start the appropriate therapy, and isolate all patients clinically suspected of post-primary disease who have AFB-positive sputum smears. In this instance theoretical objections to such measures are outweighed by practical epidemiologic considerations.

Serologic diagnostic methods using a fluorescein-tagged antibody against soluble protein fractions of the tubercle bacillus (SAFA tests) are currently under development. These are, unfortunately, not yet sufficiently reliable for routine clinical work.

Complications of Chronic Pulmonary Tuberculosis

The complications of reactivation tuberculosis are multifarious and largely beyond the scope of this discussion. They include cavitation, abscess formation, destructive emphysema, spontaneous pneumothorax, diffuse interstitial fibrosis, serous effusion, chronic pseudochylous effusion, empyema, bronchiectasis, hemoptysis, gastrointestinal ulceration, bronchopleural fistula, tuberculous pneumonia, endobronchial tuberculosis, tuberculous laryngitis, and miliary spread, among others. The last four of these are most common in debilitated individuals, the elderly, infants and in the immunosuppressed. Tuberculous laryngitis and endobronchial disease usually appear in association with advanced cavitary disease. The former may be indistinguishable from laryngeal carcinoma, even on direct inspection. For this reason a chest roentgenogram and Mantoux test should be done in all patients with chronic laryngitis suspected of having carcinoma.

Gastrointestinal ulceration, with or without terminal ileitis, tuberculoma formation, mesenteric lymphadenitis, mucosal ulceration and/or ano-rectal fistulas may occur when massive numbers of tubercle bacilli are swallowed after expulsion from an open lung abscess. This is rare.

Hemoptysis will eventually occur in only a small minority of patients with tuberculosis (approximately 10%). When present, it can take two forms: incidental or massive. The former follows superficial bronchial erosion by the tubercle bacillus and is the most frequent type. It usually consists of minimal to moderate streaking of the sputum with bright-red blood, and generally responds well to conservative therapy (*i.e.*, rest and sedation). Rarely, a tuberculous cavity will invade the wall of a major subdivision of the pulmonary artery. If the artery is sufficiently weakened, a Rasmussen's aneurysm may form. Subsequently, the aneurysm may rupture producing massive hemoptysis of dark red blood. Although usually too late to save the patient, thoracotomy with resection of the cavity and involved pulmonary artery segment is the only dependable therapy.

Treatment of Pulmonary Tuberculosis

CHEMOTHERAPY

The chemotherapy of tuberculosis has been summarized elsewhere and will not be discussed in detail here. Drugs in current use, along with their dosages, routes of administration and major toxicities are listed in Table VII–8. What is said relative to the chemical treatment of pulmonary disease also pertains for the most part to the treatment of extrapulmonary disease.

As depicted in the table, isoniazid (INH), para-aminosalicyclic acid (PAS) and streptomycin (SM), used simultaneously, are still the agents usually chosen in the therapy of newly discovered pulmonary tuberculosis. While primary drug resistance to these compounds is common in underdeveloped nations, aside from sporadic outbreaks, it is comparatively rare in the United States, Great Britain, and Canada.

Despite their added cost, both rifampin and ethambutol have been shown to be extremely effective and palatable drugs when used in conjunction with INH in the treatment of tuberculosis. The general therapeutic considerations applicable to the use of other first-line agents also apply to the use of rifampin and ethambutol. Side effects are rare, and are summarized in Table VII-8.

Drug Resistance

Disregarding disease caused by atypical organisms, most cases of drug-resistant tuberculosis are related either to lack of patient cooperation in taking the appropriate drugs, or to lack of physician expertise in administering the drugs. With regard to the latter, the chief factors involved appear to be intermittent therapy, therapy with inadequate drug dosages, and therapy with too few drugs for insufficient periods of time. When possible, treatment of resistant infection should be given by expert physicians in centers specializing in such treatment.

In any event, the following general principles should be observed:

1. Do not treat until a complete drug history has been obtained. Has the patient been taking his medicines? If so, how?

2. Do not treat without knowing the results of *all* initial drug sensitivity tests.

3. Do not unnecessarily discontinue partially effective drugs. Almost all "resistant" organisms show some susceptibility to INH. This drug should probably be incorporated into most retreatment drug regimens. In addition, tubercle bacilli may sometimes show transiently diminished *in vitro* sensitivity to any or all chemotherapeutic agents just before AFB disappear from the sputum. Such "transitional resistance" is well recognized and should not be regarded as an indication for altering therapy.

4. Whenever possible, use at least three drugs to which the tubercle bacillus has been shown to be sensitive. Second-line drugs are generally less potent than first-line drugs. Wherever possible, use two second-line agents for each first-line substitution.

5. Use first-line drugs when possible, before considering a second-line replacement.

6. Never use monotherapy.

7. Avoid intermittent therapy.

8. Make sure that the patient takes his medicines.

9. Monitor sputum closely. Cultures should be obtained at monthly intervals while sputum remains positive for AFB, and every three to four months after sputum conversion.

10. As second-line drugs tend to be more toxic than first-line agents, be on the look out for side effects; especially in atopic individuals and in patients with pre-existing renal, hepatic or CNS disease.

With proper, closely supervised care, chemotherapeutic reversal of infectiousness— if not cure of the disease—can be anticipated in almost 75% of cases of drug-resistant tuberculosis.

Indications for In-hospital Care

Since the advent of effective anti-tuberculous chemotherapy, the indications for prolonged hospitalization in the treatment of tuberculosis have become fewer in number. At present most patients should be hospitalized only during the infectious phase of their disease, provided adequate out-patient care facilities are available. That is to say, most patients may be discharged from the hospital following the demonstration of "... several consecutive (sputum) specimens of which the majority are negative and the others contain only rare acid-fast bacilli (less than 10 per slide or Gaffky grade I or II)."

Surgical Management of Pulmonary Tuberculosis

According to Shields, Streider, Neptune, and their colleagues, surgical treatment for pulmonary tuberculosis may be entertained in the following circumstances:

1. Persistent, thick-walled, open cavity (with or without positive AFB cultures) which has not responded to six months of appropriate anti-tuberculosis chemotherapy.
2. Local or diffuse caseous nodules or fibrocaseous disease (with or without positive AFB culture) which persists or progresses despite vigorous medical management.
3. Persistent pulmonary tuberculoma.
4. Persistently AFB-positive, partially drug-resistant sputum cultures associated with localized parenchymal disease.
5. Recurrent and/or life-threatening hemoptysis.
6. Symptomatic bronchostenosis, bronchiectasis or fixed atelectasis which is not amenable to medical care.
7. Chronic encapsulated tuberculous empyema associated with an unexpandable lobe.
8. Bronchopleura fistula with empyema secondary to previous therapy.
9. Prior thoracoplasty failure or removal of previous plombage.
10. Suspected neoplasm.
11. Open cavitary disease in patients who cannot or will not tolerate long-term medical therapy (*e.g.* alcoholics, schizophrenics, drug addicts).

When surgery is indicated, the preferred procedure is resection of the involved lung tissue.

Streider gives the following contraindications to resectional surgery:

1. Inadequate pulmonary or cardiac reserve.
2. Extensive bilateral pulmonary involvement.
3. Involvement of the entire lung with active disease following full-scale chemotherapy.
4. Persistently positive sputum with organisms totally resistant to all drugs. (The risk of surgical dissemination of the disease is great in such patients.)
5. Concurrent terminal disease.

One may expect 92 to 95% of patients with active pulmonary infection to have become inactive one year after resectional therapy, and approximately 79 to 87% to have become inactive after plombage. In most series peri-operative mortality from resection averages about 2% (about 1% for wedge resection or segmentectomy). Plombage mortality, which is generally performed in much sicker patients, varies from 0.8 to 4%.

Pulmonary Carcinoma vs. Pulmonary Tuberculosis

The clinician is frequently faced with the task of differentiating granulomatous disease of the lung from carcinoma. In a review of 887 cases of solitary pulmonary nodules, Steele found that 316 of these were cancer, 474 were granulomas, 65 were hematomas, 23 were assorted cysts, lymph nodes or local pneumonitis, and 9 were chest wall or pleural tumors of various types. Carcinoma was rare, but not non-existent below the age of 30.

Berroya et al. reviewed the case histories of some 6,750 patients with tuberculosis or lung cancer. They found that, of these, only 54 had concurrent disease. The conclusion drawn was that the simultaneous occurrence of carcinoma and tuberculosis was largely coincidental. From analysis of their cancer patients' clinical presentation, however, they further concluded that malignancy, with or without concomitant tuberculosis, should be strongly suspected in any patients who develop any of the following:

1. Continuous, localized chest pain.
2. Persistent hemoptysis.
3. Hectic cough with paroxysmal dyspnea.
4. Unilateral or localized wheezes or rhonchi.
5. Prolonged low-grade fever.
6. Segmental or lobular atelectasis.
7. Unilateral hilar enlargement.
8. Abrupt appearance of new chest lesions on roentgenogram.
9. Thick-walled cavity surrounded by a localized pneumonitis.

As might be inferred from the above, there are still no clear-cut, noninvasive methods of absolutely differentiating the patient with cancer from the patient with tuberculosis. In a patient with a solitary nodule or with any of the findings listed above, the definitive diagnosis must all too frequently be made at surgery.

Miliary TB should be suspected immediately in any (especially elderly) patient with a fever of obscure origin who complains of malaise, weakness, weight loss, anorexia, vague abdominal pain, or any of the symptoms of classical pulmonary tuberculosis. The diagnosis should be pursued vigorously and the diagnostic routine should include sputum cultures, urine cultures, spinal fluid cultures, and—as is usually necessary—microscopic examination of liver and bone marrow biopsy specimens. Open or percutaneous lung biopsy may be required when lung lesions are present and other diagnostic methods have proved fruitless. If after all of these studies have been performed the diagnosis is still in doubt, a therapeutic trial of chemotherapy may be reasonably entertained. The latter should be continued for at least two months before the diagnosis is abandoned.

Extrapulmonary Tuberculosis

SKELETAL TUBERCULOSIS

Skeletal tuberculosis is the most common extrapulmonary form of the disease, and occurs in approximately 1% of all cases of clinical tuberculosis. The disease may occur at any time after primary infection but (as is the case with most other types of tuberculosis) it shows its peak incidence in later life.

The most frequent sites of bony involvement are the thoracolumbar spine, hip and knee joint.

Persistent bone pain is the usual presenting complaint. When the spine is involved, pain may be diffuse or radicular in type. Signs and symptoms of paraplegia will ultimately develop in as many as 11% of patients with vertebral column involvement, if untreated. Fortunately, the latter complication will resolve in the majority of instances, if proper therapy is instituted promptly.

When extravertebral sites are involved, the usual picture is one of muscle wasting and muscle spasm around a pale, warm, "doughy" or "boggy" joint. Joint effusion and synovial thickening may be slight or marked. Cartilaginous destruction tends to develop slowly, but limitation of joint motion may be severe and may occur early in the disease. In most cases the onset and progression of the disease are subacute and extend over several weeks or months.

Fever, leukocytosis, and increased sedimentation rate may or may not be apparent. The PPD skin test is usually but not invariably positive. AFB may occasionally be seen on direct joint fluid smear, and may frequently be cultured from the joint aspirate.

Narrowing of the intervertebral space on a lateral x-ray film of the thoracic or lumbar spine is the most frequent radiologic presentation. Less commonly, an area of localized radiolucency, and rarely a focus of osteosclerosis may be seen in the vertebral bodies. Periarticular decalcification is one of the earliest signs of joint involvement. Subsequently, lytic lesions with sequestrum formation may appear. Secondary periosteal reaction with resorption of underlying bone may sometimes be seen, especially in the metacarpals and/or metatarsals of affected children.

Chemotherapy is the same as that for pulmonary tuberculosis. This is supplemented by rest and immobilization of the affected joint during the active phase of the disease and sometimes by surgical intervention.

GENITOURINARY TUBERCULOSIS

Usually included under this heading are infections involving the kidneys, ureters, bladder, prostate, epididymis and seminal vesicles. The definitive diagnosis is made by isolation of the organism.

The chemotherapy of urinary tuberculosis is essentially that recommended for the treatment of active pulmonary infection. Since it is excreted primarily in the urine, however, cycloserine is probably the second-line drug of choice in patients resistant or intolerant to first-line and alternate first-line agents. Using the standard regimen, well over 90% of patients will be urine culture negative for AFB at the end of five years.

TUBERCULOSIS OF THE CENTRAL NERVOUS SYSTEM

Neurologic tuberculosis may be insidious in its onset and protean in its manifestations. Patients may present with signs and symptoms consistent with the diagnoses of encephalitis, meningitis, communicating hydrocephalus, cerebrovascular accident, brain or meningeal tumor, primary spinal cord neoplasm, metastatic disease of the brain and spinal cord, prolapsed intervertebral disc, or organic brain syndrome. As the meninges, spinal cord and nerve roots are the usual sites of neurologic involvement, they are discussed in some detail below.

TB Meningitis. During the hematogenous phase of primary respiratory infection, tubercle bacilli may come to rest within small terminal arterioles near the surface of the brain. The resulting "Rich foci" are small granulomata within the substance of the brain. These may eventually grow, rupture into the subarachnoid space and, by direct extension, cause a classical, basilar tubercular pachymeningitis.

Of Hinman's 35 patients with tuberculous meningitis, approximately 50% had symptoms for less than one week before presentation. By contrast, almost 17% were ill for more than six weeks before seeking medical assistance. The commonest complaint in this series was fever, which was subjectively present in about two-thirds of patients, and objectively demonstrable in roughly 90% of cases. Lethargy was noted in some 63% of cases, confusion in 23%, and headache in 57%. Signs of meningeal irritation were apparent in almost 86% of cases. Thirty % of Hinman's patients had evidence of cranial nerve involvement (usually third, fourth, seventh, or eighth nerves). Coma eventually developed in 29%, and was by far the most ominous prognostic sign. One-half of the comatose patients expired—some despite intensive antituberculous chemotherapy. (This compares to an over-all mortality of 20 to 30% in most series.)

In terms of laboratory diagnosis, peripheral white blood cell count is normal in 40% of cases. The PPD skin test is usually positive but, as in other forms of the disease, it may be negative or equivocal. The chest roentgenogram is of immense diagnostic importance, as it may show signs of pulmonary involvement in up to 60% of patients with tuberculous meningitis. A substantial portion of the latter group of patients can be demonstrated to have active pulmonary infection. Examination of the cerebrospinal fluid reveals the sugar content to be less than 40 mg.% in approximately two-thirds of patients. Of these, half will have a CSF glucose of less than 20 mg.%. Acid-fast bacilli are seen on smear in roughly 20%, and are culturable in 75% of cases. Most spinal fluid samples from patients with tuberculous meningitis will contain an increased number of leukocytes, but early in the disease, the CSF cell count may be normal, or may contain mostly polymorphonuclear leukocytes rather than the classical pleomorphic lymphocytes. Spinal fluid protein content is typically elevated. Occasionally, a picture of encephalitis with normal CSF glucose, increased and minimally abnormal cell count may be observed early in the course of tuberculous meningitis. For this reason, it is well to bear in mind that more than one lumbar puncture is often necessary to make the correct diagnosis. Also recall that spinal fluid changes are especially apt to be absent or minimal in patients taking corticosteroids.

Spinal Cord and Nerve Root Tuberculosis. Direct extension from involved paravertebral lymph nodes may lead to extradural nerve root compression with its attendant signs and symptoms. The disease produced may be superficially indistinguishable from that produced by rupture of an intervertebral disc. Evidence of bony invasion (Pott's disease) may be absent on roentgenograms of the vertebral column; although ill-defined paravertebral radio-opacity may sometimes be seen. Fever, lymphadenopathy and non-specific complaints such as weight loss or malaise may be the only available clues to the diagnosis. For these reasons, tuberculosis of the spinal cord or its coverings should be considered in any person (particularly a young adult from an underdeveloped country) who presents with a puzzling myelopathy which is associated with pyrexia, radicular pain and lymphadenopathy. This is especially so since seemingly fixed neurologic deficits secondary to tuberculosis (including paraparesis) will often respond dramatically to appropriate therapy.

Treatment is, again, largely that employed in other forms of tuberculosis; namely, triple therapy and, when indicated, surgery. Intrathecal chemotherapy is no longer used. Steroids may reduce the extent of cerebral and spinal cord edema. There is little doubt that in certain instances they may also dramatically improve both the patient's sense of well-being and/or his level of consciousness.

Discrete, symptomatic tuberculomas should be removed when surgically accessible. With regard to tuberculous meningitis, one should recognize that the development of a surgically treatable hydrocephalus may be heralded by the onset of coma. In any event, and regardless of the operation contemplated, triple therapy (with or without steroids) should probably be given for a least several days prior to surgery in order to reduce edema of the involved nerve tissue and to limit the opportunities for surgical dissemination of the disease.

PERITONEAL TUBERCULOSIS

Although the disease affects both sexes and all age groups, there is a decided tendency for it to occur in young women. The most frequent chief complaint is abdominal swelling which occurs in 53 to 100% of cases. Abdominal pain is prominent in roughly 80% of cases, and is the principal complaint given by as many as 30% of patients. Virtually 100% of patients offer a history of fever, and well over half will complain of night sweats, weight loss, anorexia, intermittent chills and/or malaise. Only 6 to 10% have respiratory complaints; although as many as 50% of patients will have objective signs of concomitant thoracic tuberculosis.

On physical examination, the majority of patients can be shown to have ascites. Roughly 10% have evidence of an epigastric mass which may suggest the erroneous diagnosis of intraabdominal malignancy. In reality, the latter usually proves to be a segment of thickened omentum adherent to several loops of bowel. Occasionally, an enlarged left hepatic lobe or bowel tuberculoma will be felt as an abdominal mass. Fortunately, most of these space-occupying lesions will disappear eventually with appropriate chemotherapy. In addition to abdominal mass, hepatomegaly can be detected in almost 20% of cases. Splenomegaly occurs in only 5%. Axillary and/or supraclavicular lymph nodes are frequently enlarged. Signs of pleural (and less often pericardial) effusion are commonly present; with the control of bovine tuberculosis, primary intestinal involvement has become an increasingly rare event.

The preliminary steps used in making the diagnosis of tuberculous peritonitis are similar to those already mentioned in the previous discussion of pulmonary tuberculosis. Most patients will have a normal peripheral white blood cell count, and most (but not all) will have a positive intermediate PPD skin test. Acid-fast bacilli may be found in the ascitic fluid of more than 80% of cases if more than 1 liter of fluid is collected for examination. The ascites is almost universally transudative and it ordinarily contains an increased number of white cells, especially lymphocytes. Not infrequently, the ascitic fluid cytology will be reported as class 4 or 5, again supporting the spurious diagnosis of intraabdominal neoplasm. Perhaps paradoxically, percutaneous liver biopsy and liver enzyme studies are usually unremarkable. The previously venerated association between peritoneal tuberculosis and cirrhosis now seems somewhat tenuous.

In most series, peritoneal biopsy performed during peritoneoscopy or during open laparotomy is the most fruitful diagnostic procedure. This will disclose typical epithelioid tubercles studding the peritoneum in the vast majority of cases.

Once diagnosed, therapy is instituted along lines similar to those outlined above in earlier sections of this paper. Regardless of whether steroids are included in the drug regimen, early treatment will yield an excellent prognosis in most cases.

Hematologic Manifestations of Tuberculosis

Aside from mild anemia, hematologic abnormalities are surprisingly infrequent in uncomplicated tuberculosis of the non-disseminated type.

Idiosyncratic or toxic drug reactions (especially to PAS) should be suspected in any patient who manifests anemia, leukopenia, leukocytosis or thrombocytopenia only after beginning antituberculous chemotherapy.

Pyridoxine-responsive sideroblastic anemia is occasionally seen in patients taking INH, pyrizinamide or cycloserine. This presents as a microcytic hypochromic anemia in patients in whom no source of blood loss can be identified. In contrast to iron deficiency anemia, copious amounts of iron contained within the mitochondria of "ringed sideroblasts" are seen on iron stains of the bone marrow aspirate. In addition, serum iron is elevated, and iron saturation is increased in sideroblastic anemias; whereas, both are decreased in classical iron deficiency.

Pericardial Tuberculosis

Tuberculous pericarditis is a surprisingly prevalent, easily misdiagnosed, and easily treatable disease. It occurs most frequently in the third through the fifth decades of life, is significantly more common in males, and affects nonwhites much more often than whites. Whereas the over-all mortality for tuberculosis is generally 1 to 5%, the mortality for untreated tuberculous pericarditis approaches 40%.

Presenting symptoms of the disease are non-specific and occasionally are frankly misleading. In Rooney et al.'s excellent review, symptoms are listed in the following order of frequency: Weight loss (85%), cough (85%), dyspnea (74%), orthopnea (66%), chest pain (57%), ankle swelling (49%), night sweats (39%), hemoptysis (17%), and ascites (3%). The corresponding physical signs included: fever (97%), tachycardia (94%), roentgenographic cardiomegaly (85%), pleural effusion (71%), hepatomegaly (63%), edema (49%), jugular venous distention (46%), distant heart sounds (46%), friction rub (37%), and pulsus paradoxicus (23%). EKG findings consist primarily of low voltage and ST-segment depression with T-wave inversion. During the early phase of the illness, signs and symptoms tend to be insidious or non-specific, with those of malaise, fever, fatigue, weight loss, cardiomegaly and pericardial effusion predominating. Months or years later signs of congestive heart failure and pericardial constriction appear. More than half of those with tuberculous pericarditis have no signs of extra-cardiac tuberculosis during life. Of those patients dying with their disease, however, virtually all will have evidence of pulmonary, pleural or mediastinal disease at autopsy. Another large group of patients will be discovered at postmortem examination to have extrathoracic involvement, most notably in the liver, spleen, peritoneum and meninges.

During life, pericardial aspiration will yield culturable organisms in approximately 50% of patients. The intermediate PPD is almost invariably positive. Pericardial biopsy, likewise, is universally positive for either caseating granulomata or AFB.

From what has been said, tuberculous pericarditis should be considered in any patient who complains of malaise, weight loss, and fever in association with signs of congestive failure and/or pericardial or pleural effusion. Occasionally patients present only with mild fever and hepatomegaly. The treatment of the disease is much the same as that already described in the section on therapy of pulmonary tuberculosis. In addition, steroids appear to have a definite role in reducing the incidence of pericardial tamponade, and seem to significantly lessen over-all mortality. They should be given in a dose of 80 mg. prednisone equivalent per day for five to seven days. Thereafter the steroid dose may be tapered and then continued for five to seven weeks. Pericardiectomy should be entertained in patients whose hearts are persistently enlarged despite six months of adequate chemotherapy, and in patients who develop intractable congestive failure, or in whom central venous pressure begins to rise in the presence of decreasing heart size.

With adequate, aggressive therapy, prognosis is good and mortality falls into the 8 to 15% range.

References

Berger, H. W., and Samortin, T. G.: Miliary Tuberculosis: Diagnostic Methods with Emphasis on the Chest Roentgenogram. Chest *58*:586, 1970.

Berroya, R. B. et al.: Concurrent Pulmonary Tuberculosis and Primary Carcinoma. Thorax *26*:384, 1971.

Citron, K. M.: The Management of Tuberculosis. Brit. J. Hosp. Med. *5*:799, 1971.

Davidson, P. T., and Horowitz, I.: Skeletal Tuberculosis. Amer. J. Med. *48*:77, 1970.

Davies, P. D. B.: Clinical Presentation of Tuberculosis. Brit. J. Hosp. Med. *5*:749, 1971.

Editorial: Miliary Tuberculosis: A changing pattern. Lancet *1*:985, 1970.

Editorial: Neurologic Complications of Tuberculosis. Lancet *1*:1094, 1970.

Glasser, R. M., Walker, R. I., and Herion, J. C.: The Significance of Hematologic Abnormalities in Patients with Tuberculosis. Arch. Int. Med. *125*:691, 1970.

Gruft, H., Gaafar, A. H., and Kaufmann, W.: Identification of Mycobacteria: What Constitutes an Adequate Examination? Am. J. Pub. Health *60*:2055, 1970.

Grzybowski, S. et al.: Chemoprophylaxis for the Prevention of Tuberculosis: A statement by the ad hoc committee of the American Thoracic Society. Amer. Rev. Resp. Dis. *96*:558, 1967.

Hinman, A. R.: Tuberculous meningitis at the Cleveland Metropolitan General Hospital, 1959 to 1963. Amer. Rev. Resp. Dis., *95*:670, 1967.

Holden, M., Dubin, M. R. and Diamond, P. H.: Frequency of negative intermediate strength tuberculin sensitivity in patients with active tuberculosis. New Eng. J. Med., *285*:1506, 1971.

Horne, N. W.: Epidemiology and Control of Tuberculosis. Brit. J. Hosp. Med. *5*:732, 1971.

Hyde, H.: The Clinical Significance of the Tuberculin Skin Test. Amer. Rev. Resp. Dis. *105*:453, 1972.

Kocen, R. S. and Parsons, M.: Neurologic Complications of Tuberculosis: Some Unusual Manifestations. Quart. J. Med. *39*:17, 1970.

Lattimer, J. K., Reilly, R. J., and Segawa, A.: The Significance of the Isolated Positive Urine Culture in Genitourinary Tuberculosis. J. Urol. *102*:610, 1969.

Lester, W. et al.: Treatment of Drug-Resistant Tuberculosis: A statement by the Committee on Therapy. Amer. Rev. Resp. Dis. *94*:125, 1966.

Mitchell, R. S.: Control of Tuberculosis. New Eng. J. Med. *276*:842, 905, 1967.

Narain, R. et al.: Microscopy Positive and Microscopy Negative Cases of Pulmonary Tuberculosis. Amer. Rev. Resp. Dis. *103*:761, 1971.

Neptune, W. B., and Bookwalter, J.: Current Surgical Management of Pulmonary Tuberculosis. Amer. J. Surg. *119*:469, 1970.

Nitti, V. et al.: Rifampin in Association with Isoniazid, Streptomycin and Ethambutol, Respectively, in the Initial Treatment of Pulmonary Tuberculosis. Amer. Rev. Resp. Dis. *103*:329, 1971.

Proudfoot, A. T.: Cryptic Disseminated Tuberculosis. Brit. J. Hosp. Med. *5*:773, 1971.

Robson, K. and Emerson, P. A.: Post-primary tuberculosis. Chest Diseases p. 237, Perry, K. M. A. and Sellors, Sir T. H. (eds.). London, Butterworth and Co., 1963.

Rooney, J. L., Crocco, J. A., and Lyons, H. A.: Tuberculous Pericarditis. Ann. Intern. Med. *72*:73, 1970.

Sadler, M. R. DeL., and Beersford, O. D.: Miliary Tuberculosis Associated with Addison's Disease. Tubercle *52*:298, 1971.

Schacter, E. N.: Tuberculin Negative Tuberculosis. Amer. Rev. Resp. Dis. *106*:587, 1972.

Seal, R. M.: The Pathology of Tuberculosis. Brit. J. Hosp. Med. *5*:783, 1971.

Shields, T. W., Fox, R. T. and Lees, W. M.: The changing role of surgery in the treatment of pulmonary tuberculosis. Arch. Surg., *100*:363, 1970.

Singh, M. M., Bhargava, A. M., and Kranti, P. Jain.: Tuberculous Peritonitis. New Eng. J. Med. *281*:1091, 1969.

Smith, D. T., Conant, N. F., et al. (eds.): Zinsser Microbiology p. 564, 14th Ed. New York, Appleton-Century-Crofts, 1968.

Stead, W. W.: Tuberculosis. Harrison's Principles of Internal Medicine, 6th Ed, pp. 865–880. New York, McGraw-Hill Book Co., 1968.

Stead, W. W., and Bates, J. H.: Evidence of a "Silent" Bacillemia in Primary Tuberculosis. Ann. Int. Med. *74*:559, 1971.

Stead, W. W. et al.: The Clinical Spectrum of Primary Tuberculosis in Adults. Ann. Int. Med. *68*:731, 1968.

Steele, J. D.: The Solitary Pulmonary Nodule: with a foreword by J. Rigler p. 226. Springfield, Charles C Thomas, 1964.

Vall-Spinosa, A., and Lester, W.: Rifampin: Characteristics and Role in the Chemotherapy of Tuberculosis. Ann. Intern. Med. *74*:758, 1971.

Weed, L. A., and Macy, N. E.: Tuberculosis: Problems in Diagnosis and Eradication. Amer. J. Clin. Path. *53*:136, 1970.

4. Osteomyelitis

RICHARD H. ROTHMAN, JOHN SACK AND STEVEN ROCKOWER

Causes: Inflammation of bone from bacterial, tuberculous, fungal, or parasitic infection.

Early Manifestations: Pain and tenderness over the affected area, fever, malaise.

Treatment: Intensive antibiotic therapy, surgical debridement and drainage, immobilization.

Possible Dire Consequences without Treatment: Septicemia, necrosis of bone, amputation of extremity, and death.

The specter of osteomyelitis has become less fearful since the era of antibiotics. Prior to the advent of penicillin, a diagnosis of osteomyelitis was a grave one, often condemning the patient (usually a child) to years of disability and often death. With the discovery of antibiotics, control of osteomyelitis is now a good probability.

Osteomyelitis is defined as an inflammation of bone secondary to bacterial, tuberculous, fungal, or parasitic infection. The bacterial etiology is the most common. The disease manifests itself with pain and tenderness over the affected area. Classically, osteomyelitis is an acute disease of children, resulting from a blood-borne infection and residing in the metaphysis of long bones. Other forms of osteomyelitis differ both in acuteness of onset and location of the infection.

PATHOPHYSIOLOGY

The anatomy of the vascular supply to the metaphysis of long bones must be considered in a discussion of hematogenous osteomyelitis. The nutrient arteries and capillaries, approaching the epiphyseal plate from the metaphyseal side, execute a 180 degree turn as they become sinusoidal veins. This transition from artery to vein is accomplished by an increase in diameter of the vessel from 8 μ to approximately 15 to 30 μ. This increased diameter leads to a sluggish and turbulent blood flow through this area. These ascending capillary loops do not form anastomoses, so that any obstruction (by bacterial growth or microthrombi) results in avascular necrosis.

Hematogenous osteomyelitis has three forms, depending on the age of the patient. In infants, the epiphyseal plates are still perforated by capillaries, so that metaphyseal infection can easily spread to articular cartilage and growth plate, leading to septic arthritis. In children between age one and puberty, these capillaries have become obliterated, so that infection must spread laterally through haversian and Volkmann's canals in cortex to reside subperiosteally. This suppuration and periosteal elevation lead to formation of periosteal new bone termed involucrum. In adults, the epiphyseal growth plate has matured, with residual vascular anastomoses between metaphysis and epiphysis through which joint spaces can become infected. In addition, the junction of bone and periosteum is tighter, so that the tendency for infection to spread laterally is limited. This may lead to increased intramedullary pressure higher than local blood pressure resulting in stasis, thrombosis, avascular

145

necrosis, and sequestrum formation.   The necrosis is also a function of the pH changes, leukocytosis, and local edema resulting from the infection.   These factors contribute to the breakdown of trabeculae, the loss of calcium, and the resorption of matrix material, leading to the high incidence of pathological fractures.

In vertebral osteomyelitis, the infection usually resides in the vertebral body.   It may spread via the anastomosing Batson plexus of veins to involve adjoining vertebrae.   Alternately it may spread by direct extension of the infection through the disc space to the adjoining vertebra.

AGE AND BONE DISTRIBUTION

While hematogenous osteomyelitis is classically described as a disease of long bones of children, it has variously been reported as involving other bones (including vertebrae, mandible, calvarium and others) and adults as well.   The bones most commonly affected in acute cases were the distal femur, proximal tibia, and humerus. While chronic cases followed the same general patterns, cases arising from surgery, fracture, or other trauma involved other bones.   As mentioned before, vertebral osteomyelitis has a much greater incidence in adults, particularly of the tuberculous variety.

The morbidity and mortality of osteomyelitis have dropped since the advent of antibiotics, but resistant strains are always appearing.   Waldvogel et al. report an overall mortality rate of 2% for acute cases as compared with 15 to 25% in the preantibiotic era.   Blockey and Watson reported no deaths in 113 acute cases, but 18.6% went on to become chronic.

CLINICAL PICTURE

The earliest clinical picture includes the acute onset of high fever, pain, severe tenderness, and swelling over the affected part.   The patient appears critically ill and toxic.   However, this entire constellation of symptoms is not necessary for a diagnosis of acute osteomyelitis.   A careful history may reveal a recently healed furuncle.   Pain is the key symptom accompanied by exquisite point tenderness over the infected bone.   In postoperative or posttraumatic cases, spiking fevers, severe inflammation and edema are present as in acute osteomyelitis.   In the early stages of the disease, radiographic changes are *not* evident, save for soft tissue swelling.

LABORATORY FINDINGS

Laboratory values indicate a bacteremia.   A leukocytosis is present but does not usually exceed a count of 16,000 per cubic millimeter, with a shift to the left.   An anemia is usually noted with a drop in hemoglobin and hematocrit.   The alkaline phosphatase, normal early in the course of the disease becomes elevated later.

RADIOGRAPHIC FINDINGS

Radiographic findings are not evident until ten to fourteen days from the onset of symptoms.   As mentioned before, soft-tissue swelling is evident early.   Periosteal new bone may become evident, particularly in children where the periosteum is not so firmly bound to bone.   Local destruction of metaphyseal and cortical bone can be seen.   This is radiolucent at first and later, if reactive bone formation occurs, sclerotic.   When the joint is involved, changes similar to pyogenic arthritis are seen. Sclerosis of the bone indicates a duration of at least one month.   If the disease becomes chronic, segments of necrotic bone become evident as sequestra.   Since these sequestra are avascular, their radiographic appearance will not change once they are formed.   Also walled off pockets of infectious material may form, known as a Brodie's abscess.   At times the destruction of cortex is so great that pathological fractures may occur.

BACTERIOLOGY

Staphylococcus Aureus.   Staphylococcus aureus is implicated in 50 to 95% of all osteomyelitis lesions.   These organisms are cultured either from blood or directly from the abscess.   In acute cases, approximately half are resistant to penicillin G. Most chronic cases are resistant to penicillin, since that was usually the primary antibacterial agent used, and these usually represent failures of therapy of acute lesions. Infecting organisms include *Streptococcus, Salmonella, Escherichia coli, Proteus, Pseudomonas, Mycobacterium tuberculosis* and others.   Some lesions, however, prove to be sterile by culture, especially Brodie's abscess.

It should be noted that salmonella infections are often found in conjunction with sickle cell disease.   In one study of 117 patients with normal hemoglobin, one had salmonella osteomyelitis; whereas of 20 patients with sickling hemoglobin, 14 had salmonella.   The reason for this preponderance of salmonella in sickle cell patients is unknown.

CLINICAL COURSE AND THERAPY

The prognosis of acute cases is good when definitive treatment is started within three to five days of the onset of symptoms.   The basic principles of treatment include bed rest, elevation and immobilization of the part, correction of anemia, appropriate antibiotic therapy, and properly timed surgery.   Prompt antibiotic treatment is often all that is necessary to inhibit growth of the organism.   Duration of treatment varies depending on the promptness of treatment, host resistance and the sensitivity of the organism to antibiotics.   Often the clinical signs are improving while the radiographic picture is deteriorating.

Surgery in acute cases is not recommended unless there is no remission within forty-eight hours of treatment.   With evidence of abscess formation, surgical drainage is indicated, if the patient's condition permits.   The medullary canal is usually decompressed if there is evidence of increased pressure.   This is accomplished by removal of a cortical "window."   The marrow cavity is opened and thoroughly curetted to remove all involved tissue, and cultures are sent to determine the appropriate antibiotic therapy.   Drains are mandatory.

Chronic cases are often associated with sequestra, involucra, and draining sinuses. Injection of the sinus with methylene blue or radiopaque dye is often helpful in determining the extent of the infection.   The surgical treatment of chronic osteomyelitis is difficult and requires great judgment.   Techniques utilized include saucerization, muscle pedicle transfers, and suction-irrigation drainage.

The irrigation and suction technique is often used because of the failure of parenteral antibiotics to reach devascularized tissue, sequestra, and sclerotic new bone.

After debridement, polyethylene tubes are placed in the wound, half delivering antibiotic solution, half with suction drainage. This process is continued for a period of two to four weeks, until cultures from the suction are negative. One must be sure, however, that all areas of infection are removed at operation, or the efforts will be doomed to failure.

It must be noted that infections secondary to implantation of metal prostheses necessitate their removal.

Antibiotic treatment is critical. Until a culture is taken and the sensitivities are known, it is best to treat the patient with methicillin to cover the resistant staphylococcus and ampicillin to cover the usual gram-negative organisms. The methicillin is given intravenously, 1 gm. every six hours. Ampicillin should be given intravenously $\frac{1}{2}$ gm. every six hours. These should not be given to penicillin hypersensitive individuals.

Salmonella osteomyelitis, occurring more frequently in patients with sickle cell disease, is best treated with chloramphenicol. Erythropoietic function must be observed closely in these patients. Those receiving a dosage in excess of 100 mg. per kg. of body weight must be expected to undergo reticulocyte depression but this is reversible and entirely different from the rare irreversible pancytopenia which is not related to time or dose.

After the sensitivities are known, appropriate antibiotics are administered, with regular re-cultures to check for resistant strains. It must be stressed that the antibiotic therapy must be sufficient to completely eradicate the infecting organism. Failures in treatment can occur due to both insufficient dosage and insufficient time. In acute osteomyelitis antibiotics should be continued for six weeks after acute symptoms have subsided. In chronic osteomyelitis antibiotics should be administered for six to twelve months. Proper treatment is a harmony between antibiotic therapy and surgical debridement. It must be remembered, however, that there is often no absolute cure for osteomyelitis—only successful control: exacerbations have been reported after thirty-nine years of freedom from symptoms.

References

Anderson, C. D., and Horn, L. G.: "Irrigation-suction technic in treatment of acute hematogenous osteomyelitis, chronic osteomyelitis, and acute and chronic joint infections." South. Med. J. *63*:745, 1970.

Blockey, N. J.: "Conservative management of acute osteomyelitis." Pro. R. Soc. Med. *64*:1199, 1971.

Blockey, N. J. and Watson, J. T.: "Acute osteomyelitis in children." J. Bone Joint Surg. *52*B:77, 1970.

Crenshaw, A. H., ed.: Campbell's Operative Orthopedics, St. Louis, C. V. Mosby Co., 1971.

Coman, D. R. and deLong, R. P.: "The role of the vertebral venous system in the metastasis of cancer to the spinal colum—experiments with tumor cell suspensions in rats & rabbits." Cancer *4*:610, 1951.

Engh, C., Hughes, J., Abrams, R., and Bowerman, J.: "Osteomyelitis in patients with sickle cell disease." J. Bone Joint Surg. *53*A:1, 1971.

Hamblen, D. L.: "Hyperbaric oxygen in the treatment of osteomyelitis." Pro. R. Soc. Med. *64*:1202, 1971.

Harris, N. J.: "Some problems in the diagnosis and treatment of acute osteomyelitis." J. Bone Joint Surg. *42*B:535, 1960.

Harris, N. H. and Kirkardy-Willis, W. H.: "Primary subacute pyogenic osteomyelitis." J. Bone Joint Surg. *47*B:527, 1965.

Jones, G. B.: "Place of surgery in treatment of acute hematogenous osteomyelitis." Pro. R. Soc. Med. *64*:1200, 1971.

Kelley, P. J., Martin, W. J., and Coventry, M. D.: "Chronic osteomyelitis—II. Treatment with closed irrigation and suction." JAMA *213*:1843, 1967.

Rowling, D. E.: "Further experience in the management of chronic osteomyelitis." J. Bone Joint Surg. *52*B:302, 1970.

Taylor, A. R. and Maudsley, R. H.: "Instillation-suction technic in chronic osteomyelitis." J. Bone Joint Surg. *52*B:88, 1970.

Trueta, J.: "The three types of acute hematogenous osteomyelitis." J. Bone Joint Surg. *41*B:671, 1959.

Waldvogel, F. A., Medoff, G., and Swartz, M. N.: "Osteomyelitis: a review of clinical features, therapeutic considerations, and unusual aspects." New Eng. J. Med. *282*:198, 260, 316, 1970.

West, W. F., Kelley, P. J., and Martin, W. J.: Chronic osteomyelitis: I. "Factors affecting the results of treatment in 186 patients." JAMA *213*:1837, 1967.

Winters, J. L. and Cahen, I.: "Acute hematogenous osteomyelitis: a review of 66 cases." J. Bone Joint Surg. *52*B:428, 1970.

————: "Case records of the Massachusetts General Hospital." New Eng. J. Med. *285*:166, 1971.

5. Infections Due to Non-sporeforming Anaerobic Bacteria

ROBERT M. SWENSON

Cause: Non-sporeforming anaerobic bacteria, particularly *Bacteroides fragilis.*

Early Manifestations: Fever, chills, abscess formation with putrid smelling pus.

Treatment: Antibiotics, surgical drainage.

Possible Dire Consequences without Treatment: Continued pain and debilitation, and death.

The non-sporeforming anaerobic bacteria constitute a major part of the normal flora of the human. Although these obligate anaerobes are usually considered to be commensals, it has become clear that they are frequent causes of infection. Such infections are invariably of endogenous origin resulting from the introduction of constituents of the normal flora into areas where they are not normally present.

A number of different organisms can be classified as non-sporeforming anaerobic bacteria. Of these, the Bacteroides species, particularly *Bacteroides fragilis*, are the most frequent causes of infection. Others commonly involved include *Peptostreptococcus*, *Peptococcus* and *Fusobacterium* species. It should be noted that these anaerobic bacteria cause infection far more frequently than the *Clostridium* species.

Anaerobic bacteria are the predominant organisms in the gastrointestinal tract, vagina and upper respiratory tract. Thus, infections due to anaerobes frequently involve these areas. These are usually mixed infections. In approximately two-thirds of cases, not only are multiple anaerobic bacteria isolated but other facultative organisms as well.

SYMPTOMS AND CLINICAL MANIFESTATIONS

Although a wide variety of infections may be caused by these organisms there are certain clinical characteristics common to all. Signs of systemic infection, such as fever and chills, are usually present. Other signs and symptoms are dependent upon the location of the infection and the nature of the infecting organisms.

Some common anaerobic infections are listed in Table VII–9. Intraabdominal infections, obstetrical and gynecological infections and putrid lung abscess almost invariably involve anaerobic bacteria. Approximately 50% of brain abscesses are due to these organisms. The other infections listed are occasionally caused by anaerobic bacteria.

DIAGNOSIS

The findings are dependent upon the site of infection. However, certain findings are suggestive of the presence of anaerobic bacteria. There is usually marked tissue necrosis and abscess formation. It is not uncommon to find evidence of gas formation in infected tissues. Putrid smelling pus is present in 75% of cases. Finally, an associated cellulitis or thrombophlebitis is a common feature of these infections.

TABLE VII–9.
INFECTIONS INVOLVING NON-SPOREFORMING
ANAEROBIC BACTERIA

Site	*Mixed Flora*	*Anaerobic Bacteria*	*Associated Facultative Bacteria*
1. Obstetrical and gynecological infections (not due to gonococcus)	Frequently	*Bacteroides* spp. *Peptococcus* spp. *Peptostreptococcus* spp.	*Escherichia coli* *Proteus* spp.
2. Intraabdominal infections (peritonitis, localized abscess)	Frequently	*Bacteroides* spp. *Peptococcus* spp. *Peptostreptococcus* spp.	*Escherichia coli* *Proteus* spp.
3. Aspiration pneumonia, abscess, and empyema	Frequently	*Peptostreptococcus* spp. *Peptococcus* spp. *Fusobacterium* spp. *Bacteroides* spp. (occasionally)	*Streptococcus* spp. *Staphylococcus aureus*
4. Brain abscess	Frequently	*Peptostreptococcus* spp. *Peptococcus* spp. *Bacteroides* spp.	*Streptococcus* spp.
5. Skin and soft tissue abscesses	Frequently	*Peptococcus* spp. *Peptostreptococcus* spp.	*Staphylococcus aureus* *Streptococcus* spp.
6 Osteomyelitis	Seldom	*Bacteroides fragilis*	——
7. Endocarditis	Seldom	*Bacteroides* spp.	——

These anaerobic bacteria are frequently not isolated using the procedures employed in most hospitals. For this reason, a gram stain of specimens is absolutely essential. The presence of bacteria on gram stain with subsequent negative cultures is strongly suggestive of the presence of anaerobic bacteria.

In order to increase the possibility of isolating these bacteria and obtaining clinically reliable information, the following precautions should be taken. Every effort should be made to prevent contamination with normal flora. Whenever possible, material should be collected in an oxygen-free tube. Finally, the specimen should immediately be taken to the laboratory. These simple measures will markedly increase the frequency with which clinically significant anaerobic bacteria will be isolated.

PROGNOSIS AND COMPLICATIONS

The prognosis in these infections is dependent mainly upon the location of the infection. Another major variable is the nature of the infecting organism. The *Bacteroides* species, particularly *Bacteroides fragilis*, are the most virulent and invasive of the non-sporeforming anaerobic bacteria. Approximately 10 to 20% of patients with infections due to *Bacteroides fragilis* develop a bacteremia which may produce a picture of endotoxic shock indistinguishable from that caused by other gram-negative bacilli. Additional complications occur much less frequently with infections caused by the other non-sporeforming anaerobic bacteria.

TREATMENT

The majority of infections caused by these organisms are marked by significant abscess formation. A major part of the therapy, and in some cases the only therapy, is to provide adequate drainage of the abscess. In terms of antibiotic therapy, two major considerations must be made. First, antibiotic susceptibility tests as currently performed in the usual clinical laboratory are unreliable for anaerobic bacteria. Thus, the choice of an antibiotic must be based on knowledge of susceptibilities determined by other reliable methods. Such studies have indicated that non-sporeforming anaerobes, in general, are susceptible to Clindamycin and chloramphenicol. All anaerobes, except the *Bacteroides* species, are susceptible to penicillin and cephalothin. Tetracycline, erythromycin, lincomycin, and vancomycin are less satisfactory alternatives. Secondly, the physician should be aware of the frequent involvement of other facultative organisms in these infections and provide appropriate antibiotic coverage for these also.

References

Bodner, S. J., Koenig, M. G., and Goodman, J. S.: Bacteremic bacteroides infections. Ann. Intern. Med. *73*:537, 1970.

Bornstein, D. L. et al.: Anaerobic infections—Review of current experience. Medicine *43*:207, 1974.

6. Streptococcal Infections

Condition:
1. Streptococcal sore throat.
2. Streptococcal pyoderma (impetigo).
3. Erysipelas.
4. Streptococcal pneumonia (now a rare condition).
5. Streptococcal meningitis (nearly disappeared).

Cause: Group A Streptococcus.

Early Manifestations:
1. Fever, sore throat, tender nodes.
2. Fever, small tender pustules.
3. Often preceded by local trauma or friction.
4. Usually a sequel to pharyngitis or scarlet fever, fever, cough, chest pain, hemoptysis.
5. Fever, meningisms.

Treatment: Penicillin.

Possible Dire Consequences without Treatment: Septicemia, empyema, and death.

The organs involved are (1) nasopharynx, (2) skin, (3) skin, (4) lungs and pleura (5) meninges and brain.

Complications may include (1) latent rheumatic fever and acute glomerulonephritis, (2) complicating staphylococcal infections, (3) septicemia and possibly death, (4) lobular pneumonia bacteremia and (5) fulminating meningitis brain abscess.

Definitive diagnosis is made by finding the organism.

Lancefield, R. C.: Current knowledge of type-specific M antigens of group a streptococci. J. Immun. *89*:307, 1962.
Seegal, D. and Seegal, B. C.: Facial erysipelas: A study of 281 cases treated at the Massachusetts General Hospital from 1870–1927. J.A.M.A. *93*:430, 1929.
Stellerman, G. H. and Pearce, I. A.: The changing epidemiology of rheumatic fever and acute glomerulonephritis. Advances Intern. Med. *14*:201, 1968.

7. Meningococcal Meningitis

Cause: Meningococcus to nasopharynx, vascular endothelium, and meninges.

Early Manifestations: Upper respiratory infection. Septicemia, meningismus. May present with shock and diffuse disease as in Waterhouse syndrome. May present as fever and/or hemorrhagic rash.

Treatment: Sulfonamides.

Possible Dire Consequences without Treatment: Death from meningitis, shock, secondary to Waterhouse and Friderichsen syndrome. Polyarthritic diathesis, ocular palsies, blindness, psychoses, hydrocephalus. Mortality results from treatment delays.

Organs involved are skin, intima of blood vessels, joints, eyes, ears, lungs, pericardium, urethra, meninges, adrenals.

The vascular endothelial damage may result in necrosis, thrombosis and focal hemorrhages.

The diagnosis is made by bacterial identification usually of blood or cerebrospinal fluid.

References

Banks, H. S.: Meningococcal fever. *In* Modern Practice in Infectious Fevers. Vol. 1. New York, Paul B. Hoeber, Inc., 1951.

Feldman, H. A.: Recent development in the therapy and control of meningococcal infections. Disease-a-Month, Feb. 1966.

8. Diphtheria

ORVILLE HORWITZ

Cause: Corynebacterium diphtheriae gram-positive, preferentially aerobic, pleomorphic bacillus. Forms extremely potent and lethal exotoxin.

Early Manifestations: Incubation period usually three to five days. Pharyngitis, diphtheritic membrane, fever to 103°F., cervical lymphadenopathy. May get streptococcal superinfection.

Treatment: Supportive plus 30,000 to 80,000 units of antitoxins depending on the severity of the disease.

Possible Dire Consequences without Treatment: Suffocation, myocarditis, tubular necrosis, death.

The organs involved are mucosal surfaces of upper respiratory tract. Genital and ocular membranes are rarely involved. Nervous system and myocardium may be involved later as result of toxin.

The pathological changes are the result of the exotoxin locally causing edema of respiratory passages, and systemically, myocarditis, tubular necrosis, and myelin degeneration of the nervous system—mostly the result of interference with protein synthesis.

The eventual diagnosis is made by demonstration of organism by smear and culture.

Reference

Frost, W. H.: Infection, immunity and disease in the epidemiology of diphtheria, with special reference to some studies in Baltimore. J. Prev. Med., *2*:325, 1928 (Reprinted in Maxcy, K. F. (ed.) Papers of Wade Hampton Frost, New York, The Commonwealth Fund, 1941, pp. 447–466).

9. Pneumonia

ORVILLE HORWITZ

Cause: Pneumococcus and other organisms

Early Manifestations: Fever, chills, chest pain, dyspnea, cough, malaise, often prostration in elderly or alcoholic patients.

Treatment: Rest, proper antibiotic agent(s) and proper fluids.

Possible Dire Consequences without Treatment: Septicemia, empyema, anoxia, endocarditis, meningitis, death.

There is usually no problem for a physician to come to the conclusion that a pulmonary disorder exists which is causing a fever. Having arrived at this conclusion, a conditioned reflex as in Pavlov's dogs nearly always occurs. This results in the patient receiving penicillin or tetracycline and being ordered to bed. In a large majority of cases this represents adequate treatment. However, there is an important minority that is bound to suffer. The problem is not that the disease is not treated, but that it is not correctly or completely diagnosed and not properly treated.

There are two diagnostic procedures which will greatly reduce the possibility of error in this respect. They should ideally be employed before therapy is instituted—certainly if the patient is hospitalized. They are sputum culture with typing of the organism, if pneumococcus, and a genuine effort to rule out pulmonary infarction.

TABLE VII–10

Organism	Usual Optimal Antibiotic
Pneumococcus	Penicillin—if allergic— Erythromycin Chloramphenicol
Staphylococcus	Penicillin—if resistant— ($>$1/3) Methicillin 6 gm. daily Nafcillin parenterally Cephalothin
Beta Hemolytic Strepococcus	Penicillin G 1.2—2.4 million units/day
Klebsiella (Friedlander's)	Chloramphenicol and Kanamycin
Hemophilus Influenza	Ampicillin 2—4 gm. daily
E. Coli	Kanamycin 1.5 gm. daily
Proteus	Kanamycin and Ampicillin
Tuberculous	See Section

It is often impossible to identify the offending organism by a sputum culture taken *after* the institution of antibiotic therapy. This may lead to prolonged and inadequate therapy by an inappropriate antibiotic agent.

Table VII–10 includes some of the organisms which may cause pneumonia and the *usual* antibiotic to which the organism is most sensitive.

Pulmonary infarction may mimic pneumonia to the point that the patient will be deprived of proper treatment by heparin which should be instituted without delay.

Other conditions which may imitate bacterial pneumonia in some respects are: Mycoplasmal and viral pneumonia, neoplasms, and eosinophilic pneumonias.

Pneumonia in a host crippled by other conditions such as old age, alcoholism, epilepsy, chronic bronchitis, and emphysema deserves particularly vigorous diagnostic and therapeutic management.

In patients suffering from recurrent pneumonia a coexisting occult process should be suspected.

References

Austrian, R. and Gold, J.: Pneumococcal bacteremia with especial reference to bacteremic pneumococcal pneumonia. Ann. Intern. Med. *60*:759, 1964.

Reimann, Hobart: *The Pneumonias.* Myers, J. A. (ed.) *In* series of Modern Concepts of Chest Diseases. St. Louis, Warren H. Green, 1971.

10. Amebic Liver Abscess

Richard K. Root

Cause: Hepatic infection with *Entameba histolytica.*

Early Manifestations: Fever, persistent upper quadrant abdominal pain, weight loss.

Treatment: Metronidazole (Flagyl) or emetine and chloroquine.

Possible Dire Consequences without Treatment: Rupture leading to peritonitis, pleuritis, pericarditis and/or death.

Left untreated, amebic liver abscess can be a fatal complication of intestinal parasitization with *E. histolytica.* The disease has a striking sex prevalence in that males account for 90% of cases. The presenting symptoms are subtle and may be confused with cholecystitis, hepatitis, malignancy or vasculitis. They include fever, often hectic in course, upper quadrant abdominal pain and tenderness and weight loss in almost all cases. A remote or current history of diarrhea indicative of active intestinal infection may be found in only $\frac{1}{3}$ of cases. Jaundice is rare. The appearance of an hepatic rub is a late and ominous sign, heralding imminent rupture of the abscess.

Most abscesses are in the right lobe of the liver; these may rupture intraperitoneally, causing an acute peritonitis, intrapleurally, leading to the rapid development of a pleural effusion or even into the bronchial tree with the sudden occurrence of a cough productive of "anchovy paste" sputum. Abscesses of the left lobe can rupture into the pericardial sac causing pericardial tamponade and death. An example of pericardial effusion due to a ruptured left lobe abscess is shown in Figure VII–1. Both the abscess cavity and the effusion are delineated by an injection of contrast material. This case had been misdiagnosed as lupus erythematosus prior to the development of this complication. Most abscesses are single and will be readily detected on liver scan (Fig. VII–2). If the liver scan is positive, and particularly if a single large defect is found in either the right or left lobes, an amebic serology should be obtained. If the hemagglutination titer against antigens derived from the parasite is positive and particularly if it exceeds 1:4096, then the diagnosis is highly likely. Amebic serologies may be obtained at the National Center for Disease Control, Atlanta, Georgia. Definitive diagnosis is made by aspiration of "anchovy paste" pus, which is bacteriologically sterile in 95% of cases. Finding the organism in the aspirated material is unusual since the trophozoites reside in the abscess wall. Similarly positive stool cultures are found in only $\frac{1}{3}$ of cases. Oral administration of metronidazole (800 mg. PO t.i.d. for five days, for adults) offers a highly effective and relatively non-toxic therapeutic approach. This is also effective against the intestinal phase of the organism. Alternative more toxic therapy is provided by the combined use of chloroquine and emetine. Surgical drainage of abscesses is not essential for cure. Eradication of the intestinal parasites is necessary to prevent relapse.

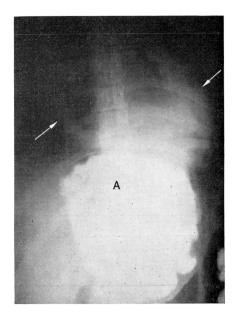

Fig. VII–1.   Injection of Hypaque into a large amebic abscess cavity (A) in the left lobe of the liver of this patient led to the appearance of dye in the pericardial sac (arrow). The abscess cavity was drained and a window created to drain the pericardium and relieve the signs of tamponade which had rapidly developed several hours before this roentgenogram was obtained. Cure was achieved after chemotherapy with emetine, chloroquine and tetracycline.

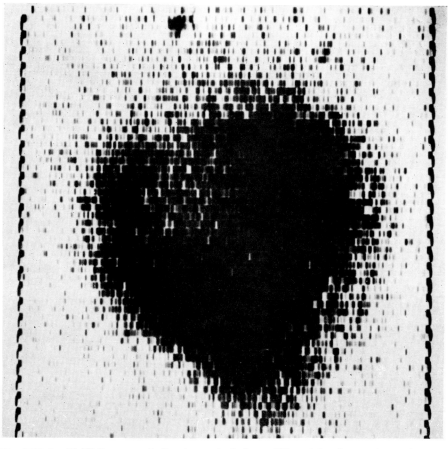

Fig. VII–2. Te^{199} liver scan indicating a single large filling defect in the right lobe of the liver. Amebic serology was positive and aspiration revealed "anchovy paste" pus. Cure was achieved with oral metronidazole.

References

Adi, F. C.: Complications, treatment and prognosis of hepatic amoebiasis. West Afr. Med. J., *15*:43, 1966.

MacLeod, I. N., Wilmot, A. J., and Powell, S. J.: Amoebic pericarditis. Quart. J. Med. *35*:293, 1966.

Maddison, S. E., et al.: Comparison of intradermal and serologic tests in the diagnosis of amebiasis. Am. J. Trop. Med. & Hyg., *17*:540, 1968.

May, R. P., et al.: Difficulties in differentiating amebic from pyogenic liver abscess. Arch. Intern. Med. *119*:69, 1967.

Powell, S. J.: Drug therapy in amoebiasis. Bull. WHO *40*:953, 1969.

Sheehy, T. W., et al.: Resolution time of amebic abscess. Gastroenterology *55*:26, 1968.

Wilmot, A. J.: Clinical Amebiasis. London, Blackwell Scientific Publications, and Philadelphia, F. A. Davis Co., 1962.

11. Cholera

ORVILLE HORWITZ

Cause: Transmitted by ingestion of bacteria vibro cholera, a gram-negative comma-shaped motile bacillus.

Early Manifestations: Severe diarrhea, abdominal pain, dehydration. Often nausea, vomiting, prostration, low mouth temperature, slightly elevated rectal temperature.

Treatment: Fluid and electrolyte balance. Tetracycline 100 mg. per liter of I.V. fluid

Possible Dire Consequences without Treatment: Dehydration, electrolyte imbalance, death.

The organs involved are the intestines, in which the pathological changes are mononuclear cell inflammation of mucosa, vascular congestion and goblet cell hyperplasia.

The diagnosis is confirmed by stool cultures and serum antibody titers.

References

Carpenter, C. C. J., Mitra, P. P., and Sack, R. B.: Clinical studies in asiatic cholera I-VI. Bull. Johns Hopkins Hosp. *118*:165, 1966.
Wallance, C. K., et al.: Optimal antibiotic therapy in cholera. Bull. World Health Organ. *39*:239, 1968.

12. Typhoid Fever

ORVILLE HORWITZ

Cause: Salmonella typhosa, a gram-negative motile aerobic bacillus which forms an endotoxin. It is transmitted by ingestion of feces.

Early Manifestations: Fever, headache, apathy, cough, prostration, splenomegaly, maculopapular rash, melena, rose spots, leukopenia. There is a relative bradycardia and a step-like increase of fever. Generalized abdominal pain and tenderness.

Treatment: Chloramphenicol, 1 gm. q.i.d., and for ampicillin, 1 gm. q.i.d. (somewhat less effective but also less toxic). Perforation is usually treated nonsurgically. Salicylates may cause hypothermia. Attention to electrolyte balance. Cholecystectomy for carrier.

Possible Dire Consequences without Treatment: Weakness, long morbidity, intestinal hemorrhage and perforation, pneumonia, cholecystitis, osteomyelitis, septic aneurysm. Ten % mortality. Septicemia is much more common in this disease than in other salmonella infections.

The organs involved are intestinal lymphoid tissue, spleen, blood, liver, lungs, gallbladder, and bone. Diverticulitis with abscess formation is not uncommon.

The pathological changes are necrosis and ulceration of lymphatic tissue (Peyer's patches) with erosion of blood vessels and hemorrhage, as well as cloudy swelling of liver and septicemia. Intestinal hemorrhage and perforation are most dreaded symptoms. Pneumonia, cholecystitis, and osteomyelitis are less frequent complications.

The diagnosis is made by stool cultures, blood cultures and Widal reaction.

References

Hornick, R. B.: Salmonella Infections—Newer perspectives of an old infection. The Jeremiah Metzger Lecture 1973. Transactions of the American Clinical and Climatological Association, *85*:164, 1973.
Keusch, G. T., Mata, L. J. and Grady, G. F.: Shigella enterotoxin: isolation and characterization. Clin. Res. (Abt). 18:422, 1970.
McCrae, T.: The symptoms of typhoid fever, chap. 4. In Modern Medicine vol. 2, Infectious Diseases, p. 104. W. Osler and T. McCrae (eds.). Philadelphia, Lea Brothers and Co., 1907.
Sprinz, H.: Pathogenesis of intestinal infections. Arch. Path., *87*:556, 1969.
Woodward, T. E., et al.: Treatment of typhoid fever with antibiotics. Ann. N.Y. Acad. Sci., *55*:1043, 1952.

13. Enteric or Paratyphoid Fever

ORVILLE HORWITZ

Cause: S. paratyphi A and B, usually less menacing than typhoid fever. There are some 1400 salmonella other than S. typhosa.

Early Manifestations: Same as typhoid fever (fever, headache, apathy, cough, prostration, splenomegaly, maculopapular rash, rose spots, leukopenia. Relative bradycardia, step-like increase of fever. Melena, generalized abdominal pain and tenderness. Bradycardia relative to fever). Diarrhea prominent, but disease is milder.

Treatment: Chloramphenicol, 1 gm. q.i.d. Attention to electrolyte balance.

Possible Dire Consequences without Treatment: Weakness, long morbidity; rarely intestinal hemorrhage and perforation, pneumonia, cholecystitis, osteomyelitis. Mortality 1 to 2%. Septicemia is rare in salmonella infections other than typhoid.

Although this disease may produce the symptoms of typhoid fever, it is a more gentle disease with lower morbidity and lower mortality.

References

Bennett, I. L., Jr. and Hook, E. W.: Some aspects of salmonellosis. Ann. Rev. Med. *10*:1, 1959.
Black, P. H., Kunz, L. J., and Swartz, M. N.: Salmonellosis—A review of some unusual aspects. New Eng. J. Med., *262*:811, 864, 921, 1960.
Hornick, Richard B.: Salmonella Infections—Newer Perspectives of an Old Infection. The Jeremiah Metzger Lecture 1973. Transactions of the American Clinical and Climatological Association, *85*:164, 1973.

14. Gonorrhea

C. W. HANSON

Cause: Inoculation of a susceptible individual with the gonococcus, an organism characterized by transmission with sexual contact, by involvement of body surfaces to an unusual degree, by the development of a low degree of host interaction and resistance so that long carriage and re-infections are frequent, and by a striking ability to develop resistance to antimicrobial agents. It is the commonest of the venereal diseases, the number one reportable disease in the United States; it is epidemic throughout the world; and it will no doubt continue to grow as a public health concern.

Early Manifestations: In the typical presentation, the male is symptomatic with dysuria, penile discharge, and a mildly septicemic picture. Because of these symptoms, he seeks medical attention within a week in an estimated 80% of instances; the basic condition is a posterior urethritis. In the female, there are many more possible sites of initial or simultaneous involvement, including as well as urethra the endocervix, fallopian tubes, and the rectum. It is estimated that only 20% of infected women seek medical attention for the classical picture of pelvic inflammation with tubal involvement, and they may do so as much as a month after inoculation. These differences occur and are relevant because as symptoms tend to be mild or absent in the woman, there is greater time between inoculation and diagnosis for potential dissemination. This delay is also true of male homosexuals, who frequently harbor the organism in peri-rectal tissues, rather than in the urethra.

Unusual Manifestations: The organism, when disseminated from a focus itself quiet or of subclinical significance, may produce difficulties in a number of ways not customarily associated with venereal disease. Awareness of "early manifestations" then must include such considerations as arthritis and synovitis, dermatitis, hepatitis and perihepatitis, peritonitis, meningitis, and cardiac involvement in all three layers. These are the result of infection disseminated by the blood stream from a classical locus. On the other hand, there are as well alternative sites of primary involvement, as the conjunctiva, the rectum, or the oropharynx, the latter giving rise to a complex including stomatitis, pharyngitis, and tonsillitis.

About 90% of gonorrhea in the female and about 12% in the male occurs asymptomatically. A high index of suspicion and aggressive searching in those who are likely candidates, such as those asking advice in a VD clinic and those named as contacts, can prevent our missing many active cases. There is a considerable margin of error associated with the Thayer-Martin culture technique.

Treatment is with antimicrobials as follows: (1972 United States Public Health Service Recommendations, subject to review and periodic change)

For *Neisseria gonorrhoeae* infection the preferred drug is pencillin or ampicillin. Physicians are cautioned to use no less than the recommended doses of antibiotics.

Possible Dire Consequences without Treatment: Urethritis, urethral stenosis, epididymitis, prostatitis, salpingitis, septicemia, arthritis, endocarditis, death.

For Treatment of Uncomplicated Gonorrhea (*Urethral, Cervical, Pharyngeal, or Rectal*)

Parenteral—Men or Women—Aqueous procaine penicillin G, 4.8 million units intramuscularly divided into at least two doses and injected at different sites at one visit, together with 1 gm. of oral probenecid, preferably given at least thirty minutes before the injection.

OR

Oral—Men or Women—Ampicillin, 3.5 gm., with probenecid, 1 gm. administered simultaneously.

Treatment of contacts: Patients with known exposure to gonorrhea should receive the same treatment as those known to have gonorrhea.

When Penicillin or Ampicillin is Contraindicated,* or When the Above Schedules Are Ineffective

Parenteral—Men—Spectinomycin, 2 gm., in one intramuscular injection.
Women—Spectinomycin, 4 gm., in one intramuscular injection.

OR

Oral—Men or Women—Tetracycline HCL, 1.5 gm. initially, followed by 0.5 gm. four times a day for 4 days, a total dosage of 9 gm. Other tetracyclines are not more effective.

FOLLOW-UP

Follow-up urethral cultures should be obtained from males seven days after completion of treatment; cervical and rectal cultures should be obtained from females at seven to fourteen days after completion of treatment.

COMPLICATIONS

Although treatment of complications (gonococcal salpingitis, bacteremia, arthritis, etc.) must be individualized, repeated large parenteral doses of aqueous crystalline penicillin G have been shown to be effective. The efficacy of alternate antibiotic regimens is unproven. Post-gonococcal urethritis can be treated with tetracycline, 0.5 gm., orally four times a day for at least seven days.

SYPHILIS

All gonorrhea patients should have a serologic test for syphilis at the time of diagnosis. Patients receiving the recommended parenteral penicillin schedule need not have follow-up serologic tests for syphilis. Patients treated with ampicillin, spectinomycin, or tetracycline should have a follow-up serologic test for syphilis each month for four months to detect syphilis that may have been masked by treatment for gonorrhea.

Patients with gonorrhea who also have syphilis should be given additional treatment appropriate to the stage of syphilis.

While long-acting forms of penicillin (such as benzathine penicillin G) are effective in syphilotherapy, they have *NO* place in the treatment of gonorrhea.

The diagnosis, however, should be made with precision first, when possible. When the organism is felt likely to exist in pure culture, as in joint or vesicle fluid, mere

* Allergy to penicillin, ampicillin, probenecid, or previous anaphylactic reaction.

inoculation of pus onto a chocolate agar plate, with incubation under carbon dioxide, should suffice for diagnosis. Where the organism may be in competition with other bacteria, specific selective differential media (the Thayer-Martin plate) must be employed, which will enable the isolation of gonococcus from among other flora, by selective inhibition of the latter. The physician seeing a young population, with high geographic mobility, and with sexual standards different from any generation heretofore (made possible by the availability of contraception, abortion, and other sociological phenomena), absolutely must have an awareness of gonorrhea in all its guises, as well as a clear idea of how to proceed about the matter of its bacteriologic diagnosis, its treatment, its reporting to Public Health authorities, and its follow-up.

Possible dire consequences of the classical picture if untreated include the well-known male sequela of posterior urethral stricture, and the female complication of tubal adhesions and sterility. Given the enlarged list of possible multi-organ involvement, however, blindness, destructive endocarditis, joint sepsis, and death from a variety of septic possibilities deserve consideration, to say nothing of the problem of communicability itself, with all that that implies.

References

Nicholas, L.: Sexually Transmitted Diseases. Springfield, Charles C Thomas, 1973.
Prariser, H.: Asymptomatic Gonorrhea. Med. Clin. N. Am., *56*:1127, 1972.
Schroeter, A. L. and Pazin, G. J.: Gonorrhea. Ann. Intern. Med. *72*:553, 1970.

15. Syphilis

C. W. Hanson

Cause: Infection with the Treponema pallidum, acquired in a variety of ways, most notably via sexual contact. There have also been reported transmission transplacentally, through direct non-venereal contact with infectious lesions, and certain forms of inadvertent passage by needle (*i.e.* injection therapy, administration of blood products, tattooing, etc.).

Early Manifestations: A complete recitation of these is far beyond the scope of this publication. It is well said that "to know syphilis is to know medicine." A simple recitation should suffice: the typical primary lesion is the chancre; the secondary lesions are a variety of mucocutaneous eruptions; tertiary involvement is particularly of the nervous system, the vascular system, and (now rare) destructive gummata. The average clinician does not see one case of infectious syphilis per year. Case detection is therefore best served when he maintains an awareness of these clinical pictures, but reinforces that type of effort with an automatic reinforcement consisting of the routine procurement of serologic tests for syphilis on hospitalized individuals, new office patients, and all persons likely to be sexually active and/or promiscuous. Serology is the cornerstone of diagnosis; it is but rarely true at this time that diagnosis will emerge from efforts with dark field identification or histology.

Treatment: A summarization of the current United States Public Health Service recommendations for the treatment of syphilis is as follows:

1. Penicillin is the drug of choice in the nonpenicillin-allergic patient. In primary or secondary syphilis, or for preventive treatment of sexual contacts of syphilis, a single intramuscular injection of 2.4 million units of benzathine penicillin G is curative in the great majority of instances.

Other acceptable regimens include procaine penicillin G, 600,000 units intramuscularly once daily for eight to ten days or procaine penicillin G with 2% aluminum monostearate, 2.4 million units intramuscularly on the first day with 1.2 on the fourth and seventh days.

In latent syphilis with a known negative spinal fluid, the same regimen is used.

In late syphilis, 6 to 9 million units of penicillin should be given in total, either by 3 million units of benzathine penicillin G weekly for three weeks, or 600,000 units of aqueous procaine penicillin G for ten to fifteen days.

Syphilis in pregnancy is treated according to the staging above.

Congenital syphilis is treated with a single injection of benzathine penicillin G in a dose of 50,000 units/kg. of body weight.

2. Secondary antibiotics if the patient is allergic to penicillin

A. Tetracycline—early syphilis—30 gm. over ten to 15 days
   late syphilis—60 to 80 gm. over thirty to forty-five days
   NOTE: Tetracycline should not be used in pregnancy or in the treatment of children less than six or seven years of age, because of adverse effects upon dentition and bone.

B. Erythromycin—generally not recommended for the treatment of syphilis, except in highly selected instances

C. Cephaloridine—approximately 10% as effective as penicillin G versus T. pallidum. 0.5 to 1.0 gm. intramuscularly once a day for ten days is probably effective, but extensive studies have not been performed.

Possible Dire Consequences if Untreated: Infectivity in the early stages, and a host of destructive lesions in critical areas at any time after the early stages, particularly involving the cardiovascular and central nervous systems.

The patient with primary or secondary syphilis should be followed clinically and with periodic VDRL titers for one to two years. Early syphilis generally converts to sero-negativity within two years. Late cases should be followed less closely, and there is a much greater expectation of sero-positivity despite adequate treatment.

All cases should be reported to Public Health authorities, regardless of stage, so that record-keeping and epidemiologic investigations can function most effectively.

References

Sparling, P. J.: Diagnosis and Treatment of Syphilis. New Eng. J. Med. *284*:642, 1971.
Syphilis, A Synopsis, Publication of the U.S. Department of Health, Education, and Welfare. Public Health Service, National Center for Disease Control, Atlanta, Georgia 30333.

16. Rickettsial Diseases

ORVILLE HORWITZ

Cause: Rickettsiaceae

Early Manifestations: Fever, malaise, headache, rash. Generally positive specific complement fixation. Weil-Felix (WF) agglutination.

Treatment: Tetracycline and/or chloramphenicol.

Possible Dire Consequences without Treatment: Prolonged morbidity and possibly death in more virulent diseases.

Chloramphenicol and the tetracyclines are highly effective in the treatment of these diseases. Certainly in the less severe conditions the exclusive use of the less toxic tetracyclines should be utilized.

References

Elisberg, B. L. and Bozeman, F. L.: Serologic diagnosis of rickettsial diseases by indirect immunofluorescence. Arch. Intst. Pasteur Tunis *43*:193, 1966.
Murray, E. S.: Rickettsial Diseases. *Textbook of Medicine*, 13th Ed., Beeson, P. B. and McDermott, W. (eds.). Philadelphia, W. B. Saunders Co., 1971.
Murray, E. S., O'Connor, J. M., and Gaon, J. A.: Differentiation of 19S and 7S complement-fixing antibodies in primary versus recrudescent typhus by either ethanethiol or heat. Proc. Soc. Exp. Biol. Med., *119*:291, 1965.
Smadel, J. E.: Status of the rickettsioses in the United States. Ann. Intern. Med. *51*:421, 1959 .

TABLE VII–11.
SUMMARY OF CERTAIN IMPORTANT EPIDEMIOLOGIC AND CLINICAL CHARACTERISTICS OF RICKETTSIAL DISEASES (Beeson & McDermott)

Disease	Epidemiologic Features					Rash	
	Geographic Occurrence	Usual Mode of Transmission to Man	Reservoir	Usual Incubation Period (Days)	Eschar	Distribution	Type
Typhus group							
Primary epidemic typhus	Worldwide	Infected louse feces rubbed into broken skin or as aerosol to mucous membranes	Man	12 (8–15)	None	Trunk to extremities	Macular, maculopapular
Brill-Zinsser disease	Worldwide	Recrudescence months or years after a primary attack of epidemic typhus	—	—	None	Trunk to extremities	Macular, maculopapular
Murine typhus	Scattered pockets, worldwide	Infected flea feces rubbed into broken skin or as aerosol to mucous membranes	Rodents	12 (6–14)	None	Trunk to extremities	Macular, maculopapular
Spotted fever group							
Rocky Mountain spotted fever	Western hemisphere	Tick bite	Ticks, rodents	6 (2–12)	None	Extremities to trunk; palms and soles	Macular, maculopapular, petechial
Tick typhus	Mediterranean littoral, Africa, Asia	Tick bite	Ticks, rodents	12 (7–18)	Frequent	Trunk, extremities, face, palms, soles	Macular, maculopapular, petechial
Rickettsialpox	USA, USSR, Korea	House mouse, mite bite	Mites, mice	12 (9–24)	Usually present	Trunk, face, extremities	Papular, vesicular
Scrub typhus	Japan, SW Asia, W and SW Pacific	Mite bite	Mites, rodents	11 (6–21)	Frequent	Trunk to extremities	Macular, maculopapular, evanescent
Q fever	Worldwide	Inhalation of dried dusts from environment of infected animals	Ticks, mammals	14 (9–20)	None	None	None

17. Malaria

John D. Eshleman

Cause: Parenteral introduction of hepatocytic and erythrocytic protozoan parasites (plasmodia) by female Anopheles mosquitoes, placental transmission, or needles.
1. P. vivax: Usual cause in civilians and in military personnel a few months after return to U.S. (Vivax tertian)
2. P. falciparum: Usual cause in southeast Asia (Malignant tertian)
3. P. malariae: Uncommon (Quartan)
4. P. ovale: Rare (Ovale tertian)

Precipitating Causes: 1. Previous malaria: Secondary hepatocytic phase may persist and induce relapse after periods up to forty-five years.
2. Travel, even for a few hours, in an endemic area.
3. Military service in Southeast Asia.
4. Congenital malaria may occur in offspring of asymptomatic mothers.
5. Needle-borne: Contaminated syringe used by addicts.
6. Needle-borne: Transfusions can cause fatal malaria.

Early Manifestations: 1. Fever though usual may be absent.
2. Anemia may be present with or without hemolytic icterus and splenomegaly.
3. Leukocyte count is usually normal despite fever and/or anemia; rarely there may be pancytopenia.
4. Headache, myalgias, chills, urticaria are common.
5. Thin smears are preferable for identification of the parasite by the inexperienced; the experienced prefer thick smears.
6. Prior tetracycline by diminishing symptoms and parasitism on smear may make diagnosis difficult but is no longer recommended for treatment.

Late Manifestations: 1. Herpes labialis.
2. Hemolytic anemia and hemolytic icterus especially with P. falciparum infections.
3. Hemoglobinuria (blackwater fever) with or without acute renal failure.
4. Non-cardiac pulmonary edema probably a manifestation of hypersensitivity pneumonitis.
5. Nephrotic syndrome following both P. falciparum and P. malariae has been reported though doubted by others.

Treatment: 1. Prohibitions upon blood donation:
    a. Travelers to endemic areas, including Vietnam veterans, who have taken antimalarial chemoprophylaxis, within three years of return to U.S.
    b. Travelers to endemic areas, who are well and who have not taken antimalarial chemoprophylaxis, within six months of return to U.S.
2. Treatment of chloroquine-resistant strains of P. falciparum from Central and South America and from Southeast Asia, or if parasite is unidentified:
    a. Diaminodiphenylsulfone (DDS) 25 mg. initially
    b. Pyrimethamine 25 mg. t.i.d. for three days.
    c. Quinine 650 mg. t.i.d. for ten days.
3. Treatment of P. vivax, malariae or ovale and of non-chloroquine resistant P. falciparum.
    a. Chloroquine 600 mg. initially
    b. Chloroquine 300 mg. six hours later.
    c. Chloroquine 300 mg. daily for seven days.
4. Treatment of secondary hepatocytic phase of P. vivax, malariae and ovale infections:
    a. Primaquine 15 mg. daily for fourteen days.
    b. Twelve % of U.S. blacks have G 6 PD deficient erythrocyte and should be screened for this trait prior to institution of primaquine therapy.

Possible Dire Consequences without Treatment: 1. Cerebral malaria may be fatal within
   hours.
   2. Disseminated intravascular coagulation.
   3. Splenic rupture.
   4. Transmission to others.

Optimum treatment of malaria depends upon specific diagnosis with identification
of parasites on a stained peripheral blood smear.   Red cells infected with P. vivax are
enlarged and pale, containing in addition to red-staining chromatin (Shuffner's)
dots, trophozoites which may be of any shape containing 12 to 24 daughter cells
(merozoites).   The trophozoites of P. malariae are ring-shaped containing 8 merozoites arranged in rosettes.   More than one trophozoite of P. falciparum may parasi-
tize the same red cell, cells of all ages and sizes being involved, up to 20% of the total
in heavy parasitism.   The trophozoites are small, containing chromatin dots and 8 to
18 merozoites, assuming a banana shape with enlargement. Merozoites released into
the circulation may reinvade liver cells or invade other red cells where they become
sexual forms (gametocytes), prey to ingestion by the definitive host, the mosquito.   In
the mosquito stomach gametocytes undergo sexual fusion to become mobile zygotes.
They then penetrate the stomach wall to encyst, yielding sporozoites which migrate
to the mosquito salivary glands.   Then they are transmitted to another human
host when the mosquito next feeds.   In the new human host the sporozoites circulate
briefly prior to entering the liver where they develop into schizonts and ultimately
merozoites which enter the circulation and gain access to red cells and platelets.
Although chloroquine is effective against the erythrocytic forms, primaquine is
necessary to eradicate merozoites of all except P. falciparum, which may reenter liver
cells where they would otherwise elude radical cure.   Reported cases of malaria in
the U.S., which had fallen to 50 per year by 1959, had reached a high point of perhaps
a 300-fold increase by the end of 1969, and the index of suspicion for this infection
should remain high.   The diagnosis requires identification on blood smear.   Serologic tests are available, costly, and not especially helpful in diagnosing acute attacks
of malaria.   Fluctuating titers of antibody may be useful in determining need for
retreatment of established cases, but fall of a titer to zero does not necessarily signify
radical cure.

References

Berger, M., Birch, L. M., and Conte, N. F.:   The nephrotic syndrome secondary to acute
   glomerulonephritis during falciparum malaria.   Ann. Intern. Med. *67*:1163, 1967.
Bick, R. L. and Anhalt, J. E.:   Malaria transmission among narcotic addicts.   Calif. Med.
   115:56, 1971.
Blount, R. E.:   Malaria: A persistent threat.   Ann. Intern. Med. *70*:127, 1969.
Brooke, M. H. and Barry, K. G.:   Fatal transfusion malaria.   Blood *34*:806, 1969.
Brooke, M. H. et al.:   Acute pulmonary edema in falciparum malaria.   New Eng. J. Med.
   279:732, 1968.
Cahill, K. M.:   Symposium on malaria.   Bull. New York Acad. Med. *45*:997, 1969.
McQuay, R. et al.:   Persistence of malarial antibody.   Am. J. Trop. Med. *16*:258, 1967.
Rees, P. H. et al.:   Possible role of malaria in the aetiology of the nephrotic syndrome in
   Nairobi.   Lancet *1*:1143, 1972.
Rieckman, K. H. et al.: Effects of tetracycline against chloroquine-resistant and chloroquine-
   sensitive falciparum malariae.   Am. J. Trop. Med. *20*:811, 1971.
Sheehy, T. W. and Reba, R. C.:   Complications of falciparum malaria and their treatment.
   Ann. Intern. Med. *66*:807, 1967.

18. Bubonic Plague

Orville Horwitz

Cause: Pasteurella pestis, which is from animals (mostly rodents) to man via fleas. It is an aerobic non-motile bacillus.

Early Manifestations: High fever, tachycardia, malaise, aching back and extremities. Buboes in 50% of cases. Hence the name. Prostration, delirium.

Treatment: Streptomycin and chloramphenicol nearly useless after fifteen hours of disease. Tetracyclines are antibiotics of choice.

Possible Dire Consequences without Treatment: Ninety % mortality without treatment; the pneumonic infection is responsible for high mortality.

The organs involved are the skin, lymph nodes, liver, mucosa, serosa, small vessels of the liver, kidneys, meninges, and lungs. The pneumonia is particularly virulent and overwhelming, being lobular and lobar. The latter may involve as many as four lobes.

The pathological changes include bubo at regional lymph node with necrosis. Hemorrhage of serous and mucosal area. Degeneration of renal tubular endothelium, cerebral edema, pneumonia and bacteremia.

The diagnosis is made by isolation of organism from bubo or sputum. There is leukocytosis of 12,000 to 15,000.

Reference

Cavanaugh, D. C. et al.: Some observations on the current plague outbreak in the republic of Vietnam. Am. J. Public Health *58*:742, 1968.

19. Spirillary Rat Bite Fever

Orville Horwitz

Cause: Dogs, cats, mice, rats, weasels, carrying spirillum minus, *not* Streptobacillus moniliformis.

Early Manifestations: Healed recent wound from animal bite. Incubation period is from four to twenty-eight days. Eventually local inflammation, fever, lymphadenitis. Possible urticarial rash occurs. White blood cell count ranges from 8,000 to 30,000.

Treatment: Penicillin and streptomycin.

Possible Dire Consequences without Treatment: Prolonged fever.

Diagnosis depends on demonstration of organism from lymph nodes by Giemsa stain or dark field microscopy. Response to treatment is prompt. Bites by above animals should be treated by local antisepsis and prophylactic penicillin.

References

Brown, T. M., and Nunemaker, J. D.: Rat-bite fever: A review of the American cases with re-evaluation of etiology; Report of cases. Bull. Hopkins Hosp. *70*:201, 1942.
Roughgarden, J. W.: Antimicrobial therapy of rat-bite fever. Arch. Intern Med. *116*:39, 1965.

20. Streptobacillary Rat Bite Fever

ORVILLE HORWITZ

Cause: Bite from dogs, cats, mice, rats, and weasels carrying Streptobacillus moniliformis.

Early Manifestations: Healed recent wound from animal bite. Incubation one day to three weeks. Then chills, fever, headache, vomiting, general aches, pains, and arthralagia. Possible petechial rash, WBC 8,000–30,000.

Treatment: Penicillin and/or tetracycline.

Possible Dire Consequences without Treatment: Long febrile illness and possibly bacterial endocarditis. Low mortality.

Diagnosis confirmed by culture of the organism. Usually good response to therapy. Bites by the above animals should be treated by local antisepsis and a prophylactic dose of penicillin.

References

McCormack, R. C., Kaye, D., and Hook, E. W.: Endocarditis due to Streptobacillus moniliformis. J.A.M.A. *200*:77, 1967.
Roughgarden, J. W.: Antimicrobial therapy of rat bite fever. Arch. Intern. Med. *116*:39, 1965.

21. Ornithosis. Psittacosis

ORVILLE HORWITZ

Cause: Microbial agent of questionable classification: "bedsonia" agent.

Early Manifestations: Headaches, malaise and myalgia. Cough may be delayed. Blood streaked sputum and pleurisy are rare. Fever may be as high as 105°F. Pulmonary physical findings sparse. Spleen may be palpable.

Treatment: Tetracyclines.

Possible Dire Consequences without Treatment: Morbidity may be prolonged. Death is uncommon, but a definite possibility.

The organ involved most frequently in man is the lung.

The pathological changes include exudates, vasculitis, small hemorrhages, inflammatory exudates with polymorph and later monocytes.

The diagnosis is made by isolation of the organism which is difficult. Complement fixation may help.

Reference

Seibert, R. H., Jordan, W. S., Jr. and Dingle, J. H.: Clinical variations in the diagnosis of psittacosis. New Eng. J. Med. *254*:925, 1956.

22. Brucella

ORVILLE HORWITZ

Cause: Brucella abortus melitosis, suis, small gram-negative aerobic non-motile coccobacillus. Brucellosis generally transmitted by infected milk. It can be transmitted via infected organs of cattle, pigs, goats and sheep.

Early Manifestations: Most often insidious with headache, fever, weakness, joint pains, insomnia, sweats, and low back pain. Splenomegaly is a later manifestation.

Treatment: Tetracycline 0.5 gm. q.i.d. for three weeks.

Possible Dire Consequences without Treatment: Morbidity, abscess formations. Mortality less than two %.

The organs involved are bone marrow, endocardium, biliary tract, liver, spleen, eye, meninges, and kidney.

The pathological changes are granulomas consisting of lymphocytes, epithelioid cells, plasma cell and giant cells. In severe cases, caseation and abscess formation may occur.

The diagnosis is made by isolation of organism and agglutination against antibody.

Reference

Spink, W. W.: The Nature of Brucellosis. Minneapolis, University of Minnesota Press, 1956.

23. Tularemia

ORVILLE HORWITZ

Cause: Francisella tularensis, small gram-negative coccobacillus carried by many mammal and arthropod vectors, classically rabbits. Invades man through skin and respiratory tract. One attack usually yields immunity.

Early Manifestations: Abrupt high fever persisting one month if untreated. Ulceroglandular type most common. May be *only fever or typhoidal nature with obscure vector contact.* May be only pneumonitis. Oculoglandular type rare. Bacteremia may give rise to pneumonia.

Treatment: Streptomycin 30 to 40 mg. per kg. body weight per day for three days injected intramuscularly.

Possible Dire Consequences without Treatment: Five % mortality without pneumonia. Thirty % mortality with pneumonia.

The organs involved are skin (ulcer), lymph nodes (drainage), lungs in man and liver in rabbits.

The pathological changes are maculo-erythematous skin lesions two days after exposure, somewhat like a positive tuberculin test. This is followed by ulceration and regional lymphadenopathy from inhalation tracheitis, bronchitis, and pneumonia. The gastrointestinal form is rare.

The diagnosis is made by isolation of organism from sputum, ulcer, lymph nodes, or blood. Skin test antigen positive in 90% of cases.

References

Farmer, J. L. and Duncan, G. G.: Tularemia: Report of six cases occurring in Pa. Bull. Ayer Clin. Lab. *3*:237, 1938.

Foshay, L.: Tularemia. Ann. Rev. Microbiol. *4*:331, 1950.

24. Anthrax, Malignant Pustule

ORVILLE HORWITZ

Cause: B. anthracis, large gram-positive and sporeforming encapsulated hemolytic aerobic microorganism, invades through the skin.

Early Manifestations: Hard edematous pustule with nonpitting edema and without adenopathy in people exposed to animals.

Treatment: Penicillin G 1 to 2 million units daily and tetracycline.

Possible Dire Consequences without Treatment: Death in 20% of patients having disseminated disease.

The organ involved is skin.   This is followed by dissemination through the blood stream with toxicity.

The pathological changes include local edema, hemorrhage, necrosis and inflammation.

The diagnosis is made by demonstration of organism from the pustule.

Reference

Brachman, P. S. et al.: An epidemic of inhalation anthrax: II. epidemiologic investigation. Med. J. Hyg. *72*:6, 1960.

25. Histoplasmosis

ORVILLE HORWITZ

Cause: Two forms of H. capsulatum: yeast and hyphal.

Early Manifestations: Cough, dyspnea, pleuritic pain, hoarseness, cyanosis, hemoptysis. Roentgenogram of the lung may show miliary effect after dissemination. Endocarditis and hepatitis may also occur early, but usually only in rare discriminated form.

Treatment: Amphotericin B intravenously in increasing doses starting with 1.0 mg. in 500 ml. 5% glucose. STEROID TREATMENT CONTRAINDICATED.

Possible Dire Consequences without Treatment: Usually benign and self-limited. Only progressive cavitary and disseminated forms require specific treatment which has reduced mortality to about 15%.

The organs involved are lungs, lymph nodes, liver, spleen, and adrenals.

The pathological changes include epithelioid histiocytic granulomas with tubercle-like nodules, caseation, necrosis, and calcification. Cavitary pulmonary disease may also be present.

The definitive diagnosis which is made by cultures from urine and sputum by special stains is often unsatisfactory. Positive histoplasmin skin test is suggestive but not confirmatory.

Reference

Sweany, H. C.: Histoplasmosis. Springfield, Charles C Thomas, 1960.

26. Botulism

ORVILLE HORWITZ

Cause: Clinical botulism types, A, B, E, and F in man. Aerobic motile, gram-positive, bacillus producing heat resistant spores. Only the vegetative form elaborates the toxins which are the most poisonous substances known.

Early Manifestations: Toxin usually ingested from contaminated food. After a period of a few hours to a week, acute descending weakness and/or paralysis beginning with cranial nerves. Mental processes are clear. There is no fever and there are no sensory disturbances.

Treatment: Intensive care. Antitoxin may be obtained from Center for Disease Control and Lederle. Center for Disease Control telephone numbers are Day: (404) 633-3311, Ext. 3751 or 3684. Night: (404) 633-2176 or (404) 633-8673. Lederle Laboratory number is as follows: (914) 735-5000.

Possible Dire Consequences without Treatment: Death.

Intoxication blocks release of acetylcholine. Cholinergic synaptic transmission halts.

A state of practical denervation persists causing aspiration pneumonia, and asphyxia due to lack of proper bulbar function.

The diagnosis is confirmed by demonstration of toxin in serum.

Reference

Rogers, D. E.: Botulism: Vintage, 1963. Editorial, Ann. Intern. Med., *61*:581, 1964.

27. Nocardiosis

ORVILLE HORWITZ

Cause: Gram-positive acid-fast filaments may prevail as either coccoid or bacillary form considered to be the aerobic counterparts of actinomycosis.

Early Manifestations: This condition is mentioned particularly because about 40% of the diagnoses are made at autopsy, particularly in patients whose resistance is lowered by other debilitating conditions. It should be suspected in patients with persistent pneumonia not yielding to conventional antibiotic treatment.

Nocardial infection of the brain is particularly difficult to diagnose. Actual brain biopsy may be necessary to establish a diagnosis and to treat properly certain desperately ill patients displaying diffuse fever and non-specific neurological signs and symptoms.

Treatment: Triple sulfonamides 75 mg./kg. body weight per day.

Possible Dire Consequences without Treatment: Death.

The organs involved are respiratory tract, the pleura, and the brain. Pathological changes that may occur are pneumonia, lung abscess and brain abscess. Organisms are difficult to culture and to isolate.

Reference

Weed, L. A. et al.: Nocardiosis: Clinical, bacteriologic and pathologic aspects. New Eng. J. Med. *253*:1138, 1955.

28. Cryptococcal Meningitis

RICHARD K. ROOT

Cause: Infection of the brain and meninges with *Cryptococcus neoformans*.

Early Manifestations: Persistent headache, mental confusion and obtundation, focal neurologic signs.

Treatment: Amphotericin-B, 5-fluorocytosine.

Possible Dire Consequences without Treatment: Death (>95%).

Meningoencephalitis due to infection by the fungus *Cryptococcus neoformans* can be easily diagnosed by appropriate cultures and with the aid of a relatively new technique to measure free polysaccharide released from the capsules of the organisms. Despite this it is not unusual for patients to go for weeks or months undiagnosed because of the subtle manner in which it may present, an example of which is demon-

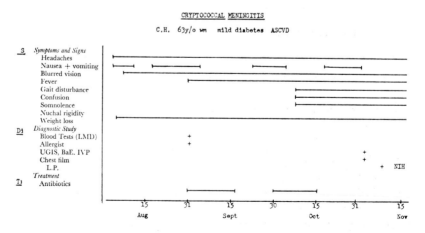

Fig. VII–3. The bars denote the duration of various symptoms and signs in this patient in relationship to diagnostic procedures (pluses) and therapeutic measures (bars). The definitive diagnostic procedure (lumbar puncture) was not performed until the patient had been symptomatic for 12 weeks.

strated in Figure VII–3. Persistent headache occurs in approximately 75% of patients with this disorder and represents the most common presenting symptom. Associated neurological symptoms vary widely from mental obtundation, psychosis and/or confusion to specific abnormalities such as hemiparesis, ataxia, aphasia, and visual disturbances. Because of the variety of this symptomatology, cryptococcal meningitis may masquerade as a space occupying lesion of the central nervous system, a demyelinating disorder or psychiatric disease. In contrast to bacterial or viral meningitis, chills and fever are relatively infrequent (~30% of cases) as are signs of meningeal irritation on physical examination (~35%). Ten to 15% of affected patients will have no symptoms referrable to the central nervous system. Furthermore, while cryptococcosis is traditionally thought of as a disease that affects impaired hosts (particularly patients with lymphoma) fully 50% of reported cases have had no underlying disease. Some of these latter patients are detected because of positive sputum cultures and chest x-ray findings indicative of pulmonary cryptococcosis. This makes examination of the cerebrospinal fluid a mandatory procedure in all patients with evidence of cryptococcosis elsewhere. A mononuclear CSF pleocytosis is found in almost all patients (>95%) with active infection, as is an elevation of protein. Depression of CSF glucose is less universal, but is found in approximately 60% of cases.

Therefore CSF findings may be confused with those of TB, viral or partially treated bacterial meningitis. Definitive diagnosis is made by demonstration of the organisms or polysaccharide in the CSF. Collection of large volumes (>10cc) of CSF will

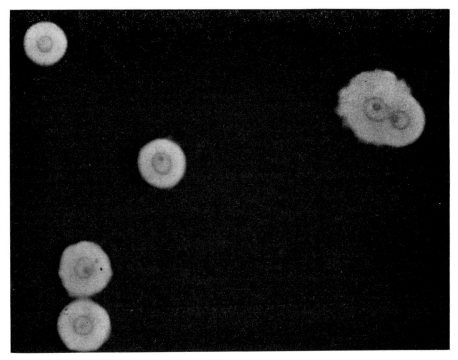

Figure VII–4. Positive India ink preparation from a patient with cryptococcal meningitis. No other fungal species has the large polysaccharide capsule which is responsible for the clear area around the central yeast form. The cell wall and nucleus of the organism are clearly visible.

enhance organism recovery, as will examination and culture of centrifuged specimens. India ink preparations are positive in about 60% of cases (Fig. VII–4). The characteristic feature is the finding of a large clear halo around the centrally located organism. Focusing the microscope up and down while observing the organism will demonstrate this more clearly and should help to distinguish it from lymphocytes that may also be present. Cultures on Sabouraud's medium are positive in more than 90% of cases; however, several specimens may be necessary to obtain a positive result. Cultures of areas outside the central nervous system may also be helpful in diagnosis, since 20 to 30% of patients will have positive urine, blood or sputum cultures and about 10% positive bone marrow cultures. No reliable skin tests or measurements of antibody response are available as diagnostic tools.

The ease of diagnosis has been greatly enhanced by the development of a serological assay for free cryptococcal polysaccharide employing either complement fixation or latex agglutination technique. Free polysaccharide is found in the CSF of 70 to 80% of patients with active meningitis, and the amount and persistence correlate roughly with disease activity. Polysaccharide may also be found in the circulation of infected patients even in the absence of positive blood cultures. The assays appear to be highly specific for *C. neoformans* and afford the most rapid way of diagnosing the disease. As such, they should be routinely performed on every case in which CSF or clinical findings may suggest the disease, but India ink preparations or cultures are negative. At the present time these assays are being performed at the National Center for Disease Control, Atlanta, Georgia, and at several university and research centers throughout the U.S. (In addition, a latex agglutination kit is now commercially available.)

The treatment of choice for cryptococcal meningitis remains intravenous amphotericin B, initially effective in about 85% of cases. Approximately 35% will relapse and require further treatment. All patients who receive therapeutic doses (1 to 1.5 mg./kg./day) of amphotericin will develop some degree of nephrotoxicity which is partially reversible. It is usually safe to continue until the BUN is 50 or the creatinine 3.0 at which time it may be necessary to stop for several days to allow these values to return toward normal. Over the long term, however, it is unwise to allow more than forty-eight hours to elapse between dosages, since almost all of the drug is metabolized in the body by that time, and if somewhat resistant organisms are present they may overgrow as the more sensitive organisms are eliminated. The duration of treatment after negative cultures are obtained has not been precisely established. One regimen calls for a total dose of at least 3 gm. of amphotericin, more if cultures remain positive. Another recommends administering enough drug to permit blood levels of twice the minimal inhibitory concentration of amphotericin, against the isolate. Treatment is continued after cultures are negative for at least several weeks, and preferably a month or more. There is no evidence to suggest that intrathecal administration of amphotericin is more effective than the intravenous route and because of frequent complications is generally contraindicated unless all other measures have failed. Recent experience with a new orally administered less toxic compound, 5-fluorocytosine in a dose of 50 to 100 mg./kg./day (4 divided doses), suggests that it will not be as effective as amphotericin. The therapeutic success rate has been only around 33% and failure has been associated with the rapid development of high-level resistance in about half. If 5-fluorocytosine and amphotericin are given together, then the dose of the former must be reduced when nephrotoxicity develops since it is excreted by the renal route, and marrow suppression may ensue.

References

Bennett, J. E., Hasenclever, H. F., and Tynes, B. S.: Detection of cryptococcal polysaccharide in serum and spinal fluid: value in diagnosis and prognosis. Trans. Assoc. Am. Physic. *77*:145, 1964.

Block, E. R., and Bennett, J. E.: Pharmacological studies with 5-fluorocytosine. Antimicrobial Agents & Chemother. *1*:476, 1972.

Butler, W. T. et al.: Diagnostic and prognostic value of clinical and laboratory findings in cryptococcal meningitis. New Eng. J. Med. *270*:59, 1964.

Drutz, D. J. et al.: Treatment of disseminated mycotic infections: a new approach to amphotericin B therapy. Am. J. Med. *45*:405, 1968.

Goodman, J. S., Kaufman, L., and Koenig, M. G.: Diagnosis of cryptococcal meningitis, value of immunologic detection of cryptococcal antigen. New Eng. J. Med. *285*:434, 1971.

Sarosi, G. A. et al.: Amphotericin B in cryptococcal meningitis. Ann. Intern. Med. *71*:1079, 1969.

Tynes, B. et al.: Variant forms of pulmonary cryptococcosis. Ann. Intern. Med. 69:1117, 1968.

29. Pneumocystis Carinii Pneumonia

Richard K. Root

Cause: Infection by the protozoan pneumocystis carinii.

Early Manifestations: Dry cough, dyspnea, anoxia, and fever in neonates and hypogammaglobulinemic patients or those receiving corticosteroids or other immunosuppressive treatment.

Treatment: Pentamidine isethionate, or pyramethamine and sulfadiazine.

Possible Dire Consequences without Treatment: Death.

In a retrospective and prospective study of patients with hematogenous malignancies and acute interstitial pneumonias, 44% were discovered to have *Pneumocystis carinii* as the causative agent. With the advent of therapy with the imidine derivative, pentamidine isethionate, this disease has been converted from a universally fatal condition to one in which cure is quite possible, despite a patient population which frequently has severe underlying disease. Thus it becomes important to recognize these cases and to be familiar with the means of diagnosis.

With the exception of sporadic disease appearing in epidemic fashion in neonates virtually all reported cases have been found in patients who have primary or therapeutically induced immune deficiencies, *i.e.*, transplantation patients and those receiving treatment for malignancies, collagen vascular disease, etc. In particular, corticosteroid therapy has been present in 60 to 80% of cases. In most patients symptoms develop rapidly and are characterized by dry cough, dyspnea, cyanosis, and fever. A minority of patients will have more chronic symptoms. The chest x-ray

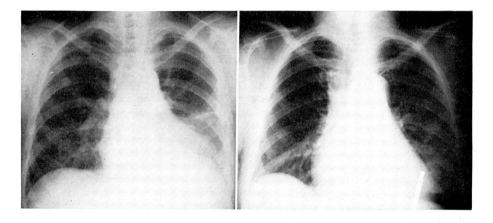

Fig. VII–5. Chest x-rays films from two renal transplantation patients with biopsy proven *Pneumocystis carinii* pneumonia. Note the fine reticulonodular infiltrates in the right-mid-lung field of the patient on the left. The patient on the right also had a pleural effusion on the left which was determined to be secondary to staphylococcal infection. Pleural effusions are *not* a feature of *Pneumocystis carinii* infection.

examination most often reveals diffuse patchy, interstitial infiltrates which can progress rapidly (Fig. VII–5). Blood gases are compatible with an "alveolar-capillary block" syndrome demonstrating hypoxia that responds to oxygen, and hypocapnia. The peripheral leukocyte response is usually unremarkable, and often obscured by treatment induced alterations. Examination of the sputum is usually unrewarding. The cellular response is scanty with mononuclear cells predominating, consistent with a nonbacterial pneumonitis. Recovery of the organisms in tracheal aspirates is so infrequent as to merit case reporting. To date the only reliable means of diagnosis has been through the use of open or percutaneous lung biopsy. The latter has been associated with significant complications in over 35% of cases, and therefore unless conditions warrant otherwise, open biopsy procedures should be pursued when the diagnosis is suspected. The material should be stained with methenamine silver or the Gram-Weigert technique to demonstrate the typical cup-shaped organisms floating in debris in the alveoli (Fig. VII–6).

Recently, the technique of deep bronchial brushing has yielded highly favorable results, and is more benign than open lung biopsy. No skin or serological tests are available for diagnosis and biopsies outside the pulmonary area are almost always negative, since in the vast majority of cases infection remains localized to the lung. Vigorous pursuit of a diagnosis prior to the institution of therapy is desirable, since pentamidine treatment is associated with an appreciable incidence of toxicity. Standard dosage is 4 mg./kg. IM for ten days. The most common toxic reactions are those of azotemia, local muscle necrosis and hypoglycemia. Companion treatment with other nephrotoxic drugs should be avoided if at all possible since their effects may be additive with pentamidine. In less critically ill patients it is probably worthwhile to treat with sulfadiazine 1 gm. q six hours and pyramethamine 25 mg., b.i.d., together with folinic acid 6 mg./day for twenty-eight days (to prevent bone marrow suppression), rather than pentamidine, since this regimen is less toxic. When treatment is successful, relapse and/or reinfection almost never occurs and most

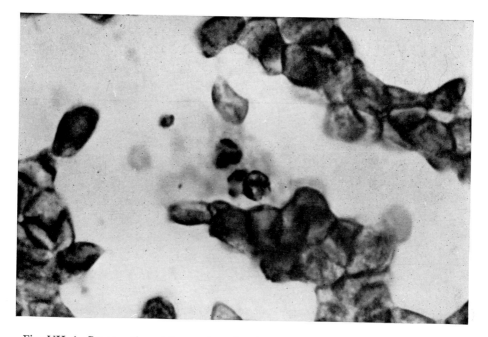

Fig. VII–6. *Pneumocystis carinii* organisms free in the alveolar space as obtained by open lung biopsy from the patient with the chest x-ray film on the left of Figure VII–5 (Gram-Weigert Stain 100×).

studies have revealed eradication of the organisms after ten days of pentamidine therapy.

As one of the few treatable interstitial pneumonias recognition of this syndrome and making the correct diagnosis become most important.

References

Goodell, B. et al.: *Pneumocystis carinii:* the spectrum of diffuse interstitial pneumonia in patients with neoplastic diseases. Ann. Intern. Med. *72*:337, 1970.

Neff, T. A.: Percutaneous trephine biopsy of the lung. Chest *61*:18, 1972.

Raskin, J. and Remington, J. S.: The compromised host and infection, I. *Pneumocystis carinii* pneumonia. J.A.M.A. *202*:96, 1967.

Repsher, L. H., Schröter, G., and Hammond, W. S.: Diagnosis of *pneumocystis carinii* pneumonitis by means of endobronchial brush biopsy. New Eng. J. Med. *287*:340, 1972.

Rifkind, D., Faris, T. D., Hill, R. B., Jr.: *Pneumocystis carinii* pneumonia: studies on the diagnosis and treatment. Ann. Intern. Med. *65*:943, 1966.

Robbins, J. B. et al.: Successful treatment of *Pneumocystis carinii* pneumonia in a patient with congenital hypogammaglobulinemia. New Eng. J. Med. *272*:708, 1965.

Western, K. A., Perera, D. R., Schultz, M. G.: Pentamidine isethionate in the treatment of *pneumocystis carinii* pneumonia. Ann. Intern. Med. *73*:695, 1970.

30. Systemic Candidiasis

RICHARD K. ROOT

Cause: Deep infection with one of the species of candida fungi.

Early Manifestations: Fever, signs of dysfunction of specifically infected organs. Peripheral embolization if endocarditis. Often involves an impaired host.

Treatment: Remove intravenous lines if an entry site. Amphotericin B and 5-fluorocytosine. Surgery.

Possible Dire Consequences without Treatment: Candidemia due to intravenous catheters is usually self-limited. Infections elsewhere progressive and often fatal unless combined medical-surgical approach taken.

Deep infection with candida species most often occurs in one of three settings: (1) As a complication of prolonged intravenous therapy, often in conjunction with antimicrobial treatment and, (2) as an opportunistic infection in the host impaired by serious underlying disease and/or immunosuppressive chemotherapeutic treatment for malignancy or organ transplantation; or (3) as endocarditis following insertion of a prosthetic cardiac valve or in narcotic addicts.

In the first setting, fungemia with candida species is heralded by the appearance of fever and leukocytosis without other more specific symptomatology. While the intravenous catheter is in place, multiple blood cultures are positive for the organism, as frequently are urine cultures, since the kidney serves as the major clearing organ for the fungus. The majority of patients will respond to discontinuing the intravenous line, and no further treatment is indicated. A small percentage of patients will continue to be febrile and have persistently positive blood and/or urine cultures despite this maneuver. They may develop signs of pyelonephritis, fluffy or miliary infiltrates in the lungs and rarely fluffy infiltrates in the retinae indicative of secondary infection in these areas. Heart valve infection is often signaled by the occurrence of large vessel embolization as outlined elsewhere in this text. Such patients will not be recognized unless appropriate cultures are obtained after discontinuing the inlying catheters and the appropriate areas examined by retinoscopy and roentgenograms. Skin tests will be of no value since over 90% of the adult population already has established delayed hypersensitivity to candida antigens. Serological tests are of limited value unless they can be related to positive clinical manifestations. Treatment is with amphotericin B or if sensitivity to 5-fluorocytosine is demonstrated (about 50% of species), then this agent has been successfully employed.

Candida infection usually appears in the second group of patients after intensive chemotherapy, which often includes corticosteroids. Concomitant broad spectrum antibiotic therapy permits resistant organisms such as the candida species to overgrow and cause infection. Mucosal candidiasis is frequently found in this setting, but may bear no relationship to deep infection with the organism. Likewise in the presence of oral candidiasis positive sputum cultures for candida are meaningless unless the material is collected by transtracheal aspiration or bronchoscopy and can be related to pulmonary infiltration and signs of an inflammatory response in the sputum. Pul-

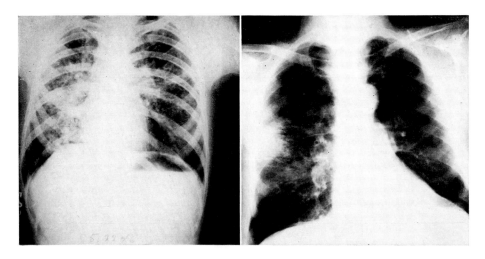

Fig. VII–7. Chest x-ray films from two patients with pulmonary candidiasis. The one on the left has miliary nodules in the right lung. The patient on the right has a single wedge-shaped dense infiltrate in the right lung which resembles a pulmonary infarct. This appearance is produced by vascular invasion with organisms and secondary thrombosis and infarction. Pulmonary infection with aspergillus species may produce x-ray pictures similar to these.

monary infiltrates (Fig. VII–7) due to candida species vary from miliary in character to modular densities. CNS infection may occur as a meningitis or brain abscess. Infection of liver and kidneys can also develop. Blood cultures are often negative. Definitive diagnosis can be made only by tissue examination since as mentioned earlier skin tests are valueless and serological data are unreliable. Because of their underlying disease these patients as a rule do poorly despite appropriate therapy. More often they develop this complication in the last few weeks of life and are discovered to have candidiasis only at autopsy.

Patients with candida endocarditis have been discussed in detail elsewhere in this text (p. 109), and will not be commented upon further here, except to emphasize that *combined* medical and surgical treatment is usually necessary to effect a cure.

References

Bodey, G. P.: Fungal infections complicating acute leukemia. J. Chron. Dis. *19*:667, 1966.
Bornstein, D. L.: Fungal Endocarditis. Specifically Treatable Diseases, 1972.
Curry, C. R., and Quie, P. G.: Fungal septicemia in patients receiving parenteral hyperalimentation. New Eng. J. Med. *285*:1221, 1971.
Eras, P., Goldstein, M. J., and Sherlock, P.: Candida infection of the gastrointestinal tract. Medicine, *51*:367, 1972.
Fass, R. J., and Perkins, R. L.: 5-fluorocytosine in the treatment of cryptococcal and candida mycosis. Ann. Intern. Med. *74*:535, 1971.
Fishman, L. S. et al.: Hematogenous candida endophthalmitis—a complication of candidemia. New Eng. J. Med. *286*:675, 1972.
Kay, J. H. et al.: Surgical treatment of candida endocarditis. J.A.M.A. *203*:621, 1968.
Louria, D. B., Stiff, D. P., and Bennett, B.: Disseminated moniliasis in the adult. Medicine *41*:307, 1962.
Preisler, H. D. et al.: Serologic diagnosis of disseminated candidiasis in patients with acute leukemia. Ann. Intern. Med. *70*:19, 1969.

31. Listeriosis

ORVILLE HORWITZ

Cause: Listeria monocytogenes, gram-positive and small aerobic motile bacillus transmitted from small animals, or from another human.

Early Manifestations: Headache, myalgia, fever, chills, nausea, vomiting, stiff neck, maculopapular rash, hepatosplenomegaly.

Treatment: Penicillin, erythromycin and tetracycline.

Possible Dire Consequences without Treatment: Stupor, convulsions, somnolence, 70% mortality without treatment.

The organs involved are the meninges most common and important, but nearly all internal organs may become involved including urethra and vagina.

The pathological changes are disseminated granulomas and focal necrosis or suppuration.

The diagnosis is made by bacterial identification in cerebrospinal fluid, but such identification is often confused with other organisms.

The distribution is world wide.

Reference

Hoeprich, P. D.: Infections due to listeria monocytogenes. Medicine *37*:143, 1958.

32. Actinomycosis

ORVILLE HORWITZ

Cause: Actinomycosis israeli into infected focus in mouth from eating and dentistry.

Early Manifestations: Fever, painful indurated swelling, sinus formation with sulfur granules. Lesions can appear in all parts of the body.

Treatment: Penicillin and tetracycline are effective.

Possible Dire Consequences without Treatment: Loss of local function, discomfort, death.

The diagnosis is easy once the pus comes out of the sinus. However, before this happens the presentation is that of a hidden abscess, and the proper diagnosis may be delayed for months.

References

Cope, V. Z.:   Actinomycosis. London, Oxford University Press, 1938.
Nichols, D. R. and Herrell, W. E.:   Penicillin in the treatment of actinomycosis.   J. Lab. Clin.
   Med. *33*:521, 1948.

33. Blastomycosis

ORVILLE HORWITZ

Cause: Blastomycosis dermatidis, a dimorphic yeast-like fungus.

Early Manifestations: Cutaneous papule or pustule.   Peripheral spread from primary
   pulmonary infection.   Also fever, night sweats, anorexia, weight loss.

Treatment: Amphotericin B 2 gm. usually sufficient.   Also less toxic and often effective 2-hydroxystilbamidine 225 mg. per day for twenty days.

Possible Dire Consequences without Treatment: Chronic progressive disease with about
   20% mortality.

The organs involved are lung, skin, bone, subcutaneous tissue, meninges prostate,
and epididymis.

The pathological changes include giant cell granulomas, bronchopneumonia and
cavitation, microabscesses and granulomata.

The diagnosis is made by demonstration of organism from the skin lesion.

Reference

Busey, J. F.:   Blastomycosis: A review of 198 collected cases in Veterans Administration
   Hospitals.   Amer. Rev. Resp. Dis., *89*:659, 1964.

34. Bartonellosis

ORVILLE HORWITZ

Cause: Bartonella bacilliformis, a small gram-negative motile bacillus. Insect borne
   disease of South America.

Early Manifestations: Intermittent high fever, muscle and joint pains, large tender
   lymph nodes, prostration from severe hemolytic anemia with resulting jaundice.

Treatment: Tetracycline.

Possible Dire Consequences without Treatment: May be over 50% mortality, especially
   when complicated by other diseases.

The organs involved are blood, blood vessels, and bone marrow.

The disease is not infrequently focused in travelers returning from South America.

The pathological changes are hemolytic anemia, dilation of capillaries of skin and proliferation of vascular endothelial cells.

The diagnosis is made by clinical picture and blood smears, showing bacteria adhered to red cells.

Reference

Weinman, D.: The bartonella group *In* Bacterial and Mycotic Infections of Man. Dubso, R. J. and Hirsch, J. G. (eds.), Philadelphia, J. B. Lippincott Co., 1965, p. 775.

35. Leprosy

ORVILLE HORWITZ

Cause: Mode of transmission not completely understood. Mycobacterium leprae. Acid-fast rod 2 to 6μ long. Less acid-fast than Tubercle bacillus.

Early Manifestations: Lepromatous: lesions on face. Tuberculoid: anesthesia of area supplied by nerve.

Treatment: Diaminodiphenyl sulfone (D.D.S.). Start with 25 mg. per week and increase gradually to 100 mg. daily.

Possible Dire Consequences without Treatment: Lepromatous, death from amyloidosis, nephrosis, and other infection. Tuberculoid, recovery with residual nerve damage.

The organs involved are skin and subcutaneous nerves.

The pathological changes manifest themselves as cutaneous, papular and nodular lepromas.

The diagnosis is made by identification of organism in an overt lesion or in nasal scrapings.

References

Fasal, P.: Leprosy Occurs Everywhere. GP. *32*:95, 1965.
Proceedings of Symposium on sulfones by the U.S.-Japan cooperative medical science program. Internat. J. Leprosy, *35*(4, pt. 2):563, 1967.

36. Coccidioidomycosis (Valley Fever)

ORVILLE HORWITZ

Cause: Coccidioides immitis, a dimorphic fungus.

Early Manifestations: Often like those of influenza: headache, backache, fever, malaise, cough, fatigue, and pleuritic pain. History of being in San Joaquin Valley.

Treatment: Amphotericin B. In meningitis, intrathecal adminstration 2 to 3 times weekly. 1.0 mg./ml. glucose solution diluted with 10 cc. cerebrospinal fluid injected slowly.

Possible Dire Consequences without Treatment: Life threatening in less than 1 in 1,000 infections, but untreated meningitis is 100% fatal.

The organs involved are lungs, skin, subcutaneous tissue, bones in disseminated form, and meninges.

The pathological changes include pneumonitis with possible cavity formation, coccidiomas (solitary nodules), fistulae and lymphadenopathy.

The diagnosis is made by isolation of fungus. Skin tests negative early in disease.

Reference

Fiese, M. J.: Coccidioidomycosis. Springfield, Charles C Thomas, 1958.

37. Schistosomiasis

EILEEN RANDALL

Cause: Schistosoma mansoni, Schistosoma haematobium, Schistosoma japonicum.

Early Manifestations: Dermatitis due to penetration of the skin by the cercariae, tissue reactions to the maturing worms inside and outside of the blood vessels and associated toxic and allergic reactions. Manifestations include dysentery, hepatic cirrhosis, splenomegaly, pneumonitis, vascular occlusion, and constitutional intoxication.

Treatment: S. japonicum: tartar emetic
S. mansoni and *S. haematobium:* Stibophen (Fuadin); Stibocaptate (Antimony dimercaptosuccinate); and Niridazole (Ambilhar).

Possible Dire Consequences without Treatment: Ascites, anemia, and portal cirrhosis which may lead to death.

Of the three human species of *Schistosoma, S. mansoni* is seen more commonly in the United States primarily due to the endemicity of the organism in Puerto Rican people. *Schistosoma japonicum* is present in the Far East and *S. haematobium* primarily in Africa. *Schistosoma mansoni* is also found in Africa, South America and the West Indies.

Schistosoma haematobium is the cause of vesical schistosomiasis, schistosomal hematuria or urinary bilharziasis. *Schistosoma japonicum* is the cause of oriental schistosomiasis or intestinal schistosomiasis. *S. mansoni* produces intestinal schistosomiasis.

Schistosomiasis can be divided into three stages: (1) developmental from the cercarial penetration of the skin to the mature adult worm, (2) active oviposition and extrusion of eggs and (3) tissue proliferation and repair. The manifestations depend upon the worm burden, the numbers of eggs laid and the site of oviposition. *Schistosoma japonicum* migrate mainly to the lower branches of the superior mesenteric veins which drain the lower ileum and cecum. *Schistosoma mansoni* migrate mainly to the colic branches of the superior and inferior mesenteric veins. *S. haematobium* migrate mainly to the vesical and pelvic plexuses. *Schistosoma mansoni* may lay as many as 300 eggs daily into the venules while *S. japonicum* may lay 3,500 eggs.

The eggs, when laid in the venules, provoke a tissue response and develop into granulomas or non-necrotizing pseudotubercles. The eggs can often be found in other parts of the body. The eggs of *S. mansoni* and *S. japonicum* are often swept into the liver to evoke pseudotubercle formation, and the eggs of *S. haematobium* may reach the lungs and sometimes the liver. Eggs have been reported from practically every site of the body including the central nervous system.

The metabolites of the organism are discharged and contribute to allergic and toxic manifestations in the patient.

Abdominal tenderness, hepatitis, anorexia, fever, headache, myalgia, dysentery, weight loss are characteristic of intestinal schistosomiasis. In vesical schistosomiasis as the mucosal surfaces become inflamed painful micturition and frequency begin with mucus and pus present in the urine. Eventually fibrosis of the entire bladder may occur.

The diagnosis of *S. mansoni* and *S. japonicum* infections are made by finding the characteristic eggs in feces or from intestinal biopsies. *Schistosoma haematobium* eggs are found in urine. The leukocyte count is increased and there is usually an eosinophilia.

Schistosoma japonicum is the most difficult to treat. This involves the intravenous administration of progressively increasing doses of 0.5% tartar emetic on alternate days until a total of about 500 ml. has been given. The initial dose is 4 ml. and the maximum single dose is 25 to 30 ml.

For treatment of *S. mansoni* and *S. haematobium* Stibophen (Fuadin) is used. This is an organic trivalent antimonial in solution in 5 ml. ampoules containing 8.5 mg. of antimony. The usual dose is 4 to 5 ml. IM daily for five days a week for four weeks; or a total dose of 80 to 100 ml. The principal toxic manifestation is vomiting. This is the drug most commonly used in the United States. Nitridazole (Ambilhar) is a nitrothiazole derivative which is effective against *S. haematobium* infections. The optimum dose seems to be 12.5 mg. per kg. twice a day for seven days. Children may require up to 40 mg. per kg. per day.

References

Brown, Harold W., and Belding, David, L.: Basic Clinical Parasitology. New York, Appleton-Century-Crofts, 1964.

Faust, Ernest, Russell, Paul and Jung, Rodney: Craig and Faust's Clinical Parasitology.
8th Ed. Philadelphia, Lea & Febiger, 1970.
Most, Harry: Treatment of Common Parasitic Infections of Man Encountered in the United
States. New Eng. J. Med. *287*:698, 1972.

38. Ascariasis

Eileen Randall

Cause: Ascaris lumbricoides, the large intestinal round worm of man.

Early Manifestations: Large numbers of migrating larvae may produce pneumonitis.
Heavy infections of adults in the small intestine lead to abdominal pain and
vomiting. Acute colicky pains in the epigastric region are at times experienced.

Treatment: Pyrantel, Hexylresorcinol Crystoids, Piperazine Citrate (Antepar) and
Thiabendazole.

Possible Dire Consequences without Treatment: In heavy infections abdominal obstruction
may occur. A worm may migrate into the appendix and cause appendicitis.
Abdominal perforation has been known to occur.

The pathology and symptomatology are divided into two types, the respiratory
manifestations produced by the migrating larvae and the manifestations produced
by the adult worms which normally reside in the small intestine.

As the migrating larvae escape from the blood vessels into the alveoli on their
way to the bronchioles trauma and petechial hemorrhage occur. Ascaris pneumonitis
may occur, especially in children.   Frequent spasms of coughing, bronchial rales and
physical signs of lobular involvement usually lasting one to two weeks are observed.

The adult worms are found in the lumen of the small intestine and feed on liquid
nutrient material present.

At times the worms may be passed spontaneously through the anus, may be vomited
or even passed through the nares. The most common symptoms provoked by the
adults are vague abdominal discomfort and acute colicky pains in the epigastric
region.

Those ascarids which wander may produce acute symptoms such as ileus caused by
many worms matted together, perforation of the bowel and acute appendicitis due to
the presence of the worm in the appendiceal lumen.   Other less common complications may be blockage of the ampulla of Vater or the common bile duct, entry into the
parenchyma of the liver by adult wandering worms and hemorrhagic pancreatitis.

A diagnosis is made by recovery of fertilized and/or unfertilized eggs or recovery
of the adult. If only male worms are present, the diagnosis is difficult. An eosinophilia of 10% or more is frequently observed.

The drugs for therapy in order of efficacy are: Pyrantel, 10 mg. per kg. single dose
(1 ml. of the suspension per 4.5 kg. and not to exceed 1 gm.); Piperazine, 50 to 75 mg.
per kg. daily (not to exceed 4 gm.) in a single dose for two days; and Thiabendazole,
25 mg. per kg. twice a day for two days.

Hexylresorcinol crystoids can be used in the dosage of 1 gm. for adults, 0.6 gm. for children under school age and 0.8 gm. for those between six and ten years of age.

Ascaris infection is more common in warm, moist areas of the world but occasionally is seen in patients in the northern areas of the United States especially in late summer and early fall.

References

Faust, Ernest, Russell, Paul, and Jung, Rodney: Craig and Faust's Clinical Parasitology, 8th Ed. Philadelphia, Lea & Febiger, 1970.
Most, Harry: Treatment of Common Parasitic Infections of Man Encountered in the United States. New Eng. J. Med. *287*:495, 1972.

39. Hookworm Infection

EILEEN RANDALL

Cause: Necator americanus or *Ancylostoma duodenale.*

Early Manifestations: Cutaneous manifestations of "ground itch" where the larvae penetrate the skin. This consists of itching and burning followed by edema and erythema of the area which develops into a papular eruption ending in vesicles. With moderate blood decompensation in hookworm disease the symptoms consist of heartburn, flatulence, feeling of fullness in the abdomen and epigastric pain. There may be low grade intermittent fever, dyspnea and palpitation of the heart.

Treatment: Tetrachlorethylene, Bephenium (Alcopara), Hexylresorcinol.

Possible Dire Consequences without Treatment: Severe untreated hookworm disease will terminate in physical exhaustion, cardiac failure and anasarca.

Light hookworm infection produces few or no symptoms. Hookworm disease is a chronic, debilitating disease which varies in individuals depending on the worm burden, the nutritional state of the patient, and the degree of anemia. As the worms attach to the small intestine and feed on blood the disease is first characterized by a hyperchromic microcytic anemia.

The pathology and symptomatology are proportional to the number of worms and nutritional intake of the patient. In adults an infection with 50 worms is subclinical, one with 50 to 125 worms is borderline and one with 500 is serious. Depending on the degree of anemia, which may be as low as 2.0 gm./100 ml. of blood, the patient experiences dyspnea on exertion, weakness, and dizziness.

A diagnosis is established by finding the characteristic eggs and/or rhabdiform larvae in the feces. These must be distinguished from *Strongyloides* which are similar in appearance. An egg count which can be used to establish the worm burden should be done so this information is available to guide therapy.

Necator is the most common species in the Western Hemisphere. However, *Ancylostoma* have been found in veterans, Peace Corps personnel or missionaries.

Infections with *Ancylostoma* are more severe and produce symptoms with fewer worms than infections with *Necator*, as the former consumes more blood.

For treatment the drug first employed is tetrachlorethylene at a dose of 0.12 ml. per kg. (maximum 15 ml.) taken in a fasting state. It may take several courses of drug to reduce the number of worms markedly. If a fair number of eggs persist, bephenium (Alcopara) in a single 5 gm. dose can be given. This drug may not be as effective for *Necator* infections as for *Ancylostoma* infections. Hexylresorcinol (Crystoids) can be used and repeated at three-day intervals. The adult dosage is 1 gm. and that for pre-school children 0.6 gm. and that for children between six and ten years 0.8 gm.

If *Ascaris* is present, it should be treated before the patient is given tetrachlorethylene. High protein food and iron supplementation should be administered.

In northern continental United States hookworm infection and/or disease is rarely seen. However, in Puerto Rican populations migrating to the north, the worm is not uncommonly found. Recently there has been a reported increase in the numbers of children in the southern United States diagnosed to be harboring hookworm eggs in their feces.

References

Faust, Ernest, Russell, Paul, and Jung, Rodney: Craig and Faust's Clinical Parasitology, 8th Ed., Philadelphia, Lea & Febiger, 1970.
Brown, Harold: Basic Clinical Parasitology, 3rd Ed., New York, Appleton-Century-Crofts, 1969.
Most, Harry: Treatment of Common Parasitic Infections of Man Encountered in the United States. New Eng. J. Med., *287*:495, 1972.

40. Visceral Larva Migrans

EILEEN RANDALL

Cause: *Toxocara canis* and *T. cati*, dog and cat ascarids.

Early Manifestations: The most consistent early manifestation is persistent eosinophilia.

Treatment: Thiabendazole.

Possible Dire Consequences without Treatment: In heavy infections hepatomegaly, pulmonary disease, cardiac dysfunction, nephrosis, evidence of cerebral lesions, or eye lesions may occur. Death may ensue.

Visceral larva migrans is a disease which results from usually dog and sometimes cat ascarid larvae involving the viscera of an abnormal host—man. It has been reported to be due also to aberrant human *Ascaris*, *Strongyloides*, and hookworm larvae.

Characteristically the lesions are in the liver which microscopically show small,

8

gray elevated areas.   Microscopically these are granulomatous lesions consisting of eosinophils, lymphocytes, epithelioid cells and foreign body type giant cells which surround the larva.   These eosinophilic granulomas may be found in practically every organ of the body.

The symptomatology depends upon the number of migrating larvae.   The lesions may be very few or miliary.   The clinical picture varies dependent upon the sites where the granulomas develop.   The most common sites involved are the liver, followed by lung, kidneys, heart, striated muscles, brain and the eyes.

A persistent eosinophilia varying from 20 to 80% is present.   No symptoms may be present or the picture may be that of one characterized by hepatomegaly, pulmonary disease, cardiac dysfunction, nephrosis, fever, hyperglobulinemia, cough, cerebral signs, and eye signs.   It has been reported that eyes of children removed because of a clinical diagnosis of retinoblastoma revealed nematode larvae in some of them.   Severe infections have resulted in death.

Diagnosis is suggested by eosinophilia, hepatomegaly, fever and asthma.   The diagnosis can be confirmed by liver biopsy and serologic tests.   Cross reactions do occur with ascariasis and strongyloidiasis.

The infection is usually seen in young children one to five years of age who practice pica.   The embryonated eggs are swallowed by the dirt-eating children and after hatching in the intestine the larvae begin their migration.

Visceral larva migrans due to dog or cat ascarid may not respond to any therapy but it has been suggested that thiabendazole may be helpful.

References

Brown, Harold: Basic Clinical Parasitology, 3rd Ed., New York, Appleton-Century-Crofts, 1969.

Faust, Ernest, Russell, Paul, and Jung, Rodney: Craig and Faust's Clinical Parasitology, 8th Ed., Philadelphia, Lea & Febiger, 1970.

Chapter VIII

Infection and Nephritis

Introduction

Man is a competitor with and provider of nutriment to diverse organisms which are ubiquitous to the point of residing in his gut, astride his food supply at its very entry. This renders the liver a ceaseless inactivator of microorganisms and of their metabolic products, which gain access via lacteals and portal capillaries to its circulation. Further upstream a similar processing function is performed by the lung which removes native and foreign proteins and peptides that come to it by the way of alveoli and returning systemic blood. But glial cells astride circulatory outreaches to the brain, which has no such processing function, rigorously exclude them. In general organs most highly endowed with an endothelial expanse also are highly "reticular," that is to say, they have a proportionate mononuclear phagocytic system. The demands placed upon such a system by the kidneys' specialized functions, that place nutrient flow in series rather than in parallel with its processing flow, are, however, unusually exacting. Some problems thus arising from this particular exposure to competing Scylla and Charybdis of the microbial world, infection and opposing immunity, are discussed in this chapter. Like problems as they affect supporting tissues and other viscera have been discussed in earlier chapters, and are considered in subsequent chapters on the lungs, endocrine organs and the heart.

Particularly relevant here are some humoral agents of host defense, especially serum proteins, that make up about 10% by weight of the globulin fraction of blood, and that collectively are termed complement. They form a highly effective protective system that is, although preformed, largely potential, becoming operational only insofar as some remainder of the globulin fraction attains specificity as immunoglobulins (Ig) (antibodies). This requires recognition of a site, usually on a cell surface as antigenic, the ensuing step being coating of the site by antibodies. One effect of this is to render the site at risk to cytotoxic attack by lymphocytes. Another is to trigger an inflammatory response (allergic inflammation, complex-mediated hypersensitivity); this begins with combination of antibody with antigen activating a circulating sialoglycoprotein (Hageman factor; blood coagulation factor XII) which glass, collagen, fatty acids, homocystine and other stimuli may activate non-specifically. Hageman factor catalyzes tissue kinins that initiate vasodilation, platelet aggregation, and the release of serotonin and of other vasoactive materials. Ratio of antibody to antigen molecules affects the magnitude of the inflammatory response, there being more local inflammation, complement activation and phagocytosis with antibody excess (Arthus reaction). With antigen excess there is formation of soluble complexes having the potentiality for distant dispersion (serum sickness reaction). This sequel may become the mechanism whereby distant immunologic responses inflict kidney damage by complex-mediated hypersensitivity with in situ activation of complement.

With attachment of antibody to an antigenic site two portions of an IgM molecule or two distinct IgG molecules can orient so as to permit attachment of a subunit of the first component of complement, which has three subunits designated C1q, C1r, and C1s. The recognition unit making this initial attachment is C1q, largest and most basic of the complement proteins, along with C8 the only one that migrates as a gamma globulin. Next added is C1r, which like most complement proteins migrates as a beta globulin, followed by C1s. This component again is iconoclastic in migrating, along with C9, the other smallest complement protein, as an alpha globulin. At this point in assembly C1 has an aggregate molecular weight of a million and is held apart from the site of Ig attachment. The C1s moiety last added then functions as an enzyme to effect union of C4 and C2 to produce a larger enzyme of 350,000 molecular weight; its activity is directed toward activation of C3, most abundant of complement proteins with a serum concentration of around 120 mg./100 ml. The activated C3 molecules, less a 4% portion of their bulk called C3b, now can fix at sites near the Ig attachment, amplifying its effect nearly a hundred fold. Complement activation to this point can be attained without prior antibody attachment, mediated by natural humoral substances such as kallikrein and plasmin. It also may begin at the stage of C3 because of the existence of other circulating proenzymes that are susceptible to activation by cobra venom components, gram-negative bacterial endotoxin, and possibly properdin. If there is enhanced C3 activation, there may be a decreased serum level due to cell attachment, detectable by decreased migration of the beta-1c component on immunoelectrophoresis, or due to abnormal breakdown, detectable by breakdown products migrating in the beta-1A and alpha-2D fractions. Abnormal breakdown is postulated in some varieties of nephritis disposed to chronicity and to persistently decreased C3 without equivalent decreases in other complement components. All of some 8 identified phenotypes of C3 appear to have similar migration characteristics, biologic properties, and molecular weights of around 185,000.

Attachment of molecules of activated C3 to cell surfaces renders them increasingly at risk from phagolysosomal enzymes, with or without engulfment. Phagocytes have receptors facilitating their attachment both to the surface Ig (opsonic adherence) and to the surface complement (immune adherence) on cell surfaces. At the same time highly basic small fragments of C3b which were discarded in the activation of C3 exhibit chemically separable chemotactic (granulocyte attracting) and anaphylotoxic (mast cell degranulating, histamine releasing and accordingly vasodilating) properties which further favor phagocyte attack. The properties of C3b are further amplified by the remaining complement components in minute concentrations within the beta globulin fraction, C5, 6, and 7. Allergic inflammation, as occurs in anaphlyactoid hypersensitivity, is characterized by ability of IgE, the antibody class evoked, to fix mast cells directly, bypassing complement activation entirely.

The kidney is exposed by the circulation to the consequences of microbial attacks elsewhere to directly assaulting microbes, with many of its ills on both accounts being inflammatory. This may be localized primarily in vessels and glomeruli, or primarily in interstitium and pelvis. Infection is most suspect in the latter, but interstitial inflammation and/or scarring additionally may occur (1) congenitally, due to dysplasia, (2) in old age, due to senescence, or (3) at any time due to immunologic reactions, to radiation, drugs, fever, obstruction, high or low perfusion pressure, caloric or specific malnutrition, electrolyte imbalance, or insolubility of phosphates or urates. In the more likely event that the cause is microbial, the most ubiquitous threat is from commensals from the nearby gut, skin and urethra. Moreover the kidney harbors commensals of its own; a good cell line for viral cultures is embryonic human kidneys, where legally available after stillbirths and hysterotomies, because they have acquired no post-natal wild viruses. If, however, kidneys of adult cynomolgus or rhesus monkeys are used, some 30 wild viruses have to be excluded, and the problem doubtless exists with the kidneys of other primates, including man. Some of the larger RNA viruses (mumps, rabies, rubella) and intermediate-sized DNA viruses (adenovirus, megalovirus) have been recovered from human urine during infections, as well as smaller RNA (entero-, arbo-) viruses.

Pasteur knew one hundred and ten years ago that the gut organisms are not fastidious in their growth requirements and that urine is a culture medium for them. They are kept out of the urine at one portal because the blood stream itself repels them and because the structurally normal kidney is a poor bacterial filter. At the other portal, normal rapid voiding prevents entry from the unsterile urethra. In the male, inhibitory seminal and prostatic secretions may restrict the flora to gram-positive cocci and rods of lesser pathogenicity.

Significant bacteriuria occurs in 0.03% of schoolboys, 1.2% of schoolgirls, 0.5% of unhospitalized men (Wales, Jamaica), 2.5% of urban women (Seattle, Jamaica), 5% of rural women (Wales, Jamaica), 6% of pregnant women, 34% of pregnant women with proteinuria, 6% of male diabetics, and 18% of female diabetics. The organisms are about 75% E. coli and 25% A. aerogenes as long as the source is endogenous. With more contact with a hospital ward or outpatient department, the pattern shifts to a "nosocomial" one: 35% E. coli, 15% A. aerogenes, 10% each proteus, pseudomonas, and staphylococcus, 5% each enterococcus and miscellaneous, and 10% negative. Bacteria can be cultured from 36% of needle biopsies and 29% of necropsies, if the histologic findings include interstitial and intratubular pleomorphic exudates with periglomerular fibrosis; and the organisms then are the same as in urine in 78% and 71% respectively of the specimens.

Cystitis may occur without upper tract and renal infection if there is (1) rapid antegrade peristalsis whenever urine enters a ureter from either end, (2) reverse peristalsis is absent, a criterion usually satisfied in the absence of particulate materials such as calculi, and (3) compression of the intramural ureter occurs during periods of high intravesical pressure (voiding). The conventional contrast urogram evaluates peristalsis poorly, because it is not dynamic, has some but limited resolution of calculi, and justifies its performance best when a post-voiding film is included.   Dye if seen in the bladder after voiding is assumed to result from one of two mechanisms: (1) failure of an incompetent or obstructed bladder to empty completely, or (2) reflux into the ureters at the height of micturition, with return to the bladder upon its cessation.   The latter is proven by means of films, taken with a fast film-changer or cine, throughout voiding, using contrast material instilled from below, rather than excreted via the kidney.   When re-examined in this way 60% of patients having (1) calyceal changes, (2) ureteral changes, or (3) residual urine are found to have reflux.

The treatment of cystitis and of pyelonephritis might in theory be different. Antibiotics like nitrofurantoin and penicillin are actively pumped into urine by the organic acid transport system of renal tubular epithelium, attaining high urine levels with minimal renal tissue concentrations.   This might be appropriate in cystitis with primarily mucosal involvement.   Practically it is so difficult to exclude pyelonephritis that choice of antibiotic and of dosage is predicated upon attaining bactericidal or bacteriostatic tissue levels.   Further difficulties occur as renal infection or other factors reduce renal function. Then the doses of antibiotics highly dependent upon elimination in the urine require revision.

1. Pyelonephritis and Urinary Tract Infections

CALVIN M. KUNIN

Cause: Bacterial colonization of the urinary tract.

Early Manifestations: Asymptomatic (bacteria in urine), or signs of lower urinary tract infection (bacteria in urine plus signs of inflammation of bladder), or signs of upper urinary tract infection (fever, flank pain, tenderness, leukocytosis, leukocyte casts, bacteria in urine; with or without concomitant signs of inflammation of the bladder).

Treatment: Antimicrobial therapy of acute infection.   Eradicative agents for short and long-term prophylaxis.

Possible Dire Consequences without Treatment: Reduced renal function.   Renal insufficiency.   Death.

Fifteen years ago an article entitled, "Asymptomatic Infections of the Urinary Tract," appeared in the Transactions of the American Association of Physicians written by Dr. Edward Kass of Boston.   Dr. Kass outlined the value of the quantitative bacterial count on clean-voided urine in distinguishing true bacteriuria from contamination during collection and provided an overall summary of the frequency of significant bacteriuria in various clinic and hospital patient populations. As with all significant advances in medical practice these observations stimulated tremendous interest, a flood of literature and an abundance of unanswered questions. Even today, after much experience and study, many well-informed physicians are still uncertain whether to consider the finding of persistent significant bacteriuria as simply an abnormal laboratory finding or as a disease requiring vigorous treatment. Does it mean that the patient has silent pyelonephritis of simple colonization of his urine with benign bacteria?

The matter becomes increasingly urgent to clarify when we reflect that we have potent antimicrobial agents to deal with the problem, if there is one, and may have to perform expensive diagnostic studies if we are not to miss some important, but occult, predisposing factors. I shall try to place bacteriuria and its role in patients with pyelonephritis in this brief review and try to clarify some of the issues.

First of all, the findings of significant bacteriuria should be considered as an abnormal laboratory test rather than a disease. As with all bacteriologic laboratory procedures the value of the test depends upon the reliability of the collection procedure. Bladder urine is ordinarily sterile but, when voided, collects small numbers of bacteria from the urethra. If these are not discounted by the quantitative count (almost invariably at levels less than 10,000 colonies per ml.) and distinguished from true urinary colonization (in the overwhelming majority of instances at greater than 100,000 colonies per ml.), the test will be misinterpreted. Many physicians have been troubled by the borderline counts of between 10 and 100 thousand and wonder why these are not considered as significant. The answer is that such counts may at times be significant if they are persistently found with recovery of the same bacterial strain. All such borderline counts should be repeated. Many people forget, however, that the counting method was designed primarily for clean-voided urines and that specimens obtained by aseptic methods such as by suprapubic aspiration or at operation are considered as significant bacteriuria if any bacteria are present, regardless of the numbers.

Now that we have reliable methods to diagnose significant bacteriuria, the question should be asked—what value does it have? This may be succinctly answered as follows:

Significant bacteriuria is the most common denominator of urinary tract infections. Therefore, when properly used, it can be an extremly reliable aid in diagnosis, an important guide to therapy and an excellent means of following patients for early evidence of recurrent infection. Unfortunately as with many other laboratory tests, the expense to the patient may at times be too great to permit routine testing, particularly in office practice. It is therefore understandable that physicians are reluctant to subject their patients to added expense.

Fortunately, there are several means to get around these economic barriers. First, examination of fresh urinary sediment in wet mount preparations at high dry magnification will often reveal numerous bacteria and be diagnostic. Similarly the absence of bacteria indicates that the patient is responding to treatment. Most important, however, is the introduction in recent years of convenient and reliable kits to perform quantitative urine cultures in the office or home. The best of these is the "dip-slide" and its many modifications (Figs. VIII–1, 2 and 3) which are widely used in Europe and are now being introduced into this country. In Wisconsin, as

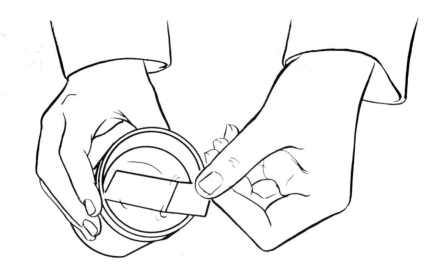

Fig. VIII–1. Using the dip slide for culture. (Kunin: Detection, Prevention and Management of Urinary Tract Infections, Lea & Febiger.)

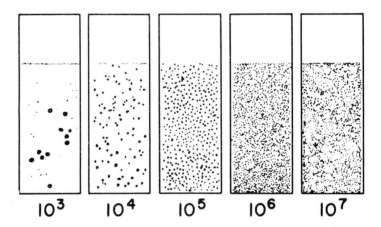

Fig. VIII–2. Interpretation of the dip slide by colony density. (Kunin: Detection, Prevention and Management of Urinary Tract Infections, Lea & Febiger.)

part of the Regional Medical Program, we distributed 3,000 slides per month, at
cost of about 65 cents to practicing physicians. The cost of a prepackaged dip slide
will vary with the manufacturer. A new device containing dehydrated media pads
and a Griess reagent pack, manufactured by the Ames Company, appears to be
most promising and may be particularly convenient for office use.

Screening for bacteriuria can be highly productive, if restricted to the population
that will most benefit and combined with a careful program of evaluation and
follow-up. These groups include young schoolgirls, sexually active girls (particularly
as part of a premarital evaluation) and pregnant women. The major goal is to detect
structural abnormalities early and prevent morbidity from symptomatic infection
which is so troublesome to many women. The literature is replete with articles
emphasizing that pyelonephritis may produce premature hypertension and renal

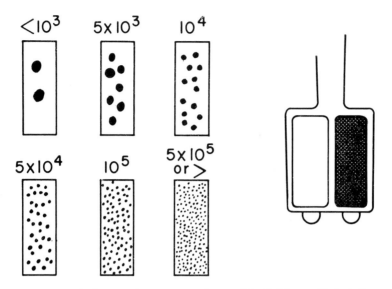

Fig. VIII–3. Bacteriuria screening test manufactured by Baltimore Biologic Laboratories. This device uses the same principle as the dip slide method. In this modification, E.-M.B. agar (blackened area) and trypticase soy agar (clear area), are layered side by side on a plastic "shovel." Only one face is used. The test is read by pattern as shown on the left. The entire device is packaged in a sterile container. The handle of the device is much larger than shown to permit easy manipulation. (Kunin: Detection, Prevention and Management of Urinary Tract Infections, Lea & Febiger.)

failure. It currently appears that, although these complications do occur, they are relatively rare. The major concern of the physician should be to make his patient with urinary infections as comfortable as possible and follow him or her closely to detect the major problem of recurrent infection and abort it by early diagnosis and treatment. As an added dividend he will prevent infection, stones, and other complications in a small, but significant, portion of the population.

In this regard, one of the most loosely used medical terms is "chronic pyelonephritis." This conjures up the image of a kidney slowly rotting from disease. In actuality it is usually used to denote that the patient may have recurrent symptomatic infection or has the radiologic finding of a calyceal distortion in the intravenous pyelogram. Neither of these findings really indicate active infection of the kidney. They may simply mean that the urinary tract is infected somewhere along the tract or that residual scars of old burned-out disease are present. In my view the diagnosis of active chronic pyelonephritis can only be suspected if the patient has upper tract signs or symptoms, fever, renal stones or evidence from localizing studies that bacteria are coming from the upper tract. Even then we do not know whether or not the renal parenchyma is infected. In the absence of a definitive method to routinely screen patients for active pyelonephritis, we should anticipate its presence by treatment directed at the organism in the urine. This is usually quite practical since the treatment of active pyelonephritis does not differ very much from that of treatment of asymptomatic bacteriuria.

The principles of therapy are based on adequate culture and sensitivity tests. Short courses of specific antimicrobial agents and frequent, routine follow-up are used to be sure that the infection is eradicated and has not silently recurred. The efficacy of antimicrobial agents depends more on *in vitro* sensitivity tests than virtues such as bactericidal versus bacteriostatic action. For the common *E. coli* infections, sulfonamides, tetracyclines and ampicillin are about equally effective and the choice of drug should depend upon sensitivity tests, relative expense and side effects. Nitrofurantoin is particularly useful for highly recurrent infections while nalidixic acid and cephalexin are usually reserved for special instances in which the organisms are not sensitive to other agents.

Prophylaxis is reserved in our practice for patients with highly recurrent, closely spaced infections. We prefer nitrofurantoin (which can be given in full dose or tried as 50 to 100 mg. at bedtime). In some patients who cannot tolerate this drug we use methenamine mandelate or hippurate together with ascorbic acid to acidify the urine. Prophylaxis is not prolonged for more than one to three months so that we can determine whether recurrences have stopped. Management of severe systemic infection is a very special problem and is beyond the scope of this article.

In sum, bacteriuria is most useful when thought of as a guide to detection and management. It is not a disease, but a useful laboratory finding. Recurrent infection or renal scars do not necessarily mean the patient has chronic pyelonephritis. The major goal of therapy, urologic evaluation and close follow-up is primarily designed to prevent morbidity and the relatively uncommon, but nevertheless important, complications of urinary tract infection—e.g. stones, reduced renal function, and their sequelae.

References

Kass, E. H.: Asymptomatic infections of the urinary tract. Tr. Am. Assn. Phys. *69*:56, 1956
Kunin, C. M.: Detection, Prevention and Management of Urinary Tract Infection, 2nd Ed. Philadelphia, Lea & Febiger, 1974.

2. Infections During Renal Failure

Joseph H. Magee

Causes: Renal and extrarenal infections.

Early Manifestations: Increased drug side effects due to uncertainties of dosage.

Treatment: Monitoring serum creatinine ([Cr]s) in high risk patients on antibiotics.

Possible Dire Consequences without Treatment: Dose related complications of antibiotic therapy.

Reduction in renal function, however effected, compromises use of the very drugs most able to eradicate infections, including those of the kidney. This dilemma affects choices among available agents, and necessitates dose adjustments for some of those selected, as pointed out by Kunin and co-workers in a series of papers beginning in 1959. The anti-infectious chemotherapeutic agents that Erhlich sought have preponderantly been syntheses from the microbiological world (antibiotics), able to interfere with growth or metabolism of other microorganisms. Out of thousands catalogued, about a hundred have known chemistry, and something is known of their manner of acting. Some inhibit protein synthesis generally and indiscriminately, some disrupt cell membranes generally by a detergent action, and some inhibit cell wall synthesis specifically in bacteria.

Inhibitors of cell wall synthesis include some of the agents most requiring dose modification when used in renal disease, especially the aminoglycoside antibiotics, including streptomycin, kanamycin, and gentamicin. With serum half lives similar to creatinine, around 2.5 hours, they are normally given q 12h so that there is little overlap of successive doses. Since alternate routes of disposal, excepting dialysis, do not emerge to compensate for decreased removal in renal disease, the usual 7 mg./kg. dose of streptomycin and kanamycin is continued as [Cr]s rises but is given at intervals of 9 times [Cr]s in hours instead of q 12h. The dose of gentamicin is continued at 1 mg./kg. and the interval lengthened to 8 times [Cr]s in hours. Unlike streptomycin and kanamycin it is not removed by peritoneal dialysis; like them it should be given following rather than preceding hemodialysis. The former can be added to peritoneal dialysis exchanges, at desired serum levels of 20 mg./ml. for the duration of the procedure as an alternative to injection elsewhere. These antibiotics are as a group associated with VIII nerve damage, a myasthenic syndrome, and postoperative respiratory paralysis. Accumulation of neomycin, which can itself cause toxic nephropathy in addition to these side effects, may occur due to absorption from bowel sterilization regimens during the course of uremia; and it should not be used for bladder sterilization.

Tetracyclines are absorbable antibiotics belonging to the group of inhibitors of microbial cell wall synthesis. They have complex intracompartmental transfers, including the formation of stable complexes with calcium in bone and enamel. Half-lives are about 3 times longer than the aminoglycosides but they are usually given q 6h, with some overlap of successive doses, to attain acceptable serum levels. Dose alterations with renal failure differ from oxytetracycline and tetracycline, where renal elimination is consequential, and for chlortetracycline and doxycycline where it probably is not. For the former where excretion is about two-thirds kidney dependent, sufficient dose overlap will continue if the dose interval is lengthened to 3 times [Cr]s in hours rather than q 6h. Doxycycline is given q 12h both normally and in renal failure. Tetracyclines of both types dialyze poorly, at about a fifth the efficiency of creatinine, but doses should follow dialyses. All are photosensitizing in some individuals and tend to raise [UN]s disparately to [Cr]s, due to their catabolic effect upon host tissues as well as upon microorganisms.

Other inhibitors of protein synthesis include the macrolide antibiotics, represented by erythromycin; and the cross-reacting Clindamycin and lincomycin. The most absorbable (estalate) salt of erythromycin is associated with cholestatic jaundice; the free base and four other salts are not. Excretion by the renal route is minimal. Chloramphenicol, if mandated in renal failure, is given in usual dosage because of rapid hepatic conjugation as the glucuronate. It is removed at half, and the conjugate at one third, the efficiency for creatinine in patients on hemodialysis. It is associated with altered ferrokinetics in a third of individuals who receive it and has in the past been associated with about 30 reported cases of aplastic anemia yearly.

Antibiotics with a detergent effect upon cell membranes include cyclic peptides such as polymyxin (polymyxin B) and colistimethate (polymyxin E). They have half-lives similar to creatinine, and about twice as long as the aminoglycoside antibiotics, and like them are usually given q 12h so that there is little overlap of successive doses. Circumoral paresthesias, facial flushing, dizziness and weakness occur

TABLE VIII–1

$T \frac{1}{2}$ hrs., Uremia			$T \frac{1}{2}$ hrs., Normal
	Metabolic Endproducts		
62	Urea	(90%)	3.1
50	Creatinine	(90%)	2.5
	Absorbable Antibiotics		
?	Cycloserine	(60%)	15
100	Oxytetracycline	(70%)	10
60	Tetracycline	(60%)	6
50	Methacycline	(55%)	8
45	Minocycline	(12%)	15
40	Demeclocycline	(45%)	10
18	Doxycycline	(35%)	18
12	Chlortetracycline	(18%)	6
25	Cephalexin	(75%)	1
10	Cephaloglycin	(25%)	1
15	Carbenicillin	(75%)	1.5
15	Ampicillin	(40%)	1.5
10	Penicillin	(75%)	0.5
10	Nitrofurantoin	(75%)	0.5
8	Lincomycin	(15%)	4
4	Clindamycin	(10%)	2
4.5	Erythromycin	(15%)	1.5
3.5	Isoniazid	(15%)	3.5
3.5	Chloramphenicol	(10%)	2.5
2.5	Rifampin	(13%)	2.5
2.5	Novobiocin	(2.5%)	2.5
2.0	Nalidixic Acid	(15%)	1.5
1.5	Nafcillin	(40%)	0.5
1.5	Dicloxacillin	(40%)	0.5
1.0	Cloxacillin	(40%)	0.5
1.0	Oxacillin	(40%)	0.5
	Nonabsorbable Antibiotics		
1800	Vancomycin	(60%)	6
80	Kanamycin	(70%)	4
80	Viomycin	(70%)	3
80	Capreomycin	(70%)	3
67	Gentamicin	(85%)	3.5
80	Streptomycin	(75%)	2.5
80	Neomycin	(75%)	2
20	Cephaloridine	(70%)	1.5
15	Cephalothin	(75%)	0.75
10	Colistimethate	(60%)	5
4	Methicillin	(40%)	0.5

(Percent urine recovery with normal renal function in parentheses)

routinely, and idiosyncratic though reversible renal insufficiency may occur in previously normal patients. Since the half-life doubles in uremia and there is no removal by hemodialysis, the dose interval should be doubled or the dose halved. The most efficient membrane-detergents are the polyene antibiotics amphotericin and nystatin, which disrupt cholesterol-containing membranes of fungal and host cells. They are ineffective against bacterial cell walls which contain no sterols.

Antibiotics which inhibit the cell wall synthesis of bacteria exploit chemically distinctive adaptations that these cells share only with some of the more primitive algae. Ordinarily one expects molecules to be smaller than cells; with bacteria it is the reverse, bacterial cytoplasm being contained within a huge single macro-molecule called murein, which constitutes its cell wall. Murein is a three dimensional assembly of sugar-containing polymers called mucocomplexes, of which there are three kinds. Techoic acid polymers contain amino acids, phosphates and polyols; mucopolysaccharides contain amino acids and ordinary sugars; and mucopeptides (glycopeptides) (peptidoglycans) contain amino acids and amino sugars. The amino sugars invariably include muramic acid and glucosamine. As few as three amino acids may be present; alanine and glutamic acid are always two of these, and lysine or diaminopimelic acid is always one of the other. Substitution of cyclo-serine results in an ineffective cell wall. Penicillin seems to prevent incorporation of mucopeptides assembled within the cytoplasm into the murein structure at the stage of crosslinking by the pentapeptide bridges. Despite the usual high renal clearance of penicillin, only slightly less for ampicillin and the penicillinase resistant semisynthetics, alternative hepatic extraction greatly mitigates the expected prolongation of half-life when renal function is wanting. The nephrotoxicity unrelated to dose which occurs rarely in patients given methicillin may occur with penicillin in doses exceeding 20 million units. Megadosage also incurs a risk of neurotoxicity and introduces 17 mM K^+ per 10 million units if the potassium salt is used. Other cell wall inhibitors of limited usefulness are bacitracin (topical) and ristocetin and vancomycin (intravenous). The latter are highly dependent upon renal elimination, dialyze poorly, and may cause fever with or without phlebitis, urticaria, VIII nerve damage and further nephropathy. Cephalexin is the preferred oral, and cephalothin the preferred injected, cephalosporin. Both cause false positive copper reduction tests in urine. The delay in excretion in renal failure is of the same order as for penicillin, with greater delay for the desacetyl conjugate of cephalothin. Dose interval can be reduced to thrice daily for patients on dialysis and twice daily for those who are not.

References

Cutler, R. E. and Orme, B. E.: Correlation of serum creatinine concentration and kanamycin half-life. J.A.M.A., *209*:539, 1969.

Greenberg, P. A., and Sanford, J. P.: Removal and absorption of antibiotics in patients with renal failure undergoing peritoneal dialysis. Ann. Intern. Med., *66*:465, 1967.

Kunin, C. M., et al.: Persistence of antibiotics in blood of patients with acute renal failure I. J. Clin. Invest., *38*:1487, 1959.

Kunin, C. M., Colazko, A. J., and Finland, M.: Persistence of antibiotics in blood of patients with acute renal failure II. J. Clin. Invest., *38*:1498, 1959.

Kunin, C. M., and Finland, M.: Persistence of antibiotics in blood of patients with acute renal failure III. J. Clin. Invest., *38*:1508, 1959.

Kunin, C. M., and Finland, M.: Persistence of antibiotics in blood of patients with acute renal failure III. J. Clin. Invest., *38*:1509, 1959.

Kunin, C. M.: A guide to the uses of antibiotics in patients with renal disease. Ann. Intern. Med., *67*:151, 1967.

Last, P. M., and Sherlock, S.: Systemic absorption of orally administered neomycin in liver disease. New Eng. J. Med., *262*:385, 1960.

McHenry, M. C., et al.: Gentamicin doses for renal insufficiency. Ann. Intern. Med., *74*:192, 1971.

New, P. S., and Wells, C. E.: Cerebral toxicity with massive intravenous penicillin therapy. Neurology, *15*:1053, 1965.

3. Tuberculous Pyelonephritis

Joseph H. Magee

Cause: Disseminated tuberculosis, with establishment of renal medullary tuberculous granulomata (tubercles) by hematogenous spread at time of primary infection, or reactivation tuberculosis, next in frequency here to lung apices; establishment of tuberculous cystitis, seminal vesiculitis and epididymitis, by urinary spread then leads to diagnosis of the renal lesions in three-fourths of cases; investigation of azotemia or routine investigation following discovery of pulmonary lesions, accounts for the remainder of cases.

Early Manifestations: Frequency, dysuria. Back, suprapubic or colicky pain. Pyuria: Smears and cultures negative for usual urinary pyogens. Hematuria: May be due either to renal or to prostate and seminal vesicle tubercles, hence is more common in males. Symptomatic epididymitis in males. Fever of unknown origin: Exceptional presentation. Nephrotomography: Through-and-through scars. Pyelography: Non-uniform contraction of calyces. Pyelography: Frequent lower ureteral and infrequent ureteropelvic strictures. Post-voiding cystogram: Vesicoureteral reflux. Cystography: Bladder dome contraction. Urine culture for Mycobacterium tuberculosis. Obtain 6 first voided A.M. specimens for culture, on at least three media plus guinea pig inoculation, prior to commitment to a treatment regime.

Treatment: Isoniazid 100 mg. t.i.d. for two years, plus pyridoxine 50 mg. b.i.d. for 2 years, plus sodium p-aminosalicylate 5 gm. t.i.d. for 2 years, plus cycloserine 250 mg. t.i.d. for 2 years.

Possible Dire Consequences without Treatment: Renal insufficiency due to bilateral involvement. Renal hypertension: Although its occurrence is rare, occasioning but 5% of nephrectomies for tuberculosis, this is the second most efficacious surgical treatment for hypertension upon indication, ranking next to correction of renal arteriovenous fistula.

References

Kauffman, J. J., and Goodwin, W. E.: Renal hypertension secondary to renal tuberculosis. Am. J. Med., *38*:337, 1965.

Lattimer, J. K.: Renal tuberculosis. New Eng. J. Med., *273*:208, 1965.

Lavender, J. P.: Hypertension and tuberculous lesions. Brit. Med. J., *1*:1221, 1957.

Wechsler, H., Westfall, M., and Lattimer, J. K.: The earliest signs and symptoms in 127 male patients with genitourinary tuberculosis. J. Urol., *83*:801, 1960.

4. Mycotic Granuloma

Joseph H. Magee

Cause: Opportunistic mycosis due to: Mucormycosis. Aspergillosis. Candidiasis.

Associated Conditions: Agranulocytosis, antibiotic therapy, cytotoxic therapy, diabetes, endocrinopathy, infancy, malabsorption, malnutrition, neoplasia, pregnancy, surgery, transplantation and trauma.

Early Manifestations: Fever, chills. Frequency, dysuria. Flank pain. Gross hematuria. Sterile pyuria. Mycelia on smear and inhibitory media. Enlarged radiographic renal shadows. Non-opacification on renal angiography and excretory urography.

Treatment: Amphotericin 25 mg./kg. in divided intravenous doses daily over five hours with 5 mg. and increasing by 5 to 10 mg./day, until daily doses of 50 mg. are given. Complications are headache, skin rash, gastrointestinal upset, fever with or without phlebitis, and hypokalemia.

Possible Dire Consequences without Treatment: Confusion with primary anastomotic failures and with rejection crises in kidney grafts. Bilateral involvement, uremia, sepsis, death.

References

Albers, D. D.: Monilial infection of kidney. J. Urol., *69*:32, 1953.
Diriart, H., et al.: Mucoviscidose à localization renale dominante paresitee par une mucoracée. Arch. Franc Pediat., *20*:220, 1963.
Ellis, C. A., and Spivak, M. L.: The significance of candidemia. Ann. Intern. Med., *67*:511, 1967.
Grezer, L. B., and Haley, D. D.: Fungous infection of the urinary tract. Yale J. Biol. and Med., *30*:292, 1958.
Louria, D. B.: Disseminated moniliosis in the adult. Medicine, *41*:307, 1962.
Louvin, D. B.: Deep seated mycotic infections. New Eng. J. Med., *277*:1025, 1126, 1967.
Prout, G. R., Jr., and Goddard, R.: Renal mucormycosis. New Eng. J. Med., *263*:1246, 1960.
Rifkind, D., et al.: Systemic fungal infections complicating renal transplantation and immunosuppressive therapy. Am. J. Med., *43*:28, 1967.
Watson, D. W., and Johnson, A. G.: The clinical use of immunosuppression. Med. Clin. N.A., *53*:1225, 1969.

5. Brucella Granuloma

Joseph H. Magee

Cause: Brucella abortus, suis or melitensis septicemia, following handling infected cattle, pigs and goats respectively (75%); or milk-borne infection (25%). It is believed that 7/8 of cases are not diagnosed. Genitourinary system is most frequent site of persistent disseminated lesions.

Early Manifestations: Frequency and dysuria. Back or suprapubic pain.

Pyuria: routine urine cultures are sterile; cultures under increased carbon dioxide tension grow in 7 to 42 days, usually less than 14; 20% of febrile melitensis cases have positive urine cultures without localizing features.

Hematuria occurs, especially in males, who frequently have epididymoorchitis but not prostatitis; 75% of cases are males aged twenty to forty years. Preceding fever, chills, night sweats, headache, anorexia, weight loss, myalgias, arthralgias, irascibility, weakness and fatigue are usual.

Positive bone marrow, blood, lymph node, stool, or spinal fluid cultures and agglutination titers of 1:100 or more may be obtained upon suspicion of the diagnosis.

Treatment: Tetracycline 500 mg q.i.d. × three weeks.

Possible Dire Consequences without Treatment: Inappropriate treatment due to confusion with genitourinary tuberculosis.

Reference

Forbes, K. A., et al.: Brucellosis of the genito-urinary tract. Urologic Survey, *4*:391, 1954.

6. Septic Infarcts of Kidneys

Joseph H. Magee

Cause: Acute bacterial endocarditis. Other infective endocarditides including candida. Pulmonary infections including streptococcal and pneumococcal. Extra-pulmonary infections with paradoxical arterial embolization. Erythrocytic infections including malaria. Bacteremic phases of typhoid, relapsing and epidemic typhus fevers.

Synonym: Focal embolic nephritis; focal suppurative nephritis.

Early Manifestations: Fever (2/3). Hypertension (1/3). Albuminuria (1/3). Hematuria (1/3). Pain (abdomen, back) (1/3). Tenderness (costovertebral angles) (1/3).

Associated Abnormalities: Splenic, cerebral and pulmonary infarcts.

Treatment: Treatment of primary focus. Consideration of kidney as an ancillary metastasizing focus if further embolization follows satisfactory control.

Possible Dire Consequences without Treatment: Abscess formation and further destruction of the kidney. Death from bacterial endocarditis.

References

Boyarsky, S., Burnett, J. M., and Barker, W. H.: Renal failure in embolic glomerulonephritis as a complication of subacute bacterial endocarditis. Bull. Johns Hopkins Hosp., *84*:207, 1949.
Hoxie, H. J., and Coggin, C. B.: Renal infarction. Arch. Intern. Med., *65*:687, 1940.

7. Renal Carbuncle

JOSEPH H. MAGEE

Cause: Blood-borne staphylococcal renal cortical abscess, usually unilateral and solitary, secondary to distant skin, dental or other focus.

Early Manifestations: Fever, chills, malaise, anorexia, nausea, vomiting. May simulate appendicitis, cholecystitis, diverticulitis, salpingitis. Localizing physical signs are usually absent until late. Right upper pole most common site. Males 2:1, especially young adults. Cocci stainable in urine sediment; culture may be negative or reported as having low colony count. WBC usually greater than 10,000/mm³. Urographic appearance may simulate renal carcinoma, especially when "sterile" due to treatment of recognized extrarenal staphylococcal infection. Signs of perinephric abscess: (*a*) muscle guarding, (*b*) warmth and rubor of overlying skin, (*c*) ipsilateral concave scoliosis, (*d*) fistulous tracts to viscera or skin, (*e*) indistinct psoas margin, (*f*) no renal motion on fluoroscopy or kine-radiography, (*g*) anterior renal displacement on lateral pyelograms, (*h*) gas in perirenal mass, (*i*) thicker wall than cysts on nephrotomography.

Treatment: If *no* extrarenal staphylococcal infective focus is known, appearance of carbuncle should be assumed to be gram-negative abscess, secondary to retrograde lymphogenous rather than hematogenous spread, especially if perinephric drainage has already occurred.

Cloxacillin (Tegopen), or dicloxacillin 2 to 6 gm./day orally; or oxacillin (Prostaphlin) 6 to 12 gm./day orally; in divided doses one hour after eating, and two hours prior to next meal; sulfonamides depress absorption of oxacillin.

In penicillin-sensitive patients Clindamycin (Cleocin) 0.6 to 1.8 gm./day orally in divided doses. Erythromycin 2 gm/day orally in divided doses may be used but entails risk of cholestate hepatitis in courses exceeding one week.

Decision to drain is conditioned by principles, including size, applicable to abscesses elsewhere, by confusion with carcinoma, or is forced by evidence of perinephric extension.

Possible Dire Consequences without Treatment: Perinephric abscess. Other extraurinary drainage (fistulization).

References

Atcheson, D. W.: Perinephric abscess with a review of 117 cases. J. Urol., *46*:201, 1941.

Bosniak, M. A., and Faegenburg, D.: The thick wall sign; an important finding in nephrotomography. Radiology, *84*:692, 1965.

Burger, R. H., Ward, J. N., and Draper, J. W.: Perinephric abscess with gas formation. Am. Surgeon, *30*:302, 1964.

Campbell, M. F.: Perinephric abscess. S.G.O. *51*:674, 1930.

Cobb, O. E.: Carbuncle of the kidney. Brit. J. Urol., *38*:262, 1966.

Colby, F. H., Baker, M. P., and St. Goar, W. T.: Renal carbuncle. New Eng. J. Med., *256*:1147, 1957.

Graves, R. C., and Parkens, L. E.: Carbuncle of the kidney. J. Urol., *35*:1, 1936.

Moore, C. A., and Grangai, M. P.: Renal cortical abscess. J. Urol., *98*:303, 1967.

Nesbit, R. N., and Dick, S. V.: Acute staphylococcal infections of the kidney. J. Urol., *43*:623, 1940.

Pearlman, J. J.: Carbuncle of the kidney. J. Urol., *65*:754, 1951.

8. Non-suppurative Kidney Syndromes

JOSEPH H. MAGEE

Cause: Extrarenal infection (bacterial): Diphtheria, hemophilus, streptococcus, typhoid.

Nonbacterial infection: Syphilis, measles, smallpox, common viral respiratory illnesses.

Immunologic events: Immunization, transfusion reactions, graft rejection crises.

Trauma: Tonsillectomy, dental extractions.

Drug and toxic reactions: (See Acute Interstitial Nephritis).

Synonyms: Benign, essential episodic or recurrent hematuria. Focal non-suppurative nephritis. Focal glomerular nephritis (proliferative, necrotizing).

Early Manifestations: No latent interval. Proteinuria scant or absent. Sediment scant; on differential staining lymphocytes may be distinguished from round epithelial cells. Hypertension absent. Nitrogen retention and oliguria characteristically absent, and where present symmetrical renal enlargement is seen on plain abdominal films or tomograms.

Treatment: Treatment of extrarenal infection. Dietary and dialytic treatment of acute renal failure if it occurs.

Possible Dire Consequences without Treatment: Combined renal and extrarenal (catabolic) azotemia.

The kidneys associated with infantile deaths from diphtheria, scarlet fever and measles were huge, 2 to 3 times normal size, and showed interstitial nephritis most prominent in three areas of the cortex: next to the capsule, next to the medulla and surrounding individual glomeruli. Except when complicating existing glomerular nephritis, however, "the glomeruli show no change" according to the classic paper of Councilman, which attributes the first description to Biermer in 1860. According to Kimmelstiel, "incidental interstitial nephritis is known to accompany almost every infectious or septic condition" including burns, food poisoning and transfusion reactions. Kannerstein found it 20 times more commonly than acute glomerular nephritis in fatal cases of scarlet fever and a high incidence was found by Mallory and Keifer.

However, the para-infectious kidney lesion in patients who survive usually is manifested by hematuria alone, without oliguria, nitrogen retention or hypertension; it may occur either during a single illness or recurrently as long as thirty-one years. Instances without pathologic correlation were reported by Baehr (14 cases), Ellis (35 cases), and Davson and Platt (19 cases) With the advent of the biopsy era the lesion is seen to be a focal proliferative one involving the glomeruli and not the interstitial areas. Bodian and his colleagues presented evidence for an immunologic mechanism. The biopsy appearance is not, however, distinctive in that progression of otherwise similar lesions to diffuse disease occurs in allergic purpura and the Goodpasture syndrome.

References

Baehr, G.: A benign and curable form of hemorrhagic nephritis. JAMA, *86*:1001, 1926.
Bates, R. C., Jennings, R. B., and Earle, D. P.: Acute nephritis unrelated to Group A hemolytic streptococcus infection. Am. J. Med., *23*:510, 1957.
Bodian, M., et al.: Recurrent hematuria in childhood. Quart. J. Med., *34*:359, 1965.
Councilman, W. T.: Acute interstitial nephritis. J. Exp. Med., *3*:393, 1898.
Davson, J., and Platt, R.: A clinical and pathologic study of renal disease. Quart. J. Med., *18*:149, 1949.
Ellis, A.: Natural history of Bright's disease. Lancet, *1*:1, 1942.
Ferris, T. F., et al.: Recurrent hematuria and focal nephritis. New Eng. J. Med., *276*:770, 1967.
Kannerstein, M.: Histologic changes in acute infectious disease. Amer. J. Med. Sci., *203*:65, 1941.
Kimmelstiel, P.: Acute hematogenous interstitial nephritis. Am. J. Path., *14*:737, 1938.
Mallory, G. K., and Keifer, C. S.: Tissue reactions in fatal cases of streptococcus hemolyticus infections. Arch. Path., *32*:334, 1941.
Ross, J. A.: Recurrent focal nephritis. Quart. J. Med., *29*:391, 1960.

9. Liver-Kidney Syndrome I

Joseph H. Magee

Cause: Spirochetes. Contact by abattoir workers, butchers, coal-miners, dairymen, fish-cleaners, pig farmers, sewer workers and others with water, soil or vegetation contaminated by animal urine (cattle, dogs, hedgehogs, hogs, mice, rats, sheep, shrews, moles), infected with Leptospira interrogans (130 serotypes, 22 of which occur in the United States), producing *leptospirosis* (Weil's disease, spirochetal jaundice, canicola fever, Fort Bragg fever). Louse-borne *relapsing fever* due to Borrelia recurrentis. Tick-borne *relapsing fever* due to Borrelia persica and related species.

Early Manifestations: Aseptic meningitis: Headache, nuchal rigidity, retrobulbar pain, photophobia, prostration, protracted vomiting.
Hemorrhages: Conjunctival, subarachnoid; macular or hemorrhagic epistaxes, hemoptyses, hematuria, hematemeses, melena.
Leukocytosis, lymphadenopathy.
Oliguria, azotemia, proteinuria, pyuria.
Jaundice, tender hepatomegaly.
Fever: Higher levels and repeated recurrences suggest relapsing fever.

Treatment: Tetracycline 0.5 gm. every six hours for five days, then 0.5 gm. every twelve hours for *relapsing fever*; value of antibiotics is questioned in *leptospirosis*, but penicillin (4 to 6 million units/day) is favored over tetracycline by some. Treatment of acute renal failure.

Possible Dire Consequences without Treatment: Relapses.

References

Edwards, G. A., and Domm, B. M.: Human Leptospirosis. Medicine, *39*:117, 1960.
Heath, C. W., Alexander, A. D., and Galton, M. M.: Leptospirosis in the United States. New Eng. J. Med., *273*:857, 1965.

10. Liver-Kidney Syndrome II

JOSEPH H. MAGEE

Cause: Ebstein-Barr (E-B) virus. Megalovirus. Rarely herpes simplex virus.

Early Manifestations: Onset with fever and/or headache without pharyngeal syndrome where caused by megalovirus and in 20% of cases where caused by E-B virus. Fever to 104° F. may occur. Antibodies against sheep (1:224 dilution or greater) and horse (1:480 dilution or greater) erythrocytes and against E-B or megaloviruses. IgM antibodies including the cold and heterophile types are raised by various infections but in 1:56 liters after guinea pig kidney absorption are characteristic of classic E-B mononucleosis. Relative and usually absolute atypical lymphocytosis; with 30 to 40% of count being typical and 10 to 20% atypical lymphocyte. Half of cases have splenomegaly. Convalescence is slow with 8% incidence of relapse. Icteric hepatic involvement occurs in 8%. Hematuria and proteinuria occur in 8%. Nephrotic syndrome has been recorded after both classic and megalovirus mononucleosis. Megaloviremia, present in a high proportion of blood donors, may induce mononucleosis without pharyngeal syndrome after multiple transfusions, especially heart surgery.

Treatment: Antibiotics, gamma globulin; usually corticosteroids are not indicated. Rest. Follow spleen size and regulate physical exertion until regression has occurred.

Possible Dire Consequences without Treatment: Splenic rupture.

References

Brun, C., Madsen, S., and Olsen, S.: Infectious mononucleosis with hepatic and renal involvement. Scand. J. Gastroent., *5*:Suppl 7:89, 1970.

De Luca, H. E.: A rare case of cytomegalic inclusion disease. Minerva Med., *16*:1164, 1964.

Greenspan, G.: The nephrotic syndrome complicating infectious mononucleosis. Calif. Med., *98*:162, 1963.

Kaarien, L., Klemola, E., and Paloheino, J.: Rise of cytomegalovirus antibodies in an infectious mononucleosis like syndrome after transfusion. Brit. Med. J., *1*:1270, 1966.

Klemola, E., et al.: Further studies on infectious mononucleosis in healthy persons. Acta Med. Scand., *182*:311, 1967.

Klemola, E., et al.: Cytomegalovirus mononucleosis in previously healthy individuals. Ann. Intern. Med., *71*:11, 1969.

Lindsey, D. C., and Chrisman, W. P.: Gross hematuria as the presenting symptom of infectious mononucleosis. JAMA, *157*:1407, 1955.

Niederman, J. C., et al.: Infectious mononucleosis. JAMA, *203*:205, 1968.

Peters, J. H.: Heterophile reactive antigen in infectious mononucleosis. Science, *157*:1200, 1967.

Taub, E. A.: Renal lesions, gross hematuria and marrow granulomas in infectious mononucleosis. JAMA, *195*:1153, 1963.

Tennant, F. S.: The glomerulonephritis of infections mononucleosis. Texas Rep. Biol. Med., *26*:603, 1968.

Thompson, W. T., and Pitt, C.: Frank hematuria as a manifestation of infectious mononucleosis. Ann. Intern. Med., *33*:1274, 1950.

Tidy, H. L., and Morley, E. B.: Glandular fever. Brit. Med. J., *1*:452, 1921.

Toghill, P. J., et al.: Cytomegalovirus infection in the adult. Lancet *1*:1351, 1967.

Utian, H. L., Fanahoff, A. A., and Plitt, M. D.: Glomerular disease in childhood. S. Afr. Med. J., *38*:162, 1964.

Wechsler, H. F., Rosenblum, A. H., and Sills, C. T.: Infectious mononucleosis. Ann. Intern. Med., *25*:113, 1946.

11. Liver-Kidney Syndrome III (Yellow Fever)

Joseph H. Magee

Cause: Mosquito-borne neurotropic and viscerotropic arbovirus infection.

Early Manifestations: Fever of unknown origin with few other manifestations. High fever to 104° F., with relative bradycardia (Faget's sign), as low as 50 per minute, accompanied by hypotension and cardiac dilatation. Encephalopathy: Headache, photophobia, prostration, restlessness, neck, back and extremity aches. Jaundice, anorexia, vomiting, hiccups, constipation. Mucocutaneous hemorrhagic rash, epistaxes, hematemeses, melena. Proteinuria 3 to 20 gm. per day, hematuria, oliguric acute renal failure.

Treatment: Supportive. Coagulation studies should be undertaken to evaluate role of consumption coagulopathy.

Possible Dire Consequences without Treatment: Hypodynamic and oligemic circulatory failure.

References

Dennis, L. H., et al.: The original hemorrhagic fever: Yellow fever. Blood, *30*:858, 1967.
Strode, G. K.: Yellow Fever. New York, McGraw-Hill Book Co., 1951.

12. Hemorrhage and Uremia

Joseph H. Magee

Cause: Microangiopathy; intravascular coagulation, consumption coagulopathy, and thrombocytopenic purpura; capillary permeability and third space formation; prerenal oliguria with or without subsequent ischemic tubular necrosis; due to mite-borne (Far East and South America), tick-borne (Eastern Europe and Asia) and mosquito-borne (Southeast Asia, Philippines) *arbovirus* infections.

Synonyms: Epidemic hemorrhagic fever (Argentinian, Bolivian, Calcuttan, Cambodian, Central Asian, Crimean, Korean, Malaysian, Omsk, Philippine, Thailand, and Vietnamese); hemorrhagic nephroso-nephritis.

Early Manifestations: Febrile phase: High fever, chills, anorexia, erythema of face and neck, conjunctivitis, palatal exanthem. Hypotensive phase: Arterial and valveless vein hypotension, hemoconcentration, with rise in hematocrit to 70% despite petechiae and ecchymoses, abdominal pain, periorbital edema, proteinuria. Oliguric acute renal failure. Exaggerated diuretic phases are common, with as many as one third of deaths occurring during this interval.

Treatment: Plasma expanders, monitored by venous pressure, and restriction of crystalloid fluids during hypotensive and oliguric phases. Dialytic treatment of hyperkalemia and uremic syndrome. Replacement therapy during diuretic phase.

Possible Dire Consequences without Treatment: Post-necrotic salt loss syndrome, oligemia, death.

References

Entwistle, G., and Hale, E.: Hemodynamic alterations in epidemic hemorrhagic fever.
    Circulation, *15*:414, 1957.
Hollinghorst, R. L., and Steer, A.: Pathology of epidemic hemorrhagic fever. Ann. Intern.
    Med., *38*:77, 1953.
Oliver, J., and MacDowell, M.: The renal lesion of epidemic hemorrhagic fever. J. Clin.
    Invest., *36*:99, 1957.

13. Hemolysis and Uremia

JOSEPH H. MAGEE

Cause: Microangiopathy; intravascular coagulation, consumption coagulopathy,
    and thrombocytopenic purpura; microangiopathic hemolytic anemia; pretubular
    (angiopathic) oliguria due to *enterovirus* infection.

Early Manifestations: Constitutional signs: anorexia, nausea, vomiting, malaise,
    fatigue, myalgias. Neurologic signs: Headache, confusion, stupor, psychotic
    behavior, focal neurologic defects. Renal signs: Hematuria, proteinuria, oliguric
    acute renal failure. Platelet and clotting factor consumption, hemolytic anemia
    with icterus and abnormal (burr) red cells on blood smear, bone marrow and
    lymphoid hyperplasia. Epidemic or sporadic occurrence with peak incidence in
    three- to ten-month-old infants.

Treatment: Treatment of acute renal failure. Heparin may be required for thrombotic
    phenomena despite concurrent hemorrhagic phenomena.

Possible Dire Consequences without Treatment: Uremic syndrome, hyperkalemia, hyper-
    volemia, hypertension, pulmonary edema. Exsanguinating hemorrhage. Hemor-
    rhagic or thrombotic stroke.

References

Gianantonio, C. A., et al.: Acute renal failure in infancy and childhood. J. Pediat., *61*:660,
    1962.
Shinton, N. K., et al.: Hemolytic anemia with acute renal disease. Arch. Dis. Child., *39*:455,
    1964.

14. Post-pharyngitic Nephritis

JOSEPH H. MAGEE

Cause: Microbial antigen in excess, from nephritogenic serotypes of Group A beta-
    hemolytic streptococci, following pharyngeal or tonsil infections, with or without
    scarlatina. Formation of complement-activating soluble complexes with immuno-
    globulin.

Synonyms: Acute diffuse glomerular nephritis. Acute hemorrhagic nephritis. Hemorrhagic Bright's disease. Active onset nephritis. Ellis Type I nephritis. Longcope Type A nephritis. Post-streptococcal nephritis. Post-scarlatinal nephritis. Pharyngitis-associated nephritis.

Early Manifestations: Peak incidence is in winter and spring in schoolchildren aged five to ten years in temperate and cold climates; rare before age three.

Common source epidemics follow direct spread from human reservoirs, probably nasal carriers.

Rheumatic fever attack rate is 3%, regardless of M type, but for nephritis varies from 0.3 to 60% depending upon virulence (resistance to phagocytosis) (M type).

Nephritogenic strains usually have 12 M antigen, occasionally 1 or 4, rarely 6 or 25. Type 49 (Red Lake), frequently associated with skin infections, also causes pharyngitis and scarlatina.

Incidence of throat infections by nephritogenic strains is underestimated because of a tendency of their blood agar colonies to produce greenish, but little or no beta, hemolysis.

Initial raised titers of antistreptolysin O (ASO) in patient's serum (to 1:333 or 8th tube dilution), or 2 tube rises (to 1:625) or falls (to 1:166) during convalescence, are useful in distinguishing infection from carrier state. Nephritogenic strains are large nicotine adenine dinucleotidase (NAD) producers, and initial raised anti-NADase titers of the same magnitudes as ASO are preferred on grounds of specificity. Initial raised titers of anti-streptokinase (ASK) (antifibrinolysin) to 1:166, of antihyaluronidase (AH) to 1:100, and of antistreptodornase B (ASD) (anti-desoxyribonucleotidase B) to 1:100 have similar significance. The 12 tube dilutions in the Rantz-Randall dilution method are 1:12, 1:50, 1:100, 1:125, 1:166, 1:250, 1:133, 1:500, 1:625, 1:833, 1:1250, and 1:2500. At least four other dilution systems in common use may be encountered, however.

Less translucent ("smoky") or Coca-Cola colored urine is noted by parent or patient. Erythrocyturia in casts is easily seen on microscopic urinalysis. Erythrocyturia may persist for months after otherwise complete recovery.

Phase of scant urine output, with low sodium salt despite high total solute content, occurs in most patients recognized as being ill and occasioning its measurement.

Increased plasma and interstitial fluid volumes, weight gain, serous effusions, periorbital and peripheral edema occur.

Filtration rate and filtration fraction (filtration to plasma flow rate ratio) fall; urea nitrogens and creatinines rise.

"The combination of azotemia with well maintained phenosulfonphthalein excretion and high urinary specific gravity is seen in few diseases of the kidney other than acute glomerulonephritis."

Arterial pulse pressure, stroke volume and cardiac output rise, due to salt retention and plasma volume expansion.

Valveless vein and atrial pressures increase without prolongation of the circulation time or increased arteriovenous oxygen difference. Pressures decrease with phlebotomy or bloodless phlebotomy.

Treatment: Treatment of streptococcal infections of pharynx or tonsils, with or without scarlatina: For a minimum of ten days with penicillin V 250 mg. q.i.d. by mouth (or by repository injection form) to prevent secondary otitis, peritonsillar abscess, etc. as well as non-suppurative complications (rheumatic fever, glomerular nephritis, streptococcal fever, scleredema, erythema marginatum). Salt and fluid restriction for duration of oliguria, edema, and congestive manifestations. Ultrafiltration peritoneal or hemodialysis for marked venous pressure elevation, with or without uremia and hyperkalemia.

Possible Dire Consequences without Treatment: Left ventricular dilatation and failure, acute pulmonary edema. Hypertensive encephalopathy. Uremic syndrome, hyperkalemia.

References

Addis, T.: Glomerular nephritis: Diagnosis and treatment   New York, The Macmillan Co., 1948.

Albert, J. J., Pickering, M. R., and Warren, R. J.: Failure to isolate streptococci from children under the age of 3 years with exudative tonsillitis. Pediatrics, *35*:393, 1966.

Brod, J.: Acute diffuse glomerulonephritis. Am. J. Med., 7:317, 1949.

Dixon, F. J.: The pathogenesis of glomerulonephritis. Am. J. Med., *44*:493, 1968.

Ellis, A.: Natural history of Bright's disease. Lancet, *1*:1, 34, 72, 1942.

Epstein, F. H.: Glomerulonephritis, acute and chronic. Lupus, scleroderma, and periarteritis, in Harrison's Principles of Internal Medicine, 6th Ed. Wintrobe, M. M., et al., Ed. New York, McGraw-Hill Book Co., 1970, p. 1411.

Longcope, W. T.: Studies of the variations in the antistreptolysis titer of the blood serum from patients with hemorrhagic nephritis II. Observations on patients suffering from streptococcal infections, rheumatic fever and acute and chronic hemorrhagic nephritis. J. Clin. Invest., *15*:277, 1936.

Michael, A. F., et al.: Acute post-streptococcal glomerulonephritis; Immune deposit disease. J. Clin. Invest., *45*:237, 1966.

Stetson, C. A., et al.: Epidemic acute nephritis. Medicine, *34*:431, 1955.

Uhr, J. W.: The streptococcus, rheumatic fever and glomerulonephritis. Baltimore, The Williams & Wilkins Co., 1964.

15. Post-impetigo Nephritis

Joseph H. Magee

Cause: Complement-activating soluble complexes of immunoglobulin with microbial antigen from nephritogenic serotypes of Group A beta-hemolytic streptococci following skin infections.

Synonyms: Impetigo-associated, pyoderma-associated nephritis; acute glomerular nephritis.

Early Manifestations: Peak incidence in summer and autumn in preschool children in warm or tropical climates.

Endemic or epidemic occurrence involves multiple sources, preceding skin lesions (chronic eczema, dermatitis, venenata, scabies, pediculosis, insect bites, abrasions) and possibly environmental reservoirs and/or mechanical vectors.

Rheumatic fever is not a sequel but nephritis attack rates are similar to those of pharyngeal infection.

Involved nephritogenic strains have unusual M antigens (31, 33, 39, 41, 43, 52), the Red Lake antigen (49M), or M antigens (2, 13, 25) with unusual T antigens; and usually are identified primarily by T agglutination rather than by M precipitation. Infecting strains identical to these, which often are followed by nephritis in children under age $6\frac{1}{2}$ years, also occur in adult skin infections, but seldom are followed by nephritis.

Initial raised titers of antistreptolysin O and anti-NADase do not reliably occur following streptococcal impetigo, although titer changes may be of some help. Antihyaluronidase (AH) titers and antistreptodormase B (ASD) (anti-desoxyribonucleotidase B) titers $\geq 1:100$ initially, and/or titer rises, are preferable in confirming the significance of streptococcal growth in cultured skin lesions, and of post-infectious complications.

Treatment: Penicillin V 250 mg. q.i.d. by mouth every ten days. Acute renal failure is managed as in preceding section.

Possible Dire Consequences without Treatment. Bacteremia. Scarlatina. Oliguric acute renal failure. Non-cardiac circulatory congestion.

References

Dillon, H. C., Jr.: Pyoderma and nephritis. Ann. Rev. Med. *12*:207, 1967.
Futcher, P. H.: Glomerular nephritis following infections of the skin. Ann. Intern. Med., *65*:1192–1210, 1940.
Wannamaker, L. W.: Differences between streptococcal infections of the throat and of the skin. New Eng. J. Med., *282*:23, 78, 1970.

16. Post-endocarditic Nephritis

Joseph H. Magee

Cause: Diffuse or focal non-embolic and non-suppurative lesions after subacute bacterial endocarditis due to α-hemolytic streptococci.

Early Manifestations: Hematuria, proteinuria, or nitrogen retention in a patient with intracardiac shunts or valve lesions, with or without fever, especially if there has been short-term antibiotic treatment of some intercurrent infection.

Hematuria, proteinuria or nitrogen retention in known subacute bacterial endocarditis of about six weeks' duration.

Hypertension and progressive renal insufficiency are considered exceptional but occurred in 10% of fatal cases analyzed by Villareal and Sokoloff.

Treatment: Lesion is reversible with eradication of bacterial antigen and consists of treatment based upon culture.

Possible Dire Consequences without Treatment: Confusion with septic infarcts (focal embolic nephritis) (See p. 204).

The lesion, a disappearing one in the antibiotic era, was sterile, seen in subacute (viridans) endocarditis, after about six weeks. Septic infarcts, seen in acute and subacute endocarditis, may occur at any time, with prominent hypertension and renal insufficiency and have not similarly disappeared.

References

Bell, E. T.: Glomerular lesion associated with endocarditis. Am. J. Path., *8*:639, 1932.
Spain, D. M., and King, D. W.: The effect of penicillin on the renal lesions of subacute bacterial endocarditis. Ann. Intern. Med., *36*:1086, 1952.
Villareal, H., and Sokoloff, L.: The occurrence of renal insufficiency in subacute bacterial endocarditis. Am. J. Med. Sci., *220*:655, 1950.

17. Shunt Nephritis

JOSEPH H. MAGEE

Cause: Complement-activating immune complexes of bacterial antigen, from Staphylococcus albus or aureus infections of ventriculocisternal or ventriculoatrial shunts for relief of hydrocephalus, with host immunoglobulins.

Early Manifestations: Heavy proteinuria, low serum proteins, nephrotic edema, nitrogen retention, hypertension usually absent. Infection may be otherwise absent. Infection may be otherwise occult.

Treatment: Antibiotic treatment based upon in vitro sensitivities; surgical shunt revision if necessary.

Possible Dire Consequences without Treatment: Purulent meningitis, brain abscess.

References

Black, J. A., Challacombe, D. N., and Ockenden, B. G.: Nephrotic syndrome associated with bacteraemia after shunt operations for hydrocephalus. Lancet, 2:921, 1965.
Kaufman, D. B., and McIntosh, R.: The pathogenesis of the renal lesion in a patient with streptococcal disease infected ventriculoatrial shunt, cryoglobulinemia and nephritis. Am. J. Med., 50:263, 1971.

18. Vaccinial Nephritis

JOSEPH H. MAGEE

Cause: Vaccination with cowpox virus.

Early Manifestations: Onset of heavy proteinuria, and of periorbital and/or generalized edema, shortly after vaccination.

Treatment: As that of idiopathic nephrotic syndrome.

Possible Dire Consequences without Treatment: Recurrence, prevented by avoiding revaccination in later life for routine or administrative reasons.

References

Metcoff, J.: The nephrotic syndrome in children. J. Clin. Invest., 30:471, 1961.
Rohmedder, H. J.: Nephrotic syndrome after smallpox vaccination. Arch Kinderheilk, 168:53, 1963.

19. Luetic Nephrosis

JOSEPH H. MAGEE

Cause: Congenital syphilis. Acquired secondary syphilis.

Early Manifestations: Antibodies to the Wassermann antigen, found in other infectious diseases (leprosy, infectious hepatitis, infectious mononucleosis), after small pox vaccination as well as in syphilis, are non-specific. Specific (treponemal immobilizing) antibodies are also present. Presentation otherwise is identical to idiopathic nephrotic syndrome. Remission with penicillin therapy.

Treatment: Benzathine penicillin G 50,000 units/kg. I.M. in infants; or 1,200,000 units I.M. in each buttock in adults.

Possible Dire Consequences without Treatment: Unrecognized syphilis, transmission of syphilis.

References

Braunstein, G. D., et al.: The nephrotic syndrome associated with secondary syphilis. Am. J. Med., *48*:643, 1970.
Falls, W. F., et al.: The nephrotic syndrome in secondary syphilis. Ann. Intern. Med., *63*:1047, 1965.
Papaioannu, A. C., Asrow, A. C., and Schuckmell, N. H.: Nephrotic syndrome in early infancy as a manifestation of early syphilis. Paediatrics, *27*:636, 1961.

20. Quartan Malarial Nephrosis

JOSEPH H. MAGEE

Cause: Complement-activating immune complexes of protozoan antigen (usually from plasmodium malariae infection) with host immunoglobulins.

Early Manifestations: Malarial parasitemia, fever. Peak incidence at age five to seven years. Massive and usually unselective proteinuria (clearance of immunoglobulin G 30% of albumin clearance, or more); hypoalbuminemia.

Treatment: Treatment of malaria takes precedence over steroid and immunosuppressive agents which have been associated with a high incidence of side effects.

Possible Dire Consequences without Treatment: Confusion with fever of unknown origin complicating primary (idiopathic) nephrotic syndrome.

References

Allison, A. C., et al.: Immune complexes in the nephrotic syndrome of African children. Lancet, *1*:1231, 1969.
Berger, M., Birch, L. M., and Conte, N. F.: The nephrotic syndrome secondary to acute glomerulonephritis during falciparum malaria. Ann. Intern. Med., *67*:1163, 1967.
Gilles, H. M., and Hendrickse, R. G.: Nephrosis in Nigerian children. Brit. Med. J., *2*:27, 1963.

Hendrickse, R. G., et al.: Quartan malarial nephrotic syndrome. Lancet, *1*:1143, 1972.

Kibukamusoke, J. W., Hutt, M. S. R., and Wilks, N. E.: The nephrotic syndrome in Uganda and its association with quartan malaria. Quart. J. Med., *36*:393, 1967.

Rees, P. H., et al.: Possible role of malaria in the aetiology of the nephrotic syndrome in Nairobi. Brit. Med. J., *2*:130, 1972.

Ward, P. A., and Kibukamusoke, J. W.: Evidence for soluble immune complexes in the pathogenesis of the glomerulonephritis of quartan malaria. Lancet, *1*:283, 1969.

21. Serum Sickness

JOSEPH H. MAGEE

Cause: Large dose of preformed antigen or hapten. Specific aggregation of immunoglobulin molecules after interaction with antigen. Allergic inflammation due to activation of complement components.

Early Manifestations: Urticaria or other skin eruption. Facial or glottal angioedema. Lymphocytosis and lymphadenitis. Arthralgia. Neuropathy. Albuminuria and transiently decreased renal function.

Treatment: Tripelennamine (100 mg. q.i.d.) or diphenhydramine (50 mg. q.i.d.). Prednisone 10 to 40 mg/day during elimination of antigen.

Possible Dire Consequences without Treatment: Repeat accelerated reaction upon re-exposure to same antigen, especially animal foreign proteins and sensitizing drugs.

References

Adams, D. A.: The pathophysiology of the nephrotic syndrome. Arch. Intern. Med., *106*:117, 1960.

Longcope, W. T.: Serum sickness from serum and from certain drugs, particularly the sulfonamides. Med., *22*:251, 1943.

22. Rhus and Venom Nephrosis (Dermatitis Venenata; Bee Sting)

JOSEPH H. MAGEE

Cause: The mechanism probably corresponds to that in serum sickness, and recurrences follow rechallenges.

Early Manifestations: Identical to those of Idiopathic Nephrotic Syndrome.

Treatment: High index of suspicion, corroboration by history, measures to eliminate re-exposure.

Possible Dire Consequences without Treatment: Continuation of symptoms.

References

Hardwicke, J., et al.: Nephrotic syndrome with pollen hypersensitivity. Lancet, *1*:500, 1959.
Rytand, D. A.: Fatal anuria, the nephrotic syndrome and glomerulonephritis as sequels to the dermatitis of poison oak. Am. J. Med., *5*:548, 1945.
Venters, H. D., et al.: Bee sting nephrosis. Am. J. Dis. Child, *102*:688, 1962.

23. Penicillamine Nephrosis

Joseph H. Magee

Cause: Recognition of an antigen of D-penicillamine (cuprimine, D-3-mercapto-valine), an amino acid derivative given in 1 to 4 gm. per day orally in divided doses for chelation of copper in Wilson's disease, and of cystine in cystinuria.
　　Combination of antigen in excess with antibody.
　　Circulation of soluble antigen-antibody complexes.
　　Nephrotic syndrome due to renal localization with or without activators of complement components.
　　Analogous train of events is not established in nephrotic episodes following bismuth, gold and mercurial compounds, perchlorates, phenindione, probenecid, paradione, tridione, sulfonamides, and trichloroethylene.

Early Manifestaions: Fever, lymphadenopathy, rash, eosinophilia. Nephrotic syndrome. Positive immunofluorescence for Ig and complement on renal biopsy.

Treatment: Discontinuance of penicillamine.
　　Alternative drugs for Wilson's disease require intramuscular (dimercaprol) or intravenous (calcium disodium edetate) adminstration, but resumption of penicillamine may provoke nephrotic syndrome repeatedly.
　　Patients should be regarded as penicillin-sensitive.
　　Anemia if present may reflect Fe^{++} chelation.
　　Optic neuritis, if present, may reflect pyridoxine deficiency.

Possible Dire Consequences without Treatment: Continuation of symptoms.

References

Adams, D. A., et al.: Penicillamine-induced nephrotic syndrome. Am. J. Med., *36*:230, 1964.
Fellers, F. X., and Shamidi, N. T.: The nephrotic syndrome induced by penicillamine therapy. Am. J. Dis. Child, *98*:669, 1958.
Hayslett, J. P., et al.: Focal glomerulitis due to penicillamine. Lab. Invest., *19*:376, 1968.
Jaffe, I. A., et al.: Nephropathy induced by D-penicillamine. Ann. Intern. Med., *69*:549, 1968.

24. Lupus Nephropathy

JOSEPH H. MAGEE

Cause: Complex-mediated hypersensitivity, fundamental cause unknown with suggested possibilities including viral, with many drugs implicated in activating latent disease:

Antibiotics: Griseofulvin, penicillin, sulfonamides, tetracycline.

Antituberculous drugs: INH, PAS, streptomycin.

Anti-epileptic drugs: Diphenylhydantoin, ethosuximide, mephenytoin, primidone, trimethadione.

Antihypertensive drugs: Hydralazine, methyldopa, thiazides.

Other: Procainamide, phenylbutazone, thiouracils, oral contraceptives.

Early Manifestations: Half as prevalent as rheumatic fever with peak incidence (age fifteen to forty) a decade later, and female predominance (8:1) greater; 10 times as prevalent as polyarteritis, which has 3:1 male predominance, and a peak incidence a decade later.

Regularly, or during exacerbations, circulating nucleotides (DNA); antinucleotide antibodies (single or double stranded DNA, double stranded RNA); circulating immune complexes detectable by precipitin technique; reduction in C1, C4 or whole serum complement; and phagocytosis of antibody-coated nuclear material (LE or Hargraves cells), are present in 80%.

Arthralgias (90%) and hematologic manifestations, (80%) may precede skin manifestations (85%) and fever not due to infection (85%), by a decade.

Skin manifestations, facial in 30%, may be precipitated by sunlight.

Hematologic manifestations include leukopenia, even in the presence of infection (70%); hemolytic anemia (10%); and thrombocytopenic purpura.

Serous membrane involvement including pleuritis and pericarditis occurs in 50% of cases.

Nervous system involvement (25%) includes polyneuritis; myelitis; cranial nerve palsies; hemiplegia; movement disorders; seizures; sensorium changes; psychotic delirium or coma; without evidence of independent associated disease.

Lung involvement, which may simulate viral pneumonia, is more common with drug-induced LE.

Renal involvement (66%), less common with drug-induced LE, is indicated by increasing proteinuria, creatininemia, and erythrocyte casts; accompanied by glomerular deposits of complement; and of Ig, comprising antibodies to single and double stranded DNA, and to RNA proteins.

Hypertension occurs in but 10%.

Treatment: Prednisone 20 mg. per M.^{2} per day on alternate days, tapering according to remission. Azothioprine 2.5 mg. per kg./day if WBC is 3000/mm.^{3} or greater. Azothioprine is otherwise withheld until count returns to 3000/mm^3 and reinstituted at 2 mg. per kg. per day. Complications include (a) bone marrow depression, (b) opportunistic infections associated with (a), and (c) gram-positive bacterial infections unassociated with bone marrow depression. Criteria of remission include (a) stabilization or improvement in renal function, (b) reduction in proteinuria raised serum albumin levels, weight loss due to mobilization of edema, (c) return of immunoelectrophoretic beta-1$_c$ globulin levels to normal values (145 ± 22 mg per 100 ml).

Possible Dire Consequences without Treatment: Exacerbations with serositis, arthralgias, hemolytic anemia, thrombocytopenia, encephalopathy. These occur less frequently with treatment. Death from renal failure or intercurrent infection.

References

Baldwin, D. S., et al.: The clinical course of the proliferative and membranous forms of lupus nephritis. Ann. Intern. Med., *73*:929, 1970.

Berlyne, G. M., Short, I. A., and Vickers, C. H. F.: Placental transmission of the L.E. factor. Lancet, *2*:15, 1957.

Comerford, R. F., and Cohen, A. S.: The nephropathy of systemic lupus erythematosus. Med., *46*:425, 1967.

Donadio, J. V., et al.: Treatment of lupus nephritis with prednisone and combined prednisone and azothioprine. Ann. Intern. Med., *77*:829, 1972.

Drinkard, J. F., Stanley, T. M., and Dornfield, L.: Azothioprine and prednisone in the treatment of adults with lupus nephritis. Med., *49*:411, 1970.

Dubois, E. L.: The effect of the LE cell test on the clinical picture of systemic lupus erythematosus. Ann. Intern. Med., *38*:1265, 1953.

Dubois, E. L., and Martel, S.: Discoid lupus erythematosus. Ann. Intern. Med., *44*:482, 1956.

Friedman, I. A.: The LE phenomenon in rheumatoid arthritis. Ann. Intern. Med., *46*:1113, 1957.

Glagov, S., and Colechman, E.: Familial occurrence of disseminated lupus erythematosus. New Eng. J. Med., *255*:936, 1956.

Harvey, A. M., et al.: Systemic lupus erythematosus. Medicine, *33*:291, 1954.

Haserick, J. R.: Modern concepts of systemic lupus erythematosus. J. Chron. Dis., *1*:317, 1955.

Hayslett, J. P., et al.: The effect of azothioprine in systemic lupus erythematosus. Med., *51*:393, 1972.

Heller, P., et al.: The L.E. cell phenomenon in chronic hepatic disease. New Eng. J. Med., *254*:1160, 1956.

Israel, H. L.: The pulmonary manifestations of disseminated lupus erythematosus. Am. J. Med. Sci., *226*:387, 1953.

Lee, S. L., Rivers, I., and Siegal, M.: Activation of systemic lupus erythematosus by drugs. Arch. Intern. Med., *117*:620, 1966.

Michael, S. R., et al.: The hematologic aspects of disseminated (systemic) lupus erythematosus. Blood, *6*:1059, 1951.

Muehrcke, R. C., et al.: Lupus nephritis. Medicine, *36*:1, 1957.

Russell, P. W., Haserick, J. R., and Zucker, E. M.: Epilepsy in systemic lupus erythematosus. Arch. Intern. Med., *88*:78, 1951.

Scheinberg, L. and Hudson, L. P.: Polyneuritis in systemic lupus erythematosus. New Eng. J. Med., *255*:416, 1956.

Shearn, M. A.: Normocholesterolemic nephrotic syndrome of systemic lupus erythematosus. Am. J. Med., *36*:250, 1964.

Shearn, M. A.: Mercaptopurine in the treatment of steroid-resistant nephrotic syndrome. New Eng. J. Med., *273*:943, 1965.

Shelp, W. D., Bloodworth, J. M. B., and Reiselbach, R. E.: Effect of azothioprine on renal histology and function in lupus nephritis. Arch. Intern. Med., *128*:566, 1971.

Siegal, M., and Lee, S. L.: The epidemiology of systemic lupus erythematosus. Seminars in Arthritis Rheum., *3*:1, 1973.

Simenhoff, M. L., and Merrill, J. P.: The spectrum of lupus nephritis. Nephron *1*:348, 1965.

Sztejnbok, K., et al.: Azothioprine in the treatment of systemic lupus erythematosus. Arthr. Rheum., *14*:639, 1971.

Walsh, J. R., and Zimmerman, H. J.: The demonstration of the "L. E." phenomenon in patients with penicillin hypersensitivity. Blood, *8*:65, 1953.

25. Hypocomplementemic Persistent Nephritis

Joseph H. Magee

Synonyms: Mesangiocapillary glomerular nephritis. Membranoproliferative glomerular nephritis.

Cause: Cytotoxic hypersensitivity associated with consumption of third component (C3) of complement, despite maintained levels of other complement components; progressive renal disease associated with interstitial (mesangial) proliferation of mononuclear phagocytes and mesangial matrix.

Early Manifestations: Peak incidence in older children, adolescents, young adults, in whom it constitutes 25% of progressive renal disease, females predominating.

Presentation may be hematuric, mimicking acute glomerular nephritis, nephrotic, or routine with discovery of proteinuria on urinalysis.

Serum beta 1_c globulin (C3) is reduced on immunoelectrophoresis. C1, 4, and 2 measured by specific antisera are not decreased, suggesting an alternate path of complement activation, decreased synthesis, increased destruction, or a combination of these mechanisms.

C3 breakdown products are demonstrable in fresh plasma. Serum at this time contains a heat labile, transferable "nephritic C3 factor" which is able to break down C3 in normal plasma but not in pure form, unlike the preformed "nephritic C3 convertase" activity occurring in poststreptococcal cases which can do both. It is believed that the latter convertase activity is complex-mediated following the path of classical complement activation but that the bypass convertase in MCGN arises by an alternate pathway. Some C3 breakdown by the classical pathway is however required to activate the bypass convertase (specifically the 4% remnant not surface attached, discussed in the introduction) and exposure to normal plasma supplies this need.

Course is persistently nephrotic with declining renal function and fluctuating beta 1_c globulin levels, usually below 100 mg./100 ml. Ten-year survivals without instituting regular dialysis are not uncommon.

Electron microscopy of renal biopsy sections shows proliferation of the interstitial phagocytes (mesangial cells) of the glomerulus. This gives a separation of the lobules of the glomerulus at its hilus on light microscopy similar to that seen following streptococcal infection. Here, however, there is much more proliferation on both sides of the capillary basement membranes, narrowing their lumina and giving the spurious impression of membrane thickening on light microscopy.

Histologic examination reveals enlargement of glomeruli and separation of lobules at the hilus, seen on electron microscopy to be due to proliferation of mesangial cells and mesangial matrix on both sides of capillary basement membranes, narrowing their lumina and giving the spurious impression of membranes thickening on light microscopy.

Treatment: Response to glucocorticoid, cytotoxic and anticoagulant therapy is not to be expected; if assignment to this entity is borne out by histology and serial estimations of C3 or whole complement, they should be held.

Dietary treatment and regular dialysis with onset of uremia. Disease recurs posttransplant in some but not all cases.

Possible Dire Consequences without Treatment: Uremia.

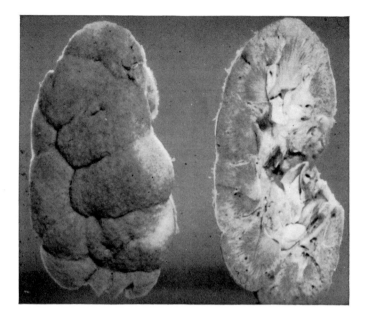

Fig. VIII–4.   Gross appearance of kidney of Edward Morgan originally described by Bright. (Courtesy of Guy's Hospital Museum.)

References

Cameron, J. S., Glasgown, E. F., Ogg, C. S., and White, R. H. R.   Membranoproliferative glomerulonephritis and persistent hypocomplementemia.   Brit. Med. J., *4*:7, 1970.

Herdman, R. C., et al.:   Chronic glomerulonephritis associated with low serum complement activity (chronic hypocomplementemic glomerulonephritis).   Medicine *49*:207, 1970.

Lewis, E. J., Carpenter, C. B., and Schur, P. H.:   Serum complement component levels in human glomerulonephritis.   Ann. Intern. Med., *75*:555, 1971.

Ogg, C. S., Cameron, J. S., and White, R. H. R.:   The $C^1$3 component of complement (B_{1c}-globulin) in patients with heavy proteinuria.   Lancet, *2*:78, 1968.

Spitzer, R. E., et al.:   Serum C3 lytic system in patients with glomerulonephritis.   Science, *164*:436, 1969.

Weller, R. O., and Nester, R.:   Histologic reassessment of three kidneys originally described by Richard Bright.   Brit. Med. J., *2*:761, 1972.

West, C. D., et al.:   Immunosuppressive therapy in persistent hypocomplementemic glomerulonephritis and in lupus nephritis.   J. Pediat., *67*:1113, 1965.

West, C. D., et al.:   Hypocomplementemic and normocomplementemic persistent (chronic) glomerulonephritis: clinical and pathological characteristics.   J. Pediat., *67*:1089, 1965.

Williams, D. G., et al.:   Role of C3b in the breakdown of C3 in hypocomplementemic mesangiocapillary glomerulonephritis.   Lancet, *1*:447, 1973.

Williams, D. G., et al.:   C3 breakdown by serum from patients with acute post-streptococcal nephritis.   Lancet, *2*:360, 1972.

9

26. Cryoglobulinemic Nephritis

Joseph H. Magee

Cause: Complex-mediated hypersensitivity associated with disseminated macroglobulin (IgM) antibodies, having both rheumatoid factor and incomplete cryoglobulin activity in combination with antigen (IgM).

Early Manifestations: Females predominate 8:1 as in lupus nephropathy; and antinuclear antibodies and reduced whole complement levels are usually found. Extrarenal manifestations precede renal disease by months to years.
  (*a*) Purpura, chiefly lower limbs
  (*b*) Arthralgia without arthritis
  (*c*) Anemia
Cryoglobulins require twenty-four hours at $0°$ C. for precipitate to occur and electrophoretic pattern is not distinctive.
Renal presentation may be as acute renal failure without preceding proteinuria; histology reveals proliferative diffuse glomerular nephritis with some exudation and little necrosis.

Treatment: Same as for lupus nephropathy.

Possible Dire Consequences without Treatment: Progressive renal failure.

Reference

Meltzer, M., and Franklin, E. C.: Cryoglobulinemia: A clinical and laboratory study of cryoglobulins with rheumatoid factor activity. Am. J. Med., *40*:837, 1966.

27. Neoplastic Nephrotic Syndromes

Joseph H. Magee

Cause: Complement fixing soluble complexes of antibody (IgG, IgM) with antigens of malignant cells.

Early Manifestations: Nephrotic syndrome may precede discovery of neoplastic disease and should raise index of suspicion for it. Incidence of neoplastic disease in adult nephrotic syndromes may be as high as 10%.

Treatment: Treatment of neoplasm may ameliorate nephrotic syndrome.

Possible Dire Consequences without Treatment: Confusion with renal vein thrombosis, inappropriate heparin therapy.

References

Brodowsky, H. S., et al.: Chronic lymphocytic leukemia, Hodgkin's disease and the nephrotic syndrome. Arch. Intern. Med., *121*:71, 1968.
Lee, J. C., Yamauchi, H., and Hopper, J.: The association of cancer and the nephrotic syndrome. Ann. Intern. Med., *64*:41, 1966.
Loughridge, L. W., and Lewis, M. G.: Nephrotic syndrome in malignant disease of non-renal origin. Lancet, *1*:256, 1971.
Miller, D. G.: The association of immune disease and malignant lymphoma. Ann. Intern. Med., *66*:507, 1967.
Plager, J., and Stutzman, L.: Acute nephrotic syndrome as a manifestation of active Hodgkin's disease. Am. J. Med., *50*:56, 1971.

28. Skin Purpura with Nephritis (Allergic or Anaphylactoid Purpura) (Schoenlein-Henoch Purpura)

Joseph H. Magee

Cause: Allergic inflammation (vasculitis) involving skin, mucosa and synovia. Lungs are never involved and resemblance of kidney lesions (focal to diffuse with local fibrinoid necrosis of tufts, worse in males and in adults) to those of the lung-kidney syndromes may be superficial.

View since Osler as immediate hypersensitivity (anaphylactoid, IgE mediated) to extrinsic allergens (microbial, drug, serum, venom and food) or cold may require revision to delayed hypersensitivity, mediated by T-lymphocyte-bound antibodies to macrophage-processed allergens.

Two-thirds of attacks follow upper respiratory infections by one to three weeks, but ASO (antistreptolysin), ASD (antistreptodornase) and antiDNase titers do not differ from control populations. Numerous analgesic, antibiotic, antiepileptic, antihistamine, diuretic, and other drugs, especially meprobamate, penicillin, chlorothiazide and heavy metals (Bi, Hg, Mg) have also been incriminated, encouraging profound conservatism in medicating these patients.

Early Manifestations: Attacks are more frequent in spring and fall with peak incidence at age five, twice as common in boys, rare after age twenty and under age two.

Skin rash (Willan, 1808) occurs in 100% of cases but may not always precede abdominal and/or joint involvement. Lesions are symmetrical and centripetal, in clusters, especially on extensor surfaces; initially urticarial, including angioneurotic edema of extremities in 46% and scalp in 24%; next papular; and finally purpuric (confluent petechiae).

Fever, 75%; with granulocytosis, eosinophilia; platelets normal, erythrocyte sedimentation rapid, anemia absent.

Joint pains (Schoenlein, 1837): Multiple with distal joints most involved, but not centripetal (migratory), with effusion but little heat or rubor and without residual deformity; in 68%.

Abdominal crises (Henoch, 1874): Colicky abdominal pain (53%) due to subserous inflammation, usually with bleeding (49%), usually frank melena (38%), with significant risk of intussusception, requiring exploration when doubt exists; hypoproteinemia due to protein-losing enteropathy may occur.

Episodic hematuria (Johnson, 1852) (38%) due to renal tract bleeding of focal glomerular nephritis (33%), with transient nitrogen retention and/or oliguria in 3% of children, more often in adults. Hematuria may recur with relapses but urine findings are normal a year later in 84% of children.

Progressive renal failure due to diffuse glomerular nephritis occurs in 4% of adults.

Treatment: Glucocorticoid therapy (20 mg per M^2 on alternate days) controls joint and abdominal manifestations and may lessen risk of intussusception. It is ineffectual in skin involvement and in preventing hematuria or other evidence of renal involvement.

Possible Dire Consequences without Treatment. Intussusception. Protein-losing enteropathy.

References

Ackroyd, J. F.: Allergic purpura, including purpura due to foods, drugs and infections. Brit. Med. Bull., *11*:28, 1955.

Allen, D. M., Diamond, L. K., and Howell, D. A.: Anaphylactoid purpura in children (Schoenlein-Henoch syndrome). Am. J. Dis. Child. *99*:833, 1960.

Anderson, A. B.: Anaphylactic purpura following intramuscular penicillin therapy. Med. J. Austral., *1*:305, 1947.

Burke, D. M., and Jellinek, H. L.: Nearly fatal cases of Schoenlein-Henoch syndrome following insect bite. Am. J. Dis. Child, *88*:772, 1954.

Gairdner, D.: The Schoenlein-Henoch syndrome (anaphylactoid purpura). Quart. J. Med., *17*:95, 1948.

Jensen, B.: Schoenlein-Henoch's purpura: Three cases with fish or penicillin as antigen. Acta Med. Scand. *152*:61, 1955.

Sterky, G., and Thilen, A.: A study on the onset and prognosis of acute vascular purpura (The Schoenlein-Henoch syndrome) in children. Acta Paed., *49*:217, 1960.

Urijar, R. E., and Herdman, R. C.: Anaphylactoid purpura III. Am. J. Clin. Path., *53*:258, 1970.

Urijar, R. C., et al.: Anaphylactoid purpura II. Lab. Invest., *119*:437, 1969.

Vernier, R. L., et al.: Anaphylactoid purpura I. Pediatrics, *27*:181, 1961.

29. Lung Purpura without Nephritis (Idiopathic Pulmonary Hemosiderosis)

Joseph H. Magee

Cause: Juvenile variant of next entity (lung purpura or Goodpasture syndrome p. 225) with infrequent and inconspicuous renal involvement, equal predilection for boys and girls, duration of years rather than months, with remissions more frequent but still exceptional.

Early Manifestations: Fever. Cough and dyspnea with or without hemoptysis. Confluent, slowly resolving, symmetrical radiographic shadows giving way to nodularity. Eosinophilia occurs in a minority. Hemosiderin in macrophages of Prussian blue stained smears of sputum. Anemia. Focal glomerular nephritis may be found on biopsy of cases with proteinuria and erythrocyturia.

Treatment: Prednisone 20 mg/M^2 on alternate days, with remission of anemia and hemoptyses as end points, continuing for a year beyond attainment of full remission.

Possible Dire Consequences without Treatment: Fatal pulmonary hemorrhage. Renal involvement.

References

Anspach, W. E.: Pulmonary hemosiderosis. Am. J. Roent., *41*:592, 1939.

Brannan, H. M., McCaughey, W. T. E., and Good, C. A.: The roentgenographic appearance of pulmonary hemorrhage associated with glomerulonephritis. Am. J. Roent., *90*:83, 1963.

Bruwer, A. J., Kennedy, R. L. J., and Edwards, J. E.: Recurrent pulmonary hemorrhage with hemosiderosis. Am. J. Roent., *76*:98, 1956.

Heptinstall, R. H., and Salmon, M. V.: Pulmonary hemorrhage with extensive glomerular disease of the kidney. J. Clin. Path., *12*:272, 1959.

O'Connel, E. J., et al.: Pulmonary hemorrhage-glomerulonephritis syndrome. (Initial pulmonary manifestations preceded renal involvement by one year in an 8-year-old girl). Am. J. Dis. Child., *108*:302, 1964.

Ognibene, A. J., and Johnson, D. E.: Idiopathic pulmonary hemosiderosis in adults. Arch. Intern. Med., *111*:503, 1967.

Soergel, K. H.: Idiopathic pulmonary hemosiderosis. Pediatrics, *19*:1101, 1957.

Soergel, K. H., and Sommers, S. C.: Idiopathic pulmonary hemosiderosis and related syndromes. Am. J. Med., *32*:499, 1962.

Sprecase, G. A.: Idiopathic pulmonary hemosiderosis. Am. Rev. Resp. Dis., *88*:330, 1963.

30. Lung Purpura with Nephritis (Membrane Disease of Lung and Kidney) (Goodpasture's Syndrome)

Joseph H. Magee

Cause: Unknown but possibly more frequent following influenza epidemics, initiated by minimal lung damage and maintained by allergic inflammation due to hypersensitivity and mediated by transferable, complement-fixing antibodies to lung and glomerular capillary membrane antigens, probably glycoproteins.

Early Manifestations: Male predominance (3/4 cases) throughout age range nine to seventy-eight with most cases in late adolescence, the twenties and early thirties. Fever (22%). Hemoptysis (82%) with or without cough, dyspnea and chest pain. Symmetrical radiographic infiltrates (89%). Lung manifestations may precede diffuse renal involvement by six weeks to six months. Serial biopsies where recorded indicate rapid progression, focal to diffuse, of glomerular lesions. Anemia.

Treatment: Prednisone 40 to 240 mg. per day. Supportive care for hemoptyses and for restrictive ventilatory insufficiency due to massive intraalveolar hemorrhage. Repetitive dialysis for renal failure. Pre-transplant nephrectomy.

Possible Dire Consequences without Treatment: Death, equally divided between pulmonary hemorrhage and uremia; steroid therapy, tentatively, has been efficacious respecting the former but not the latter.

The first patient bilaterally nephrectomized, prior to transplant, by Hume's surgical group, incidentally was regarded as an instance of "Goodpasture's syndrome." Hemoptyses had ceased spontaneously three months earlier. In 1965 Walton performed a renal allograft in a patient with this diagnosis, reported by Siegel in 1970. Upon graft rejection four weeks later, the patient's own kidneys were removed along with the graft. An immediate improvement in the patient's arterial pO_2 lung radiographic findings, ventilatory function, serum iron, and hematocrit occurred; and intermittent hemoptyses did not recur. Other instances of improvement in hemoptyses and in intraalveolar hemorrhage have been reported.

Siegel has proposed that necrotizing glomerulitis, with declining renal function, makes the kidney a source for disseminating both membrane antigen and soluble complexes of antigen with the membrane-specific antibody via the circulation, inflicting complex-mediated as well as direct cytotoxic pulmonary capillary injury. Earlier removal of kidneys, whose function is irretrievably lost, appears to be advisable whenever the mechanism of renal failure appears to be via the mechanism of direct immunologic attack as postulated here.

References

Benoit, F. L., et al.: Goodpasture's syndrome: A clinicopathologic entity. Am. J. Med., *37*:424, 1964.

Heptinstall, R. H., and Salmon, M. V.: Pulmonary hemorrhage with extensive glomerular disease of the kidney. Am. J. Clin. Path., *12*:272, 1959.

Hume, D. M., et al.: Renal homotransplantation in man in modified recipients. Ann. Surg., *158*:608, 1963.

Lerner, R. A., McPhaul, J. J., and Dixon, F. J.: Soluble glomerular basement membrane antigens in normal urine—possible autoimmunogens in man. Ann. Intern. Med., *68*:249, 1968.

Maddock, R. K., et al.: Goodpasture's syndrome: Cessation of pulmonary hemorrhage after bilateral nephrectomy. Ann. Intern. Med., *67*:1258, 1967.

Munro, J. F., Geddes, M. A., and Lamb, W. L.: Goodpasture's syndrome: Survival after acute renal failure. Brit. Med. J., *4*:95, 1967.

Proskey, A. J., et al.: Goodpasture's syndrome: A report of 5 cases and review of the literature. Am. J. Med., *48*:162, 1970.

Rusby, N. L., and Wilson, C.: Lung purpura with nephritis. Quart. J. Med., *53*:501, 1960.

Saltzman, P. W., West, M., and Chomet, B.: Pulmonary hemosiderosis and glomerulonephritis. Ann. Intern. Med., *56*:409, 1962.

Shires, D. L., Pfaff, W. W., and De Quesada, A.: Pulmonary hemorrhage and glomerulonephritis: Treatment of two cases by bilateral nephrectomy and renal transplantation. Arch. Surg., *97*:699, 1968.

Siegel, R. R.: The basis of pulmonary disease resolution after nephrectomy in Goodpasture's syndrome. Am. J. Med. Sci., *259*:201, 1970.

Stanton, M. D., and Tange, J. D.: Goodpasture's syndrome (pulmonary hemorrhage associated with glomerulonephritis). Aust. Ann. Med., *7*:132, 1958.

31. Polyarteritis with Lung Involvement (Allergic Granulomatous Arteritis) (Allergic Granulomatosis)

Joseph H. Magee

Cause: Unknown. However in some patients with polyarteritis, Australia antigen has been detected in vessel walls of muscle biopsies, and antigen, antigen-antibody complexes, and episodic low complement levels have been detected in serum.

Early Manifestations: Obstructive pulmonary disease precedes other systemic involvement. Precedent upper respiratory involvement, seen in two out of three of patients with Wegener's granulomatosis, does not occur. Pulmonary involvement is a granulomatous and necrotizing alveolitis and arteritis, characterized by infiltration, consolidation and cavitation, as a Wegener's granulomatosis. Also in common with Wegener's granulomatosis, extrapulmonary lesions are eosinophilic, granulomatous, necrotic, both in and without vessels, both arterial and venous; and glomerulitis occurs in three-fourths of patients.

Treatment: Same as that of Wegener's granulomatosis (p. 239).

Possible Dire Consequences without Treatment: Stroke, uremia, coronary arteritis, myocardial or pericardial involvement, abdominal catastrophe, mononeuritis multiplex.

References

Carrington, C. B., and Liebow, A. A.: Limited forms of Wegener's granulomatosis. Am. J. Med., *17*:168, 1966.

Cassan, S. M., Coles, D. T., and Harrison, E. G., Jr.: The concept of limited forms of Wegener's granulomatosis. Am. J. Med., *49*:366, 1970.

Churg, J.: Granulomatosis and granulomatous-vascular syndromes. Ann. Allergy, *21*:619, 1963.

Churg, J., and Strauss, L.: Allergic granulomatosis, allergic angitis and periarteritis nodosa. Am. J. Path., *27*:277, 1951.

Davson, J., Ball, R., and Platt, R.: The kidney in periarteritis nodosa. Quart. J. Med., *17*:175, 1948.

Parkin, T. W., et al.: Hemorrhagic and interstitial pneumonitis with nephritis. Am. J. Med., *18*:220, 1955.

Rose, G. A., and Spencer, H.: Polyarteritis nodosa. Quart. J. Med., *26*:619, 1957.

Zeek, P. M.: Periarteritis nodosa and other forms of necrotizing angiitis. New Eng. J. Med., *248*:764, 1953.

Zeek, P. M., Smith, C. C., and Weeter, J. C.: Studies on periarteritis nodosa. Am. J. Path., *24*:889, 1948.

32. Wegener's Granulomatosis

Joseph H. Magee

Cause: Generally regarded as a variant of polyarteritis.

Early Manifestations: Male predominance is less than the 3:1 usually cited for polyarteritis, neurologic complications are less frequent and hypertension less characteristic.

Treatment: See p. 239.

Possible Dire Consequences without Treatment: Death from uremia.

33. Pneumonia with Nephritis

JOSEPH H. MAGEE

Cause: Pneumonia (influenza, parainfluenza, respiratory syncytial virus, adenovirus, mycoplasma pneumoniae, ornithosis, Q fever, bacterial).

Early Manifestations: Non-oliguric acute renal failure. Episodic proteinuria and erythrocyturia.

Treatment: Supportive, for pneumonia. Fluid monitoring by weights and calculation of balances. Early ambulation to minimize catabolic response to illness and immobilization.

Possible Dire Consequences without Treatment: Confusion with Goodpasture's syndrome if hemoptysis has been a feature during pneumonia.

The several fates of the lung in epidemic influenza include: (1) primary influenza virus pneumonia, (2) combined influenza virus and bacterial pneumonia, and (3) influenza complicated by bacterial pneumonia. The criteria for primary influenza virus pneumonia include: (1) cytopathogenic changes in the respiratory epithelium extending down to the respiratory bronchioli and alveolar ducts, (2) cytopathogenic changes in the fixed alveolar cells, (3) capillary thrombosis and necrosis with focal leukocytic exudates, (4) capillary aneurysms and capillary hemorrhages, (5) exudative hyaline membranes, (6) regeneration of the epithelium of the respiratory bronchioli and alveolar ducts after five to seven days, and (7) regeneration of alveolar epithelium.

Goodpasture wrote an article in 1919 citing evidence for a distinctive pathologic condition of the lung in epidemic influenza of fatal issue, citing two cases where the lungs had been bacteriologically sterile at post mortem. "The clinical histories of these two cases leave little doubt that they represent instances of fatal influenzal pneumonia, caused by an infectious agent of which we are totally ignorant, and without invasion of the lungs by any of the pathogenic bacteria commonly found associated with it. Granting that they are examples of influenzal pneumonia, the presence of the hyaline membrane on the walls of the dilated alveolar ducts is further evidence of the specificity of the lesion. The pathology of the lungs in the second case is strikingly suggestive of persistence of the infecting agent in this tissue from the time of the initial attack one month previously, with a final and fatal exacerbation."

Influenza viruses are myxoviruses with core antigens made up of protein and single-stranded ribonucleic acid which are responsible for their differentiation as influenzas A, B, and C, identified respectively in 1933, 1940, and 1950. Surface or envelope components, having hemagglutinating and sialidase (neuramidase) activities, are the antigens responsible for host susceptibility and immunity. Influenza A appears to be responsible for pandemics which have occurred about every fifteen years for the past four hundred and fifty years and for urban epidemics about every two or three years. Major changes in the antigenic determinants of influenza A were associated with pandemics in 1946–47, 1957–58 and 1967–68. Influenza **B** appears to cause urban epidemics about every three to four years, with antigenic changes having been apparent in 1954 and 1962.

Soon after the 1954 increment in influenza B cases, Parrish and colleagues reported cases of acute renal failure after pulmonary infections, emphasizing the then new technique of renal biopsy introduced by them into this country. An important implication, disclosed not by the morphologic but by the physiologic studies of these cases, was that a criterion of tubular function, aminohippurate excretory maximum or Tm_{pah}, returned to normal rapidly and in disproportion to glomerular function (inulin clearance). Far more physiologic observations of this character are urgently needed.

The second case alluded to by Goodpasture was an eighteen-year-old hospital corpsman whose illness began with fever, continued with malaise, cough and weight loss for six weeks, and then culminated in right pleuritic pain, right and then left pneumonia, and death two days prior to the 1918 armistice. He had a white cell count of 17,600 with 58% polymorphonuclears, expectorated both frank blood and bloody sputum, and had a right pleural effusion at autopsy, with hemorrhagic consolidation of all of the right and of the lower left lung. "A guinea-pig inoculated intraperitoneally with ground lung died in forty-eight hours . . . its blood culture was sterile."

Additional findings were that the spleen had foci of necrosis "situated about the small arteries," and that "hemorrhagic points in the intestine show focal lesions in the walls of the arterioles," which were bacteriologically sterile. The kidneys showed "fibrinous exudate in Bowman's capsule and cellular proliferation of glomerular tufts; some urinary tubules are filled with erythrocytes." There was no record of urea retention but it had been observed that "the urine showed a trace of albumin." Presciently, Goodpasture went on to observe, "the presence of lesions in the kidney and spleen may be regarded as evidence that this case does not represent a pure influenzal infection," adding that "it does not seem inconceivable although rare, that the virus of influenza might persist within the body for six weeks with the production of lesions of the character found in this man."

The eponym "Goodpasture's syndrome" cannot be applied to pneumonia with nephritis, for the best of reasons, having been preempted in another cause. During the decade 1958–1968 it appeared 25 times in the titles of articles dealing with lung purpura with nephritis (membrane disease of lung and kidney). Attaching Goodpasture's name to this entity has conferred a prodigious paternity and a heady immortality upon a prosecutor who merely asked a question. The question turns rather baldly upon whether or not either of these two 1918 patients had pneumonia which in that case was primary influenza virus pneumonia, at all; it is an important one if "we may assume that in the second wave of this pandemic the high mortality was caused by a strain which had developed within a few months a high human pneumotropic virulence" In 1889 and 1957 this virulence is believed to have been low except as "enhanced by pre-existing chronic congestion of the lung, lung disease pregnancy, and perhaps also by secondary bacterial infection." The possibility remains that lung-kidney syndromes due, as in the entity now bearing Goodpasture's name, to aggressive immunity, are periodically to be matched with counterpart lung-kidney syndromes due to aggressive infectivity by influenza virus or other microorganisms.

References

Abernethy, T. J., and Farr, L. E.: Renal physiology in pneumonia. J. Clin. Invest., *16*:421, 1937.

Bell, E. T., and Kuntston, R. C.: Extrarenal azotemia and tubular disease. J.A.M.A., *134*:441, 1947.

Goodpasture, E. W.: The significance of certain pulmonary lesions in relation to the etiology of influenza. Am. J. Med. Sci., *158*:863, 1919.

Hers, J. F., Masurel, N., and Mulder, J.: Bacteriology and histopathology of the respiratory tract and lungs in fatal Asian influenza. Lancet, 2:1141, 1958.

Jeghers, H., and Bakst, H. J.: The syndrome of extrarenal azotemia. Ann. Intern. Med., *11*:1861, 1937–8.

Louria, D. B., et al.: Studies of influenza in the pandemic of 1957–1958, II. Pulmonary complications of influenza. J. Clin. Invest., *38*:213, 1959.

McIntosh, R., and Reimann, H. A.: Kidney function in pneumonia. J. Clin. Invest., *3*:123, 1926.

Parrish, A. E., and Howe, J. S.: Needle biopsy as aid in diagnosis of renal disease. J. Lab. & Clin. Med., *42*:152, 1953.

Parrish, A. E., Rubenstein, N. H., and Howe, J. S.: Acute renal insufficiency associated with respiratory infections. Am. J. Med., *18*:237, 1955.

Chapter IX

Lungs and Metabolism

Introduction

The ventilating apparatus of a young and smallish (1.73 M^2) healthy male accommodates with maximum effort 6 liters of air. He can expel (vital capacity) all but a fifth of this, leaving as residual volume 1200 ml., all but 150 ml. of it in the lungs themselves. With usual expiratory effort, twice as much (functional) residual capacity is left behind, after expelling but 1200 ml. inspired air. At inspirations of 1200 ml. each it would take but 5 cycles to exchange his instantaneous lung capacity completely in a minute. This would be hyperventilation with respect to depth, and more usual ventilation would be inspirations of 500 ml. performed 12 times per minute; delivering as much O_2 and removing as much CO_2 per minute, but diluting the alveolar phase of the latter less per cycle. When he lies down he is able to accommodate only about 5.5 liters maximally but with his ability to expel all but a fifth of it essentially unimpaired; both residual volume and functional residual now, however, are less. Less outward record of the chest boundaries lessens the vacuum opposing undiminished inward recoil of the lungs. Inspirations of 500 ml. now would have to be performed but 11 times per minute to completely exchange this instantaneous lung capacity. The mythical ward patient who regularly breathes 20 times per minute must be reducing the depth (tidal volume) of each breath considerably or else he has some need for additional minute volume due to fever, activity or equivalent metabolic demand.

Nourishment of the musculo-elastic elements of the lung and the larger components of its vascular tree takes place by way of the bronchial circulation, which receives about 1% of the cardiac output (blood previously oxygenated by passage through alveolar capillaries). The alveoli, which both process and receive subtrates for their metabolism from the entire cardiac output, occupy in this respect a pre-eminent position among viscera. Some 5% of the body's oxygen uptake is diverted to their metabolic activities rather than being carried to the periphery. Among these activities is preservation of constant alveolar wall surface tension with changing volumes throughout the respiratory cycle, believed to be a function of surfactant secreted by the pneumonocytes and removed by alveolar macrophages. Lung mast cells and their circulating counterparts are the sources of the mediators of immunologic reactions. These reactions bind and prevent the absorption of specific inhalants. Being astride the circulation as it converges for gas exchange, the metabolically active endothelium appears to be remarkably specialized, as expected, for ordered procession of the agent cells of gas transport through channels, surrounding the alveoli; and further for processing a returning

TABLE IX–1.
LUNGS AND METABOLISM

Normal Values

Oxygen Capacity = the capacity of blood to carry oxygen which is chemically combined rather than physically dissolved = a measure of oxyhemoglobin availability, carrying oxygen (mole = 22.4 1.):

		Arterial	Venous	Difference
Males:	mM/l.	9.3	7.1	2.2
Males:	ml./100 ml.	21.2	16.2	5.0
Females:	mM/l.	8.2	6.3	1.9
Females:	ml./100 ml.	18.2	14.3	3.9

Oxygen Content = the content of both chemically combined and physically dissolved oxygen in blood handled without loss to atmosphere = a measure of oxygenation in lungs and tissue extraction:

Males:	mM/l.	9.1	6.9	2.2
Males:	ml./100 ml.	20.3	15.3	5.0
Females:	mM/l.	8.0	6.1	1.9
Females:	ml./100 ml.	17.9	13.7	4.2

Oxyhemoglobin Content or Saturation = the content of chemically combined oxygen per unit blood volume or of hemoglobin = a measure of oxygen transfer and hemoglobin affinity:

Males:	mM/l.	8.8	6.7	2.1
Males:	ml./100 ml.	20.0	15.2	4.8
Females:	mM/l.	7.9	6.0	1.9
Females:	ml./100 ml.	17.6	13.6	4.0
Males:	% Saturation	98.0	73.5	24.5
Females:	% Saturation	98.0	73.5	24.5

Carbon Dioxide Content = the content of both chemically combined and physically dissolved carbon dioxide in blood handled without loss to atmosphere = a measure of diffusion from tissues and lungs and of bicarbonate formation:

Males:	mM/l.	21.9	23.8	1.9
Males:	ml./100 ml.	49.0	53.1	4.1
Females:	mM/l.	21.1	22.6	1.5
Females:	ml./100 ml.	48.0	51.4	3.4

pH = a measure of the concentration of free protons in solution, in logarithmic mass units of solvent per unit available protons (hydrions) $[H^+]$ = conventional activity of protons, compared to standards at same ionic strength and temperature, as determined coiorimetrically or electrometrically:

	Arterial	Capillary	Venous	Difference
pH	7.405	7.395	7.365	0.040
pCO_2 = partial pressure (tension) of carbon dioxide mm Hg:	40 ± 2.5	41 ± 2.5	44 ± 2.5	4
pO_2 = partial pressure (tension) of oxygen mm Hg:	96 ± 5.0	90 ± 5.0	39 ± 2.5	57

Vital Capacity = maximum volume that can be expired after maximum inspiration = a measure of the elastic properties of the lungs, helpful in evaluating the treatment of asthma, emphysema and heart failure.

Males: 3–5 liters (2.5–3.0 liters per square
Females: 2.5–4 liters meter body surface area.)

Functional Expiratory Volume = timed vital capacity

Males: 83% or 2.5–4.2 liters in 1 second (FEV_1)
Males: 97% or 2.9–4.9 liters in 3 seconds (FEV_3)
Females: 83% or 2.1–3.3 liters in 1 second (FEV_1)
Females: 97% or 2.4–3.9 liters in 3 seconds (FEV_3)

mixed plasma phase, containing a heterogeneous array of mostly non-volatile substances from diverse peripheral sites. Finger-like out-pouchings, which contain ribosomes and pinocytotic vesicles (alveoli), enormously increase surface area. The alveoli are believed to be particularly important as sites of extraction of adenine nucleotides and peptide hormones from plasma. The same lung hydrolase which splits off a phenylalanyl-arginine dipeptide to inactivate bradykinin also splits off a histadyl-leucine to activate angiotensin I, as angiotensin II. Other physiologically active agents such as serotonin and prostaglandins E and F are nearly quantitatively removed in transit through lung capillaries.

1. Acute Respiratory Distress Syndrome

H. L. Israel

Causes: Infantile respiratory distress syndrome. Oxygen toxicity. Smoke and gas inhalation. Radiation. Radiomimetic agents. Viral pneumonia. Aspiration pneumonia. Drug narcosis. Fat embolism. Disseminated intravascular coagulation. Acute renal failure. Septicemia. Burns. Postperfusion lung. Shock lung. Neurogenic pulmonary edema.

Early Manifestations: Physical signs of pulmonary edema. Minimal radiographic findings early. History of precipitating event. Absent evident cause for acute cardiac pulmonary edema.

Late Manifestations: Progressive dyspnea. Tachypneic grunting respiration with prominent intercostal and suprasternal retractions. Progressive cyanosis unresponsive to oxygen therapy without ventilatory assistance.

Treatment: Volume respirator providing large tidal volumes and maintenance of positive end-expiratory pressures *without* prolonged administration of high oxygen concentrations. Corticosteroids are often given in high doses but proof of their efficacy is lacking. Infection is a major problem in patients in whom survival of initial phase occurs.

Possible Dire Consequences without Treatment: Progressive respiratory failure is the invariable outcome of the condition if not recognized and treated early.

Oxygen may be life saving in direct pulmonary insults such as aspiration pneumonia, contusions, and hyaline membrane disease of the newborn. Identical physiologic and pathologic changes may occur in severe illnesses and injuries accompanied by shock and septicemia. The frequency and importance of respiratory failure accompanying such conditions have not until recently been appreciated, the causes are extremely diverse and collectively are often designated the respiratory distress syndrome. It is important to recognize that by definition acute cardiac pulmonary edema is excluded from the list of causes, and to emphasize the distinction between pulmonary edema that is purely circulatory in origin from that due to pulmonary injury. The pulmonary injury may be the consequence of ischemia during low flow periods in shock. With stasis, leukocyte aggregation and release of lysosomes may also cause damage. Loss of surfactant has been observed but whether this is cause or effect is not established. Prostaglandins may be involved in the vascular injury. In infants the lungs are small and airless at autopsy. In adults they are relatively airless, heavy, congested and red. After prolonged therapy, fibrosis and emphysematous blebs are prominent. Microscopically there is intraalveolar exudate and hemorrhage, with interstitial hemorrhage and edema. The pathologic changes are not specific and the diagnosis of respiratory distress syndrome is not usually made by the pathologist.

Treatment has become more successful with wider availability of skilled personnel and of respiratory intensive care units. Successful use of membrane oxygenators has recently been reported, and it is possible that development and simplification of the necessary equipment when they occur will play a decisive role in treating the respiratory distress syndrome.

References

Ashbaugh, D. G., et al.: Continuous Positive Pressure Breathing in Adult Respiratory Distress Syndrome. J. Thor. and Cardiovasc. Surgery., *57*:39–41, 1969.

Kumar, A., et al.: Continuous Positive Pressure Ventilation in Acute Respiratory Failure. New Eng. J. Med. *283*:1430, 1970.

Lutch, J. S., and Murray, J. F.: Continuous Positive Pressure Ventilation: Effects on Systemic Oxygen Transport and Tissue Oxygenation. Ann. Intern. Med., *76*:193, 1972.

2. Asthma Disguised as Emphysema

H. L. ISRAEL

Cause: Hypersensitive state.

Early Manifestations: Shortness of breath. Physical signs of severe airway obstruction. Radiographic signs of hyperaeration attributed to emphysema.

Treatment: Prednisone, as detailed in the case summarized below. A dramatic response to prednisone identified the patient's disease as asthma. The differentiation of asthma from emphysema is impossible without a trial of corticosteroid therapy.

Dire Consequences without Treatment: Ineffective treatment for emphysema.

Case Report: An eighty-one-year-old female seen October 26, 1971 had been well until the previous January. Cough had persisted after a severe respiratory infection and chest radiography in February indicated emphysema. Cough, wheezing and dyspnea which had lessened during the summer recurred in autumn. The patient who looked well coughed incessantly and rhonchi were present at both bases. Radiography revealed flattened diaphragms and hyperaeration. Vital capacity was 1.1 liters, 0.4 liter in one second, with no improvement after inhalation of isoproterenol. Leukocyte count was 10,300 mm³ with 37% eosinophils; sputum grew mixed flora. During an initial month's prednisone treatment cough abated gradually and vital capacity increased to 2.0 liters. When prednisone was reduced to 5 mg. daily symptoms recurred, and 10 mg. daily were given from January to April 1972. She remained free of cough and wheezing from April to August 1972 on 5 mg. prednisone daily, vital capacity attaining 2.1 liters, 1.9 liters in one second.

Differentiation of asthma and emphysema is difficult in older patients. Symptoms may be persistent rather than paroxysmal, and a radiographic appearance of marked hyperaeration and diminished vascularity may lead to an impression that chronic emphysema is present. Severe airway obstruction on spirogram may be unresponsive to inhalation of bronchodilators, and diffusing capacity may show reduction. There may be minimal wheezing. A dramatic response to corticosteroid therapy established nevertheless that airway obstruction and hyperaeration have not been the consequence of anatomic change. It is a reasonable routine in distinguishing the various types of chronic obstructive pulmonary disease (COPD) with onset in adult life to determine the response to prednisone treatment before arriving at a conclusion as to whether airway obstruction is reversible or fixed.

Reference

Bates, D. V., and Christie, R. V.: Respiratory Function in Disease. Philadelphia, W. B. Saunders Co., 1964, p. 140.

3. Allergic Bronchopulmonary Aspergillosis

H. L. Israel

Cause: Atopic reaction to aspergillosis.

Early Manifestations: Allergic pneumonia. Bronchial obstruction.

Late Manifestations: Proximal bronchiectasis. Atelectasis.

Treatment: Prednisone.

Dire Consequences without Treatment: Repeated thoracotomies. Death.

Case Report: A forty-four-year-old engineer was seen October 20, 1970, because a third thoracotomy had been recommended for suspected neoplasm. He had had asthma as a child and during adolescence and early adult life, but more recently had been symptom free while residing in New Mexico. In 1965 symptoms recurred when he moved to Philadelphia. Wheezing, cough, and expectoration exacerbated each summer. In 1967 he had an attack of such severity that he received corticosteroids for the first time. In January 1968 he developed a febrile illness. A right lung lesion (Fig. IX–1A) was seen on plain chest radiograph and bronchography showed bilateral bronchiectasis. There was improvement in surrounding inflammatory conditions but a right upper lobectomy was done based upon a diagnosis of lung abscess. The pathologic examination revealed chronic granulomatous inflammation with abscess formation and Aspergillus fragments. Asthma again was severe during the summer of 1968 and allergic reactions to all molds were demonstrated by skin sensitivity tests. Desensitization was carried out. He again developed a febrile illness in December 1969, chest radiograph showing complete collapse of the left upper lobe (Fig. IX–1B). Thoracotomy was performed because of concern about neoplasm. The lobe was not resected, biopsy showing eosinophilic inflammation. He was started on prednisone with rapid improvement in symptoms and in appearance of the chest radiograph (Fig. IX–1C). During the spring, prednisone therapy was stopped, and in the summer there was recurrence of left upper lobe atelectasis. Bronchoscopy disclosed a patent upper lobe bronchus but because of concern about neoplasm resection was again advised. When seen in October 1970 he was not wheezing and was in no distress. Vital capacity was 4.2 liters before isoproterenol and 4.5 liters after, one second timed vital capacity being 3.2 liters. There was segmental collapse of the left upper lobe roentgenographically. Because of the report of hyphae in the first operative specimen, serologic studies for aspergillus antibodies were performed, being slightly positive in November and negative in December. A sputum specimen grew Aspergillus fumigatus. There was no blood eosinophilia. Treatment with prednisone resulted in prompt clearing of the left upper lobe density, and it was continued in dosage of 10 mg. daily. There have been no additional episodes of asthma, pneumonia, or atelectasis.

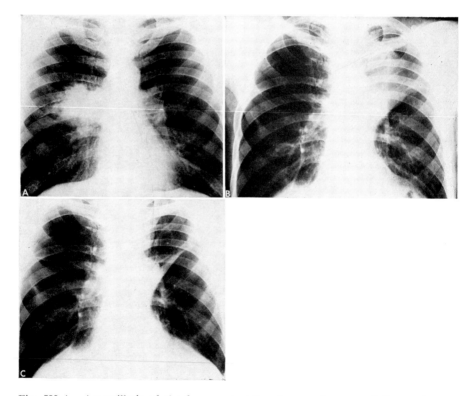

Fig. IX–1. Aspergillosis of the lungs. A, Chronic granulomatous inflammation with abscess formation and Aspergillus fragments. B, Collapse of left upper lobe developed later. C, Improvement following prednisone treatment (see Case Report in text).

This condition has been infrequently recognized in the United States and a 1969 report described it as "a North American rarity." Greater familiarity with the entity is now leading to more frequent recognition. Knowledge of its etiology, pathogenesis and morbid anatomy emanates from Great Britain where it has long been recognized. A similar illness has been induced in asthmatics by sensitivity to Candida species. Recurrent pneumonia is the usual clinical pattern but in cases such as the preceding there may be simulation of abscess or neoplasm. With slow and spontaneous recovery there may be considerable damage to proximal bronchi with bronchography demonstrating a characteristic pattern of bronchiectasis. Prompt diagnosis and corticosteroid therapy result in prompt clearing with less residual damage, often with quick expectoration of the obstructing plugs responsible for atelectasis of distal segments. Masses of hyphae of Aspergillus species are demonstrable in the plugs. Cultures are frequently negative since fungi that are no longer viable may perpetuate an allergic bronchial reaction and direct treatment of Aspergillus organisms may be unavailing. Corticosteroids reduce the inflammatory reaction, permit evacuation of the plug, and distal pneumonia then resolves.

References

Hoene, J., Reed, C., and Dickie, H.: Allergic bronchopulmonary aspergillosis is not rare. J. Lab. Clin. Med., *78*:1007, 1971.
Scadding, J. G.: The bronchi in allergic aspergillosis. Scand. J. Resp. Dis., *48*:372, 1967.
Slavin, R. G., et al.: Allergic bronchopulmonary aspergillosis: A North American rarity. Am. J. Med., *47*:306, 1969.

4. Pulmonary Sensitivity to Nitrofurantoin

H. L. Israel

Cause: Nitrofurantoin (Cyantin, Furachel, Furadantin, Macrodantin, Trantoin). History of nitrofurantoin therapy.

Early Manifestations: Fever. Episodic dyspnea. Chronic dyspnea. Pulmonary infiltrates simulating pulmonary embolism, pneumonia, or chronic interstitial fibrosis. Pleural effusion may occur. Delayed eosinophilia.

Treatment: Withdrawal of implicated drugs, occasioned by high index of suspicion. Drugs used in treatment of urinary tract infections, including both sulfonamides and nitrofurantoin, appear to be a particularly fruitful line of inquiry. Thirty-five additional instances of pulmonary sensitivity to nitrofurantoin have been reported since our original case was recorded.

Dire Consequences without Treatment: No deaths have been reported but a number of patients have been critically ill upon admission.

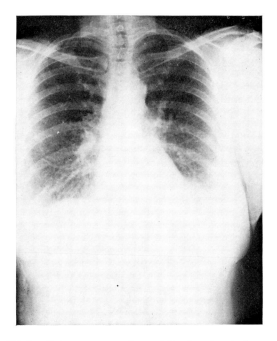

Fig. IX–2.   Pulmonary reaction to Nitrofurodantin (see text).

Instances of hypersensitivity to this drug probably greatly exceed the incidence as reported.   In some cases cyanosis and dyspnea are sufficiently severe to make death appear imminent.   The list of respiratory illnesses simulated by these hypersensitivity reactions is a varied one: pulmonary embolism, tracheobronchitis, pneumonia, pulmonary edema and chronic interstitial fibrosis.   The onset of respiratory symptoms is usually explosive but may be insidious.   The latter group may develop irreversible fibrosis.   There are clinical and radiologic similarities to farmer's lung, but the speed with which acute lesions disappear suggests that the pathologic changes are those of edema and pneumonia rather than granulomatous inflammation.   (See Fig. IX–2.)

An unusual feature of nitrofurantoin lung disease is delayed eosinophilia, which has been observed in over 50% of cases.   In the first few attacks, or early in the course of the attack, eosinophilia is usually absent, but subsequent blood counts may reveal eosinophilia of 25 to 50%, and provide strong support for the diagnosis of a hypersensitivity reaction.

References

Cortez, L. M., and Pankey, G. A.: Acute pulmonary hypersensitivity to furazolidine. Amer. Rev. Resp. Dis., *105*:823, 1972.

Editorial: Pulmonary sensitivity to nitrofurantoin. Brit. Med. J., 2:704, 1969.

Israel, H. L., and Diamond, P.: Recurrent pulmonary infiltration and pleural effusion due to nitrofurantoin sensitivity. New Eng. J. Med., *267*:1024, 1962.

Ngan, H., Millard, R. J., and Lant, A. F.: Nitrofurantoin lung. Brit. J. Radiol., *44*:21, 1971.

Rosenow, E. C., De Remee, R. A., and Dines, D. E.: Chronic nitrofurantoin pulmonary reaction. New Eng. J. Med., *279*:1258, 1968.

Rosenow, E. C., II.: The spectrum of drug-induced pulmonary disease. Amer. Inter. Med., *77*:977, 1972.

5. Wegener's Granulomatosis

H. L. ISRAEL

Cause: Unknown.

Early Manifestations: Multiple chronic pulmonary nodules resembling metastases, acute migratory consolidations, destructive lesions of upper respiratory tract.

Treatment: Cytotoxic drugs. Chlorambucil (0.1 to 0.2 mg./kg. body weight) best tolerated.

Dire Consequences without Treatment or with *Corticosteroid Therapy:* Death from upper respiratory tract, renal or pulmonary damage.

Until recently this disorder, a rare form of granulomatous inflammation with vasculitis most often involving lungs (Fig. IX–3A & B), upper respiratory tract and kidneys, was regarded as invariably and rapidly fatal. In 1966 a limited form with predominately pulmonary involvement was recognized. About the same time the effectiveness of cytotoxic drug therapy was noted. Interest stimulated by these developments has led to the recognition of 17 cases in Philadelphia in the last few years.

The disease is of unknown nature, resembling lymphoma in some respects. The characteristic pathologic appearance is of necrotizing inflammation with angiitis in the surrounding parenchyma. The lungs appear to be most commonly affected, with sinuses, larynx, pituitary gland, kidneys, skin and subcutaneous tissues less often involved. It differs from polyarteritis which as a rule involves liver, kidney and musculature with equal intensity.

Age, sex, race, occupational or geographic influences have not been demonstrated in the genesis of the disease.

The course may be explosive in onset and rapidly fatal. Growing use of lung biopsy has demonstrated the frequent existence of torpid and asymptomatic forms. It is evident that the pulmonary forms of this disease were often not correctly identified, even after biopsy, in the past.

A review of the 17 pulmonary cases seen in Philadelphia revealed several features which should facilitate the diagnosis. One almost pathognomonic feature is the slow resolution of massive densities in one lung while progression is occurring in the other lung. This sequence eliminates the possibility of neoplasm which would otherwise be suggested by the mass lesions. In other cases the lesions appear as nodular masses, typical of metastases, which may persist for months or years without deterioration of health. A third characteristic which may lead to recognition of this disease is the occurrence of subcutaneous nodules which on biopsy examination will show necrotizing inflammation with angiitis and no pathogenic organisms. Upper respiratory tract involvement has occurred in 4 cases, none showed renal involvement.

A Lancet editorial hailed the advance in treatment of Wegener's granulomatosis as "The therapeutic success story of the sixties." At the beginning of the decade, prednisone was the recommended therapy but improvement was infrequent and transient. By the end of the decade, consistent improvement had been reported with use of chlorambucil, imuran, methotrexate and cyclophosphamide. Not

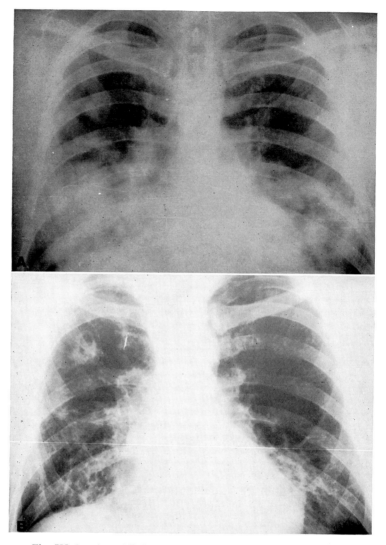

Fig. IX–3. A and B, Wegener's granulomatosis involving lungs.

infrequently a six-month course of any of these agents sufficed for prolonged remission or cure. In other cases, more prolonged therapy was needed, and fatalities continued to occur as a result of drug toxicity and infections or from the results of irreversible damage incurred before the start of treatment. Chlorambucil appears to be best tolerated of the cytotoxic drugs and this agent should be tried first, particularly in disease confined to the lungs. Cyclophosphamide appears to be more effective and should be used in patients with severe extrapulmonary involvement.

References

Carrington, C. B., and Liebow, A. A.: Limited forms of angiites and granulomatosis of
    Wegener's type. Am. J. Med., *41*:497, 1966.
Editorial: Wegener's granulomatosis. Lancet, *2*:519, 1972.

Israel, H. L., and Patchefsky, A. S.: Wegener's granulomatosis of lung. Diagnosis and treatment. Experience with 12 cases. Ann. Intern. Med., *74*:881, 1971.

Wolff, S. M., Fauci, A. S., Horn, R. G., and Dale, D. C.: N.I.H. Conference on Wegener's granulomatosis. Ann. Intern. Med., *81*:513, 1974.

6. Echinococcus Cyst of Lung

Robfrt K. Brown

Cause: Echinococcus granulosus. Transmitted from sheep, via dogs. Human infestation follows ingestion of ova contained in dog feces.

Early Manifestations: Often no symptoms; discovered on routine or survey chest roentgenogram.

Treatment: Surgical excision.

Possible Dire Consequences without Treatment: Pulmonary and/or pleural suppuration, hemorrhage.

Echinococcus disease is endemic in Australia, Argentina, North Africa, the Near East, and some European countries, including England and Wales. In the United States human cases, though rare, occasionally do occur. There is recognized

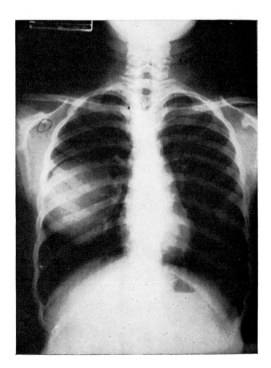

Fig. IX–4. Male, age eighteen: large single cyst involving three lobes, right lung.

widespread infestation of sheep and various animals here.   The avenue of transmission is from sheep via dogs to man.   In the countries of high incidence, dogs eat fresh infected viscera discarded during butchering of sheep.   The parasite ova are excreted in the dogs' feces, to be picked up by man as he handles or pets the dog and then touches mouth while eating.   The ingested ova hatch in the human stomach and the larvae go via duodenum and portal vein to liver, then via blood stream to lung, forming large thin-walled cysts.   In some cases transmission may be direct from stomach to lung by lymphatics, without involving liver.   Each of the pulmonary cysts contains thousands of tiny daughter cysts which appear grossly as a sandy particulate sediment in the clear fluid of the cyst.

Diagnosis of pulmonary echinococcus cyst is usually radiologic.   Chest roentgenogram will show rounded opaque mass or masses, occasionally up to 4 or 5 inches in diameter.   (Fig. IX–4.)   Often there will be a thin semilunar radiolucency in the top of the sphere.   Complicated cases may show pleural effusion or pneumothorax, due to rupture and subsequent infection.   As to symptoms, the patient may have none, or he may complain of cough, occasional mild chest pain, or small hemoptysis.   If history indicates a possibility of earlier exposure to the parasite, and if neoplasm is reasonably ruled out, a diagnosis of hydatid cyst must be considered.   There is a skin test antigen (Casoni), and a complement fixation test.

References

Sarsam, Adnan: Surgery of Pulmonary Hydatid Cysts.   J. Thorac. Cardiovasc. Surg., *62*:663, 1971.
Steele, J. D.:   The Solitary Pulmonary Nodule.   Springfield, Charles C Thomas, 1964, p. 226.
Thomas, D. M. E.:   Hydatid Disease of the Lung (chapter 14 in *Clinical Surgery—Thorax*, ed. d'Abreu).   Washington, Butterworths, 1965.
Wolcott, M. W., et al.:   Hydatid Disease of the Lung, J. Thorac. Cardiovasc. Surg., *62*:465, 1971.

7. Spontaneous Pneumothorax

ORVILLE HORWITZ

Cause: Ruptured emphysematous bullae or congenital pleural blebs.

Early Manifestations: Dyspnea with or without pain.   Agonizing pleuritic pain may occur.   Asphyxia (low pO_2 and high pCO_2).   Absent breath sounds and tympany on affected side.   Displacement to affected side in ordinary pneumothorax.   Displacement to opposite side in tension pneumothorax.

Treatment: Suction by chest tube and water seal in severe cases.   For pressure (tension) pneumothorax at a distance from a hospital, introduction of a large intravenous needle between the ribs will stop embarrassing mediastinal shift until proper suction can be instituted.   Resolution of pneumothorax should be complete before air travel is permitted.   Sea level gas volumes are doubled at 18,000 feet (379 mm. Hg) and tension pneumothorax will occur in the absence of pressurization.   Artificial symphysis of visceral and parietal pleura for recurrent pneumothoraces.

Possible Dire Consequences without Treatment: Recurrences are common and unprovoked by exertion in three-fourths of cases.   Severe mediastinal shift.   Death, especially with background of emphysema.

References

Blumer, H. M.: Ten year review of spontaneous pneumothorax in armed force hospitals. Am. Rev. Resp. Dis., *90*:261, 1964.
Pepper, O. H. P.: The insidious onset of pneumothorax. Am. J. Med. Sci., *142*:522, 1911.

8. Malignant Hyperthermia

Chandra M. Banerjee

Cause: Familial trait in which muscle contractures, catabolism and heat production are induced by caffeine, muscle relaxants and volatile anesthetics.

Early (Pre-Anesthetic) Manifestations: Generalized muscularity. Localized weakness, especially face, spine, articular, abdominal muscles. Localized cramps or contractures potentiated by caffeine are relieved by Procaine or tetracaine but not lidocaine. Elevated serum creatine phosphokinase levels are seen in most but not all families. Trismus or fasciculations may have been seen after previous otherwise uneventful anesthesias. History of operative deaths in family members.

Late (Anesthetic) Manifestations: Tachypnea, tachycardia, hypotension. Tremors, warmth, cutaneous flush. High pCO_2 and low pO_2 (asphyxia). Lactic acidosis, hyperglycemia. Raised [K]s and [Mg]s with later preterminal fall in [K]s and [Ca]s. Myoglobinemia and myoglobinuria.

Treatment: Preoperative interview as to familial occurrence of muscle disorders, anesthetic accidents. Creatine phosphokinase determinations in suspected individuals. Avoid preoperative digoxin, lidocaine, mepivacaine, muscle relaxants, halothane. Procaine, tetracaine, barbiturates, nitrous oxide are agents of choice.

Treatment of Acute Pyrexia: Ice mattress, lavage, external applications. Hyperventilate with new tubing and mask to eliminate volatile anesthetic. Oxygen. Monitoring ECG, give Procaine or procainamide 0.5–1.0 mg./kg./min. Undiluted 44 mM Na bicarbonate ampules intravenously for lactic acidosis, monitoring blood pH. Insulin in 50% dextrose for hyperkalemia, monitoring [K]s. Monitor urine flow rate and myoglobinuria.

Dire Consequences without Treatment: Acute left ventricular failure. Massive muscle swelling. Consumption coagulopathy. Pigment nephropathy, oliguria. Two thirds of cases are fatal. Amentia following encephalopathy.

References

Moulds, R. F. W., and Denborough, M. A.: Biochemical basis of malignant hyperpyrexia. Brit. Med. J., 2:241, 1974.
Ryan, J. F., et al.: Cardiopulmonary bypass in the treatment of malignant hyperthermia. New Eng. J. Med., *290*:1121, 1974.

Chapter X

Metabolism and Kidney

Joseph H. Magee

Introduction

Catabolism (metabolic heat production) is the oxidation of foodstuffs to produce heat, carbon dioxide, and water. Oxygen from the atmosphere is required for this and the process is affected by diseases of hemoglobin, the lungs, or the circulation. Dissipation of the heat of metabolism is the responsibility of skin and lungs; carbon dioxide is eliminated by the lungs; and loss of water is the function of skin, lungs, and kidney. A still greater involvement of the kidney concerns special products of metabolism.

The lungs eliminate small amounts of ammonia which escape neutralization as carboxylic residues of amino acids are consumed. Most other amino acid transformations produce residues that the kidneys must eliminate. Sulfuric acid arises from oxidation of sulfhydryl (dithiol) groups, and phosphoric acid from metabolism of phospholipids, phosphoproteins, and nucleoproteins. If the liver produces too many keto from fatty acids, these accumulate, and some keto acids (pyruvic and α ketoglutaric) and hydroxy (lactic and succinic) acids from anaerobic muscle metabolism escape neutralization. These catabolites share the property of carbon dioxide, in its hydrated state, of being acids, without its virtue, in a reverse reaction, of becoming volatile. Since the lungs cannot accordingly eliminate them, the kidneys must. Exogenous sources of excess organic or mineral acids are methanol, glycols, salicylates and chloride (NH_4, Ca, K). These metabolic problems are considered in an initial section addressed to acid and base disturbances.

Additionally treated in this chapter are some faults of the kidneys, not as consequences of infection, not especially characterized by hypertension, and not simulating any of the endocrine errors. Diagnostic leading points of these conditions are proteinuria, oliguria, and isosthenuria. At the hands of pathologists, these conditions formerly had a degree of unity that the reader may no longer be willing to accord them. The earliest designation of protein-losing kidneys was nephrosis, by which was meant changes in tubular morphology. The finding of changes in tubular morphology, in connection with oliguric states, then occasioned their designation by terms such as hypoxic nephrosis, hemoglobinuric nephrosis, toxic nephrosis and lower nephron nephrosis. Finally various obstructive nephropathies are subsumed under the term hydronephrosis, literally tubular changes due to hydrostatic pressure.

TABLE X–1 ABBREVIATIONS

pH	= a measure of the concentration of free protons in logarithmic mass units of solvent per equivalence unit of proton (hydrion) = a measure of conventional activity, respective to standards of same ionic strength and temperature, determined electrometrically or colorimetrically.
pH_c	= capillary blood pH = 7.39–7.42
pH_a	= arterial blood pH = 7.38–7.41
pH_v	= venous blood pH = 7.35–7.38
pCO_2	= partial pressure (tension) of CO_2 in capillary blood = 38.5–43.5 mm. Hg
$[HCO_3]s$	= serum concentration of bicarbonate = 24–30 mM/l
$[Cl]s$	= serum concentration of chloride = 100–106 mM/l
$[\Delta]s$	= serum concentration of undetermined anions = 11.5–19.5 mM/l
$[Na]s$	= serum concentration of sodium = 135–142 mM/l
$[K]s$	= serum concentration of potassium = 3.8–4.3 mM/l; spuriously elevated in thrombocytosis in which case plasma concentration, $[K]_p$, should be used.
$[H]$	= sample concentration of free protons = 10^{-pH} moles/liter assuming an activity coefficient of unity.

ACIDS AND BASES

"Once perhaps the atmosphere of the earth consisted chiefly of water and carbon dioxide, but cooling had caused the condensation of most of the water, and geologic processes . . . have removed nearly all of the carbon dioxide . . . . Today carbon dioxide makes up only a little more than 0.03 percent by volume of the whole atmosphere . . . when water is in contact with air, and equilibrium has been established, the amount of free carbonic acid in the water is almost exactly equal to the amount in the air. The extraordinary capacity of carbonic acid to preserve neutrality in aqueous solution, which is explained by its strength and solubility in water, is a well-established experimental fact, and no other known substance shares this power . . . ordinarily it is quite accurate enough to speak of any solution containing both free carbonic acid and a bicarbonate, when the disparity between the concentrations of the two substances is not very great, as of constant neutral reaction. This characteristic of carbonic acid is of the utmost significance, first by regulating one of the most fundamental of physicochemical conditions, and secondly by preserving throughout nature the chemical inactivity of water, which disappears whenever the reaction becomes either appreciably acid or appreciably alkaline. . . . Almost wholly through this mechanism the oceans are always nearly neutral. Chiefly with its aid protoplasm and blood possess an unvarying reaction. . . . The present ratio between bicarbonate and carbonic acid in sea water has not been accurately estimated but it is perhaps 50:1 or 100:1." "In blood and protoplasm the concentration of bicarbonates must be from ten to twenty times as great as the concentration of carbonic acid, for these are the relationships at hydrogen in concentrations corresponding to those found in normal blood. . . . It is evident that wherever free carbonic acid exists, alkalinity of any real intensity is impossible, for by the action of the free acid all excess of alkali must be speedily and completely converted into bicarbonate; therefore, in such a case the hydrogen ion concentration is defined by the equation $[H\pm] = k\ (H_2\ CO_3/NaHCO_3)$, in which k varies with the temperature. . . . We may then write as an approximation sufficiently accurate for our present purposes the equation $(H\pm) = k/0.8 \times HA/NaA$, that is to say in the solution of a weak acid and its sodium salt, the concentrations of hydrogen ions is equal to the ionization constant of the acid divided by 0.8, approximately the degree of ionization of the salt, and multiplied by the ratio between the total amounts of acid and salt in the solution . . . ." "The average normal hydrion concentration of the blood plasma lies near the slightly alkaline point $(H+) = 4 \times 10^{-8}$ or pH 7.4. This figure was estimated by L. J. Henderson in 1909 and has been confirmed by the electrometric determinations of Lundsgaard."

Hydrogen occurs in the physical world as hydrogen gas, in the biologic world as organic compounds, and in both as a solvent, called water, with peculiar properties. A surprising aspect of familiar watery milieu is a lesser prevalence of ionized hydrogen than in the atmosphere, despite an abundance of other ionizations, water's dielectric constant being 75 times that of the atmosphere. Water's blandness toward this ionic species is owed, as Henderson surmised, to the ready availability, but scant ionization, of carbon dioxide in common solution with strong electrolytes. Most solutes occur in biologic fluids in tenth to thousandth molar amounts; the ratio of their aggregated numbers, respective to solvent molecules, is among the most vigorously guarded of biologic norms. The usual variance of about $\pm 1.25\%$ is maintained by an overall regulation of water economy, independently of solute partition, with osmotic gradient between adjacent fluid phases being exceptional. Hydrogen ions occur in far smaller (billionth molar) amounts but with a greater variance of around $\pm 12.5\%$, and steep gradients occur from interstitial fluid to cytoplasm, from cytoplasm to mitochondria, and in the formation of urine and gastrointestinal fluids.

Both the least and the most abundant solutes of body fluids are charged particles. Exceptions abound, however, in an intermediate range (about 5 millimolar each), as seen with glucose and urea. Essentially unaffected by the presence of other particles in the same solution, these substances exhibit ideal thermodynamic behavior. If an increment of these substances occurs it does not matter whether you measure their concentrations or their effects, which classically are raised osmotic pressure and boiling point, or lowered vapor pressure and freezing point. If it is of relevance to identify the substance causing solvent effects, a measurement is of course chosen based upon a principle such as light absorbance that yields particles numbers for the specific compounds in solution. Analogous measurements of electrolytes, when not in infinitely dilute solution, are more uncertain as to the correspondence of their particles numbers and their solution effects; that is to say we do not know unambiguously the solute activity (corrected or effective concentration). A reverse query of course applies when specific ion measurements are initially based upon activity, based upon effective rather than actual concentration, as in the electrometric determination of hydrogen ion.

The hydrogen electrode dates from 1909, the quinhydrone electrode from 1921, the glass electrode from 1923, and the Sanz microelectrode from 1957. Following the last development, direct determinations of a blood sample's reaction have been increasingly available in medical practice. If blood were a buffered single-phase system, knowledge of pH would tell one directionally how to treat the patient (give alkali or give acid). Speculatively, with both pH and a titration curve, one would know how to treat quantitatively (titrate the patient to normal pH). Since we actually deal with a two-phase system (gas dissolved in blood), we need to know both pH and pCO_2. Let us say that these are available. We know that with acidity and hypercapnia (or with alkalinity and hypocapnia) we have a carbonic acid disturbance (respiratory). With acidity and hypocapnia (or alkalinity and hypercapnia) we have a disturbance of the non-volatile phase of the system, called metabolic, and reflected in a primary change in bicarbonate. Again we know how to treat directionally. We refrain, however, from projecting quantitative aspects of treatment, especially in unsteady states, due to the large differences in distribution volumes of the volatile and non-volatile components of the system.

When pH is determined electrometrically, the response of the galvanic cell to the hydrogen ions in test solution is changed electrical potential, which can be read out on a meter. The meter can be calibrated to read instead in units of chemical potential, a thermodynamic quantity which at a given temperature is a logarithmic function of available hydrogen ions. Sorensen's pioneer applications of the hydrogen electrode had to do with production problems of the Danish beer industry and here a wide range of hydrogen ion concentrations were encountered. Accordingly, as another byproduct of this endeavor, the pH nomenclature emerged as an operationally successful method of dealing with some very small numbers.

One way of dealing with small numbers is to convert them to large numbers. This can rather readily be rationalized in solution chemistry, since one may elect to speak of the solvent to solute ratio of a solution instead of its conventional reverse. Thus, where the ratio of hydrogen ions to solvent molecules is four in a hundred million, or 4×10^{-8}, the reverse ratio of solvent molecules to hydrogen ions is a hundred millions to four, or $10^8 \div 4$. So far there is no practical advantage in facilitating memory or preventing errors, unless one maintains that large numbers are inherently easier to remember than small ones. Conceptually, should it seem more elegant to stress the changed behavior of a solvent rather than its solute, it will indeed be satisfying to have this in the numerator. The practical advantage is, however, that it becomes easier to use mathematical operators. Say that we wish to take the logarithms, something our electrochemical cell already does inherently, of the hydrogen ions in solution. Here this is done not primarily to ease subsequent multiplying and dividing, but because of the numerical reduction that is achieved. Thus, the quotient of $10^8 \div 4$, becomes a matter of subtracting 0.6 (the logarithm of 4) from 8 (the logarithm of 10^8), yielding a most manageable 7.4.

There are alternate ways of handling very small numbers, without inverting them, that are serviceable though scarcely as powerful as pH. If the ratio, in plasma, of creatinine to solvent molecules is one in ten thousand, or 1×10^{-4}, use may be made of a unit, the micromole, which indicates a concentration of one part in a million, or 1×10^{-6}. In this unitage the concentration of creatinine is 100 micromolar. This is of a similar order of magnitude to that of hydrogen ions in the most acid of possible urines, which is about 40 micromolar. Since micromoles designate a concentration of one part in a million, there are 40×10^{-6} hydrogen ions or 4×10^{-5}. As in the previous instance, pH is the quotient of $10^5 \div 4$ found by subtracting 0.6 (the logarithm of 4), from 5 (the logarithm of 10^5), pH of the urine being 4.4.

Creatinine in urine may attain concentrations 100-fold that in plasma, or of the order of 10,000 micromolar. This is, of course, more conveniently expressed as 10 millimolar. This attains a magnitude corresponding to the lower range in which undissociated (titratable) acid occurs in the same urine.

The paucity of dissociated acids in most biologic fluids is disproportionate to known challenges in terms of invading acids. This is not wholly due to the circumstance that the major potential acid resulting from the combustion of foodstuffs is carbon dioxide, a substance in heterogeneous equilibrium from its cellular origins, via the circulating fluids, with the atmosphere, that has in this transit a slow uncatalyzed reaction rate with water. These attributes become subordinate, however, in view of the enormous amounts of the substances formed, with direction though not the velocity, of the reaction continuously determined by availability of the reactants. The reason that fluids outside cells contain abundant water but operationally contain little carbon dioxide is that the latter is rapidly shuttled into red cells, hydrated there, and disposed of by processes designated buffering.

The most abundant buffers are either polyelectrolytes (amphoteric proteins) or poorly ionized mineral acids (such as phosphoric and carbonic), in each instance paired with their conjugate bases. The first two substances enumerated occur predominantly though not exclusively in cells. A ubiquitous substance, carbonic acid everywhere accompanies water; when its origin is in protoplasm it is paired with bicarbonate ions which characteristically permeate their cells of origin and attain high concentrations outside them.

Each body fluid phase attains at equilibrium a distinctive reaction wherein $[H+]^*$ is a constant and the whole becomes describable as a mixture of isohydric solutions. In a sample of venous blood with $[H+]$ reportedly 40 nanomoles per liter the description would be:

$$[H+] = k_1 r_1 = k_2 r_2 = k_3 r_3 = k_4 r_4 = k_5 r_5$$

In the appended table numerical values are assigned for the r's which are dimensionless ratios. The k's are apparent dissociation constants of weak acids in the presence of their conjugate bases. The dimensions for k_{1-3} are nanomoles per liter plasma and for k_{4-5} nanomoles per liter blood. R is an alkali metal cation, either sodium or potassium, Pr is plasma protein, and Hb hemoglobin.

---

* It is recommended that when $[H+]$ is read in a sentence, it be articulated as "aitch" or "hydrion," according to preference.

r_1	r_2	r_3	r_4	r_5
$\dfrac{HHCO_3}{RHCO_3}$	$\dfrac{RH_2PO_4}{R_2HPO_4}$	$\dfrac{HP_r}{RP_r}$	$\dfrac{HHbO_2}{RHbO_2}$	$\dfrac{HHb}{RHb}$
$\dfrac{1.2}{24}$	$\dfrac{0.3}{1.5}$	$\dfrac{2.0}{6.25}$	$\dfrac{8.0}{14}$	$\dfrac{2.0}{2.5}$
k_1	k_2	k_3	k_4	k_5
800	200	125	70	50

If this system were single phase (wholly fluid), extending throughout plasma and red cells, but otherwise closed, the constituent solutions most effective in resisting change in their common [H+] would be those with the lowest k's and reciprocally the highest r's (ratios of weak acid to base). As the latter increase toward unity, the k's decrease toward numerical identity with [H+]. The buffers outside plasma, conforming most nearly to this ideal, affect [H+] within it. The total of so-called buffer bases in plasma, summing the denominators, is a little over 30 mM/l; their total for whole blood is about 48 mM/l, about twice the bicarbonate concentration.

How much of this information is medically useful? It is pertinent to ask because the design capability to make all of this information generally available, with little labor, undoubtedly exists. As an extension such a program could generate additional questions to ask the patient as, for example, regarding recent ingestions of soda and aspirin. As a central datum we have [H+] as 40 nanomoles per liter in a representative body compartment (plasma). This is known from ions in adjacent plasma which permeated the glass electrode; those in the interior of the red cell where their concentration was more nearly 63 nanomoles per liter were less accessible. From this datum for the plasma compartment, assuming no change in the values we assigned the thermodynamic variables (k's), we assume normality of buffer ratios generally.

On occasion the values making up some of the functions may appear a little strange, implying adjustments due to disease. Even so as long as the overall values of r remain undisturbed, [H+] also is unchanged. So far our view of how [H+] behaves and our equations representing this have been analogous to plotting values of r on one axis and those of k on another using them as Cartesian coordinates of a point to obtain values of [H+].

Originally we represent the coordinates as extraneous to the equation, ascertaining the position of points [H+] metrically. We can do the same thing parametrically. Plotting [H+] establishes a function since a rule exists whereby k can be determined for any r. Various other functions emerge as [H+] is plotted. For example, a rule is found determining $HHCO_3$ for any value of $RHCO_3/k_1$ and one determining $RHCO_3$ for any value of k ($HHCO_3$). The [H+] plot thus generates a variety of intrinsic coordinates on its own able to locate the same points. If the availability of data changes so that we now lack [H+], we have been told our business. We derive it from measurements of $HHCO_3$ and $RHCO_3$.

Such permutations are often justified, with much of the blame falling upon Gauss, as follows. Each pairing of r and k from external coordinates creates

unique values of [H+], generating a number line. The line is a one dimensional subspace and any member of its set of points can potentially be specified
by a single number or parameter. A two dimensional subspace is a surface,
with two numbers or parameters necessary and sufficient to specify the
position of each member point. In particular as r and k run through a
range of the numbers previously inscribed on axes, functions relating them
take on numerical values. As they do so [H+] now moves on a surface
having many equations in terms of r and k. Two numbers or parameters
(lines in space, intrinsic coordinates) are all that is needed to specify its
position. The same now applies if it is now decided to make RHCO₃/k or
k (HHCO₃) parameters of the surface; there simply is a transformation of
coordinates.

This notion of surface suffices particularly well for the isohydric equation
with its numerous k and r pairs:

$$[H+] = k_1r_1 = k_2r_2 = k_3r_3 = k_4r_4 = k_5 r_5$$

which suffice as parameters of a solution surface for equations of [H+]. A
little more now needs to be said about the isohydric equation. It tells us
rather more than we want to know about analytically available red cell
buffers which have but a small volume of distribution. Their buffering

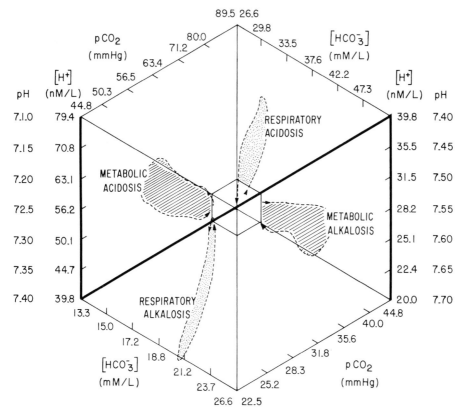

Fig. X–1.   Diagram of the relationship of the acidoses, metabolic and respiratory,
and the alkaloses, metabolic and respiratory.

capacity for the open system carrying carbon dioxide to the alveoli is enormous, effectively minimizing [H+] increases in surrounding fluids. Even as we are aware of how much we are left to surmise about k_6 r_6, etc., within cells beyond the purview of our measurements, we perforce have to scrutinize most regularly the most dynamic element of the system, the equilibrium expression for the heterogeneous buffer pair (carbonic acid-bicarbonate), k_1 r_1.

For this it is better to return to the Cartesian rendering of a surface by one equation among three coordinates $ax + by + cz + d = 0$. Here x, y, and z become pH, log pCO_2 and $1/\log RHCO_3$. A graph which flattens this out by putting the axes at 60 instead of 90 degrees to one another is that of Shock and Hastings, for which available triaxial coordinate paper can be used. Note that the non-respiratory acid-base disturbances show hysteresis, with their pathways of return differing from those of displacement.

References

Henderson, L. J.: The Fitness of the Environment. New York, The Macmillan Co., 1913. Reissued, Boston, Beacon Press, 1958, p. 134.
Henderson, L. J.: The theory of neutrality regulation in the animal organism. J. Biol. Chem., *21*:427, 1908.
Peters, J. P., and Van Slyke, D. D.: Quantitative Clinical Chemistry, Vol. I. Baltimore, The Williams & Wilkins Co., 1931, p. 940.

1. Alkaluric Alkalosis (Non-Respiratory)

Joseph H. Magee

Cause: Absorbable alkali therapy.

Therapy of cystinuria to attain urine pH 8.0, renal tubular acidosis to attain urine pH 7.0, and uric acid lithiasis to attain urine pH 6.0, using sodium bicarbonate, sodium citrate, Shohl's or Harrison's solution.

Formerly sodium bicarbonate or calcium carbonate therapy of peptic ulcer, still prominent in self-medication (Milk-alkali or Burnett's syndrome).

Formerly to promote alkaluria during sulfonamide therapy.

Early Manifestations: "That the syndrome of alkalosis which may complicate the treatment of peptic ulcer was recognized initially by Sippy and later described in detail by numerous observers ... symptoms usually begin in 3 to 8 days ..."

"Hardt and Rivers ... noted nausea, headache, distaste for milk, apathy and drowsiness, and some of their patients developed albuminuria ... the 'Sippy regime' which Hardt and Rivers employed involved frequent gastric aspiration as well as milk and alkali by mouth."

"The observations recorded here show that alkalosis *per se* has no injurious effects, at least for periods up to three weeks ... an important distinction is that in pyloric stenosis quite a moderate degree of alkalosis is commonly associated with gross depletion of body fluids and disturbance of renal function; if however, the fluid depletion is corrected, renal function improves, even if alkalosis becomes worse." (Burnett, et al.)

Treatment: Non-absorbable alkalis should be substituted in Sippy regimens and body fluid depletion should be corrected primarily.

Dire Consequences without Treatment: Nephrocalcinosis.

References

Burnett, C. H., Burrows, B. A., and Commons, R. R.: Studies of alkalosis. J. Clin. Invest., *29*:199, 1950.

Cooke, A. M.: Alkalosis in the alkaline treatment of peptic ulcer. Quart. J. Med., *1*:527, 1932.

Gatewood, L. C.: The essential safeguards in the alkali treatment of peptic ulcer. Illinois Med. J., *48*:491, 1925.

Hardt, L. L., and Rivers, A. B.: Toxic manifestations following the alkaline treatment of peptic ulcers. Arch. Intern. Med., *31*:171, 1923.

Jeghers, H. J., and Lerner, H. H.: The syndrome of alkalosis complicating the treatment of peptic ulcer. New Eng. J. Med., *214*:1, 236, 1936.

McCance, R. A., and Widdowson, E. M.: Alkalosis with disordered kidney function. Lancet, 2:247, 1937.

Steele, J. M.: Renal insufficiency developing during prolonged use of alkalis. JAMA, *106*:2049, 1936.

Van Goidsenhoven, G. M., et al.: The effect of prolonged administration of large doses of sodium bicarbonate in man. Clin. Sci., *13*:383, 1954.

10

2. Alkaluric Alkalosis (Respiratory)

JOSEPH H. MAGEE

Cause: Primary hypocapnia (primary hyperventilation).

Arterial unsaturation (Anoxic anoxia).

(*a.*) High altitude.

(*b.*) Alveolar diffusion block including pulmonary edema and pulmonary fibrosis.

(*c.*) Congenital cardiac veno-arterial shunting.

(*d.*) Acquired esophageal veno-pulmonary shunting in hepatic cirrhosis.

(*e.*) Congenital met- and M-hemoglobinopathies.

(*f.*) Acquired met-sulf-, cyan-, and carboxy-hemoglobinopathies.

Anemic anoxia.

Histotoxic anoxias including beriberi and thyrotoxicosis.

Fever, exercise, emotion, alcohol, paraldehyde, and salicylates.

Hypoglycemic coma, increased intracranial pressure, brain stem infarcts.

Ventilatory assistance in neuromuscular respiratory failure.

Early Manifestations: Vertigo, syncope; tongue, circumoral and extremity paresthesias.

Decreased pCO_2

Decreased [HCO_3]s, seldom below 15 mM per L., concomitant metabolic acidosis is suspected if lower.

Raised [Cl]s, not completely compensatory for the decreased [HCO_3], indicating that some lactic-pyruvic acidosis is universally present.

Blood pH normal or raised; if much raised in presence of minimal [HCO_3]s change, suspect combined disturbance such as metabolic alkalosis, due to vomiting, etc., in hyperventilating patient.

Alkaluria (urine pH 7.0 or more).

Treatment: Removal of responsible pharmacologic agents, especially salicylates. Alkaluria enhances salicylate elimination; urine pH should be monitored, since fall into acid range may indicate systemic organic acidosis, especially in children; in which case intravenous sodium bicarbonate therapy is indicated and acetazolamide is not. About one ampule (44 mM/50 ml) sodium bicarbonate per hour is given adults if serum salicylate level is 60 mg./ml. or more, in isotonic dextrose, fructose, or mannitol to maintain urine flow rate of 10 ml./min. or more, and continued until serum salicylate level is less than 40 mg./100 ml. Serum potassium may fall markedly and should be supplemented in each infusion bottle made up. Acetazolamide 250 mg. intravenously may be given and repeated in two hours.

Rebreathing of expired carbon dioxide, by means of a bag, is useful in some patients having anxiety-associated hyperventilation to the point of carpopedal spasm.

In most other entities removal of the underlying cause is the only step indicated; hyperventilation in many states is mediated by increased sensitivity to CO_2, which raising pCO_2 by CO_2 inhalations will not alleviate.

Possible Dire Consequences without Treatment: Confusion with metabolic acidosis with secondary hyperventilation. Underestimation of concomitant metabolic acidosis.

References

Cawley, E. P., Peterson, N. T., and Wheeler, C. E.: Salicylic acid poisoning in dermatologic therapy. J.A.M.A., *151*:372, 1953.

Cohen, A. S.: Differential diagnosis of salicylate intoxication and diabetic acidosis. New Eng. J. Med., *254*:457, 1956.

Halle, M. A., and Collipp, P. J.: Treatment of methyl salicylate poisoning by peritoneal dialysis. New York J. Med., *69*:1788, 1969.

Kallen, R. J., et al.: Hemodialysis in children. Medicine, *45*:1, 1966.

Lawson, A. A., Proudfoot, A. T., and Brown, S. S.: Forced diuresis in the treatment of acute salicylate poisoning in adults. Quart. J. Med., *38*:31, 1969.

Morgan, A. G., and Polak, A.: Acetazolamide and sodium bicarbonate poisoning in adults. Brit. Med. J., *1*:16, 1969.

Proudfoot, A. T., and Brown, S. S.: Acidaemia and salicylate poisoning in adults. Brit. Med. J. 2:547, 1969.

Prowse, K., et al.: The treatment of salicylate poisoning using mannitol and forced alkaline diuresis. Clin. Sci., *38*:327, 1970.

Singer, R. B.: Acid-base disturbances in salicylate intoxication. Medicine, *33*:1, 1954.

3. Appropriate Alkaluria (Respiratory)

Joseph H. Magee

Cause: Correction of hypercapnia.

Early Manifestations: Relief of chronic obstructive pulmonary disease by removal of secretions, pressure or volume controlled respirators, and other measures. Fall in [HCO_3]s follows decrease in pCO_2, mediated by increased urine HCO_3 excretion, with urine pH 7.0 or more.

Treatment: Treatment is primarily anticipatory since bicarbonaturia is a homeostatically useful response. If bicarbonaturia does *not* ensue or is curtailed, equivalent lowering of pCO_2 and of [HCO_3]s will not have occurred; with the patient suffering *post-hypercapnic alkalosis.* This is a potentially dangerous situation, and if respiration is being controlled, more gradual lowering of pCO_2 may become necessary.

Possible Dire Consequences without Treatment: Severe alkalosis, hypokalemia, death.

Post-hypercapnic alkalosis is likely if maximal reabsorption of sodium salts by the kidney is occasioned by factors in the patient's illness such as circulatory failure, due either to cardiac factors or to volume contraction. The propensity to increased bicarbonate in the reabsorbate, compared to the filtrate, derives from high capacity, low gradient hydrogen ion secretion linked to inward sodium movement having the same characteristics. The driving force to hydrogen ion secretion decreases if whole body pCO_2 and renal tubular cell pCO_2 fall as the respiratory ailment is treated. This may suffice to vary hydrogen ion secretion independently of sodium reabsorption, even though the latter remains maximal, provided (1) there is sufficient counterforce to hydrogen secretion in terms of chloride entering from the lumen, and (2) that other influences upon tubular cell pH (such as potassium deficit) do not continue to stimulate hydrogen ion secretion directly. Consequently oral liquid potassium chloride supplementation by tube, or in palatable ingested form, is widely used to minimize the tendency to alkalosis.

References

Cochran, R. T., Jr.: Pulmonary insufficiency and hypercapnia complicated by potassium-responsive alkalosis. New Eng. J. Med., *268*:521, 1963.

Koralnik, O.: Acidose respiratoire surcompensée, alcalose prolongée. Helvet Med. Acta, *27*:753, 1961.

Murray, J. F.: Carbon dioxide retention without acidosis. Am. Rev. Resp. Dis., *86*:126, 1962.

Pokak, A., et al.: Effects of chronic hypercapnia on electrolyte and acid-base equilibrium I. J. Clin. Invest., *40*:1223, 1961.

Refsum, H. E.: Hypokalemic alkalosis during recovery from compensated respiratory acidosis. Scand. J. Lab. & Clin. Invest., *14*:545, 1962.

Refsum, H. E.: Hypokalemic alkalosis with paradoxical aciduria during artificial ventilation of patients with pulmonary insufficiency and high plasma bicarbonate concentrations. Scand. J. Lab. Clin. Invest., *13*:481, 1961.

Robin, E. D.: Abnormalities of acid-base regulation in chronic pulmonary disease, with special reference to hypocapnia and extracellular acidosis. New Eng. J. Med., *268*:917, 1963.

Schwartz, W. B., et al.: Effects of chronic hypercapnia on electrolyte and acid-base equilibrium II. J. Clin. Invest., *40*:1238, 1961.

Schwartz, W. B., Jenson, R. L., and Relman, A. S.: Acidification of the urine and increased ammonium excretion without change in acid-base equilibrium. Sodium reabsorption as a stimulus to the acidifying process. (Maximum reabsorption of sodium ions, without chloride to decrease hydrogen counter-flow, acidified the urine to pH 4.0 in the absence of direct stimulus to hydrogen ion secretion by systemic acid-base change.) J. Clin. Invest., *34*:676, 1955.

Van Yypersele de Storihoks, C. Gulyassy, P. F., and Schwartz, W. B.: Effects of chronic hypercapnia on electrolyte and acid-base equilibrium III. J. Clin. Invest., *41*:2246, 1962.

4. Contraction Alkalosis

Joseph H. Magee

Cause: Sodium chloride losses by repeated vomiting or suctioning of upper gut fluids with average pH less than 7.0.

Early Manifestations: Virtual disappearance of sodium and chloride from urine, pH of which ranges 5.0 to 6.4 (paradoxic or inappropriate aciduria). Raised [HCO_3]s 30–50 mM/l. Thirst, water ingestion despite vomiting, renal water conservation, hyponatremia. Tetany. Decreased [Ca]s, [Mg]s, [K]s.

Treatment: Contraction and alkalosis are treated in that order. With saline volume replacement, increased urine sodium is accompanied by reappearance of bicarbonate in addition to chloride, with urine pH's greater than 7.0.

Restitution of [Cl]s to normal value, in 95 to 100 range, is useful endpoint as to adequacy of volume replacement. [K]s may have fallen during replacement. Supplemental K and Mg should be provided until resumption of complete diet is possible.

Possible Dire Consequences without Treatment: Alkalosis, tetany, hypokalemia, death.

References

Gamble, J. L., and Ross, S. G.: The factors in the dehydration following pyloric obstruction. J. Clin. Invest., *1*:430, 1925.

Haden, R. L., and Orr, T. G.: Chemical changes in the blood of the dog after pyloric obstruction. J. Exper. Med., *37*:377, 1923.

Hartmann, A. F., and Smyth, F. S.: Chemical changes in the body occurring as a result of vomiting. Am. J. Dis. Child., *32*:1, 1926.

Roberts, K. E., et al.: Changes in the extracellular water and electrolytes and the renal compensations in chronic alkalosis. Surgery, *6*:599, 1954.

VanSlyke, K. K., and Evans, E. I.: The paradox of aciduria in the presence of alkalosis caused by hypochloremia. Ann. Surg., *126*:545, 1947.

5. Potassium Deficiency

JOSEPH H. MAGEE

Cause: Loss of gastrointestinal fluids.
- (*a.*) Cessation of intake, with negative balance due to continuing renal losses, may have preceded overt G.I. fluid loss, since adaptive renal compensation for diminished intake is accomplished slowly and incompletely.
- (*b.*) Direct loss via G.I. fluids is 5 to 20 mM/l depending upon source.
- (*c.*) If gastric fluids are lost, alkalosis increases the urinary K^+ loss for any given level of [K]s.

Renal tubular acidosis.

Exogenous and endogenous mineralocorticoid and glucocorticoid excess syndromes.

Early Manifestations: Skeletal muscle weakness.
- (*a.*) This may progress exceptionally to quadriplegia and neuromuscular respiratory paralysis. Generally muscular weakness is not readily correlated with [K], as illustrated by several variants of periodic paralysis where rapid [K] changes may be observed.
- (*b.*) Increased neuromuscular irritability may be seen in K^+ depletion, without concomitant Ca^{++} depletion, but always in a setting of alkalosis.

Ileus.

Effects upon cardiac muscle and conduction tissue: loss of T wave amplitude, occurrence of positive after-potentials (U-waves) at the end of the T waves in limb leads, finally presence of U waves alone, with measurement of QU intervals as apparently prolonged QT intervals.

Renal effects
- (*a.*) Inability to concentrate the urine, an observation which should be made at frequent intervals in intubated patients, who usually have every reason to put out a concentrated urine. Both polyuria and specific gravities below 1.015 should be viewed with suspicion as possibly signifying inadequate potassium repletion.
- (*b.*) Polydipsia. This may be disproportionate to the concentrating defect and has been noted especially in primary aldosteronism, but also in K^+ depletion studies in volunteers.
- (*c.*) Vulnerability to pyelonephritis is increased by K^+ depletion.

Expansion of extracellular fluid volume and frank edema have been noted with K^+ depletion, which may aggravate the condition of the already edema-prone patient. It is sometimes noted with beginning K^+ repletion, ameliorating with further repletion. A complicated interaction of renal sodium retention and a reinfusion of cell bound sodium into extracellular spaces may be responsible.

Treatment: Administration of K^+ either parenterally or orally depending on the urgency of the need.

Possible Dire Consequences without Treatment: Inability of kidneys to concentrate urine, frank edema, paraplegia and respiratory paralysis.

6. Saline-Resistant Alkalosis

JOSEPH H. MAGEE

Cause: Renal potassium-wasting usually due to administration of, or autonomous production of, corticosteroids. Absence of body fluid contraction. Altered extra-intracellular cation equilibria with hydrion shifts into K^+ depleted cells, including renal tubular cells. High steady-state hydrion excretion, despite urine pHs in 6.0–7.0 range, due to increased ammoniagenesis. High reabsorbate bicarbonate concentration without reciprocal aciduria.

Early Manifestations: Raised blood pH, [HCO_3]s. Low [K]s. Paradoxic aciduria maintaining alkalosis, though usually with urines no more acid than pH 6.0 to 7.0.

Treatment: The [K]s is not a reliable indicator of bodily depletion since patients with 10% and 30% depletions may have identical [K]s, which may be between 2 and 3 mM/l but exceptionally may be within normal range.

"Paradoxic aciduria" with urine pH less than 6.0 due to increased [H], reciprocally to low [K] of the renal tubular cells, is seen early in K^+ depletion, returning with repletion, urine pH usually being fixed between 6.0 and 7.0 during chronic and severe K^+ depletion.

Alkalosis is resistant to volume expansion in the severe grades of K^+ depletion due to corticosteroid excesses and "repair" of alkalosis helps gauge adequacy of repletion.

Possible Dire Consequences without Treatment: Weakness, polyuria, thirst, neuromuscular irritability.

In patients presenting with an intercurrent gastrointestinal disturbance, hypokalemia and alkalosis may be ascribed to contraction alkalosis and so treated. Saline repair of circulatory contraction usually removes the stimulus to sodium resorption, and without independent acid secretory drive, bicarbonaturia occurs. In mineralocorticoid excess states neither of these conditions may be satisfied; sodium reabsorption may continue unabated, and may fail to diminish the bicarbonate pool because the urine may remain somewhat acid, with bicarbonate in the reabsorbate reciprocally high. The cause of the continued acid secretory drive is presumed to be protonation of cation deficient renal tubular cells.

Since failure of saline correction should arouse suspicion of mineralocorticoid excess, potassium repletion should precede studies of aldosterone excretion, since these may be spuriously low in extreme potassium depletion.

References

Atchley, D. W., et al.: On diabetic acidosis: Detailed studies of electrolyte balances following withdrawal and reestablishment of insulin therapy. J. Clin. Invest., *12*:297, 1933.

Evans, B. M., et al.: Electrolyte excretion during experimental potassium depletion in man. Clin. Sci., *13*:305, 1954.

Fourman, P. A.: The ability of the normal kidney to conserve potassium. Lancet, *1*:1042, 1952.

Kleeman, C. R. and Maxwell, M. H.: Contributory role of extrarenal factors in the polyuria of potassium depletion. New Eng. J. Med. *260*:268, 1959.

Kunau, R. T., et al.: Micropuncture study of the proximal tubular factors responsible for the maintenance of alkalosis during potassium deficiency in the rat. Clin. Sci., *34*:223, 1968.

Leather, M. H., and Honey, H. J.: Hypokalemia, uremia and tetany. Brit. Med. J., *2*:293, 1964.

Luke, R. G., and Levitin, H.: Impaired renal conservation of chloride and acid-base changes associated with potassium depletion. Clin. Sci., *32*:511, 1967.

Schwartz, W. B., Levine, H. D., and Relman, A. S.: The electrocardiogram in potassium depletion. Am. J. Med., *16*:395, 1954.

Schwartz, W. B., and Relman, A. S.: Metabolic and renal studies in chronic potassium depletion resulting from the overuse of laxatives. J. Clin. Invest., *32*:258, 1953.

Scribner, B. H., and Burnell, J. M.: Interpretation of the serum potassium concentration. Metabolism, *5*:468, 1956.

Seldin, D. W., Welt, L. G., and Cort, J. H.: The role of sodium salts and adrenal steroids in the production of hypokalemic alkalosis. Yale J. Biol. Med., *29*:229, 1956.

Womersley, R. A. and Darragh, J. H.: Potassium and sodium restriction in the normal human. J. Clin. Invest. *34*:456, 1955.

7. Carbonic Acidosis

Joseph H. Magee

Cause: Non-removal of carbon dioxide (Respiratory acidosis).

(*a.*) Non-carrying (pCO_2 raised in tissue phase only), theoretically may occur with sufficient red cell carbonic anhydrase inhibition (no CO_2 transport) or sufficient methemoglobinemia (no CO_2 or O_2 transport).

(*b.*) Non-perfusing ⎫ pCO_2 raised in tissue and fluid phases but not in
(*c.*) Non-diffusing ⎭ alveolar phase.

(*d.*) Non-ventilating: pCO_2 raised in tissue, fluid and alveolar phases:

    1. Primary   :CNS
    2. Costal   :Non-moving, flail-moving, deformation
    3. Diaphragmatic   :Non-moving, rupture, elevation, paradox
    4. Pleural   :Fluid, air, cortication
    5. Pulmonary   :Loss of elasticity and surface

Non-vaporizing (Hypothermic acidosis).

(*a.*) Cool blood hydrates more CO_2 than warm blood, equilibrium between the reaction of dehydration and hydration being shifted slightly to the right, so more H_2CO_3 than usual is present for a given pCO_2 even though pCO_2 itself is lower. To this complicated relation also is added a decrease in the anion value of the blood proteins. This permits additional trapping of CO_2 as bicarbonate, paralleling the gain in H_2CO_3, and minimizing the tendency to carbonic acidosis:

$$KPrOH + H_2CO_3 \longrightarrow Pr + HOH + KHCO_3$$

The same end is served as in the renal generation of bicarbonate in chronic respiratory acidosis, but it occurs at some expense to the ability of these proteins to buffer stronger invading acids such as lactic.

$$KPrOH + HX \longrightarrow Pr + HOH + KX$$

Non-compensating (dilutional acidosis)

A result of giving bicarbonate free fluids into which CO_2 becomes dissolved. This commonest acidosis in medicine is ordinarily produced knowingly and treated, expectantly and successfully, by letting the kidneys generate the bicarbonate not given, in response to normal or augmented filtration. If the recoverable rate of filtration is too low, the treatment will be unsuccessful. The pCO_2 of tissue, fluid and alveolar phases remains normal, but the proportion of bicarbonate accompanying it falls. If bicarbonate has been diluted more than sodium, as when the expanding solution has been isotonic NaCl, there will be a reciprocal hyperchloremia.

Early Manifestations: Non-removal.
 (*a.*) Due to methemoglobinemia:
 — pO_2 decrease and cyanosis disproportionate to increase in pCO_2.
 — Central origin of cyanosis evident from dark red to reddish-brown blood tint which does not brighten with aeration of sample.
 — History of congenital and/or familial cyanosis or of exposure to chemicals (Acetanilid, acetophenetidin, analgesics, benzocaine, chlorates, chromates, cuprates, nitrates, nitrites, primaquin, quinones, sulfonamides), crayons, stenciled diapers, or well water.
 (*b.*) Non-perfusion of ventilated lungs:
 — Potential source(s) of thromboemboli, fat emboli.
 — Tachypnea, tachycardia, air hunger, pleuritic pain, breath sound suppression, electrocardiographic axis shifts, arrhythmias or P pulmonale, hyperaeration radiographically.
 — pO_2 decrease disproportionate to pCO_2 increase.
 (*c.*) Diffusion block:
 — Predominant restrictive over obstructive physical signs and functional test patterns.
 — pO_2 decrease disproportionate to pCO_2 increase.
 — further pO_2 decrease with exercise.
 (*d.*) Hypoventilation:
 — pCO_2 increase disproportionate to pO_2 decrease.
 — pO_2 decrease not linearly reflected in arterial O_2 unsaturation, as measured; or as observable cyanosis.
 — in both primary (CNS) and chest-disease hypoventilation, cyanotic threshold is approached as blood production is stimulated and hematocrit increases.
 — signs of obstruction, restriction and pulmonary hypertension aid in recognition of hypoventilation secondary to chest disease.
Non-vaporizing carbonic acidosis (hypothermia):
 — A specialized team problem, where lactic rather than carbonic acidosis is highly likely.
 — Since pCO_2 underestimates H_2CO_3 of cool blood because temperature dependent equilibrium of hydration reaction has changed, simultaneous pH values are required.
 — pH's done at patient's actual temperature, corresponding roughly to room temperature (neutral point $= 7.0$), overestimate blood alkalemia when they correspond to previous pH's at usual body temperature (neutral point $=$ pH 6.8).
 — Many laboratories therefore do preoperative, operative and rewarming values at same temperature throughout, rather than following Δ pH (pH minus neutral point).
Non-compensating (Dilutional acidosis).
 — low [HCO_3]s and blood pH.
 — low [Na]s if non-saline fluids given.
 — reciprocally raised [Cl]s if saline fluids given.

Treatment: Respiratory Acidosis: Occurs in neuromuscular respiratory failure which is becoming less common, in chronic pulmonary failure which is becoming more common, and theoretically in impaired red cell CO_2 transport.
 (*a.*) Non-carrying (Methemoglobinemia):
 — discontinue toxic agent.
 — O_2 administration if stuporous or methemoglobin exceeds 40%.
 — Methylene blue 1–2 mg/kg q 2h $\times$ 24 hours unless markedly less stuporous and cyanosed. It is not helpful in individuals with hemoglobin nor with G6PD deficiency.

(*b.*) Neuro-muscular respiratory failure.
— rocking bed, drinker or bellows respirator intermittently or continuously to decrease metabolic CO_2 production incident to work of breathing.
— Removal of secretions.
— Treatment of intercurrent infections.
(*c.*) Chronic pulmonary failure.
— pressure or volume cycled intermittent pressure respirator, intermittently or continuously.
— humidification and removal of secretions.
— decreased dead space (tracheostomy).
— treatment of intercurrent infections.
(*d.*) Combined disturbances.
— sodium bicarbonate administration in respiratory acidosis has the disadvantage of volume expansion in those subjects with diminished cardiac reserve; removal of gastric HCl may supplement renal bicarbonate generation and raise blood pH without sodium addition. However, in general, measures that raise pH without lowering pCO_2 are not indicated, the exceptions being concomitant metabolic acidosis (diabetic, renal, etc.).

Possible Dire Consequences without Treatment: Confusion with cardiac failure, reliance upon O_2 therapy to neglect of ventilatory assistance in patients in whom raised pCO_2 is not suspected. Hyperkalemia, ventricular escape rhythms.

References

Anthonisen, N. R., and Smith, H. J.: Respiratory acidosis as a consequence of pulmonary edema. Ann. Int. Med., *62*:991, 1965.

Eldridge, R.: Blood lactate and pyruvate in pulmonary insufficiency. New Eng. J. Med., *274*:878, 1966.

Robin, E. D.: Abnormalities of acid-base regulation in chronic pulmonary disease with special references to hypercapnea and extracellular alkalosis. New Eng. J. Med., *268*: 917, 1963.

8. Hydrochloric Acidosis

Joseph H. Magee

Cause: Hydrochloric acid, a strong endogenous acid which, unlike carbonic acid, is completely dissociated, immediately protonating available acceptors (bases) of body fluids according to their strength. Insofar as this is bicarbonate, the surviving acid is carbonic acid so that the net effect of the invading acid is measured as lowered [HCO_3]s.

Portal of Entry: Contraluminal: loss of gut $NaHCO_3$ due to enteritis, suctioning, or fistulous loss of enteric, pancreatic or biliary fluids. Gut bicarbonate pairs HCO_3^- formed intracellularly with luminal cation R^+, shifting luminal Cl^- inward to be paired with proton. Hence its formation is coupled to continuous invasion of body fluids by HCl which is later neutralized by reabsorption of the secreted fluids. With loss of the latter both acidosis and a volume deficit ensue.

Contraluminal: Loss of $NaHCO_3$ due to reaction with urine from a ureteroenterostomy. Acidosis occurs due to the HCl secreted contraluminally and not subsequently neutralized by reabsorbed gut fluids, despite little external fluid loss. Ammonium ion formed and absorbed as NH_4Cl.

Hepatic: Metabolism of salts with an HCl residue such as NH_4Cl, arginine HCl and lysine HCl.

Luminal: Ion exchange with salts with HCl residue, such as oral $CaCl_2$ and KCl.

Systemic: Ion exchange with salts with HCl residue, such as intravenous $CaCl_2$ and KCl.

Renal: See renal tubular acidosis.

Treatment: Gut fluid loss: Estimation of volume of losses and replacement by intravenous route.

Ureteroenterostomy: Periodic emptying of rectum during day, rectal tube at night.

Oral acidifying salts: Decrease dose.

Intravenous salts: Give with metabolizable anion.

Renal tubular acidosis.

Possible Dire Consequences without Treatment: Growth failure in infants. Nephrocalcinosis, nephrolithiasis. Metabolic bone disease.

References

Ferris, D. O., and Odel, H. M.: Electrolyte pattern of the blood after bilateral ureterosigmoidostomy. J.A.M.A., *142*:634, 1950.

Lapides, J.: Mechanism of electrolyte imbalance following ureterosigmoid transplantation. Surg. Gyn. Obst., *93*:691, 1951.

McDermott, W. V., Jr.: Diversion of urine to the intestines as a factor in ammoniagenic coma. New Eng. J. Med., *256*:460, 1957.

Relman, A. S., Shelburne, P. F., and Talman, A.: Profound acidosis from ammonium chloride in previously healthy subject. New Eng. J. Med., *264*:848, 1961.

Sjoerdsma, A., and Melmon, K. L.: The carcinoid spectrum. Gastroenterology, *47*:104, 1964.

Stoker, D. J., and Wynn, V.: Pancreatic islet cell tumor with watery diarrhea. Gut, *11*:911, 1970.

Wear, J. B., and Barquin, O. P.: Ureterosigmoidostomy. Urology, *1*:192, 1973.

Williams, E. D.: Diarrhea and thyroid carcinoma. Proc. Roy. Soc. Med., *59*:602, 1966.

9. Acidosis from Disease and from Ingested Toxins

JOSEPH H. MAGEE

Cause: Mineral and organic acids, including lactic, in hereditary and acquired renal diseases (uremic acidosis).

Organic acids, including lactic, from exogenous agents (Ethanol, methanol, ethylene glycol, metformin, phenformin, paraldehyde and salicylate ingestion; fructose infusion).

Keto and lactic acids (Diabetic ketoacidosis).

Keto and lactic acids (Type I glycogenosis).

Lactic acid (Convulsions, exercise, fever, hyperventilation, infection, liver disease, normal and toxemic pregnancy).

Lactic acid with arterial unsaturation and hypoperfusion of tissues generally (Cardiopulmonary bypass, cardiac resuscitation).

Early Manifestations: Hyperventilation, which may be precipitous in onset.

Hypocapnia unaccompanied by hypotension, arterial unsaturation and cyanosis.

Low blood pH; except where hyperventilation is primary, rather than due to the acidosis, and where (adult salicylism) blood pH may be high initially.

Low $[HCO_3]$s, with $[Cl]$s increased proportionately.

Raised [lactate]s to the order of 20 to 30 mM./l may account for raised $[\Delta]$s where azotemia and creatininemia, and urine ketones and salicylates, are not found.

Drowsiness, stupor, or coma may occur depending upon rapidity of onset of acidosis.

Anorexia, nausea, abdominal pain, myalgias, weakness, and leukocytosis to 50,000 mm^3 without documentation of infection may occur.

Treatment: Salicylate removal while patient is still alkalotic, in salicylate ingestion.

Administration of sodium bicarbonate, without volume overload, by peritoneal or hemodialysis, in uremic acidosis; and where necessitated by a failing circulation in lactic acidosis.

Volume replacement, often without alkalinizing solutions, in potassium depleted subjects with diabetic ketoacidosis.

At the other extreme in cardiac resuscitation one 44 mM ampoule of NaHCO$_3$ may be necessary for every three to five minutes of artificial systole.

Search for endotoxin-producing infections, including cultures for anaerobes, in unexplained hypotension and acidosis.

Possible Dire Consequences without Treatment: Hyperkalemia due to extra-intracellular cation shifts with egress of potassium from skeletal muscle and other tissues. Lactic acidosis complicating hyperventilation. Dilutional acidosis complicating fluid expansion with bicarbonate free fluids. Irreversible neuronal damage in prolonged acidosis with coma.

Case Report: A thirty-eight-year-old habitual drinker was found stuporous in his garage. On a previous occasion he had attempted to drink permanent antifreeze but had vomited. Some antifreeze of the ethylene glycol type was found nearby. His face was florid and he was hyperventilating stertorously. Calcium oxalate crystals were present in the urine. On hemodialysis with bath bicarbonate 27 mM./l, $[HCO_3]$s fell from 4 to 2 mM./l. With bath bicarbonate 100 mM./l it rose to 15 mM./l. Infusions of CaCl$_2$ were necessary to control laryngeal and orofacial spasm and limb tetany. Pupillary dilatation and decerebrate posturing preceded death a few hours later.

Cation and chloride are alpha and beta in the alphabet of acid-base disorders. Cation always exceeds chloride because some of it is also associated with a third component (gamma) which is bicarbonate. If there were no fourth (delta) components, reciprocal changes in chloride would always accompany changes in bicarbonate, as indeed they usually do. When bicarbonate increases, as it may do in compensation for carbonic acidosis, there is a reciprocal chloride change; even though, if the compensation were exact, neither alkalosis nor acidosis would then be present. When chloride is the invader, in hydrochloric acidosis, bicarbonate is reciprocally decreased.

Where chloride and bicarbonate do not change reciprocally, evidence exists for an invading acid other than carbonic or hydrochloric. The fourth or delta fraction (undetermined anions or anion gap) is raised.

In situations where both Na and K are measured, and, as is usually the case where Ca and Mg are not, this is computed as $[Na + K]-[Cl + HCO_3]$, the normal value being 15.91 ± 4.60 mM/l. If a K measurement is not included, the value computed as $[Na]-[Cl + HCO_3]$ is about 4 mM/l lower. The delta fraction, where other evidence of acidemia (pH change) exists, is helpful in ascertaining the nature of an acidosis; it is relatively insensitive in its detection. Sometimes a peculiar delta fraction detects a gross error in one or more of the determinations used to compute it, usually $[HCO_3]$s, which has five times the coefficient of variation of $[Cl]$s in automated procedures.

References

Barnardo, D. E., Cohen, R. D., and Iles, R. A.: "Idiopathic" lactic and B-hydroxybutyric acidosis. Brit. Med. J., *4*:348, 1970.
Bennett, I. L., Jr., et al.: Acute methyl alcohol poisoning. Medicine, *32*:431, 1953.
Berman, L. B., Schreiner, G. E., and Feys, J.: The nephrotoxic lesion of ethylene glycol. Ann. Intern. Med., *46*:611, 1957.
Daughaday, W. H., Lipky, R. J., and Rasinski, D. C.: Lactic acidosis as a cause of non-ketotic acidosis in diabetic patients. New Eng. J. Med., *267*:1010, 1962.
Hayward, J. N., and Boshell, B. R.: Paraldehyde intoxication with metabolic acidosis. Am. J. Med., *23*:977, 1957.
Howell, R. R., Ashton, D. M., and Wyngaarten, J. B.: Glucose-6-phosphate deficiency glycogen storage disease. Pediatrics, *29*:553, 1962.
Huckabee, W. E.: Abnormal resting blood lactate I & II. Am. J. Med., *30*:833, 1961.
Johnson, H. K., and Waterhouse, C.: Lactic acidosis and phenformin. Arch. Intern. Med., *122*:367, 1968.
Marliss, E. B., et al.: Altered redox state obscuring ketoacidosis in diabetic patients with ketoacidosis. New Eng. J. Med., *283*:978, 1970.
Mulhausen, R., Eichenholtz, A., and Blumenthals, A.: Acid-base disturbances in patients with cirrhosis of the liver. Medicine, *46*:185, 1967.
Palmer, W. W. and Henderson, L. J.: A study of the several factors of acid excretion in nephritis. Arch. Intern. Med., *16*:109, 1915.
Peters, J. P.: Diabetic acidosis. Metabolism, *1*:223, 1952.
Sahebjami, H., and Scarletter, R.: Effect of fructose infusion on lactate and uric acid metabolism. Lancet, *1*:366, 1971.
Singer, R. B.: Acid-base disturbances in salicylate intoxication. Medicine, *33*:1, 1954.
Strauss, P. G., and Sullivan, M. A.: Phenformin intoxication resulting in lactic acidosis. Bull. Johns Hopkins Hosp., *128*:278, 1970.
Tranquada, R. E., Bernstein, S., and Martin, H. E.: Irreversible lactic acidosis associated with phenformin therapy. J.A.M.A., *184*:37, 1963.
Woods, H. F., and Alberti, K. G., M. M.: Dangers of intravenous fructose. Lancet, *2*:1354, 1972.

10. Newborn Nephrotic Syndromes

JOSEPH H. MAGEE

Cause: Postulated causes include maternal antibodies against the fetus and recessively inherited renal dysplasias.

Early Manifestations: Onset of nephrotic syndrome prior to one year of age (which occurs only in about 2% of cases of the classic nephrotic syndrome) and usually prior to three months of age.

Occurrence of nephrotic syndrome in siblings, especially where one of them is less than one year of age.

Low incidence among total births, as distinguished from the epidemic of secondary nephrotic syndrome due to mercurous chloride teething powders discovered by Arneil.

Treatment: Generally unavailing, including corticosteroids and renal transplantation.

Possible Dire Consequences without Treatment: Confusion with the classic nephrotic syndrome.

References

Arneil, G. C.: Treatment of nephrosis with prednisolone. Lancet, *1*:409, 1956.

Fanconi, G., Kousmine, C., and Frischknecht, W.: Die konstitutionelle Bereitschaft zum nephrosesyndrom. Helv. Paed. Acta, *6*:199, 1951.

Farquahar, M. G., Vernier, R. L., and Good, R. A.: Studies on familial nephrosis II. Am. J. Path., *33*:791, 1957.

Giles, H. M., et al.: The nephrotic syndrome in early infancy. Arch. Dis. Child., *32*:167, 1957.

Hallman, N., and Hjelt, L.: Congenital nephrotic syndrome. J. Paed., *55*:152, 1959.

Hallman, N., Hjelt, L., and Ahrenainen, E. K.: The nephrotic syndrome in new born and young infants. Ann. Paed. Tenn., *2*:227, 1956.

Hoyer, J. R., et al.: The nephrotic syndrome of infancy. Pediatrics, *40*:233, 1967.

Kouvalainen, K., et al.: Behavior of skin grafted from infants to mother in congenital nephrosis families. Ann. Paed., *8*:173, 1962.

Novro, R.: The nephrotic syndrome and heredity. Human Heredity, *19*:113, 1969.

Vernier, R. L., Worthen, H. G., and Good, R. A.: Studies on familial nephrosis I. Am. J. Path., *33*:791, 1957.

Worthen, H. G., Vernier, R. L., and Good, R. A.: Infantile nephrosis. Am. J. Dis. Child., *98*:731, 1959.

11. Common Nephrotic Syndrome

Joseph H. Magee

Synonyms: Nephrosis (Muller 1905). Genuine nephrosis (Volhard and Fahr 1914). Lipoid nephrosis (Munk 1916). Chronic nephrosis (Epstein 1917). Epithelial cell disease (Earle 1959). Nil disease, minimum change nephropathy.

Cause: Unknown.

Result: Massive, primarily selective proteinuria. Inverse hypoproteinemia. Hypovolemia. Secondary aldosteronism. Non-osmotic vasopressinism.

Early Manifestations: Rare before age one, peak incidence at age three, seen in older children and adults but unusual after age eight.
Peak incidence in spring and summer, males 2:1, history of recent infection in 60% or immunization in 10%, previous history of allergy in 10%.
Family history of diabetes in 30% and of allergy in 30%.
Variably selective heavy proteinuria usually without erythrocyturia, azotemia and hypertension.
Inverse hypoproteinemia with low serum albumin, raised serum beta-lipoprotein and cholesterol levels.
Generalized edema and serous effusions.
Accumulations of anisotropic lipid (cholesterol esters) are seen in the cortical microvasculature and convoluted tubules of the kidneys in numerous conditions but especially those characterized by heavy proteinuria. They are easily seen in the exfoliated cells of acid concentrated urine specimens, where they exhibit the Maltese cross phenomenon under microscopy with polarized light using suitable filters in the condenser and eyepieces. Neutral lipid is also present, appears deep orange on supravital staining with Sudan III, is less variable from day to day, depends less upon pH and prompt examination, but is seen in a broader spectrum of renal disease than is anisotropic lipid.

Treatment: The protocol of the International Cooperative Study of Nephrosis is as follows:
Prednisone 60 mg./M²/day for twenty-eight days, or 80 mg./day, whichever is smaller.
Prednisone 40 mg./M² every other day for twenty-eight days, or 60 mg./day whichever is smaller, whether or not a remission has occurred at this point.
If remission occurs between twenty-eight and fifty-six days, a further twenty-eight days of the every other day schedule is given.
Eighty % of 189 patients had remissions prior to fifty-six days' (eight weeks) therapy. A second aspect of the study, evaluating the efficacy of azothioprine in non-responders indicated that this agent is valueless. Subsequent studies have suggested that cyclophosphamide may be the preferred drug in non-responders. Dose is 3 mg./kg. per day initially and is increased if necessary to produce reduction in blood leukocyte counts to below 4000/mm³. Treatment is usually continued for a minimum of four months; remission of varying duration occurs in about 85% of the patients. Alopecia which occurs in three-fourths of patients remits with cessation of therapy.

Possible Dire Consequences without Treatment: Protein loss, edema, susceptibility to infection.

The common or classic nephrotic syndrome is a distinctive epidemiologic entity of unknown etiology and nondescript pathology. It cannot satisfactorily be called the childhood nephrotic syndrome, although two-thirds of cases are in pre-school children. It is with difficulty distinguished from congenital (prior to three months), familial (prior to one year) and secondary (throughout life) varieties of the nephrotic syndrome, all of which have less favorable prognoses. Nor is the term idiopathic nephrotic syndrome satisfactory; the entity next described in section 13 is of equally mysterious but perhaps different origin since it differs so markedly in natural history and in response to treatment.

The common nephrotic syndrome occurs twice as commonly in boys as in girls, but this ratio is reversed when the histologic appearance includes membranoproliferative change. Two-thirds of affected individuals succumbed to infection or other cause in the era preceding introduction of the sulfonamides in 1936. After this two-thirds survived to ultimately become free of proteinuria. The advent of corticosteroid therapy has raised this figure to 90%.

References

Abramowicz, M., et al.: Controlled trial of azothioprine in children with the nephrotic syndrome. Lancet, *1*:959, 1970.
Arneil, G. C., and Lam, C. N.: Long-term assessment of steroid therapy in childhood nephrosis. Lancet, *2*:819, 1966.
Barness, L. S., Moll, G. H., and Janeway, C. A.: Nephrotic syndrome in children. Pediatrics, *5*:486, 1950.
Barnett, H. L., Forman, C. W., and Lauson, H. D.: Nephrotic syndrome in children. Adv. Pediat., *5*:33, 1952.
Churg, J., Habib, R., and White, R. H. R.: Pathology of the nephrotic syndrome in children. Lancet, *1*:1299, 1970.
Connolly, M. E., Wrong, O. M., and Jones, N. F.: Reversible renal failure in idiopathic nephrotic syndrome with minimal glomerular changes. Lancet, *1*:665, 1968.
Cornfeld, D., and Schwartz, M. W.: Nephrosis: A long-term study of children treated with corticosteroids. J. Pediat., *68*:507, 1966.
Friedmann, M., and Strang, L. B.: Effects of long-term corticosteroids and corticotropin on the growth of children. Lancet, *2*:568, 1966.
Meadow, S. R., Weller, R. O., and Archibald, R. W. R.: Fatal systemic measles in a child receiving cyclophosphamide for nephrotic syndrome. Lancet, *2*:876, 1969.
Moncrieff, M. W., et al.: Cyclophosphamide therapy in nephrotic syndrome in childhood. Brit. Med. J., *1*:666, 1969.
Qureshi, M. J. A., et al.: Cyclophosphamide therapy and sterility. Lancet, *2*:1290, 1972.
Scheinman, J. I., and Stamler, F. W.: Cyclophosphamide and fatal varicella. J. Pediat., *74*:117, 1969.

12. Focal Glomerular Sclerosis

Joseph H. Magee

Cause: Unknown, possibly a variant of the classic nephrotic syndrome, which culminates in renal insufficiency and which recurs in grafted kidneys.

Early Manifestations: Age incidence is identical to classic nephrotic syndrome. Of 20 patients reported by Rich, 17 were aged one and one-half to eight years, 2 were age sixteen and one was age twenty-four. A high incidence has recently been found in young adult heroin users.

Average survival from onset to death from uremia was 2.2 years (0.8 to 0.5 years). Manifestations are initially identical to those described in section 11; erythrocyturia, azotemia, and hypertension appear after an interval varying from two months to two years, occasionally longer.

Biopsy is insensitive in distinguishing these cases, due to sampling error; characteristic changes first appearing in the deeper glomeruli.

Treatment: A trial of prednisone to differentiate from chronic nephrotic syndrome is indicated. There usually is no response in focal glomerular sclerosis.

Possible Dire Consequences without Treatment: Protein loss, edema, susceptibility to infection.

Rich reconstructed the changes in glomerular pathology in the classic nephrotic syndrome on the eve of the biopsy era, which began for children in about 1960. The kidneys were studied in 9 patients aged one and a half to eight years, who died of infection an average of 0.92 years (0.1 to 4.5) after onset of the disease; and in 11 patients, aged one and a half to sixteen years who died of renal failure, an average of 2.2 years (0.8 to 5.0) after onset. Even in glomeruli that "appear essentially normal on cursory inspection" "slight, focal thickening of some of the capillary basement membranes can be discerned; with the passage of time, however, glomerular alterations of a more definite type may occur." The latter were focal intercapillary hyaline deposits "leading gradually to the complete obliteration of the normal glomerular architecture," although "proliferation of the endothelial and epithelial cells of the tuft is slight or absent." All patients with renal failure, and half those dying of infection, had the lesions; but in the latter only juxtamedullary glomeruli were affected. "An adequate understanding of the glomerulosclerosis should account for the peculiar susceptibility of the juxtamedullary glomeruli." A new fact, adduced by Hoyer, is that recurrent disease, with an identical distribution of lesions, has been seen in the grafted kidneys of 3 patients in whom the original disease had progressed to renal failure. Thus possibly 10% of nephrotic patients who have both nondescript findings on renal biopsy and steroid resistance may constitute a group difficult of identification but in whom transplantation may not be beneficial.

References

Cameron, J. S.: Histology, protein clearances, and response to treatment in the nephrotic syndrome. Brit. Med. J., *4*:352, 1968.

Dodge, W. F., et al.: Percutaneous renal biopsy in children III. Ped., *30*:459, 1962.

Hoyer, J. R., et al.: Recurrence of idiopathic nephrotic syndrome after renal transplantation. Lancet, *2*:343, 1972.

McGovern, V. J.: Persistent nephrotic syndrome. Austral. Ann. Med., *13*:306, 1964.

Rao, T. K., Nicastri, A. D., and Friedman, E. A.: Natural history of heroin associated nephropathy. New Eng. J. Med., *290*:19, 1974.

Rich, A. R.: A hitherto undescribed vulnerability of the juxtamedullary glomeruli in lipoid nephrosis. Bull. Johns Hopkins Hosp., *100*:173, 1957.

White, R. H. R.: Cytotoxic therapy in steroid-resistant glomerulonephritis. Proc. Roy. Soc. Med., *60*:1164, 1967.

13. Toxic Nephrotic Syndromes

Joseph H. Magee

Cause: Heavy metals (Au, Bi, Hg), including mercurial teething powders and salves, and the organomercurial diuretics.

Chlorinated hydrocarbons: Trichlorethylene.

Heterocyclic: Sulfonamides, including oral hypoglycemic agents; phenindione, trimethadione, paramethadione.

Salts: Potassium, perchlorate.

Aromatic acids: Probenecid.

Early Manifestations: Identical to classic nephrotic syndrome of idiopathic origin.

Treatment: Drug withdrawal.

Possible Dire Consequences without Treatment: Continued intoxication, death.

References

Berger, H., and Zoole, J.: The relief of nephrosis after hepatitis. J.A.M.A., *145*:228, 1951.

Cameron, J. S., and Trounce, J. R.: Membranous glomerulonephritis and the nephrotic syndrome appearing during mersalyl therapy. Guy's Hosp. Rep., *114*:101, 1965.

Ferris, T. F., Morgan, W. S., and Levitin, H.: Nephrotic syndrome caused by probenecid. New Eng. J. Med., *265*:381, 1961.

Haugen, H. N.: Tridione nephropathy. Acta Med. Scand., *159*:375, 1957.

Lee, R. E., Ulstrom, R. A., and Vernier, R. L.: Nephrotic syndrome as a complication of perchlorate treatment of thyrotoxicosis. New Eng. J. Med., *264*:1221, 1961.

Mandema, E., et al.: Mercury and the kidney. Lancet, *1*:1266, 1963.

Nabarro, J. D. N., and Rosenheim, M. L.: Nephrotic syndrome complicating tridione therapy. Lancet, *1*:1091, 1952.

Rigdon, R. H., Siddon, W. H., and Fletcher, D. E.: Consideration of glomerular nephritis in relation to sulfonamide therapy. Am. J. Med., *6*:177, 1949.

Schnall, C., and Wiener, J. S.: Nephrosis occurring during tolbutamide administration. J.A.M.A., *167*:214, 1958.

Tart, G. B.: Nephropathy during phenindione therapy. Lancet, *2*:1198, 1960.

White, J. C.: Nephrosis occurring during trimethadione therapy. J.A.M.A., *139*:376, 1949.

Wren, J. C., and Nutt, R. L.: Nephrotic syndrome occurring during paramethadione therapy. J.A.M.A., *153*:918, 1953.

14. Adult Nephrotic Syndromes

JOSEPH H. MAGEE

Causes: Diverse (Table X–2).

Early Manifestations: Less selective proteinuria, and is more frequently accompanied by hypertension, hematuria, azotemia, and hypocomplementemia at outset as compared to Common or Classic Nephrotic Syndrome, characteristically a disease of the preschool child, which accounts for but 20% of cases of the nephrotic syndrome in adults.

Treatment: Fluid and electrolyte balance, corticosteroids, and treatment of associated extrarenal disease.

Possible Dire Consequences without Treatment: Edema, continued nephrotic syndrome and further renal damage.

Twenty % of adults with the nephrotic syndrome demonstrate on renal biopsy a nondescript histologic appearance, resembling that seen in most children and infants so affected. They thus may have the same disease, though this assumption of course involves risk similar to that involved in saying that all invisible people look alike. However, the similarity also includes the same tendency to spontaneous remission and to steroid-induced remissions as manifested in the childhood disease.

TABLE X–2. ADULT NEPHROTIC SYNDROMES

	PERCENT
1. Common nephrotic syndrome (nil disease): Adult occurrence of disease with peak incidence in preschool children (age three), 90% recovery with glucocorticoid therapy.	20
2. Glomerular (hemorrhagic) nephritis: Active onset (Ellis I, Longcope A), post-infections and proliferative, peak incidence in school children (age six), 95% recovery with supportive therapy.	30
3. Glomerular (hemorrhagic) nephritis: Latent onset (Ellis II, Longcope B), not obviously related to infections episode, age incident ten to sixty without obvious peaks, low recovery rate, around 10%.	30
4. Associated with extrarenal disease	20

4. Associated with extrarenal disease
   (*a.*) Diabetic nephropathy.
   (*b.*) Autoimmune: Lupus, polyarteritis, Sjögren's.
   (*c.*) Postimmune: Lymphoma, myeloma, hypernephroma.
   (*d.*) Postimmune: Penicillamine.
   (*e.*) Postimmune: Serum, pollen, bee and snake venom, rhus toxin.
   (*f.*) Para-Infectious: Syphilis, malaria, tuberculosis, leprosy, diphtheria, typhus, jejunoileitis, bacterial endocarditis, megalovirus mononucleosis.
   (*g.*) Myxedema nephropathy.
   (*h.*) Amyloidosis with or without renal venous hypertension.
   (*i.*) Renal venous hypertension.
   (*j.*) Genetic: Newborn nephrotic syndromes, sicklemia.

The other 80% have some other variety of renal disease, usually without so good a prognosis, and with histologic abnormality to go along with it. In 60 of the 80%, the disease is glomerular nephritis (hemorrhagic nephritis), which has either active onset (Ellis I, Longcope A) or latent onset (Ellis II, Longcope B). The two varieties are variably represented. Least likely to be the responsible renal disease are arteriolar nephrosclerosis and pyelonephritis.

The final 20% of the 80 who do not have "nil disease," are accounted for by a bewildering variety of diseases. The two most common are diabetic nephropathy and lupus nephropathy.

References

Black, D. A. K., Rose, G. A., and Brewer, D. B.: Controlled trial of prednisone in adult patients with the nephrotic syndrome. Brit. Med. J., *3*:421, 1970.

Bloom, W. L., and Selgal, D.: The nephrotic phase; its frequency of occurrence and its differential diagnostic value in determining the nature of the renal lesion in 120 patients who died of renal failure. Ann. Intern. Med., *25*:15, 1946.

Kark, R. M., et al.: The nephrotic syndrome in adults. Ann. Intern. Med., *49*:751, 1958.

Nesson, H. R., Sproul, L. E., and Relman, A. S.: Adrenal steroid in the treatment of idiopathic nephrotic syndrome in adults. Ann. Intern. Med., *58*:268, 1963.

Pollak, V. E., et al.: Natural history of lipoid nephrosis and of membranous glomerulonephritis. Ann. Intern. Med., *69*:1171, 1968.

Sharpstone, P., Ogg, C. L. S., and Cameron, J. S.: Nephrotic syndrome due to primary renal disease in adults (2). A controlled trial of prednisone and azothioprine. Brit. Med. J., *2*:535, 1969.

Spencer, A. G.: Recent advances in renal disease. Post. Grad. Med. J., *35*:612, 1959.

15. Diabetic Nephropathy

Joseph H. Magee

Cause: Diabetes Mellitus.

Early Manifestations: The nephrotic syndrome is a late manifestation of diabetes mellitus. Frequently in the usage of the Joslin Clinic, "triopathy" is present with the patient presenting retinopathy and raised spinal fluid protein, in addition to nephropathy. Among the universe of adult nephrotics, diabetic nephropathy represents a considerable proportion of the final 20% of patients in Table X–2. Hence, if the patient is even a latent diabetic, the chances that his nephrotic syndrome may be diabetes-related are great, probably far greater than his chance of having "nil disease" as an adult.

Treatment: Treatment of diabetes with diet and/or insulin.

Salt restriction, avoiding chloruretic sulfonamides if possible.

For reasons given above, trial of glucocorticoids is generally inadvisable on a probability basis; the more so if nitrogen retention and/or "triopathy" is present. With evolution of uremic syndrome, timely shunting for maintenance hemodialysis is advisable.

Treatment of visceral neuropathy: Includes Credé maneuver after each voiding, where detrusor function is impaired.

Treatment of urinary tract infections.

Possible Dire Consequences without Treatment: Acidosis, renal insufficiency, uremia, death.

References

Marble, A., Wilson, J. L., and Root, H. F.: Diabetic nephropathy: A clinical syndrome. Tr. Am. Ass. Phys., *64*:353, 1951.

Runyan, J. W., Jr., Hurwitz, D., and Robbins, S. L.: Effect of Kimmelstiel-Wilson syndrome on insulin requirements in diabetes. New Eng. J. Med., *252*:388, 1955.

16. Renal Venous Hypertension

Joseph H. Magee

Underlying Causes: Pericardial constriction (quiet heart, venous hypertension, and ascites, in addition to proteinuria, hypoproteinemia, and peripheral edema).

Tricuspid valve disease (active heart, venous hypertension, pulsatile liver, and ascites; in addition to usual nephrotic manifestations).

Vena caval thrombosis or obstruction (demarcating edema; out of proportion to usual nephrotic generalized edema).

Renal venous thrombosis or obstruction, in infantile dehydration, amyloidosis, hypernephroma, and ileofemoral phlebitis.

Early Manifestations: Lumbar abdominal or groin pain. Radiographic enlargement of one or both kidneys. Hematuria, proteinuria, edema. In pericardial disease, hypoproteinemia may be a consequence both of heavy protein urea and of exudative enteropathy. Fever, leukocytosis. Thromboses elsewhere. Superficial collateral veins.

Treatment: Heparinization if acute onset is detected or if pulmonary embolization is suspected.

Thrombectomy if involvement is limited to larger vessels.

Possible Dire Consequences without Treatment: Renal vein thrombosis, oliguria, uremia, fluid retention, death.

References

Derow, H. A., Schlesinger, M. J., and Savitz, H. A.: Chronic progressive occlusion of the inferior vena cava and the renal and portal veins with the clinical picture of the nephrotic syndrome. Arch. Intern. Med., *63*:625, 1939.

McCarthy, L. J., Titus, J. L., and Daugherty, G. W.: Bilateral renal vein thrombosis and the nephrotic syndrome in adults. Ann. Intern. Med., *58*:837, 1963.

Morris, J. F., Ginn, H. E., and Thompson, D. D.: Unilateral renal vein thrombosis associated with the nephrotic syndrome. Am. J. Med., *34*:867, 1963.

Pollak, V. E., et al.: Renal vein thrombosis and the nephrotic syndrome. Am. J. Med., *21*:496, 1956.

Rosenman, E., Pollak, V. E., and Pirani, C. L.: Renal vein thrombosis in the adult. Medicine, *47*:269, 1968.

Introduction: Physiologic Oligurias

Oliguria, the most characteristic feature of acute renal failure, must be differentiated from oligurias due to pre-renal and post-renal factors. Oliguria is defined as less than 480 ml. urine per day (less than 20 ml. per hour) (less than 1/3 ml. per minute). Hourly recordings are practical and preferred in the patient in whom oliguria is questioned. Chemical findings in the urine may be indicative of a role of intact tubular mechanisms in causing the oliguria.

If enhanced reabsorption of filtrate is operative in causing oliguria, as in the prerenal or pretubular oligurias (Table X–3), the final urine will show reduced Na, Cl and HOH, respective to non-electrolyte solids. Na and Cl determinations have lost much of their value because patients are so routinely given mannitol or furosemide as therapeutic tests prior to other investigations into the nature of the oliguria.

Specific gravity (SG) is the ratio of the mass of a solution to the mass of an identical volume of water. It will be falsely high if there is glycosuria, if the patient has been given mannitol, if there is proteinuria of nephrotic proportions, or if done when urine is at body instead of room temperature; in each case by a factor of about 0.003. There will be an even greater overestimation if some radiographic contrast material has recently been given.

Refractometry is popular in pediatric practice because relative water removal from filtrate can be measured in small urine samples, collected in 0.02 ml. capillary pipettes. Similar cautions apply respecting unusual urinary particles, which affect this determination not according to their number or mass, but according to the arrangement of their constituent atoms. Colloids, including proteins, have higher refractive indices than crystalloids. The refractive index (RI) of concentrated urines, without proteinuria, increases to 85 to 134, and total solids to 5.8 to 8.5 gm./100 gm. urine. When SG is fixed, RI is less than 44, and total solutes less than 2.8 gm./100 gm., correlating reasonably well with the figure for "Roberts' Rule" at room temperature given by: $Sg - 1.000 (260) = 2.6$ gm./100 gm.

Osmometry (cryoscopy) is preferable to both. It measures numbers rather than any other attributes of solutes, their aggregate numbers having a dependable effect upon chemical potential or escaping tendency of the solvent, water in the case of urine. This depends upon temperature and pressure during measurement, plus a quantity called activity, which is proportional to the number of particles dissolved. Compared with other techniques which measure the extent of water removal incident to urine formation somewhat more grossly, there can be an estimation of the uncoupling

TABLE X–3. DIFFERENTIATION OF OLIGURIC STATES

	$\frac{[Na]_u}{[K]_u}$	Ratio	$[Cl]_u$	SG	RI	Osm	$[Osm]\,u/p$	$[Cr]\,u/p$	$\frac{[UN]_u}{[UN]_p}$	Ratio
PHYSIOLOGIC OLIGURIAS "Prerenal"	3–20								1000–1800	
		0.3–1.5	15–50	1.018 or >	45 or >	345 or >	1.3 or >	5–15		20–60
ANGIOPATHIC OLIGURIAS "Pretubular"	20–45								30–50	
INTRINSIC OLIGURIAS "Tubular"	30–90								500–1000	
		1.5–6.0	50–100	< 1.018	< 45	< 345	< 1.3	2–8		2–10
EXTRINSIC OLIGURIAS "Pretubular"	10–30								50–150	

of water and solute reabsorption from paired urine and plasma determinations. This U/P ratio will retain some of its value even as the differential value of urine electrolyte concentrations has been lost as a result of therapeutic exertions; and it often can be had more quickly than U/P comparisons for urea N and creatinine.

17. Oligemic Reaction

JOSEPH H. MAGEE

Result: Hypoperfusion of organs generally, including the kidney; increased sympathetic activity; secondary aldosteronism; non-osmotic vasopressinism; and in the first group of causes enumerated below, osmotic vasopressinism.

Causes: Non-renal aqueous volume loss.
(*a.*) Decreased intake: No thirst.
(*b.*) Decreased intake: Stupor.
(*c.*) Decreased intake: Water unavailable.
(*d.*) Lung loss: Thermal, pharmacologic.
(*e.*) Skin loss: Thermal, pharmacologic.
Non-renal saline volume loss.
(*a.*) Skin loss: Heat exhaustion, burns.
(*b.*) Gut loss: Vomiting, suctioning, internal fistulas.
(*c.*) Gut loss: Enteritis (salmonella, shigella, cholera).
(*d.*) Gut loss: Pancreatic cholera (pancreatic adenoma).
(*e.*) Gut loss: Villous adenoma (colon).
(*f.*) Peritoneal loss: Paracenteses, dialyses.
(*g.*) Third space loss: Peritonitis ascites, major vein thromboses, burns, hypodermoclyses, toxic megacolon.
Circulating protein loss.
(*a.*) Kidney loss.
(*b.*) Gut loss.
(*c.*) Inadequate synthesis.
(*d.*) External hemorrhage.
(*e.*) Concealed hemorrhage.

Early Manifestations: Oliguria is accompanied and often preceded by extrarenal signs and symptoms of decreased circulating volume and of specific conditions occasioning it.
Valveless vein hypotension.
Postural arterial hypotension.
Recumbent arterial hypotension.
Decreased arterial pulse pressure, stroke volume and cardiac output
Normal circulation time.
Plasma volume decreased with or without RBC volume decrease.
Edema absent except in protein loss and third space formation.
Tissue volume decreased regionally (eyeballs).
Scant salivation, dry mucous membranes.
Thirst when alert in absence of specific lesions.
Restlessness.
Corroborative urine findings.

Treatment: Fluid replacement. (Restoration of venous and arterial pressures, and augmentation of urine flow are criteria of adequacy); urine composition should be monitored for duration of oliguria.

Possible Dire Consequences without Treatment: Ischemic tubular necrosis.

References

Danowski, T. S., Winkler, A. W., and Ellington, J. R.: Biochemical and hemodynamic changes following the subcutaneous injection of glucose solution. J. Clin. Invest., *26*:887, 1947.

Fishberg, A. M.: Pre-renal azotemia and the pathology of renal blood flow. Bull. N.Y. Acad. Med., *13*:710, 1937.

McCance, R. A., and Widdowson, E. M.: The secretion of urine in man during experimental salt deficiency. J. Physiol., *91*:222, 1937.

Waugh, W. H.: Functional types of acute renal failure and their early diagnosis. Arch. Intern. Med., *103*:686, 1959.

18. Hyperviscosity States

JOSEPH H. MAGEE

Result: Hypoperfusion of organs generally including the kidney.

Causes: High hematocrit states. Hyperglobulinemic (usually IgM) states. Hyperosmolar (usually hyperglycemic) states.

Early Manifestations: Oliguria preceded by signs and symptoms varying with the responsible entity.
High hematocrit states.
(*a.*) Hematocrit 50 to 80%; accompanied in primary polycythemia by leukocytosis and thrombocytosis.
(*b.*) Whole blood viscosity, normally 2 to 6 times that of water, increased to 6 to 14 times that of water.
(*c.*) Normal serum viscosity and protein concentration.
(*d.*) Circulation: Arterial and valveless vein hypertension may occur.
(*e.*) Complexion: Florid or dusky rather than pale.
(*f.*) Symptoms of visual disturbances and pruritus.
(*g.*) Splenomegaly.
(*h.*) Onset of oliguria is evaluated.
Hyperglobulinemic states.
(*a.*) Hematocrit 20 to 30%. Granulocytopenia and thrombocytopenia with relative or absolute lymphocytosis.
(*b.*) Whole blood viscosity high with low hematocrit.
(*c.*) Serum viscosity, normally 1.4 to 1.8 times water in range 4 to 7 or more.
(*d.*) Monoclonal hypergammaglobulinemia.
(*e.*) One third of IgM are cryoglobulins which precipitate with cooling
(*f.*) Most IgM and some IgG are euglobulins which precipitate with dilution by water (Sia test).
(*g*). Some IgM (irreversibly) and light chains (reversibly) are pyroglobulins which precipitate upon heating serum or urine respectively to 50 to 60° C.
(*h.*) Some IgM are warm antibodies which coat red cells causing rouleaux formation, agglutination, cross matching difficulties, positive Coombs reactions, and complement fixation.
(*i.*) Signs and symptoms include purpura, epistaxes, gum bleeding, fever, neurologic and visual disturbances.
(*j.*) Appearance of oliguria evaluated.
Hyperosmolar states.
(*a.*) Valveless vein hypotension.

(*b.*) Postural arterial hypotension.

(*c.*) Recumbent arterial hypotension.

(*d.*) Thirst.

(*e.*). Restlessness.

(*f.*) Scant salivation and sweating.

(*g.*) Soft eyeballs.

(*h.*) Hyperglycemia is a provocative test for the evaluation of oliguria, just as might be performed with mannitol. Accordingly, the oliguric response to pre-renal circulatory factors should have been abolished; and oliguria while hyperglycemia and glycosuria are still present is an untoward development.

(*i.*) Evaluation of oliguria present after correction of hyperglycemia and glucosuria may be made according to urine findings.

Treatment: High hematocrit states. Every other day 250 to 500 ml. phlebotomies until hematocrit is less than 50%.

Hyperviscosity states. Plasmapheresis of 4 to 6 units of plasma, and determination of the relative viscosity below which patient is asymptomatic and not oliguric.

Hyperosmolar states.

Possible Dire Consequences without Treatment: Oliguria, uremia, death.

References

De Wardener, H. E., McSwiney, R. R., and Miles, B. E.: Renal hemodynamics in primary polycythemia. Lancet, *2*:204, 1951.

Fahey, J. L., Barth, W. F., and Solomon, A.: Serum hyperviscosity syndrome. J.A.M.A., *192*:464, 1965.

Kopp, W. L., Beirne, G. J., and Burns, R. O.: Hyperviscosity syndrome in multiple myeloma. Am. J. Med., *43*:141, 1967.

Lewis, C. S., et al.: Chronic lung disease, polycythemia and congestive failure. Circulation, *6*:874, 1952.

Morel-Maroger, L., et al.: Pathology of the kidney in Waldenström's macroglobulinemia. New Eng. J. Med., *281*:256, 1969.

Wells, R.: Current concepts: Syndromes of hyperviscosity. New Eng. J. Med., *283*:183, 1970.

19. Altered Cardiac Dynamics

JOSEPH H. MAGEE

Results: Hypoperfusion of organs generally including the kidney. Increased sympathetic activity. Aldosteronism. Non-osmotic vasopressinism.

Causes: Decreased return to heart.
  (*a.*) Venular pooling: neurogenic.
  (*b.*) Venular pooling: Pharmacologic, including anesthesia.
  (*c.*) Venous obstruction: Portal, hepatic, caval.
  Decreased filling of right heart.
  (*a.*) Pericardial tamponade.
  (*b.*) Pulmonary artery obstruction.
  (*c.*) Rightward shunting of aortic or left chamber blood.
  (*d.*) Rapid arrhythmias.
  Decreased filling of left heart.
  (*a.*) Atrial myxoma, thrombus on pedicle.
  (*b.*) Valvular mitral stenosis.
  Decreased emptying of heart.
  (*a.*) Conduction failure.
  (*b.*) Contraction failure (toxic, ischemic, intrinsic, endocrine).
  (*c.*) Valvular failure.

Early Manifestations: Oliguria is accompanied and often preceded by extrarenal signs and symptoms of decreased cardiac output.
  Venous pressure may be raised (2 to 4).
  Low arterial pulse pressure, stroke volume and cardiac output.
  Circulation time may be increased.
  Arteriovenous oxygen difference may be increased.
  Plasma volume may be increased with or without RBC volume increase (2 to 4).
  Edema may be present (2 to 4).

Treatment: Non-specific such as bed rest and saluretic agents.
  Specific such as inotropic agents for contraction failure.
  Day time oliguria and nocturnal diuresis characterize circulatory failure and may be favorably affected by treatments.
  Overnight or worsening oliguria raises question of ischemic tubular necrosis and embolization.

Possible Dire Consequences without Treatment: Oliguria, uremia, death.

References

Ganer, O. H., Henry, J. P., and Sieker, H. O.: Cardiac receptors and fluid volume control. Prog. Cardiovasc. Dis., *4*:1, 1961.

Merrill, A. J., and Cargill, W. H.: Effect of exercise in renal blood flow and filtration rate of normal and cardiac subjects. J. Clin. Invest., *27*:272, 1948.

20. Altered Peripheral Dynamics

Joseph H. Magee

Result: Decreased perfusion and/or oxygenation of organs generally including the kidney despite regionally and/or generally increased flow. Increased sympathetic activity. Secondary aldosteronism. Non-osmotic vasopressinism.

Causes: General flow increase.
(*a.*) Hypoxia (Anoxic, anemic, histotoxic).
(*b.*) Hypermetabolism (Thyrotoxicosis, dinitrophenol).
(*c.*) Hyperactivity (Status epilepticus, tetanus).
Peripheral flow increase: A-V Fistulas.
(*a.*) Multiple: Paget's disease, hepatic cirrhosis.
(*b.*) Local: Traumatic.
(*c.*) Renal: Traumatic, surgical, hypernephroma.

Early Manifestations: Venous pressure may be raised. High arterial pulse pressure, stroke volume and cardiac output. Circulation time normal. Arteriovenous oxygen difference normal or low. Plasma volume may be increased with or without RBC volume increase. Edema may be present.

Treatment: Oliguria in high output circulatory states, as in those with low output, bespeaks decompensation, *i.e.*, inadequate perfusion of target organs. Cardiac and renal pharmacology, including agents opposing increased sympathetic, aldosterone and vasopressin activity, is subordinate to such non-specific measures as diet, rest and air conditioning, and to specific correction of the underlying abnormality.

Possible Dire Consequences without Treatment: Left ventricular failure, pulmonary edema, right ventricular failure, passive circulatory congestion, thromboembolic complications.

References

Baldus, W. P., Feichter, R. N., and Summerskill, W. H. J.: Kidney in cirrhosis. Ann. Intern. Med., *60*:365, 1964.

Berkowitz, H. D., Miller, L. D., and Rosato, E. F.: Renin substrate depletion in hepatorenal syndrome. New Eng. J. Med., *289*:1155, 1973.

Eichna, L. W.: Circulatory congestion and heart failure. Circulation, *22*:864, 1960.

Goldstein, H., and Boyle, J. D.: Spontaneous recovery from the hepatorenal syndrome. New Eng. J. Med., *272*:895, 1965.

Hecker, R., and Sherlock, S.: Electrolyte and circulatory changes in terminal liver failure. Lancet, *2*:1121, 1956.

Keefer, C. S.: The beriberi heart. Arch. Intern. Med., *45*:1, 1930.

Papper, S., Belsky, J. L., and Bleifer, K. H.: Renal failure in Laennec's cirrhosis of the liver. Ann. Intern. Med., *51*:759, 1959.

Introduction

In the oligurias considered up to this point the cause of decreased perfusion was extrinsic, not in or even in the vicinity of the kidneys. The decreased perfusion was general with the specific hypoperfusion of the kidney being physiologic and under the circumstances advantageous to whole body homeostasis.

TABLE X–4. ANGIOPATHIC (PRETUBULAR) OLIGURIAS

Aortic Obstructions	Subcutaneous Collaterals Notched Ribs, Aortography
Renal Artery Obstructions	Difference in Kidney Size Angiography
Lobular Artery Obstruction	History of Vasoconstrictor Drugs History of Pregnancy, Abruptio Placentae
Glomerular Obstructions	RBC Casts, Proteinuria; Antistreptococcal Antibodies; Antinuclear Antibodies
Venous and Caval Obstructions	Heavy Proteinuria; Demarcating Edema; Cutaneous Collaterals

In the next group of conditions chemical findings in the urine again may indicate return of a substantial share of (a generally reduced) filtrate to the circulation by intact tubular mechanisms. One must decide on other grounds (Table X–4) whether or not perfusion of the kidneys is regionally decreased rather than a response to generalized circulatory stress. If so, the prognosis may be less good.

21. Macroangiopathy (Aortic Lesions)

JOSEPH H. MAGEE

Result: Hypoperfusion affecting the renal circulation disproportionately.

Characteristic: Angiopathic oliguria renin-dependent (de novo or accentuated).

Causes: Aortic obstructions with inadequate collateral reentry above kidneys:
Abdominal coarctation with occlusion.
Retrograde aortic obstruction, extending Leriche syndrome due to intimal (nodular) arteriosclerosis.
Antegrade aortic obstruction, extending Takayasu syndrome due to cryptogenic arteritis.
Aortic dissection.

Early Manifestations: Abdominal coarctation: Preceding hypertension, symmetrical leg and buttock claudications, reduced femoral and pedal pulses, abdominal and lumbar bruits, absence of radiographic evidence of collaterals and of a hypoplastic aortic arch.
Retrograde aortic obstruction: Preceding hypertension may have been absent; symmetrical or asymmetrical leg claudications and atrophy; impotence; decreased femoral and pedal pulses.
Antegrade aortic obstruction: Preceding hypertension may have been absent; predilection for females; masseteric, neck and shoulder claudications and weakness; ocular pareses, syncopal or convulsive episodes, decreased carotid and radial pulses.
Aortic dissection: Preceding hypertension; severe thoracic and abdominal pain; anterior spinal artery syndrome; widened aortic shadow; decreased hematocrit.

Late Manifestations: Oliguria to anuria.
Earliest urines may have [Na]u less than 2 mM/l, less or no more than 1.5 times [K]u; progressing to a high [Na]u which is over 1.5 times [K]u; thence to anuria.
Progressively raised [UN]s, [Cr]s, [K]s, acidemia.

Treatment: The onset of renal involvement forces the issue of surgery. Hypotensive therapy is indicated in dissection, prior to undertaking surgery, which may be further deferred if oliguria proves to be transient.
Pre-surgical dialysis: Peritoneal dialysis, although not inconceivable, is seldom elected with greater availability of hemodialysis.

Possible Dire Consequences without Treatment: Aortic rupture. Involvement of spinal cord and other viscera. Uremia.

References

Daimon, S., and Kitamura, K.: Coarctation of the abdominal aorta. Jap. Heart J., *5*:562, 1964.
Leriche, R.: Le syndrome d'obliteration termino-aortique par arterite. Press Med., *48*:601, 1940.

22. Microangiopathy (Lobular Artery Lesions)

Joseph H. Magee

Result: Hypoperfusion affecting the renal circulation primarily, diffusely and bilaterally, with cortical atrophy or cortical necrosis.

Cause: Visceral scleroderma (progressive systemic sclerosis).
Neurogenic vasoconstriction.
(*a.*) Vascular crises: Pregnancy hypertension.
(*b.*) Vascular crises: Established hypertension.
(*c.*) Oligemic reaction (Blood loss shock in non-toxemic pregnancy).
(*d.*) Oligemic reaction (Infant dehydration).
Circulating vasoconstriction.
(*a.*) Catecholamines.
(*b.*) Serotonin.
(*c.*) Angiotensin.

Early Manifestations: Oliguria to anuria.
Earliest urines may have [Na]u less than 20 m M/l, less or no more than 1.5 times [K]u; progressing to a high [Na]u which is over 1.5 times [K]u; thence to anuria.
Consumption coagulopathy.
Progressively raised [UN]s, [Cr]s, [K]s, acidemia.

Treatment: Maintenance hemodialysis. Treatment of precipitating condition.

Possible Dire Consequences without Treatment: Continued hypertension, uremia, cerebrovascular accident.

References

Lauler, D. P., and Schreiner, G. E.: Bilateral renal cortical necrosis. Am. J. Med., *24*:519, 1958.
Rodman, G. P., Schreiner, G. E., and Black, R. L.: Renal involvement in progressive systemic sclerosis. Am. J. Med., *23*:445, 1957.

23. Microangiopathy (Arteriolar Lesions)

Joseph H. Magee

Result: Hypoperfusion affecting the renal circulation primarily, diffusely and bilaterally, with cortical atrophy.

Synonyms: Malignant nephrosclerosis.

Cause: Vasospasm, with secondary hyperplastic changes in lobular arteries and fibrinoid vasonecrosis of afferent arterioles, in:

Primary hypertension	40%
Pregnancy hypertension	3%
Endocrine hypertension	3%
Multiple systems disease	7%
Primary renal disease (unilateral)	7%
Primary renal disease (bilateral)	40%

Early Manifestations: Preceding mild or moderate hypertension. Preceding unexplained weight loss. Diastolic pressures exceed 130 mm. Hg. Retinal hemorrhages and exudates, with visual impairment, with or without papilledema. Twice as common in men reversing the female preponderance in primary hypertension. Proteinuria is heavy regardless of etiology. Hematuria may be gross as well as microscopic.

Late Manifestations: Oliguria to anuria. Sustained high diastolic pressures.

Treatment: Control of hypertension. Regulation of acid-base balance if necessary.

Possible Dire Consequences without Treatment: Hypertension encephalopathy with or

without cerebral hemorrhage.	20%
Pulmonary edema	10%
Aortic rupture, aortic dissection, myocardial infarction	10%
Uremia	60%

Reference

Kincaid-Smith, P., McMichael, J., and Murphy, E. A.: The clinical course and pathology of hypertension with papilledema. Quart. J. Med., *27*:117, 1958.

24. Microangiopathy (Glomerular Lesions)

Joseph H. Magee

Result: Bilateral renal cortical necrosis as sequel of glomerular nephritis.

Cause: Proliferative glomerulitis. Intravascular coagulation.

Occurrence: Post-pharyngitic nephritis. (Acute diffuse glomerular nephritis). (Acute hemorrhagic nephritis). (Active onset nephritis). (Ellis type I nephritis). (Longcope Type A nephritis). (Post-streptococcal nephritis). (Post-scarlatinal nephritis).

Early Manifestations: Oliguria to anuria.

Treatment: Maintenance hemodialysis. Pre-transplantation nephrectomy may be elected for uncontrollable hypertension.

Possible Dire Consequences without Treatment: Ellis thought that about 10% of post-pharyngitic nephritis ran a desultory course, contributing cases ultimately to the pool of chronic nephritics. Of the remainder, 82% got well and 8% died of the original infection, acute circulatory overload, accelerated hypertension, and/or uremia.

Case Report: A six-year-old boy had fever, nausea, vomiting, sore throat, adenitis, diarrhea briefly, and one episode of hematemesis. He was found to be anuric, prior to which there had not been hematuria, flank pain, edema or hypertension. One year previous he had had a tonsillectomy for frequent sore throats. On admission to the hospital, he was afebrile and alert. Blood pressure was 150/110 and there was periorbital edema, and retinal arterial constriction without exudates. There was a left peritonsillar abscess with marked adenopathy of the left anterior cervical lymph nodes. There was a right basilar pleural effusion. Apical impulse was displaced to the left with no murmur or gallop; neck veins were flat when recumbent. There was tenderness of the right upper abdominal quadrant and over both costovertebral angles. [Urea N] was 207 mg./100 ml., [Cr]s 11.1 mg./100 ml. Antistreptolysin titer was 625 Todd units, using to 120 units. Scant urine revealed 2-plus proteinuria, hemoglobin casts and [Na]u 78 mM/l. No augmentation of urine flow occurred during three months' maintenance by periodic hemodialysis. At postmortem, following death from a ventricular escape rhythm, there was bilateral cortical narrowing with mottled calcification.

Reference

Ellis, A.: Natural history of Bright's disease. Lancet, *1*:1, 34, 72, 1942.

283

25. Microangiopathy (Postglomerular)

Joseph H. Magee

Result: Papillary necrosis.

Cause: Intravascular sickling. Intravascular coagulation.

Occurrence: Infections (especially diabetics). Sickle cell trait. Analgesic nephropathy.

Early Manifestations: Hematuria. Abdominal or lumbar pain. Fever chills. Oliguria.

Treatment: Specific infectious treatment. Control of diabetes. Dialysis for multiple papillary involvement.

Possible Dire Consequences without Treatment: Ureteral obstruction. Hydronephrotic atrophy. Metastatic infection. Uremia.

References

Mandel, E. E.: Renal medullary necrosis. Am. J. Med., *13*:322, 1952.
Muirhead, E. E., Vanatta, J., and Grollman, A.: Papillary necrosis of the kidney. A clinical and experimental correlation. J.A.M.A., *142*:627, 1950.

26. Microangiopathy (Embolic)

Joseph H. Magee

Result: Hypoperfusion affecting the renal circulation disproportionately.

Causes: Fluid emboli (radiopaque solutions). Fluid emboli (amniotic fluid). Fat emboli. Atheromatous emboli. Neoplastic emboli.

Early Manifestations: Hematuria. Oliguria. Azotemia.

Treatment: Conservative management with restriction of fluid intake to 20 ml./kg./day plus output. Dialysis if necessary.

Possible Dire Consequences without Treatment. Uremia. Consumption coagulopathy.

References

Lynch, M. J.: Nephrosis and fat embolism in acute hemorrhagic pancreatitis. Arch. Int. Med., *94*:709, 1954.
McAfee, J. G., and Willson, J. K. V.: A review of the complications of translumbar aortography. Am. J. Roent., *75*:965, 1956.
Thurlbeck, W. M., and Castleman, B.: Atheromatous emboli to the kidneys after aortic surgery. New Eng. J. Med., *257*:442, 1957.

27. Microangiopathy (Thrombotic)

Joseph H. Magee

Result: Hemolysis and Uremia II.

Cause: Intravascular coagulation. Microangiopathic hemolytic anemia.

Synonyms: Hemolytic uremic syndrome. Generalized Shwartzman reaction.

Occurrence: Cortical necrosis (lobular). Cortical necrosis (glomerular). Neoplastic emboli. Polyarteritis nodosa. Systemic lupus erythematosus.

Early Manifestations: Platelet consumption. Clotting factor consumption. Hemolysis, hemolytic icterus. Bone marrow hyperplasia. Lymphoid hyperplasia. Constitutional signs (malaise, fatigue, myalgia). Neurologic signs (headache, confusion, stupor, psychotic behavior, focal neurologic defects). Renal signs: Oliguria, hematuria, proteinuria.

Treatment: Heparin. Dialysis.

Possible Dire Consequences without Treatment: Stroke. Uremia. Hemorrhage.

References

Brain, M. C.: The hemolytic-uremic syndrome. Seminars Hemat., 6:162, 1969.

Gasser, C., et al.: Hemolytic-uremic syndrome. Schweiz. Med. Woch., 85:905, 1955.

Hensley, W. J.: Haemolytic anaemia in acute glomerulonephritis. Austral. Am. Med., 1:180, 1952.

Piel, C. F., and Phibbs, R. H.: The hemolytic-uremic syndrome. Ped. Clin. N.A., 13:295, 1966.

Introduction: Intrinsic Oligurias ("Tubular")

In the tubular oligurias urine volume is diminished not as a result of high reabsorption but due to suppressed filtration. In some of the toxic tubular injuries there may be a combination of decreased filtration and passive backflow which vitiates, to a much greater degree than usual, the formation of filtrate. Urine sodium is not low, as in under-perfusion of intact nephron units, but high and about 3 times the simultaneous potassium content. This may be, however, unhelpful diagnostically if mannitol or furosemide has been given. Then the U/P ratio of creatinine or of urea N, becomes a more useful distinguishing feature.

11

28. Pigment Nephropathy (Myolysis)

Joseph H. Magee

Result: Decreased urine flow due to suppressed filtration without substantial modification by tubular mechanisms (Table X–3).

Causes: Atrophy, myalgia and myoglobinuria:
- (*a.*) Primary myoglobinuria (Myophosphorylase deficiency) (McArdle syndrome).
- (*b.*) Alcoholic polymyopathy.
- (*c.*) Polymyositis (Dermatomyositis).

Exertion, myalgia and myoglobinuria.
- (*a.*) Primary myoglobinuria (Paroxysmal myoglobinuria) (Meyer-Betz syndrome).
- (*b.*) March myoglobinuria (Anterior tibial compartment syndrome) (Pretibial syndrome).
- (*c.*) Squat-jump myoglobinuria (Quadriceps femoris syndrome).
- (*d.*) Convulsions, convulsive therapy, induction of anesthesia, tetany, tetanus.

Injury, myalgia and myoglobinuria.
- (*a.*) Crushing injuries.
- (*b.*) Arterial injuries.
- (*c.*) Electrical injuries.
- (*d.*) Hyperthermic injuries.
- (*e.*) Toxic injuries (Harbor disease, Haffkrankheit) (venoms).
- (*f.*) Hypokalemia.

Early Manifestations: Fever, malaise, myalgia, local swelling and weakness.
Supernatant phase of spun urine is red.
Plasma in spun blood obtained at the same time may not be red (over 40 mg./100 ml. gives visible redness). Myoglobin, which is not bound to haptoglobin, appears in urine at plasma concentrations insufficient to tint it.
Urine myoglobin is not precipitable by ammonium sulfate.

Treatment: Urine alkalinization, augmentation of urine flow (mannitol).
Potassium repletion if not oliguric and [K]s low.
Dialysis for oliguria and hypercatabolism.

Possible Dire Consequences without Treatment: Oliguria, hyperkalemia, uremic syndrome.

References

Berlin, R.: Haff disease in Sweden. Acta Med. Scand., *129*:560, 1948.

Blondheim, S. H., Margoliast, E., and Shafoir, E.: A simple test for myohemoglobinuria. J.A.M.A., *167*:453, 1958.

Bowden, D. H., et al.: Acute recurrent rhabdomyolysis. Medicine, *35*:335, 1956.

Bywaters, E. G. L., and Stead, J. K.: Thrombosis of femoral artery with myohaemoglobinuria and low serum potassium concentration. Clin. Sci., *5*:195, 1945.

Doolan, P. D., et al.: Acute renal insufficiency following aortic surgery. Am. J. Med., *28*:895, 1960.

Fischer, H.: Pathologic effects and sequelae of electrical accidents. J. Occup. Med., 7:564, 1965.

Hed, R.: Myoglobinuria in man with special reference to a familial form. Acta Med. Scand., *151*:Suppl 3:301, 1955.

Hed, R., Lundmark, C., Fahlgren, H., and Ovell, S.: Acute muscular syndrome in chronic alcoholism. Acta Med. Scand., *171*:585, 1962.

Heitzman, E. I., Patterson, J. F., and Stanley, M. M.: Myoglobinuria and hypokalemia in regional enteritis. Arch. Intern. Med., *110*:117, 1962.

Hinz, C. F., Drucker, W. R., and Larner, J.: Idiopathic myoglobinuria. Am. J. Med., *39*:49, 1965.

Javid, J., Fisher, D. S., and Spaet, T. H.: Inability of haptoglobin to bind hemoglobin. Blood, *14*:683, 1959.

Kontos, H. A., et al.: Exertional idiopathic paroxysmal myoglobinuria. Am. J. Med., *35*:283, 1963.

Leach, R. E., Zohn, D. A., and Stryker, W. S.: Anterior tibial compartment syndrome. Arch. Surg., *88*:187, 1964.

Lucke, B.: Lower nephron nephrosis. Mil. Surgeon, *99*:371, 1946.

Rowland, L. P., et al.: Myoglobinuria. Arch. Neurol., *10*:537, 1964.

Schmid, R., and Mahler, R.: Chronic progressive myopathy with myoglobinuria. J. Clin. Invest., *38*:2044, 1959.

Stahl, W. C.: March hemoglobinuria. J.A.M.A., *164*:1458, 1957.

Vertel, R. M., and Knochel, J. P.: Acute renal failure due to heat injury. Am. J. Med., *43*:435, 1967.

29. Pigment Nephropathy due to Intravascular Hemolysis

Joseph H. Magee

Results: Decreased urine volume due to suppressed filtration without substantial modification by tubular mechanisms (Table X–3).

Causes: Incompatible blood. Distilled water (I.V. or transurethral). Parasitism: Falciparum malariae. Enzyme deficiency (G6PD): Primaquinism, favism. Chemicals: Arsine, chlorates, mushrooms, venoms. March hemolysis. Cold hemolysis. Nocturnal hemolysis.

Early Manifestations: Chest and low back paresthesias, nausea, vomiting, fever, hypotension.

In operating room, differential diagnosis includes air embolism, anaphylactic reactions, bacterial contamination of blood.

In multiple transfusions differential diagnosis includes citrate intoxication, febrile reactions to platelets and leukocytes.

In hemolysis, supernatant plasma in spun blood specimen is red. This may occur within ten minutes after transfusion of 50 ml. incompatible blood; over 40 mg. hemoglobin/100 ml. plasma gives visible redness. Hemoglobin is bound to plasma haptoglobin and does not appear in urine until bound-plus-unbound concentration reaches 150 mg./100 ml.

Red tint in urine may be precipitable by adding 2.8 gm. ammonium sulfate to 5 ml. urine.

Myoglobinuria rather than hemoglobinuria is implicated (*a*) by red urine or Hemastix positive urine after addition of ammonium sulfate to urine or (*b*) urine tinted when simultaneous plasma is not.

Treatment: Urine alkalinization, augmentation of urine flow (mannitol). Dialysis for oliguria and hypercatabolism.

Possible Dire Consequences without Treatment: Oliguria, hyperkalemia, uremic syndrome.

References

Barry, K. G., and Crosby, W. H.: The prevention of renal failure following transfusion reaction. Transfusion, *3*:34, 1963.
Borden, C. W., and Hall, W. H.: Fatal transfusion reactions from massive bacterial contamination of blood. New Eng. J. Med., *245*:760, 1951.
Brittingham, T. E., and Chaplin, H., Jr.: Febrile reactions caused by sensitivity to donor leucocytes and platelets. J.A.M.A., *165*:819, 1957.
Bunker, J. P., et al.: Citric acid intoxication. J.A.M.A., *157*:1361, 1955.
Dukes, D. C., Sealey, B. J., and Forbes, J. I.: Oliguric renal failure in blackwater fever. Am. J. Med., *45*:899, 1968.
Fudenberg, H., and Allen, F. H., Jr.: Transfusion reactions in the absence of demonstrable incompatibility. New Eng. J. Med., *256*:1180, 1957.
Ingram, G. I. C.: Editorial Review: The bleeding complications of blood transfusion. Transfusion *5*:1, 1965.

30. Microcrystalline Nephropathy

JOSEPH H. MAGEE

Cause: Intratubular and/or interstitial precipitation of sulfonamides, urates, cystine, immunoglobulin light chains.

Results: Diffuse tubular obstruction.

Early Manifestations: Oliguria or anuria.
   Crystalluria on microscopic examination: Cystine crystals are colorless hexagons, less soluble in acid urine. Sodium urates are amorphous and pink. Uric acid crystals are yellow or brown wedges, rosettes, or dumbbells. They occur in acid urines but redissolve in acetic acid.
   Bence Jones proteinuria: Precipitate albumin and globulins of tubular origin by heating to 100° C. and filter while hot. To 4 volumes of filtrate add 1 volume of buffer.* Observe for turbidity for fifteen minutes in a 56° C. water bath. If turbidity decreases either on transferring to a 100° C. water bath or on cooling, a heat labile (Bence Jones) protein is present. If there is no change, seal some filtrate in a capillary tube (1.3 mm. × 75 mm.) and boil in beaker of mineral oil and again observe for decreased turbidity. Not all Bence Jones are labile in the classic 50 to 100° C. range. The significance of the finding well justifies this evaluation particularly in puzzling oliguria without known precipitating event.

References

Bartels, E. D., et al.: Acute anuria following intravenous pyelography in patients with myelomatosis. Acta Med. Scand., *150*:297, 1954.
Leucotia, T.: Multiple myeloma and intravenous pyelography. Am. J. Roent., *85*:189, 1961.
Levi, D. F., Williams, R. C., and Lindstrom, F. D.: Immunofluorescent studies of the myeloma kidney with special reference to light chain disease. Am. J. Med., *44*:922, 1968.

* 2M acetate buffer, pH 4.9: Equal parts (1) HAc, glacial 56.3 and q.s. 500 ml. and (2) NaAc, trihyd. 136.09 q.s. 500 ml. or (3) NaAc, anhyd. 82.04 q.s. 500 ml.

Mac Kenzie, M. R., et al.: Rapid renal failure in a case of multiple myeloma. Clin. Exp. Immun., *3*:593, 1968.

Myhre, J. R., Bradwall, E. K., and Knutsen, S. B.: Acute renal failure following intravenous pyelography in cases of myelomatosis. Acta Med. Scand., *156*:263, 1956.

Perillie, P. E., and Conn, H. O.: Acute renal failure after intravenous pyelography in plasma cell myeloma. J.A.M.A., *167*:2186, 1958.

Vix, V. A.: Intravenous pyelography in multiple myeloma. Radiology, *87*:896, 1966.

Wochner, R. D., Strober, W., and Waldmann, T. A.: The role of the kidney in the catabolism of Bence-Jones proteins in multiple myeloma and in patients with renal disease. J. Exper. Med., *126*:207, 1967.

31. Acute Interstitial Nephritis

Joseph H. Magee

Cause: Delayed Hypersensitivity to: Large doses (20 to 60 million units) of penicillin and (20 to 24 gm.) of methicillin.
Antituberculous antibiotics: Isoniazid, rifamycins.
Other antibiotics: Nitrofurantoin, polymyxins, sulfonamides.
Acetophenetidin in ordinary doses.

> Buff-A-Comp, Empiral, Empirin, Emprazil, Fiorinal, Novahistine, Phenaphen, Soma, Tetrex.

Phenindione.

> Athromban, Bindan, Cronodione, Danilone, Diadilan, Dinderan, Dineval, Diophinaden, Fenhydrin, Fenilin, Hedulin, Hemolidione, Indema, Indon, PID, Rectadione, Thrombasal

Diphenylhydantoin.

> Alepsin, Antisacer, Citrullamon, Dentyl, Difhydran, Dilantin, Diphantoine, Diphenamine, Diphentoin, Epanutin, Eptoin, Hidantal, Lepitoni, Minetoin, Solantoin, Solantyl, Tacosal, Zentropil.

Result: Drug becomes cell surface antigen in target tissue.
Cell surface antibodies, of circulating small lymphocytes of thymic origin, combine with antigen.
Local reaction produced with activation of macrophages, infiltration of monocytes, induration, and edema.

Early Manifestations: Elicitation of recent exposure to drugs in patient with azotemia of known recent or unknown duration.
Enlarged symmetrical kidneys seen radiographically.
Hematuria universally and gross in two-thirds of patients.
Skin rash, blood eosinophilia and fever.

Treatment: Intercurrent dialyses if oliguria or toxic. Seven day trial of cortisone 100 mg./day.

Possible Dire Consequences without Treatment: Hyperkalemia, uremic syndrome.

References

Baldwin, D. S., et al.: Renal failure and interstitial nephritis due to penicillin and
    methicillin. New Eng. J. Med., *279*:1245, 1968.
French, A. J.: Hypersensitivity in the pathogenesis of the histopathologic changes asso-
    ciated with sulfonamide chemotherapy. Amer. J. Path., *22*:679, 1946.
Melnick, P. J.: Acute interstitial nephritis with uremia. Arch. Path., *36*:499, 1947.
Simenhoff, M. L., Guild, W. R., and Dammin, G. J.: Acute diffuse interstitial nephritis.
    Am. J. Med., *44*:618, 1968.

32. Toxic Tubular Necrosis

JOSEPH H. MAGEE

Synonym: Nephrotoxic Nephropathy (Oliver).

Causes: Organic Poisons.
    (*a.*) Solvents ($CHCl_3$, CCl_4).
    (*b.*) Reagents (Oxalic, Tartaric).
    (*c.*) Antibiotics (Neomycin, Kanamycin).
    (*d.*) Antifreezes (Mathanol, Ethylene Glycol).
    (*e*). Pesticides.
    Inorganic Poisons.
    (*a.*) Al, P, As, Ag, Cd, Sb, Au, Hg, Bi, Ur.

Treatment: Intercurrent dialysis if oliguric or toxic.

Possible Dire Consequences without Treatment: Hyperkalemia. Uremic syndrome.

In intratubular obstructions and in acute interstitial nephritis, it is believed that raised intratubular pressure suppresses filtration. With the tubular poisons it is believed (on the basis of identity of creatinine and inulin clearances with the normally lower urea clearance) that passive backflow of filtrate may be a pathogenetic factor in the oliguria. There may be widespread exfoliation of tubular cells from a relatively intact basement membrane (Oliver).

References

Reidenberg, M. M., et al.: Acute renal failure due to nephrotoxins. Am. J. Med. Sci.,
    247:25, 1964.
Schreiner, G. E., and Maher, J. F.: Toxic nephropathy. Am. J. Med., *38*:409, 1965.

33. Ischemic Tubular Necrosis

Joseph H. Magee

Synonym: Ischemuric Nephropathy (Oliver).

Causes: Hypoperfusion of organs generally.
(*a*). Arterial hypotension.
(*b*.) Arterial hypotension plus increased sympathetic activity (shock syndrome).
(*c*.) Without arterial hypotension, with disproportionate renal vasoconstriction (anesthesia, norepinephrine infusion).
Hypoperfusion of kidney disproportionately.
(*a*.) Especially aortic x-clamping, atheromatous emboli.
Hypoperfusion plus systemic infections.
(*a*.) Pneumonia (especially lobar).
(*b*.) Septicemias, septic abortions.
(*c*.) Pylephlebitis, cholecystitis.
Disturbed tonicity, reaction, viscosity of body fluids, including hyperthermia.

Early Manifestations: History of precipitating event. Oliguria. See Table X–3.

Treatment: Fluid restriction. Maintain calories. Timely dialysis especially in postoperative, infectious or hypercatabolic circumstances.

Possible Dire Consequences without Treatment: Hyperkalemia. Uremic syndrome. Susceptibility to infection.

According to Oliver, the necrosis is patchy, with areas where continuity of basement membranes is lost. Radiographically the kidneys enlarge, at necropsy their weight is increased and the cut surfaces bulge. Microscopically there are more cells, as manifested by more nuclei; and in both biopsy and necropsy material encroachments of proliferating epithelial cells into Bowman's space are found. On microdissection, there are outpouchings of tubular epithelium into the interstitium. An "epithelial proliferative reaction," pathogenetic in the oliguria, appears to predominate over "interstitial edema" which is variably present as well.

References

Biber, T. U. L., et al.: A study by micropuncture and microdissection of acute renal damage in rats. Am. J. Med., *44*:664, 1968.
Muehrcke, R. C.: Acute Renal Failure: Diagnosis and Management. St. Louis, The C. V. Mosby Co., 1969.

34. Hemorrhagic Tubular Necrosis

JOSEPH H. MAGEE

Cause: Intravascular coagulation (renal vein thrombosis).

Occurrence: Oligemic reaction (infant dehydration).
Altered cardiac dynamics (congestive heart failure).
Thrombophlebitis.
Surgical handling.
Extrarenal neoplasia.
Renal disease.
(*a.*) Polyarteritis nodosa.
(*b.*) Idiopathic nephrotic syndrome.
(*c.*) Papillary necrosis.
(*d.*) Hypernephroma.
(*e.*) Amyloidosis.

Early Manifestations: Acute: lumbar pain, hematuria, proteinuria, oliguria.
Chronic: Uremic syndrome.
Chronic: Nephrotic syndrome if occlusion is gradual and/or partial.
Caval thrombosis: Venous collaterals, demarcating edema.

Treatment: Heparinization in intervals between dialyses. Thrombectomy where involvement limited to larger vessels.

Possible Dire Consequences without Treatment: Progressive renal insufficiency, uremia, death.

References

Cohn, L. H.: et al.: The treatment of bilateral renal vein thrombosis and nephrotic syndrome. Surgery, *64*:387, 1968.

Deodhar, K. P., et al.: Inferior vena caval obstruction. J. Postgrad. Med., *15*:64, 1969.

Duffy, J. L., et al.: Renal vein thrombosis and the nephrotic syndrome. Am. J. Med., *54*:663, 1973.

Harrison, C. V., Milne, M. D., and Steiner, R. E.: Clinical aspects of renal vein thrombosis. Quart. J. Med., *25*:285, 1956.

Jackson, B. T., and Thomas, M. L.: Post-thrombotic inferior caval obstruction. Brit. Med. J., *1*:18, 1970.

Lieberman, E., et al.: Thrombosis, nephrosis and corticosteroid therapy. J. Pediat., *73*:320, 1968.

McCarthy, W., Titus, J. L., and Daugherty, G. W.: Bilateral renal vein thrombosis and the nephrotic syndrome in adults. Ann. Intern. Med., *58*:837, 1963.

Menon, I. S., Dewar, H. A., and Newell, D. J.: Role of the kidney in fibrinolytic activity of the blood. Lancet, *1*:785, 1968.

Morris, J. F., Ginn, H. E., and Thompson, D. D.: Unilateral renal vein thrombosis associated with the nephrotic syndrome. Am. J. Med., *34*:867, 1963.

Pilgeran, L. O., and Pickert, L. R.: Control of fibrinogen biosynthesis. J. Atherosclerosis Res., *8*:155, 1968.

Pollak, V. E., Kark, R. M., and Pirani, C. L.: Renal vein thrombosis and the nephrotic syndrome. Am. J. Med., *21*:496, 1956.

Rosenman, E., Pollak, V. E., and Pirani, C. L.: Renal vein thrombosis in the adult. Medicine, *47*:269, 1968.

35. Non-Oliguric Acute Renal Failure (Ketotic Coma)

Joseph H. Magee

Cause: Uncontrolled diabetes with polyuria, hyperviscosity, renal hypoperfusion.

Early Manifestations: Elevated urea N for a period after an episode of ketoacidosis, peaking at day 4 to 6. (Trever and Cluff reviewed the records of 476 patients admitted once or more for ketoacidosis to the Johns Hopkins Hospital, 1934–1955, finding 3 such cases).
Ages were eighteen, twenty and sixty-three.
Blood sugar was 410, 500, 744 mg./100 ml.
Blood bicarbonate was 6.9, 6.9, 10.1 mM/l.
Initial urea N was 68, 32, 108 mg./100 ml.
Peak urea N was 163, 150, 147 mg./100 ml.

Treatment: Conservative, avoiding attribution of chronic renal disease until time course of non-oliguric renal failure elapses. Continued attempt to control diabetes.

Dire Consequences without Treatment: Oliguric acute renal failure.

About a third of cases of acute renal failure are never recognized as being oliguric. This includes postanesthetic and postoperative acute renal failure. Despite absence of recorded hypotension, normotension may have been achieved by vasoconstriction of some regions of the circulation of which the kidney may have been one. About half the instances of acute renal failure on burn services occur without an intervening period of oliguria, despite careful observations that make it unlikely that an oliguric phase has been missed.

References

Reubi, F.: Glomerular filtration rate, renal blood flow and blood viscosity during and after diabetic coma. Circ. Res., *1*:410, 1953.
Trever, R. W., and Cluff, L. E.: The problem of increasing azotemia during the management of diabetic acidosis. Am. J. Med., *24*:369, 1958.

36. Non-Oliguric Acute Renal Failure (Hyperosmolar Coma)

Joseph H. Magee

Cause: Uncontrolled diabetes with polyuria, hyperviscosity, renal hypoperfusion.

Early Manifestations: Average admission urea N is 85 mg./100 ml. (range 18 to 150), compared to 30 mg./100 ml. in ketotic coma.
Average blood sugar is 95.2 mg./100 ml. (range 400 to 2200).
Average [HCO_3]s is 23.2 mM/L. (range 15 to 36.8); somewhat a function of a definition that excludes ketotic cases.
Average age is sixty-three years (range 36 to 81).
Women predominate 2:1.
80% are previously unknown diabetics.
Fatality rate is 43%.

Treatment: The occurrence of non-oliguric renal failure may be a circumstance further increasing glycosemia because of inability to augment external glucose losses. Peritoneal dialysis, with insulin lowering of blood sugar as required to maintain a gradient with the rinsing fluid, is conservative, if age, sepsis, devitalized tissue, or poor cardiac status are factors.

Dire Consequences without Treatment: Oliguric acute renal failure.

Uncontrolled diabetes occasions large saline volume losses. The agency of loss is osmotic diuresis due to glucose. Since it is a hypotonic diuresis respective to saline, large deficits of plain water are incurred as well. To this, in the present syndrome, are added large sequestered losses. A third of body water is normally extracellular, with its glucose concentration 90 mg./100 ml. or 5 mM/l. One third liter of body fluid thus owes its extracellular position to the effect of this solute. If this is increased ten-fold to 900 mg./100 ml. or 50 mM/l, this amount increases to 3 liters. Due to this increment, the measurement of [Na]s is rendered spuriously low (diabetic pseudohyponatremia), despite the great actual deficit of water incurred at the expense of cells.

Rising hematocrit and [Pr]s although they occur may also by this sequestering effect be underestimates of fluid deficit.

References

Ehrlich, R. M., and Bain, H. W.: Hyperglycemia and hyperosmolality in an 18 month old child. New Eng. J. Med., *276*:683, 1967.

Macarrio, M., Messis, C. P., and Soscia, I. L.: Focal seizures as a manifestation of hyperglycemia without ketoacidosis. Neurology, *15*:195, 1965.

Root, H. F., and Leeck, R.: Diabetic stupor and hyperglycemic stupor compared. Med. Clin. N. A., *30*:115, 1946.

Sament, S., and Schwartz, M. B.: Severe diabetic stupor without ketosis. S. Afr. Med. J., *31*:893, 1957.

Chapter XI

Certain Endocrine Disorders and Their Mimics

Hormones and Bones

Like the direct regulation of blood sugar by opposing insulin and glucagon feedback, without trophic hormone control, blood calcium is regulated by parathormone and by calcitonin. The parathormone defense of blood calcium remodels bone; calcitonin has the opposite role, lowering blood calcium, its effect upon bone being, theoretically, osteosclerosis. Both are, like glucagon, single-chained polypeptides that are considerably smaller than insulin but larger than the neurohypophyseal peptides or angiotensin. The cellular participation of parathormone, as is now known for a variety of hormones, is in conferring critical configurations upon key steroid and nucleotide molecules.

Steroidal substances affected by parathormone are provitamins D, which arise from photochemical cleavage of the B ring of 7-dehydrocholesterol in epidermal cells, or are ingested. Two hydroxylations, at the 25 position by liver cells, and at the 1 position by kidney cortex cells, the latter requiring parathormone, are necessary to produce vitamin D optimally effective in synthesizing the calcium-transporting protein of the gut, and in remodelling bone. Parathormone has two incidental effects, independent of vitamin D, upon the kidney, causing phosphaturia and increased reabsorption of calcium. If parathormone is turned off, the calcium level in blood falls both by decreased delivery from bone and an increased leak by the kidney; thus, there may be hypercalciuria without hypercalcemia. If calcitonin is turned on at the same time, lowering the blood level is further favored, outweighing any calcitonin effects upon the kidney, which upon the whole seem to mimic parathormone weakly. The particular significance of calcitonin has to do with the greater speed with which blood calcium may fall thereby as compared to the effect of turned-off parathormone alone. If one drinks a gallon of milk a day, calcitonin forms the principal defense against both extra-osseous deposition of the calcium, and the acute hypercalcemic syndrome (Table XI–1).

TABLE XI–1.

CHRONIC HYPERCALCEMIC SYNDROME	
1. Bone Disease:	Pain, fractures
2. Stone Disease:	Colic, hematuria
3. Nephropathy:	Dilute polyuria and nocturia, progressive creatininemia
4. Enteropathy:	Constipation, anorexia, nausea, vomiting
5. Dermatitis:	Pruritus
6. Conjunctivitis:	Tearing
ACUTE HYPERCALCEMIC SYNDROME	
7. Encephalopathy:	Malaise, irrascibility, overt psychosis, lethargy, somnolence, coma, death.
8. Cardiopathy:	(1) Shortened mechanical and electrical systole (QT less than 0.40; Q-oTc 0.16 or less)
	(2) Vagal effect with prolonged PR or overt atrioventricular block.

Since 99% of calcium resides in the skeleton, aberrations in blood calcium are likely to represent bone disease; exceptionally diet can serve as a bone surrogate. Raised values for [alk ptase]s and for hydroxyproline excretion are indicators of increased bone turnover, but they are unhelpful in discriminating amongst causes. Finding a raised [Ca]u by Sulkowitch's or another method suggests decreased Ca reabsorption, because parathormone has been turned off by a sufficient signal, raised [Ca]s, or that reabsorptive capacity has been exceeded by load despite parathormonism, or that the patient is receiving calciuric saluretics (thiazides).

Reference to Table XI–2 shows that a number of conditions are characterized both by hypercalcemia and by hypercalciuria. Normal or elevated levels of cyclic adenosine monophospate (cAMP) in urine favor parathormonism, the levels in other hypercalcemic conditions tending to be lower than in controls. The finding of phosphaturia also tends to incriminate parathormonism rather specifically, with the exception of the tubular defect syndromes where the phosphaturia is intrinsic rather than hormonal.

One does not usually come upon phosphaturia deliberately but in the course of evaluating a low [P]s. The latter may have become a concern as a consequence of serendipity, a word which found its way into medical parlance due to parathyroid disease and to Mayo Clinic authors. In the other causes of a low [P]s, P excretion may be reduced or absent, and this is evaluated by simultaneous determinations of P in serum and in urine. If the urine flow rate is 1 ml./min., typically [P]u will be about 40 mg./100 ml. or 10 times a normal value of 4 mg./100 ml. for [P]s. Hence the U/S ratio is 10, and at the flow rate just given, phosphorus (orthophosphate) clearance is 10 ml./min. If inulin clearance is 100 ml./min. concurrently, the rejection fraction for urine P is 10%, and the reabsorption fraction is 90%. A low [P]s can occur without change in these fractions; if the patient takes aluminum hydroxide gel, or is on exclusive glucose alimentation, [P]s may fall to 2 mg./100 ml., and along with it [P]u to 20 mg./100 ml. At the same urine flow rate, the clearance of P is still 10 ml./min. If the patient is a child with physiologically increased growth hormone, [P]s will be more nearly 5 mg./100 ml. If [P]u

TABLE XI–2.

Hypercalcemic States	[Ca]		[Alk Ptase]	[P]	
	Decrease in serum level following cortisone administration	Urine	Serum	Serum	Urine
Paget's Disease With Immobilization	→	↑	↑	↑ →	→ ↓
Thyrotoxicosis	→	↑	→	↑ →	→ ↓
Dietary Calcium	→	→	→	↑ →	→ ↓
Vitamin D Excess	↓	↑	→	↑ →	→ ↓
Cortisol Lack	↓	↑	→	↑ →	→ ↓
Bone Metastases	↓	↑	→	↑ →	→ ↑
Ectopic Parathormone	20% ↑ of cases	↑	↑	↓	↑
Autonomous Parathormone	rarely, and < 2 mg./100 ml.	↑	↑	↓	↑

is still 40 mg./100 ml. at the same urine flow rate, the clearance of P is 8 ml./min. At the same inulin clearance the rejection fraction is now 8% and the reabsorption fraction 92%.

Now if [P]s is 5 mg./100 ml. because of renal filtration failure, [P]u may be only 25 mg./100 ml. at the same flow rate. The U/S ratio will be 5 and the clearance of P only 5 ml./min. If inulin clearance is reduced to 25 ml./min., the rejection fraction, however, is a high 20%; the reabsorption fraction is a low 80%.

Using creatinine rather than inulin as a filtration marker, the test lends itself to office or to hospital laboratory performance, the latter likely to entail an automated analysis system. The value of these tests hinges entirely on the urine and serum values being simultaneous. The two fractions arrived at are ratios of two clearances and the volume term common to both clearances drops out; urines then need not be timed as to interval, but only with regard to when the blood was obtained for serum. The arithmetic for the rejection fraction is:

$$\frac{(Creatinine)s \times (phosphorus)u}{(Creatinine)u \times (phosphorus)s}$$

The reabsorption fraction is obtained by subtracting this quotient from unity; both are multiplied by 100 if expressed as percent. This is equivalent to expressing the rejection or reabsorption fractions at a standard filtration rate of 100 ml./min.

The procedure needs to be "de-routinized" in several ways in order to make it useful. In the first place it is better to request [P]p rather than [P]s, the plasma then to be obtained with sodium fluoride as anticoagulant, or else with immediate separation of the cells. (The P released by red cell glycolysis can spuriously raise [P]s by about 25% with two hours' standing on a laboratory bench.) Furthermore, the urine specimen should be the second voided A.M. specimen. P excretion is normally maximal around midnight and minimal on awakening and cumulative urines hence can be maximally misleading. Three glasses of water on awakening will hasten the second specimen and help the chemist dilute it. The urine specimen will be run amidst blood filtrates, but the chemist may arrange for the paired specimens to be run together in duplicate, after and before readings of standard phosphate solution. Finally ask for the actual P and creatinine values for your own calculations.

Figure XI–1 shows that the rejection fraction rises continuously, at standard filtration rate, as [P] in serum or plasma rises; presumably parathormonism develops pari passu as [P] rises. The transport maximum, for P reabsorption is about 4.5 mg./min. normally, but either with marked splay, or a labile maximum, so that P appears in urine at much lower loads than this, the threshold being around 2.5 mg./min. at standard filtration rate. In hypoparathyroidism the transport maximum may be changed, but with no splay, so that P may be absent from urines below the transport maximum.

The top panel in Figure XI–1 makes it appear that the rejection fraction rises asymptotically, so that, at infinite load, rejection would be complete. This is an artifact of plotting P against its reciprocal, which appears in the ordinate term. In the middle panel this plot is changed by multiplying both the rejection and reabsorption fractions through by P; the dimensions then become mg./100 ml. of rejectate or reabsorbate. This gives a better separation of normal from hyper- and hypoparathyroid values than do the rejection and reabsorption fractions. The arithmetic for rejectate concentration is:

$$\frac{(Creatinine)s \times (phosphorus)u}{(creatinine)u}$$

Reabsorbate concentration is obtained by subtracting this quotient from filtrate (serum or plasma) concentration. When [P]p is 4.0 mg./100 ml., the normal value for rejectate concentration is 0.75 $\pm$ 0.5 mg./100 ml.; for reabsorbate concentration it is 3.25 $\pm$ 0.5 mg./100 ml. For each value of [P]p,

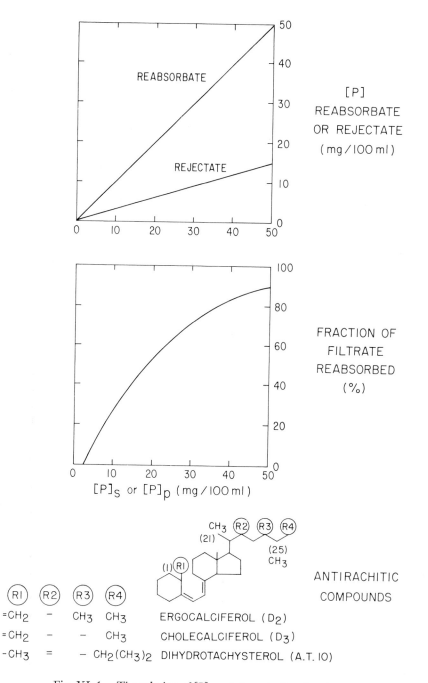

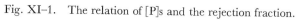

Fig. XI–1.   The relation of [P]s and the rejection fraction.

rejectate concentration should be within 0.5 mg./100 ml. of the value obtained substituting into the slope formula 0.5 [P]p–1.25, according to Nordin and Bulusu. Hypoparathyroid values uniformly fall below the lower limit and hyperparathyroid values generally are above the upper limit thus obtained. Reabsorbate concentration should be within 0.5 mg./100 ml. of the value obtained by substituting into the slope formula's reciprocal, 0.5[P]p + 1.5. In practice, rejectate values are nearly always used.

Certain clinical features accompanying hypercalcemia generally are summarized in Table XI–2. Treatment of hypercalcemia, discussed under the individual entities, is directed toward increasing renal elimination or decreasing intestinal absorption of calcium or decreasing osteoclastic activity in bone. Increased renal elimination of calcium is accomplished by saline infusions. Steroids appear to decrease the biologic availability of vitamin D, thereby decreasing bone remodelling effect of usual amounts of parathormone and decreasing calcium absorption by the gut. Both calcitonin and mithramycin decrease osteoclastic activity. Although administration of phosphate lowers [Ca]s effectively both osseous and extraosseous precipitation of calcium phosphate are consequences.

In Table XI–3, chemical features of the normocalcemic and hypocalcemic varieties of bone disease are summarized.

TABLE XI–3

Normocalcemic or Hypocalcemic States	[Ca]s		[Alk Ptase]	[P]	
	Serum	Urine	Serum	Serum	Urine
Osteoporosis	→	→	→	→	→
Phosphate Diabetes	→	→	↑	↓	↑
Tubular Acidosis	→	↑	↑	↓	↑
Calcitoninism	↓	↓	→	↓	↑
Parathormone Resistance	↓	↓	→	↑	↓
Parathormone Lack	↓	↓	→	↑	↓
Azotemic Rickets	↓	↓	↑	↑	↓
Dietary Rickets	↓	↓	↑	↓	↓

→ no significant alteration   ↑ increase   ↓ decrease

Normal Values

[alk ptase]s = serum concentration of alkaline phosphatase
 = 0.8–2.3 units (Bessey-Lowry), normally in adults.
 = 2.0–4.5 units (Bodansky)
 = 2.2–8.6 units (Shinowara)
 = 3.0–10.0 units (Gutman)
 = 5.0–13.0 units (King-Armstrong)
 = 21–91 units/L. (International) at 37° C.

[Ca]s = serum concentration of calcium
 = 4.5–5.5 mEq./L.
 = 9–11 mg./100 ml.

[Ca]u = urine concentration of calcium, graded by Sulkowitch reaction.

Ca excretion = excretion/24 hours on 10 mEq. or 200 mg. Ca diet
 = 7.5 mEq./24 hours
 = 150 mg./24 hours

cAMP = cyclic adenosine monophosphate

[P]s or [P]p = serum or plasma concentration of inorganic phosphorus
 = 1–1.5 mEq./L.
 = 3.0–4.5 mg./100 ml.

QT = interval from origin of Q wave to end of T wave

Q-otc = interval from origin of Q wave to origin of T wave.
 corrected to standard rate 60/min.

q.i.d. = four times daily

t.i.d. = three times daily

serum urea N = serum concentration of urea nitrogen = 4.66 (serum concentration of
 urea)
 = 8–19 mg./100 ml.

[Cl]s = serum concentration of chloride = 100–106 mM/L.

Reference

Nordin, B. E. C., and Bulusu, L.: A modified index of phosphate excretion. Postgraduate Med. J., *44*:93, 1968.

1. Hypercalcemic Bone Disease: Paget's Disease

George Ross Fisher, III and Joseph H. Magee

Cause: Autonomous bone remodeling.

Early Manifestations: Regularly raised [alk ptase]s, unlike simple osteoporosis.
Bone pain; pathologic fractures, and bulbar, spinal or nerve compression syndromes; despite normal [Ca]s.
Increased Ca excretion with immobilization may anticipate symptomatically raised [Ca]s levels.

Treatment: Avoidance of immobilization during intercurrent illness or surgery.
Early sitting, standing, walking if possible.
Rocking bed if these are impossible.
High index of suspicion for parathyroid adenoma in instances of raised [Ca]s not explainable as consequences of immobilization.
High fluid intake, intravenous saline. Oral Fleet's phosphosoda, tsp. q.i.d. in juice.
Enemas of above, up to t.i.d., in nauseated patients.
Avoidance of corticosteroid therapy, except for complications due to high cardiac output state.
Arthroplasties and osteotomies for deformity and pain.

Possible Dire Consequences without Treatment: Hypercalcemic syndrome.

References

Nagant de Deuxchaimes, C. and Krane, S. M.: Paget's Disease of bone. Medicine, *43*:322, 1944.
Reifenstein, E. C., Jr., and Albright, F.: Paget's Disease. New Eng. J. Med., *231*:343, 1944.
Woodhouse, N. J. Y., et al.: Radiological regression of Paget's disease treated by human calcitonin. Lancet, *2*:922, 1972.

2. Hypercalcemic Bone Disease: Osteoporosis and Thyrotoxicosis

Joseph H. Magee and Laurence G. Wesson, Jr.

Cause: Osteoporosis due to thyrotoxicosis.

Result: Predominant bone-to-blood calcium transfers with decreasing bone mass (osteoporosis).

Manifestations: Normal [alk ptase]s. Raised [Ca]s and Ca excretion. Normal [P]s and P excretion prior to nephrocalcinosis. Signs of hypothyroidism.

Treatment: Corticosteroids are ineffective. Treatment of thyrotoxicosis.

Possible Dire Consequences without Treatment: Confusion with parathyroid disease or malignant neoplasm.

Calcium and phosphorus excretions are sensitive to altered activity patterns. Calcium excretion is lowest toward the end of sleep and rises to its highest point before midday; the peak is less sharp than those for sodium, potassium and chloride which have similar patterns. Phosphorus excretion is lowest where calcium is highest and becomes maximal around midnight. Despite the hemodynamic stresses and altered activity status brought on by endocrinopathy, timing of these variations is little altered in some patients.

References

Albright, F., Bauer, W., and Auf, J. C.: Studies of calcium and phosphorus metabolism VIII. The influence of the thyroid gland and the parathyroid hormone upon the total acid base metabolism. J. Clin. Invest., *10*:187, 1931.

Aub, J. C., et al.: Studies of calcium and phosphorus metabolism III. The effects of the thyroid hormone and thyroid decrease. J. Clin. Invest., 7:97, 1929.

Epstein, F. H., Freedman, L. R., and Levitin, H.: Hypercalcemia, nephrocalcinosis and reversible renal insufficiency associated with hyperthyroidism. New Eng. J. Med., *258*:782, 1958.

Follis, R. H.: Studies on hypervitaminosis D. Am. J. Path., *51*:568, 1955.

Krane, S. M., et al.: The effect of thyroid disease on calcium metabolism in man. J. Clin. Invest., 35:874, 1956.

Rose, E., and Boles, R. S., Jr.: Hypercalcemia in thyrotoxicosis. Med. Clin. N.A., *37*:1715, 1953.

Stanley, M. M., and Fazekas, J.: Thyrotoxicosis simulating hyperparathyroidism. Am. J. Med., 7:262, 1949.

3. Hypercalcemic Nephrocalcinosis (Dietary Calcium)

George Ross Fisher, III and Joseph H. Magee

Cause: Milk and/or calcium carbonate of peptic ulcer. Calcium carbonate therapy of raised [P]s in dialyzed uremic patients. Congenital predisposition may be necessary.

Result: Increased calcium transfers from gut-to-blood (hypercalcemia), blood-to-bone (osteosclerosis) and blood-to-soft tissue (metastatic calcification), with maintained bone mass.

Synonyms: Milk-alkali syndrome. Milk poisoning. Milk drinker's syndrome. Chalk poisoning. Burnett's syndrome.

Early Manifestations: Normal [alk ptase]s.
Raised [Ca]s up to 14 mg./100 ml., with or without alkalosis, and despite azotemia.
Low Ca excretion, paralleling azotemia, rising to hyperparathyroid levels or azotemia improves.
Raised [P]s when azotemic, not falling below normal range when azotemia improves.
Metastatic calcifications (coma, conjunctivae, vessels).
Dilute or salt-wasting polyuria.

Treatment: Cessation of intake of calcium salts.

Possible Dire Consequences without Treatment: Nephrocalcinosis; nephrolithiasis; confusion with parathyroid adenoma.

References

Burnett, C. H., et al.: Nephrocalcinosis without hypercalciuria or hypophosphatemia, calcinosis and renal insufficiency, a syndrome following prolonged intake of milk and absorbable alkali. New Eng. J. Med., *240*:787, 1949.

Dworetsky, M.: Reversible metastatic calcification (milk drinker's syndrome). J.A.M.A., *155*:830, 1954.

Ginsburg, D. S., Kaplan, E. L., and Katz, A. I.: Hypercalcemia after oral calcium carbonate therapy in patients on chronic hemodialysis. Lancet, *1*:1271, 1973.

Hardt, L. L., and Rivers, A. B.: Toxic manifestations following the alkaline treatment of peptic ulcers. Arch. Intern. Med., *31*:171, 1923.

Henneman, P. H., and Barker, W. H.: Two mechanisms of sustained hypercalcemia following hypervitaminosis D and the milk-alkali syndrome. J. Clin. Invest., *36*:899, 1957.

Katz, A. I., Hampers, C. L., and Merrill, J. P.: Secondary hyperparathyroidism and renal *osteodystrophy* (?) in chronic renal failure. Medicine, *48*:333, 1969.

Lowe, C. E., Bird, E. D., and Thomas, W. C., Jr.: Hypercalcemia in myxedema. J.C.E.M., *22*:261, 1958.

McMillan, D. E., and Freeman, R. B.: The milk-alkali syndrome. Med., *44*:485, 1965.

McQueen, E. G.: Milk poisoning and calcium gout. Lancet, *2*:67, 1952.

Rifkind, B. M., Chasan, B. I., and Aitchison, J. D.: Chronic milk-alkali syndrome with generalized osteosclerosis after prolonged intake of "Rennies" tablets. Brit. Med. J., *1*:317, 1960.

Steele, J. M.: Renal insufficiency developing during prolonged use of alkalis. J.A.M.A., *106*:2049, 1936.

4. Hypercalcemic Nephrocalcinosis (Dietary Vitamin D Excess)

GEORGE ROSS FISHER, III AND JOSEPH H. MAGEE

Cause: Excess vitamin D intake. Hyperresponsiveness in sarcoidosis to normal vitamin D effect.

Result: Enhanced gut-to-blood calcium transfers, and despite normal parathormone levels, of bone-to-blood, kidney-to-blood, and blood-to-soft tissues, with maintained bone mass.

Early Manifestations: Normal [alk ptase]s.
Raised [Ca]s, persisting up to one year after ceasing vitamin D, responsive to cortisone administration.
Azotemia due to nephrocalcinosis.
Normal or raised [P]s, despite direct phosphaturic effect of vitamin D and enhancement of parathormone effects.
Raised Ca excretion, up to 1000 mg./day, despite nephrocalcinosis with azotemia.
Urine acidification not impaired as in absolute parathormone excesses.
Anorexia; nausea vomiting, weight loss.
Metastatic calcification (cornea, conjunctivae, nail beds, subcutaneous tissues).

Treatment: Eliminate all multivitamin sources of vitamin D. Cortisone 25 to 50 mg./day, as needed to control hypercalcemia. Intravenous saline. Oral Fleet's phosphosoda.

Possible Dire Consequences without Treatment: Nephrocalcinosis, nephrolithiasis, coma, disorientation.

Reference

Avioli, L. V., Birge, S. J., and Lee, S. W.: Chronic pancreatitis. Ann. Intern. Med., *74*:264, 1971.

5. Hypercalcemic Bone Disease: Osteolytic Metastasis

George Ross Fisher, III and Joseph H. Magee

Causes: Osteolytic bone metastases. Myeloma, lymphoma, leukemia. Sarcomas. Breast and other carcinomas.

Result: Acute hypercalcemic syndrome, with predominance of bone-to-blood (osteoporosis, osteolysis) over blood-to-bone (osteosclerosis) calcium transfers, due to direct replacement of osseous tissue by tumor, with reduced bone mass.

Early Manifestations: Raised [alk ptase]s. Raised [Ca]s with [P]s normal or high. [Ca]s falls with 150 mg. cortisone/day × 7.

Treatment: Treatment of neoplasm by surgery, chemotherapy, radiation. Interim treatment with prednisone, using [Ca]s as guide to dose reduction. Mithramycin 15 μg./kg./week. I.V. is usually treatment of choice, and may not be required more than a few times.

Dire Consequences without Treatment: Osteoporosis, osteolysis, fractures, death.

References

Dent, C. E., and Watson, L.: The hydrocortisone test in primary and tertiary hyperparathyroidism. Lancet, *2*:662, 1968.
Follis, R. H., Jr., and Park, E. A.: Some observations on the roentgenographic changes in childhood leukemia. Bull. Hosp. Joint Dis., *12*:67, 1961.
Gutman, A. B., Tyson, T. L., and Gutman, E. B.: Serum calcium, inorganic phosphorus and phosphatase activity in hyperparathyroidism, Paget's disease, multiple myeloma and neoplastic disease of bone. Arch. Intern. Med., *57*:379, 1936.
Katakow, B., Mines, M. F., and King, F. H.: Hypercalcemia in Hodgkin's disease. New Eng. J. Med., *256*:59, 1957.

6. Hypercalcemic Bone Disease: Ectopic Parathormone

GEORGE ROSS FISHER, III AND JOSEPH H. MAGEE

Cause: Ectopic Parathormone

Epidermoid carcinoma (lung)	30%
Epidermoid carcinoma (other)	18%
Adenocarcinoma (kidney)	30%
Adenocarcinoma (other)	18%
Lymphomas	4%

Result: Unbalanced transfers from bone-to-blood (osteitis cystica) and blood-to-bone (osteitis fibrosa), with reduced and remodelled bone mass; phosphaturic but absent anaciduric effect of ectopic parathormone helps differentiate from that due to native hormone; feedback parathyroid atrophy does not occur.

Early Manifestations: Raised [alk ptase]s, without radiographic evidence of periosteal reabsorption and/or cystic bone lesions. The primary cancer may be unsuspected. Associated liver metastases accompanying in 75%.
Raised [Ca]s and low [P]s.
Fall in [Ca]s follows cortisone 150 mg./day $\times$ 7 in about 40% of cases but not in the two most common neoplasms (lung, kidney).
Phosphaturia.
Normal urine pH minimum and titrable acidity.

Treatment: Oral sodium phosphate, mithramycin may have good effect.

Possible Dire Consequences without Treatment: Acute hypercalcemic syndrome. Confusion with parathyroid adenoma.

TABLE XI–4.

	Ectopic Parathormone	Autonomous Parathormone
Female	30%	60%
Renal Calculi	8%	50%
Osteitis Fibrosa	6%	25%
[Ca]s over 14 mg./100 ml.	75%	25%
[Alkaline Phosphatases]s over 16 K-A units	50%	Rare
Anemia	75%	None
Weight Loss	20–50 #	Rare
Symptoms	2–6 months	2–25 years

References

Case records of the Massachusetts General Hospital #27461. New Eng. J. Med., 225:789, 1941.
Lafferty, F. W.: Pseudohyperparathyroidism. Medicine, 45:247, 1966.
Plimpton, C. H., and Gellhorn, A.: Hypercalcemia in malignant disease without evidence of bone destruction. Am. J. Med., 21:750, 1956.
Snedecor, P. A., and Baker, H. W.: Pseudohyperparathyroidism due to malignant tumors. Cancer, 17:1492, 1964.

7. Hyperparathyroidism

GEORGE ROSS FISHER, III

Cause: Parathyroid adenoma, also parathyroid hormone secreted by an occult malignancy.

Early Manifestations: Usually none. Multiple kidney stones, multiple fractures, low serum phosphorus, high serum calcium, high serum parathyroid hormone level. The most usual form of presentation is the discovery of unsuspected hypercalcemia on multiphasic blood chemistry screening.

Treatment: Sometimes watchful waiting. Successful surgery.

Possible Dire Consequences without Treatment: Multiple fractures, kidney stones, possibly death.

It formerly was thought that hyperparathyroidism was a rare condition, found among a few (1 to 5%) patients who passed multiple kidney stones, and also might rarely present in a patient with multiple fractures of the bones. It now appears that the condition is relatively common with the majority of patients having hardly any specific symptoms at all. This new point of view emerges from the wide-spread use of laboratory screening procedures like the SMA-12. We have had the complete history and physical examination as an ideal routine for many years. Now clinical medicine is moving toward the "complete" laboratory examination on a routine basis.

Another factor which has prompted the early recognition of many relatively asymptomatic cases is the appreciation that the most reliable laboratory manifestation is a consistent elevation of the serum calcium value. Patients so discovered may complain of fatigue or mild anorexia, and possibly polyuria; however, there must have been some reason for the patient to visit a doctor, so these symptoms are not helpful. An elevated serum parathyroid hormone level is of assistance, provided the specimen is drawn in the morning while the patient is in a fasting state. The serum calcium level must be unequivocably elevated, however. The parathyroid glands normally oversecrete in response to a low calcium level, and the serum calcium level has diurnal fluctuations. Both calcium concentration and parathyroid hormone level must be simultaneously high to suggest hyperparathyroidism.

In addition to these findings, it is confirmatory if the serum phosphorus is low, or if the urinary phosphate reabsorption is low, if a lump can be felt in the neck (or seen on barium swallow). It is helpful to the diagnosis if subperiosteal bone resorption is seen on x-ray films, especially of the hands and feet. But hyperparathyroidism is often present without these features, and the complete investigation may only be a form of procrastination. There have been cases where the diagnosis was quite unequivocal, but the academic endeavors have shaken the confidence of the surgeon who was called in consultation. Sometimes the right thing is done for the wrong reason; a fair number of patients with hyperparathyroidism have harmless thyroid nodules which precipitate the required surgery.

The diagnosis of hyperparathyroidism is on firm grounds when the serum parathyroid hormone level is elevated in the face of repeatedly high serum calcium values. This combination of findings eliminates a wide variety of other hypercalcemic states, all of which will demonstrate a low or absent serum parathyroid hormone level. At present, this determination is only available through sending the serum to a few commercial reference laboratories. This is only a minor inconvenience, however, and is probably even preferable to reliance upon local inexperienced laboratories.

However, the problems are not completely resolved even at that point, since all that is established is that too much parathyroid hormone is circulating.

It can be regarded as the surgeon's problem to decide whether one parathyroid adenoma is present or (in 3 to 5%) more than one. Or whether all four parathyroids are hyperplastic. Or whether the tumor is in the mediastinum. The internist must decide before surgery whether the parathyroid hormone is coming from the parathyroid glands at all. In an appreciable number of cases, the parathyroid polypeptide is being secreted by an occult malignancy. The common primary sites are lung, kidney and pancreas. Hard experience reveals that these malignancies may sometimes give no sign of their presence except hypercalcemia.

Only one test is available to the internist, and that is to wait. The delay of six months before surgery in an asymptomatic case will avoid many problems.

References

Aurbach, G. D.: Hyperparathyroidism: Recent studies. Ann. Intern. Med., *79*:566, 1973.
Ballard, H. S.. Frame, B., and Hartsock, R. J.: Familial multiple endocrine adenoma—peptic ulcer complex. Medicine, *43*:481, 1964.
Canterbury, J. M., and Reiss, E.: Multiple immunoreactive molecular forms of parathyroid hormone in human serum. Proc. Soc. Exper. Biol. and Med., *140*:1393, 1972.
Cutler, R. E., Reiss, E., and Ackerman, L. V.: Familial hyperparathyroidism. New Eng. J. Med., *270*:859, 1964.
Koppel, M. H., et al.: Thiazide induced rise in serum calcium and magnesium in patients on maintainence hemodialysis. Ann. Intern. Med., *72*:895, 1970.
Parfitt, A. M.: Chlorothiazide induced hypercalcemia in juvenile osteoporosis and hyperparathyroidism. New Eng. J. Med., *281*:55, 1969.
Steiner, A. L., Goodman, A. D., and Powers, S. R.: Study of a kindred with pheochromocytome, medullary thyroid carcinoma, hyperparathyroidism and Cushing's Disease, multiple endocrine neoplasia-type 2. Medicine, *47*:371, 1968.
Strott, C. A., and Nugent, C. A.: Laboratory tests in the diagnosis of hyperparathyroidism and hypercalemic states. Ann. Intern. Med., *68*:188, 1968.
Wills, M. R., et al.: Normocalcemic primary hyperparathyroidism. Am. J. Med., *47*:384, 1969.

8. Normocalcemic Bone Disease (Osteoporosis)

George Ross Fisher, III, Joseph H. Magee and Laurence G. Wesson, Jr.

Causes: Unstimulated anabolism due to decreased gonadal steroids and/or decreased postural stress. Antianabolism due to increased endogenous or exogenous glucocorticoids. Prolonged decreased calcium intake.

Result: Unbalanced bone-to-blood calcium transfers, usually not reflected in clinical measurements, with decreased bone mass.

Early Manifestations: Bone pain, rarefaction, kyphosis.

Treatment: Early ambulation. Withdraw glucocorticoid therapy of articular disorders. Increase dietary calcium and vitamin D. If reasonable, supply deficient sex hormones. Encourage ambulation.

Possible Dire Consequences without Treatment: Vertebral compression fractures with paraplegia.

References

Nordin, E. E. C.: Osteoporosis and calcium deficiency, p. 46. In Bone As A Tissue: Proceedings Of A Conference, October 30–31, 1958. Rodahl, K., Nicholson, J. T., and Brown, E. M., Jr. (eds.). New York, McGraw, Blakiston Division, 1960.

Rabinowitz, D. and Bledsoe, T.: Metabolic bone disease. p. 949, Chapter 85 in The Principles and Practice of Medicine. Harvey, A. M., Johns, R. J., Owens, A. H., Jr. and Ross, R. S. (eds.). New York, Appleton-Century-Crofts, 1972.

9. Normocalcemic Bone Disease (Renal Phosphaturia)

George Ross Fisher, III and Joseph H. Magee

Cause: Defective renal tubular reabsorption of phosphate, heritable as an x-linked dominant trait.

Phosphoglucoaminoaciduria (Fanconi syndrome without tubular acidosis), of diverse etiology.

Synonyms: Phosphate diabetes, phosphate-losing rickets, familial hypophosphatemic vitamin D resistant rickets, hypophosphatemic vitamin D resistant osteomalacia (adults).

Glucosuric rickets, phosphoglucoamine diabetes.

Results: Primary hypophosphatemia with decreased blood-to-bone calcium transfers, with normal bone mass, and with defective osseous mineralization during growth (rickets) and/or after (osteomalacia).

Early Manifestations: Low [P]s with or without bone disease.

Slightly shortened stature and inactive postrachitic deformities in asymptomatic adults.

Raised [alk-ptase]s in adults with deformities and active osteomalacia.

Low [Ca]s associated with active rickets.

Glucosuria and glycinuria may occur in the x-linked syndrome but generalized aminoaciduria does not.

Renal function usually is unimpaired in the x-linked syndrome but microscopic nephrocalcinosis may follow vitamin D therapy.

Ca absorption by the gut is impaired, responding to phosphate repletion plus normal amounts of vitamin D, or to large doses of vitamin D alone.

Treatment: Phosphate repletion: Oral neutral phosphate solution (to 1 quart water add 1 teaspoon each of monosodium and disodium phosphate plus another 2 tablespoons disodium phosphate), up to 150 ml./day in divided doses.

Usual doses of vitamin D: 2000 to 4000 units (1 mg. = 40,000 units) of ergo calciferol or cholecalciferol (vitamin D_2 or D_3), the former being less expensive.

Usual doses of dihydrotachysterol (AT10) (Hytakerol) (125 μg. = 15,000 units).

Large doses of vitamin D, 10 to 100 fold greater than in dietary rickets may be necessary, especially if phosphate is not supplemented, beginning with 20,000 units/day and increasing monthly with careful observation for hypervitaminosis D; 3+ or 4+ urine Sulkowitch urine test* suggests a [Ca]s of 10.5 mg./100 ml. which should be verified.

Possible Dire Consequences without Treatment: Deformities, short stature.

---

* 5 ml. reagent is added to 5 ml. urine in a test tube and the precipitate graded 1+ to 4+. The reagent is:

Oxalic acid	2.5 gm.
Ammonium oxalate	2.5 gm.
Glacial acetic acid	5.0 gm.
Distilled water q.s. ad.	150 ml

References

Chisholm, J. J., et al.: Aminoaciduria, hypophosphatemia, and rickets in lead poisoning. Am. J. Dis. Child., *89*:159, 1955.

Cogan, D. G., Kuwabara, T., and Hurlburt, C. S., Jr.: Further observations on cystinosis in the adult. J.A.M.A., *160*:1725, 1958.

Costell, D. O., and Sparks, H. A.: Nephrogenic diabetes insipidus due to demethyl tetracycline hydrochloride. J.A.M.A., *193*:237, 1965.

Czerwinsky, A. W., and Ginn, H. E.: Bismuth nephrotoxicity. Am. J. Med., *37*:969, 1964.

Dawson, J., et al.: Evidence for presence of amphoteric electrolyte in urine of patients with "renal tubular acidosis." Metabolism, *2*:225, 1953.

Engle, R. L., Jr., and Wallis, L. A.: Multiple myeloma and the adult Fanconi syndrome. Am. J. Med., *22*:5, 1957.

Follis, R. H., Jr., et al.: Prevalence of rickets in children between 2 and 14 years of age. Am. J. Dis. Child., *66*:1, 1943.

Frimpter, G. W., et al.: Reversible Fanconi syndrome caused by degraded tetracycline. J.A.M.A., *185*:111, 1963.

Halvorson, S., Pande, H., and Rohem, A. C.: Tyrosinosis. Arch. Dis. Child., *41*:328, 1966.

Jonxis, J. H. P., Smith, P. A., and Huisman, T. J. H.: Rickets and aminoaciduria. Lancet, *2*:1015, 1952.

Juilliard, E., and Piguet, C.: Glucosuria and aminoaciduria familiale. Ann. Paed., *183*:247, 1954.

Morris, R. C., Jr.: The clinical spectrum of Fanconi syndrome. California Med., *108*:225, 1968.

Myerson, R. M., and Pastor, B. H.: Fanconi syndrome and its clinical variants. Am. J. Med. Sci., *228*:378, 1954.

Nicaud, P., et al.: Les lesions osseuses de l'intoxication chronique par le cadmium. Bull. et Mem Soc. Med. Hop. Paris, *19*:204, 1942.

Rampini, S., et al.: Effect of hydrochlorothiazide on proximal tubular acidosis in a patient with idiopathic "DeToni-Debre-Fanconi Syndrome." Helvet. Ped. Acta, *23*:13, 1968.

Spencer, A. G., and Franglen, G. T.: Gross aminoaciduria following a lysol burn. Lancet, *1*:190, 1952.

Stowers, J. M., and Dent, C. E.: Studies on the mechanism of the Fanconi syndrome. Quart. J. Med., *16*:275, 1947.

Uzman, L., and Denny-Brown, D.: Aminoaciduria in hepatolenticular degeneration. Am. J. Med. Sci., *215*:599, 1948.

Wallis, L. A., and Engle, R. L., Jr.: The adult Fanconi syndrome. Am. J. Med., *22*:13, 1957.

Wilson, D. R., et al.: Studies in hypophosphatemic vitamin D refractory osteomalacia in adults. Medicine, *44*:99, 1965.

Winters, R. W., et al.: A genetic study of familial hypophosphatemia and vitamin D resistant rickets. Medicine, *37*:97, 1958.

10. Normocalcemic Bone Disease (Combined Defects)

GEORGE ROSS FISHER, III AND JOSEPH H. MAGEE

Causes: Phosphaglucoamino aciduria accompanying heritable or acquired tubular acidosis.

Renal Inborn Errors

(*a.*) Recessive Inheritance. (Fanconi 1931, DeToni 1933, Debre 1934, Milkman 1934, Stowers and Dent 1947, DeToni 1956).

(*b.*) Atypical phenotype of genotype heretofore presenting as heritable tubular acidosis in probands.

(*c.*) X-linked recessive inheritance. (Lowe 1952).

(*d.*) Dominant inheritance. (Luder and Sheldon 1955).

Non-Renal Inborn Errors.

(*a.*) Cystinosis. (Aberhalden 1903, Lignae 1924, Fanconi 1936).

(*b.*) Wilson's Disease. (Von Gierke 1929, Fanconi 1949).

(*c.*) Cori Type I Glycogenosis. (Wilson 1912, Cooper 1950).

(*d.*) Tyrosinosis. (Zetterstrom 1963).

Endogenous Agents.

(*a.*) Soluble proteins: Transplant rejection, neoplasia.

(*b.*) Circulating proteins: Amyloidosis, Sjögren's syndrome.

(*c.*) Filtrable proteins: Harrison-Blainey syndrome.

(*d.*) Filtrable proteins; Myelomatosis.

(*e*). Unselective proteinuria; Amyloidosis.

(*f.*) Variably Selective Proteinuria: Classic Nephrotic Syndrome.

Exogenous Agents.

(*a.*) Heterocyclic: Old tetracycline, 6-mercaptopurine.

(*b.*) Aromatic: Phenols, diacromone.

(*c.*) Metallic; Cd, Hg, Pb, Ur.

Deficiency States

(*a.*) Vitamin C lack.

(*b.*) Vitamin D lack (dietary or malabsorption rickets).

(*c.*) Vitamin D resistance (azotemic rickets).

Result: Defective high capacity, low gradient (proximal) renal cortical hydrion secretion ("rate defect").

Massive episodic bicarbonate wasting.

Increased urine mineral cation excretion.

Secondary parathormonism and aldosteronism, and non-osmotic vasopressinism.

Increased bone-to-blood calcium and sodium transfers, with maintained but demineralized bone mass, due to parathormonism, and to intrinsic tubular phosphate reabsorptive defect.

Increased bone-to-bone calcium transfers due to acidemia.

Early Manifestations: Low [P]s with or without bone disease.

Renal glycosuria with negative blood studies for pancreatic diabetes.

Raised [alk ptase]s due to active osteomalacia with or without skeletal deformities.

Low [HCO_3]s and blood pH with urine pH usually 7.0.

Azotemia (preventable) follows nephrocalcinosis and/or lithiasis in patients with bicarbonaturia or other forms of microcrystalline deposition when secondary to non-renal inborn errors.

Treatment: 48 mM (4 gm.) (1 tsp) sodium bicarbonate t.i.d. or
45 mM (45 ml) 10% sodium citrate t.i.d., or
45 mM (45 ml) Shohl's solution* t.i.d., or
45 mM (45 ml) Harrison's solution† t.i.d.
These doses are much larger than needed in the distal variety of tubular acidosis (Butler-Albright syndrome).
Oral neutral phosphate solution‡ up to 150 ml./day in divided doses.
Vitamin D in large doses may ameliorate aminoaciduria and tubular acidosis as well.

Possible Dire Consequences without Treatment: Oligemic circulatory failure. Rickets, late rickets or osteomalacia. Nephrocalcinosis.

References

See references for Chapter XII, #9.

* Citric acid monohydrate 140 gm. and trisodium citrate dihydrate 98 gm./l.

† Citric acid monohydrate 70 gm., trisodium citrate dihydrate 98 gm. and tripotassium citrate monohydrate 108 gm./l. in non-alcoholic fruit-flavored syrup base.

‡ To 1 quart water add 1 teaspoon each of monosodium and disodium phosphate plus another 2 tablespoons disodium phosphate.

11. Normocalcemic Bone Disease (from Tubular Acidosis)

George Ross Fisher, III and Joseph H. Magee

Cause: Tubular Acidosis Syndromes.

Defective high capacity, low gradient (proximal) renal cortical hydrion secretion ("rate defect"), with episodic sodium bicarbonate wasting, usually in conjunction with Fanconi syndromes in older children and adults.

Defective low capacity, high gradient (distal) renal hydrion secretion ("gradient defect") with constant decreased weak acid and ammonium salt and increased mineral salt excretion, in the Butler-Albright syndrome.

Result: Increased bone-to-blood calcium transfers, with maintained but demineralized bone mass, due to parathormonism.

Increased bone-to-blood calcium and sodium transfers due to acidemia.

Aldosteronism due to renal sodium salt loss.

Phosphaturia and kaliuria despite low serum levels.

Metabolic bone disease.

Early Manifestations: Metabolic bone disease.

(*a.*) Raised [alk. ptase]s.

(*b.*) Normal or even raised [Ca]s unlike deficiency and azotemia rickets.

(*c.*) Bone pain, rarefaction, and pathologic fractures with normal [Ca]s.

(*d.*) Normal or low [P]s prior to azotemia.

Azotemia (preventable) follows nephrocalcinosis and/or lithiasis in Butler-Albright syndrome, is relentless in instances of Fanconi syndrome due to non-renal inborn erros such as cystinosis, remediable in others, such as Wilson's disease.

Hyperchloremic acidosis.

(*a.*) Blood: Low blood pH and [HCO_3]s with reciprocally raised [Cl]s prior to azotemia.

(*b.*) Urine: Inappropriate alkaluria with urine pH minimum 5.5 at low blood pH or at 8 hours after ammonium chloride loading (0.5 gm./kg.) in Butler-Albright syndrome.

(*c.*) Urine: Inappropriate alkaluria with urine pH seldom below 6.0–7.1 at [HCO_3]s 18–22 mM/l. in Fanconi syndromes. With profounder systemic acidosis and no bicarbonaturia, weak acid excretion and titration of urine to normal minima may occur.

(*d.*) Hyperpnea, anorexia, intermittent nausea and/or vomiting.

Sodium-wasting syndrome:

(*a.*) Low arterial and venous pressure.

(*b.*) Pre-renal azotemia.

(*c.*) Anorexia, vomiting, weight loss.

(*d.*) Raised aldosterone secretion and excretion.

(*e.*) Raised plasma renin activity and concentration.

Low [K]s with periodic paralyses, ileus, or cardiac arrhythmias.

Other urinary abnormalities in proximal tubular syndromes.

(*a.*) Glucoaminophosphaturia (Fanconi triad).

(*b.*) Uricosuria.

(*c.*) Lysozymuria and raised excretion of low molecular weight globulins with or without albuminuria.

Age of onset of Butler-Albright syndrome is from two years to middle age with females predominating 2:1 and history of occurrence in previous generations frequently obtainable.

Age of onset of Fanconi syndrome may be earlier where due to non-renal inborn errors such as cystinosis apparent at around four months and with death by ten years. In acquired errors such as myeloma or amyloid, may present in adulthood.

Treatment: 12 mM (1g.) sodium bicarbonate t.i.d., or 15 mM (15 ml.) 10% sodium citrate t.i.d., or 15 mM (15 ml.) Shohl's solution t.i.d., or 15 mM (15 ml.) Harrison's solution t.i.d.

In the proximal variety of acidosis, associated in whole or in part with the Fanconi triad, threefold these amounts may be required. Urine pH in these cases may fall below the 5.5 that is the minimum attainable in the Butler-Albright syndrome. The objective of therapy is a urine pH 7.0; use of Shohl's or Harrison's solution results in a doubled excretion of citrate which is advantageous in solubilizing cystine and uric acid particularly in certain etiologic varieties of the Fanconi syndrome. Aminoaciduria is generalized with amounts of cystine that are on the whole modest, but marked uricosuria may occur in Wilson's disease and in the renal inborn error in the families that Ben-Ishay and colleagues reported. Edathamil calcium (EDTA) treatment of Pb intoxication.
Penicillamine treatment of Wilson's disease.
Treatment of dysproteinemias.

Possible Dire Consequences without Treatment: Oligemic circulatory failure. Growth failure. Periodic paralysis. Nephrocalcinosis.

Reference

Rabinowitz, D. and Bledsoe, T.: Metabolic bone disease. p. 949, Chapter 85 in The Principles and Practice of Medicine. Harvey, A. M., Johns, R. J., Owens, A. H., Jr. and Ross, R. S. (eds.). New York, Appleton-Century-Crofts, 1972.

12. Hypocalcemic Bone Disease

George Ross Fisher, III and Joseph H. Magee

Cause: Calcitoninism,
- (*a.*) Medullary carcinoma of thyroid.
- (*b.*) Multiple endocrine neoplasia syndrome #2 (MENS–2); Parathyroid adenoma and/or pheochromocytoma in associating with medullary carcinoma of the thyroid.

Hypocalcemia due to calcitonin mediated decrease in osteoclastic activity.
Secondary parathormonism.

Early Manifestations: Asymptomatic members of the family of proven cases of medullary carcinoma should have periodic assays of serum calcitonin, and total thyroidectomy if the test is positive. Normal bones and normal serum calcium values should be ignored if the calcitonin level is elevated.

Late Manifestations: Low [Ca]s; tetany, if not sufficiently compensated by parathormonism.
Detectable osteosclerosis seldom occurs.
Thyroid enlargement, regional lymph node enlargement.
Hoarseness.
History of neck surgery in kindred.
Onset after fifty, earlier in familial aggregates.
Manifestations of pheochromocytoma may be present.

Treatment: Surgery, including parathyroid exploration.

Possible Dire Consequences without Treatment: Hypocalcemic tetany, laryngeal spasm, convulsions, death from metastases.

References

Aliaponlos, M. A., and Munson, P. L.: Thyrocalcitonin. Surg. Forum, *16*:55, 1965.
Hirsch, P. F., and Munson, P. L.: Thyrocalcitonin. Physiol. Rev., *49*:548, 1969.
Pechet, M. M.: Symposium on thyrocalcitonin. Am. J. Med., *43*:645, 1967.
Sipple, J. H.: The association of pheochromocytoma with carcinoma of the thyroid gland. Am. J. Med., *31*:163, 1961.
Williams, E. D.: A review of 17 cases of carcinoma of the thyroid and pheochromocytoma. J. Clin. Path., *18*:288, 1965.

13. Parathormone Resistance

George Ross Fisher, III and Joseph H. Magee

Cause: Inherited Disorder (x-linked dominant).

Early Manifestations: Dyschondroplasia (rounded face, short stature, short metacarpals and metatarsals) with or without mental deficiency and resistance to parathormone. Endorgan unresponsiveness to parathormone due to dysplasia of ectodermal tissues including bone.

Low [Ca]s and raised [P]s with normal [alk ptase]s despite compensatory parathyroid hyperplasia.

Ectopic calcification of soft tissues including basal ganglia, lenses, cornea, and conjunctivae.

Overt tetany.

Latent tetany.

Alopecia.

Predilection to severe moniliasis.

Treatment: Vitamin D 50,000 μ/day.

Possible Dire Consequences without Treatment: Cataracts.

References

Albright, F., Forbes, A. P., and Henneman, P. H.: Dyschondroplasia with soft tissue calcification and ossification, and normal parathyroid function (pseudopseudohypoparathyroidism). Tr. Am. Assn. Phys., *65*:357, 1956.

Chase, L. R., Melson, G. L., and Aurbach, G. .D: Pseudohypoparathyroidism: Defective excretion of 3'5' AMP in response to parathyroid hormone. J. Clin. Invest., *48*:1832, 1969.

14. Parathormone Lack

GEORGE ROSS FISHER, III AND JOSEPH H. MAGEE

Cause: Surgical removal. Post-surgical atrophy. Idiopathic atrophy.

Early Manifestations: Low [Ca]s and raised [P]s with normal [alk ptase]s.
Overt tetany.
Latent tetany.
   (*a.*) Observe breathing; laryngeal stridor is characteristic even in patients who are breathing noisily due to other disturbances.
   (*b.*) Tap or press motor nerves over bony places. If patient can cooperate, ask to hyperventilate, and repeat.
   (*c.*) For facial nerve irritability, watch muscles of expression, not mastication, especially corners of mouth; patient may "fishmouth."
   (*d.*) For brachial nerve, enough manual compression of brachial artery against humerus to shut off pulse is better than inflating a blood pressure cuff.
   (*e.*) For plantar nerves, try simple stimulation (jerking the sheets back) fast; or tap just lateral to patella, rather than inferiorly over its tendon.
Tetany may be confused with epilepsy in children and electroencephalograph abnormalities may be present.
Electrocardiographic interval from Q wave to origin of T is prolonged (QoT). It is corrected to rate 60 by dividing QoT by $\sqrt{RR}$, obtaining Qotc. Mean value in hypoparathyroidism is 0.32 (0.16–0.40) compared to 0.24 (0.16–0.29) in normals.
Chronic weakness in adults.
History of neck surgery.
Dense bones and poor dentition in children.
Cutaneous moniliasis.
Alopecia.
Surprisingly asymptomatic adjustment can be made to chronic state.

Treatment: 2000 to 4000 units (1 mg. = 40,000 units) ergocalciferol or cholecalciferol (vitamin D_2 or D_3)/day. Some patients respond better to dihydrotachysterol (AT10) (Hytakerol).
Prophylaxis of tetany: 30% oral calcium chloride solution, 10 ml. diluted 3 times/daily.
Treatment of tetany: 0.2% oral calcium chloride 55 ml. by drip over one hour.

Possible Dire Consequences without Treatment: Confusion with epilepsy. Laryngeal spasm. Cataracts.

References

Bronsky, D., Kushner, D. S., Dubin, A., and Snapper, I.: Idiopathic hypoparathyroidism and pseudohypoparathyroidism. Medicine, *37*:317, 1958.
Litvak, J., et al.: Hypocalcemic hypercalciuria during vitamin D and dihydrotachysterol therapy of hypoparathyroidism. J. Clin. End. Metab., *18*:246, 1958.

15. Renal Rickets

George Ross Fisher, III and Joseph H. Magee

Cause: Renal disease. Defective renal 1-hydroxylation of 25-hydroxycholecalciferol. Defective intestinal absorption of calcium. Hypocalcemia. Defective osseous mineralization (osteomalacia). Secondary parathormonism. Osteitis fibrosa.

Synonym: Azotemic Renal Osteodystrophy.

Early Manifestations: Low [Ca]s and raised [P]s and [alkaline phosphatase]s. Bone and articular pain.

Treatment: 0.5 to 2.0 mg. (20,000 to 80,000 units) ergocalciferol (vitamin D_2) or cholecalciferol (vitamin D_3)/ day.
Raised [alkaline phosphatase]s indicates inadequate dosage.
Raised [Ca]s, anorexia, lassitude, thirst, and worsening azotemia indicate excess dosage.
Wrist and knee x-ray films are used to observe increase in stature of children.

Possible Dire Consequences without Treatment: Tertiary Parathormonism.

References

Albright, F., Drake, T. G., and Sulkowitch, H. W.: Renal osteitis fibrosa cystica. Bull. J. Hopkins Hosp., *60*:377, 1937.
Albright, F., Sulkowitch, H. W., and Bloomberg, E.: A comparison of the effects of vitamin D, dihydrotachysterol (A.T. 10) and parathyroid extract on the disordered metabolism of rickets. J. Clin. Invest., *18*:165, 1939.
Brickman, A. S., Coburn, J. W., and Norman, A. W.: Action of 1,25 dihydroxycholecalciferol, a potent, kidney-produced metabolite of vitamin D, in mnemic man. New Eng. J. Med., *287*:891, 1972.
Curtis, J. R., et al.: Maintenance hemodialysis. Quart. J. Med., *38*:49, 1969.
Dent, C. E., Harper, C. M., and Philpott, G. R.: The treatment of renal-glomerular osteodystrophy. Quart. J. Med., *30*:1, 1961.
Dudley, F. J., and Blackburn, C. R. B.: Extraskeletal calcification complicating oral neutral phosphate therapy. Lancet, 2:628, 1970.
Jaffe, H. L., Bodansky, A., and Chandler, J. P.: Ammonium chloride decalcification as modified by calcium intake. J. Exp. Med., *56*:823, 1932.
Katz, A. I., Hampers, C. L., and Merrill, J. P.: Secondary hyperparathyroidism and renal osteodystrophy in chronic renal failure. Medicine, 48:333, 1969.
Kaye, M., et al.: Bone disease in renal failure with particular reference to osteosclerosis. Medicine, *39*:157, 1960.
Liu, S. H., and Chu, H. I.: Studies of calcium and phosphorus metabolism with special reference to pathogenesis and effect of dehydrotachysterol (AT 10) and iron. Medicine, *22*:103, 1943.
Mack, R. S., and Rutishauser, E.: Les osteodystrophies renales. Helvet Med. Acta, *4*:423, 1937.
Stanbury, S. W., and Lumb, G. A.: Metabolic studies of renal osteodystrophy. Medicine, *41*:1, 1962.
Townsend, C. M., Jr., Remmers, A. F., Jr., and Sarles, H. E.: Intestinal obstruction from medication begun in patients with renal failure. New Eng. J. Med., *288*:1058, 1973.

16. Dietary Rickets

Geoge Ross Fisher, III and Joseph H. Magee

Cause: Vitamin D deficiency.
  (*a.*) Inadequate photochemical conversion of skin 7-dehydrocholesterol to chole-calciferol (vitamin D_2) due to insufficient exposure to sunlight or
  (*b.*) Insufficient solubilization of irradiated ergosterol (vitamin D_2) or 7-dehydro-cholesterol (vitamin D_3) by bile acids in biliary steatorrhea, or
  (*c.*) Inadequate absorption of solubilized vitamin D_2 or D_3 in intestinal steatorrhea, or
  (*d.*) Inadequate vitamin D_2 or D_3 in diet.
  The minimal adult requirement for vitamin D is ordinarily well supplied by exposure of the skin to the sun, and therefore, no dietary vitamin D is required by adults.
  Decreased intestinal absorption of calcium.
  Secondary parathormonism due to low [Ca]s.
  Raised [alk ptase]s and phosphaturia.
  Bone remodelling with decreased mineralization of increasing bone mass.

Early Manifestations: Skeletal deformities prior to epiphyseal closure. Persistent generalized skeletal pain after epiphyseal closure. Widened osteoid seams on radiography or bone biopsy. Delayed dentition. Muscular hypotonia.

Treatment: 2,000 to 4,000 units (1 mg. = 40,000 units) ergocalciferol or cholecalciferol (vitamin D_2 or D_3)/day $\times$ six to twelve weeks.
  Prophylaxis of tetany: 30% oral calcium chloride solution, 10 ml. diluted 3 times/day.
  Treatment of tetany: 0.2% intravenous calcium chloride solution, 55 ml. by drip over one hour.

Possible Dire Consequences without Treatment: Hypocalcemic tetany, laryngeal spasm, convulsions, death.
  Dystrophic rickets, general growth impairment, anemia, weight loss, pathologic fractures.

References

Jonxis, J. H.: Aminoaciduria and rickets. Helvet. Ped. Acta, *10*:245, 1955.
Loomis, W. F.: Skin pigment regulation of vitamin D biosynthesis in man. Science, *157*:3788, 1967.

Disorders of Thyroid Function

Like carriage lamps and bed warmers, the BMR machine is largely an antique. There do remain a few situations where it can be useful, but as a practical matter the test is now unobtainable. The prevailing thyroid tests are the chemical determination of serum thyroxin content, either bound to protein (serum T-4), or unbound (free T-4). It can generally be assumed that the bound and unbound fractions exist in fixed ratio, and at the moment it is considerably cheaper to determine the bound portion than the unbound. For a time, it was cheaper to determine the bound thyroxin by column separation (T-4 by column) than to determine it directly by immunoassay after the method of Murphy and Pattee. But, at present, the Murphy-Pattee method of competitive binding assay is automated, accurate, and cheap. Until such time as the determination of free thyroxin becomes equally cheap and accurate, the Murphy-Pattee type of test for bound T-4 is the test of choice in thyroid disorders.

And until such time as the free thyroxin determination becomes more practical, it will generally be better to use ancillary tests in situations where the bound T-4 determination is ambiguous or undependable. Such ancillary tests would be the radioactive iodine uptake by the gland, the protein-bound iodine, the butanol-extractable protein bound iodine, and the tri-iodo-thyronine saturable serum residual (T-3 uptake).

All of these tests have their problems, and none of them is as useful alone as when determined in parallel with the serum T-4 (bound). The T-3 uptake of serum is particularly prone to inaccuracy, often causing patients to be referred to consultants. On the other hand, the routine parallel determination of T-4 and T-3 (as the jargon goes) does usually prevent the unwary from being trapped by the commonest diagnostic error: the nervous woman who is taking birth control pills. Such a woman will have an elevated protein-bound iodine level because the protein is increased by estrogens, and a somewhat less but still elevated T-4 level. Taking the T-4 and T-3 levels together in a calculation misleadingly called the T-7 calculation, the outcome in the face of estrogens will usually be normal, if the thyroid function is normal. The same situation is present in the pregnant woman to an exaggerated degree, and in this latter instance it may be better to go to the expense of free T-4 determination. The T-3 uptake test is rather gross, and there is a certain error inherent in multiplying an inaccurate test by an accurate one, since the error of the result is dependent on the least accurate ingredient of the equation. A nervous woman taking estrogens can usually be safely observed for several weeks while she takes tranquilizers, whereas the presence of pregnancy can force the physician into drastic and inappropriate overreaction.

The T-3 test was first offered as a means of unravelling the thyroid situation in a person who had recently had a cholecystogram or intravenous urogram, or who otherwise had elevated serum iodine levels because of iodine ingestion. The measurement of thyroxin by competitive protein binding, however, is not usually affected by such artifacts; and the problem is avoided by using the newer test routinely. The butanol-extractable protein-bound iodine determination (BEI) was also employed as a way of correcting the protein-bound iodine level (PBI) in the face of iodine contamination. Like the BMR, these two tests are rapidly passing from the scene.

The considerable prevalence of acute and chronic thyroiditis presents a different set of problems. Formerly a rarity, thyroiditis is now more common then thyrotoxicosis. Patients pass through stages of thyrotoxicity (as the stored hormone is suddenly released) into a stage of hypothyroidism. Therefore, the serum T-4 level can be high, low, or normal; and repeat tests will often be in conflict. However, the radioactive iodine uptake by the inflamed gland is usually low in all stages. The disorganized storage products are released into the circulation, and a high protein-bound iodine level will often be found in conjunction with a normal or low serum T-4. Far from being an artifact, this discrepancy can have considerable diagnostic value, since it represents a demonstration that abnormal, non-thyroxin, iodinated elements are bound to serum protein. It will probably only be a matter of time before the PBI determination becomes unavailable, however; and the low radioactive iodine uptake of the gland will be the diagnostic identification of thyroiditis. The patients with Hashimoto's thyroiditis will often have elevated levels of antithyroglobulin antibody, it is true. Unfortunately, this determination appears to have so many technical pitfalls that it can be misleading. It should be kept in mind that a high serum T-4 with a low uptake by the gland is a combination also seen in malingering patients who secretly take excessive doses of thyroxin.

We are thus led to a consideration of tests which may monitor treatment of recognized thyroid disorders. Consider that the diagnosis is firm and secure: how, then, may we decide that the dosage of thyroxin or antithyroid drug is too much, too little, or just right? The question is so common and so natural that it is difficult to accept the answer that no modern test has completely filled the role formerly held by the Basal Metabolism Test, although the serum T-4 test in combination with T-3 will cover most situations. Intuition, experience and common sense still have a role in interpreting thyroid test results.

After all, thyroid disorders are not contagious and generally not fatal unless they are extreme. Therefore, if the patient says he feels well, it is fair to say his thyroid function is good enough for him. The problem does remain in the few people who continue to complain of symptoms in the face of standard doses and reasonably normal physical examination. In such a situation, the doctor is not facing a need to monitor dosage, but rather he had a second diagnostic problem. Is this a neurotic chronic complainer? Is this a patient with chronic hyperhidrosis, or a dry skin for dermatologic reasons? Does he have some cardiac cause of bradycardia or tachycardia? Was the thyroid diagnosis wrong in the first place? Does he fail to take his medication, or does he take too many?

Probably the easiest way to determine whether the hypothyroid patient is taking roughly enough thyroxin is to see whether his pituitary gland has been suppressed by it. This can be determined directly by measuring serum TSH levels (they should be low) or indirectly by performing a radioactive iodine uptake of the gland (the result should also be low). If the results are consistent with the average response to an average dosage, the dosage can only be normal or too high. It can be lowered if this seems necessary, and the test repeated. But by far the better management is to be familiar with the average dose of a reliable preparation, and make a clinical titration within a moderate range of variation from the average dose.

The management of thyrotoxicosis, on the other hand, depends on familiarity with the (sluggish) response to antithyroid drugs. Doctor Frank Leahy coined the useful maxim that the BMR falls about 1% per day. So, while we do not generally have the BMR test available, it is reasonable to expect the average case of thyrotoxicosis to be in reasonable control in two or three months, and approaching myxedema in three or four months. Some physicians will reduce the dosage of antithyroid drug at about that time (particularly if the T-4 level is normalized), but there is a simpler way. It is far easier to continue the full dose of antithyroid drug, while adding an average dose of tri-iodo-thyronine (25 to 50 mcg. per day). This combination may confuse the druggist, but it simultaneously maintains complete suppression of the thyroid gland and also holds the metabolic rate in normal range.

If the patient is going to have surgery or radioiodine therapy, he is ready for it at the time that his symptoms are controlled. But if there is the intent of managing the thyrotoxicity with drugs until the disease goes into remission, there is the problem of deciding when the remission has taken place. It generally requires about a year of therapy to achieve remission, and the goiter usually shrinks at the time of remission. At this point of decision, advantage can be taken of the paradoxical fact that the serum T-4 is lowered by tri-iodo-thyronine therapy, but only if the thyrotoxicosis has gone into remission. That is, the toxic gland is non-suppressible. Therefore, when anti-thyroid therapy is reduced or stopped (but tri-iodo-thyronine continued) the serum T-4 will rise if the gland is still overactive, but the serum T-4 will remain low if the gland has returned to normal. Occasionally, it is useful to employ this suppression test as a diagnostic maneuver to make the diagnosis of thyrotoxicosis in the first place.

Another situation calls for employing the same physiological principle. Many patients have been taking thyroid preparations for such a long time that their history becomes cloudy. Naturally, one can periodically stop the thyroid medication and see if myxedema recurs. However, myxedema is a bitterly uncomfortable condition, and patients rightfully resent its capricious re-establishment. Therefore, it is much better to substitute tri-iodo-thyronine therapy for several weeks until the serum T-4 is quite low. If tri-iodo-thyronine is then discontinued, the T-4 level will rise in two weeks in normal patients, or the radioactive iodine uptake will return to normal. Since thyroxin takes six weeks to disappear while tri-iodo-thyronine takes ten days, the period of discomfort is much less. Or, an even neater maneuver is to give the patient TSH or TSH-stimulating hormone, and test the serum T-4 or radioiodine uptake without discontinuing the tri-iodo-thyronine therapy at all. Once you are satisfied that the patient really has an active thyroid gland, the proper dose is a matter of comfort and preference, rather than tests.

The drug manufacturers have tried to adjust their products to the clinical testing environment. Tri-iodo-thyronine medication lowers the serum T-4, pure thyroxin therapy elevates the level disproportionately. Some thyroid extracts contain disproportionate ratios of the two. Therefore, "physiological" mixtures of pure hormones are advanced as a means of permitting the monitoring of doses by serum T-4 determinations. It remains to be proven that the cost of such preparations can be reduced to equal whole desiccated thyroid which has been the standard drug for fifty years.

Two other diagnostic traps remain. An occasional patient produces excessive tri-iodo-thyronine without comparable amounts of thyroxine—a condition called "T-3-toxicosis." It may be that every case of thyrotoxicosis begins in this form. Therefore, the measurement of free serum T-3 in suspicious cases may reveal thyrotoxicosis even though the serum T-4 is normal. It must be emphasized that the free T-3 determination is entirely different from the "T-3 uptake" more commonly available. The free T-3 test is still quite expensive.

The other point is that myxedema may be caused by pituitary or hypothalamic failure, and thus be secondary or tertiary hypothyroidism. A skull roentgenogram, including the sella turcica, is mandatory in every case of myxedema. It becomes a matter of judgment and expense to decide whether to test the response to TSH and TRF in a myxedematous patient with a normal sella turcica. It surely is a good idea, although the possibility of discovering a remediable condition is fairly small.

17. Apathetic Thyrotoxicosis and Related Atypical Forms of the Disease

George Ross Fisher, III

Cause: Unknown

Early Manifestations: Tachycardia. Enlarged thyroid ("goiter"). Venous Hum.

Treatment: Antithyroid drugs. Radioiodotherapy in post-reproductive individuals.

Possible Dire Consequences without Treatment: Congestive heart failure. Inanition.

Apathetic thyrotoxicosis is a term which is both useful and deceptive. It is useful because it reminds the clinician that not every thyrotoxic patient is a nervous sweaty young woman. But it is deceptive to the degree that it might suggest that there are thyrotoxic patients whose complaint is apathy, or who are totally lacking in any features of thyrotoxicosis.

For the most part, diagnostic problems arise from the fact that most thyrotoxic patients are young women who bring their complaints to the doctor in a reasonably early stage. Since their complaint is usually nervousness, we tend to assume that elderly patients will complain of the same thing. In fact, the arteriosclerotic patient will often develop congestive heart failure as a presenting complaint. The situation is further complicated by the kyphosis of old age, which tends to drop the larynx to the level of the manubrial notch, and thus the goiter into the chest cavity. Without goiter, exophthalmos or nervousness to alert the doctor, management can easily be diverted to a conventional treatment of heart failure.

Young patients are not totally immune to atypical thyrotoxic presentation. Occasionally, the outstanding feature is muscle wasting, and a presumptive diagnosis may be carcinomatosis. It may be hard to interpret muscle tremor, since the muscular atrophy leads to gross tremor rather than fine tremor, and in the extreme situation there may be no tremor at all. Perhaps the easiest way to understand this phenomenon (I cannot be certain it is the correct way, however) is to visualize the behavior of people in mass famines. In India or other places where people are starving, they lie very quietly, trying to conserve energy. In my experience, this reaction has never proceeded to the point of slowing the heart rate, and the apathetic thyrotoxics have continued to have tachycardia. If the starvation analogy is correct, however, even the heart rate might eventually succumb to the energy needs of survival.

Generally, a goiter in a young person will immediately alert the clinician to the possibility of some sort of thyroid disease. Thus, it is usually enough to be aware that there is something called apathetic thyrotoxicosis, and the goiter will trigger the correct line of investigation. A thyroid gland which is producing enough hormone to bring the patient to extreme states of debility and exhaustion will usually be a large gland. However, a violently overactive gland may so deplete its colloid content that it is too soft to be felt. This may be true even if the gland is located high in a thin neck. The venous hum in the supraclavicular space is extremely loud, however, and in any event such a soft gland is rather rare. By far the commonest cause of "non-goiterous" thyrotoxicosis is descent of the gland into the chest, where it can be palpated if an effort is made while the patient swallows.

It may be apathetic thyrotoxicosis in perspective to look at the problem in children, where tremor is also uncommon. The usual nervous muscular reaction of children is total body hyperactivity. Thyrotoxic children cannot sit still or behave the way their parents order them to, and give the impression of "mechanical mice" with their sudden purposeless movements.

If we wish to think of it that way, we can look at our typical young woman thyrotoxic as "nervous" in the sense that she has the same impulse to rush about purposelessly as a child would have, but she forcibly inhibits the impulse. Thus she presents the picture of sitting on the edge of her chair, trembling, and looking as though she might at any moment get up and run. The elderly thyrotoxic lacks the muscle tone either to rush about or to inhibit the impulse, and thus may sometimes present a gross tremor (as contrasted with a fine tremor) or little tremor at all.

References

Gurney, C., et al.: Newcastle thyrotoxicosis index. Lancet, 2:1275, 1970.
McLarty, D. G., et al.: Self-limiting episodes of recurrent thyrotoxicosis. Lancet, 1:6, 1971.

18. Hot Nodules of Thyroid

GEORGE ROSS FISHER, III

Cause: Unknown.

Early Manifestations: Typical or apathetic thyrotoxicosis may be present. Neck enlargement is asymmetrical or overtly nodular. Nodule has increased activity on $Na^{131}I$ scintiscan compared to remainder of the gland, which may be completely suppressed.

Treatment: Antithyroid drugs. Radioiodotherapy in post-reproductive individuals uncontrolled by antithyroid drugs.

Possible Dire Consequences without Treatment: Thyrotoxicosis.

About 25% of women develop a 50% enlargement of the thyroid gland during the third trimester of pregnancy. Usually but not invariably it is appreciated as being both uniform and symmetrical. About 4% of random non-pregnant women have some enlargement, which often is slightly asymmetrical or appreciated as one or several nodules. Almost all elderly women have multiple nodules of the thyroid at autopsy. The average physician must see some three to five enlargements per year, discovered incidentally by himself or by the patient, treating a large proportion of them by judicious neglect.   Does this reflect a shocking widespread deficiency among practitioners, to be remedied by publicity, coercion, and continuing education, or are things about as they should be?   Answers are usually sought in statistics.

In some years in Philadelphia, deaths from primary carcinoma of the small bowel, considered almost a medical rarity, exceed those from carcinoma of the thyroid. The latter causes about 15 among some 30,000 deaths yearly, mostly due to the highly refractory undifferentiated variety of carcinoma.   With an approach to thyroid nodules as aggressive, in the future, as present policy is haphazard, this still might be adjudged an irreducible endpoint.

Reference

Selenkow, H. A. and Ingbar, S. H.:   Diseases of the thyroid.   Chapter 89, p. 462 in Harrison's Principles of Internal Medicine, Wintrobe, M. M., et al. (eds.).   New York, McGraw-Hill Book Co., 1970.

19. Cold Nodules of Thyroid

David L. Paskin

Cause: Thyroid adenoma or carcinoma.

Early Manifestations: Carcinoma peak incidence is early in fifth decade, similar to nodules in general which also have a fifth decade peak; but with overall incidence from first decade to ninth.
Both carcinoma and nodules generally have a predilection for the right lobe.
Nodules are from 4 to 8 times more prevalent in women than in men, with higher incidence of malignancy in man.
Known long duration of a nodule is not helpful in excluding malignancy.
Rapid enlargement rarely calls attention to malignant evolution of a nodule and may be simulated by hemorrhage into a cyst.

Late Manifestations: Firm fixed nodule. Regional lymph nodes. Distant metastases, especially lung and bone.

Treatment: Sometimes none. Sometimes surgical removal.

Possible Dire Consequences without Treatment: Metastasis.

Forty % of clinically apparent solitary nodules of the thyroid gland are really a dominant nodule in a multi-nodular goiter.   Twenty-five % are adenomas, the most common type being follicular adenomas.   Thyroiditis is present in less than 10%. Other types of cysts represent about 10%.   The remainder represent carcinoma of which the most common type is papillary followed by follicular and then mixed papillary-follicular and lastly the dreaded undifferentiated carcinoma.

The treatment must then be governed by the above stated facts.   Two modalities are presently used for the treatment of solitary nodules.   The first modality, that of the use of desiccated hormone, is given with the hope of reducing the TSH stimulation of nodular growth and therefore hoping that the nodule will regress. This treatment has been successful in reducing the size of the nodule in at least 50% of cases. However, nodules which are indeed carcinoma can and will reduce in size with desiccated thyroid therapy. Is this then an effective treatment? Is the fact that the nodule reduces its size considered adequate treatment for carcinoma?

The second modality of treatment is surgery. Surgery upon the thyroid gland has become quite sophisticated. The complications of thyroid storm, longstanding or permanent hypoparathyroidism and damage to the recurrent laryngeal nerves with vocal cord paralysis are problems of morbidity whose incidence is almost non-existent today, especially in surgery performed for removal of solitary nodules. The mortality approaches 0%.

Since the incidence of carcinoma in solitary nodules is as high as 30% and since the morbidity and mortality rate from operative attack on the thyroid gland in a euthyroid patient is so low, all thyroid nodules that are solitary and cold should be surgically excised. Warm nodules should be observed closely.

The operation is that of removal of that lobe of the thyroid in which the nodule is present along with the isthmus. This is considered adequate treatment for papillary and follicular carcinoma. If, unfortunately, the pathologic diagnosis is undifferentiated carcinoma, at least total thyroidectomy should be performed. Although the five-year survivals from undifferentiated carcinoma are quite low, most series quoting less than 10%, the five-year survivals following surgical treatment of papillary and follicular carcinoma are excellent with most series quoting survivals of 90%. If the lymph nodes appear to be clinically involved with carcinoma at the time of surgery, neck dissection on the ipsilateral side, along with the removal of the entire thyroid gland, is the procedure of choice.

Following lobectomy, patients usually maintain a euthyroid state without the use of replacement thyroid therapy. Some authorities state that thyroid replacement therapy should be administered to patients following thyroid lobectomy in whom the diagnosis of papillary or follicular carcinoma has been made. This is done so that stimulation for growth from endogenous TSH will be diminished. However, long-term clinical evidence justifying this use has not been substantiated.

The morbidity of thyroid surgery is low. The mortality rate of thyroid surgery approaches that of anesthesia itself (very low). Thyroid hormone does not adequately treat carcinoma of the thyroid. The incidence of carcinoma of the thyroid in solitary nodules is between 5 and 30%. Therefore, when managing a patient with a cold nodule in the thyroid gland, especially in the fifth decade and younger, and in all males with thyroid nodules, surgery is the treatment of choice. No clinician's fingers are more accurate than the pathologist's eyes looking through a microscope at a permanently stained section of thyroid gland. Untreated thyroid cancer kills. The results of surgical treatment for thyroid carcinoma are excellent.

References

Liechty, R. D., Graham, M., Freemeyer, P.: Benign Solitary Thyroid Nodules. Surg. Gyn. & Ob., *120*:571, 1965.

Robinson, E., Horn, Y., Hochmann, A.: Incidence of Cancer in Thyroid Nodules. Surg. Gyn. & Ob., *122*:1025, 1966.

20. Myxedema Coma and Myxedema Madness

George Ross Fisher, III

Cause: Previous surgery, drugs or radiotherapy for a thyroid condition. Thyroiditis. Idiopathic.

Early Manifestations: Puffiness. Hoarseness. Deafness. Loss of lateral eyebrows ("Queen Anne's sign").

Treatment: Thyroxin in small initial doses.

Possible Dire Consequences without Treatment: Vegetative existence—coma and death.

Unless some of the newer gadgets displace the clinical thermometer, a technical problem is going to continue to obscure the diagnosis of severe hypothyroidism. Almost all severely hypothyroid patients have a subnormal body temperature, but the finding is often obscured by failure to shake down the thermometer below a normal reading before putting it in the patient's mouth.

On the other hand, the report that a severely obtunded patient has a slow heart rate and a subnormal temperature should be a great help in suggesting the diagnosis of myxedema coma. The presence of a goiter (in the case of Hashimoto's disease) or a scar on the neck would probably confirm the suspicion. Unfortunately, an increasing proportion of cases of myxedema are caused by therapeutic doses of radioactive iodine, which leaves no tell-tale scar.

Myxedema is a far more serious disease than most physicians realize. It can eventually lead to death (the nineteenth century term was "cachexia thyroprivis"). Even non-fatal cases experience great unpleasantness, and it is an unusual patient who will permit his physician to withdraw treatment a second time after he experiences the sensation. Two misconceptions need continued exorcism: the patients are usually *not* fat, and they do *not* have low blood pressure. Puffiness is the most reliable feature, with hoarseness and deafness.

Statements can be found in the medical literature that some appreciable proportion of patients in mental hospitals have myxedema. It would be important to search among patients with mental retardation or apparent senility, rather than among schizophrenics or neurotic patients, since the term "madness" is a little too graphic for the mental obtundity of myxedema. Myxedema can indeed produce an organic mental syndrome; furthermore, when an elderly patient with myxedema is given unwisely large beginning doses of thyroid, agitated dementia results.

Reference

Billewicz, W. Z., et al.: Statistical methods applied to the diagnosis of hypothyroidism. Quart. J. Med., *38*:255, 1969.

Dysfunction of Sex Hormones (Also See Chapter XII)

21. Klinefelter's Syndrome and Other Eunuchoid Situations

GEORGE ROSS FISHER, III

Cause: Congenital presence of XXY chromosome constitution. Hyposecretion of interstitial cells of testes.

Early Manifestations: Gynecomastia at puberty. Failure of testicular development. Confirmation by laboratory procedures.

Treatment: Plastic surgery to breasts; testosterone administration.

Possible Dire Consequences without Treatment: Lack of potency, muscle strength, aggressiveness. Undeveloped secondary male sex characteristics.

The spectacular intersex situation in this condition makes it easily remembered, and makes it a standard lecture subject in medical genetics, endocrinology, embryology and pathology. Thus it is not likely that any doctor has escaped having lectures on the subject, complete with the dramatic photographic slides, likely accompanied by wry remarks.

On the other hand, there are statistical studies which indicate that the condition is far more common than it is clinically recognized. If the condition is really found in 1 male birth in 500, every doctor ought to have several cases in his practice. My own experience has been that when doctors in practice come across a case they are usually confused, and the patient will usually relate that he has seen several doctors in the past without comment being made.

The classical case is a boy who develops gynecomastia at the time of puberty, and that gynecomastia may assume the full size of a female breast. The probable diagnosis is then confirmed by discovering distinctly small atrophic testes. If laboratory confirmation is required, a urine gonadotropin determination will be elevated to menopausal levels. A "pap" test of the scrapings of the buccal mucosa will demonstrate 20 to 40% of the cells with Barr bodies (normally only seen in females). A karyotype of the chromosomes of white blood cells will reveal 47 instead of the normal 46 chromosomes, with an XXY sex chromatin pattern.

So what is the problem? In the first place, the prepubertal patient has no gynecomastia, and many adult cases will have only moderate gynecomastia buried in the pectoral obesity. Some cases have so little gynecomastia that it could be said they have none. Secondly, the testicular size of the prepubertal patient is normal for his age, and only appears to be small by failure to undergo the normal enlargement of adolescence. The judgment about testicular size in adolescence is not so easy. The Leydig cells ordinarily produce large amounts of testosterone for a considerable period of time before the seminiferous tubules enlarge to make up the majority of the bulk of the adult organ. Thus, it might be said that final enlargement of the testicle is the last stage of puberty, frequently appearing as late as age eighteen. The resulting variability in size may make it difficult for a doctor to judge whether the size is normal or not, particularly if he does not have reason to pay much attention to the testicular variability of teenagers. Beyond this, it would have to be said that a great many doctors have abandoned the habit of examining testicles. The organ seldom has much the matter with it, and it is easy to slip into the habit of examining the genitalia only to the extent of inspection, and probing for hernia.

The difficulty in diagnosis thus has to do with the situation that there is nothing abnormal for the pediatrician to notice, and no painful complaint to take the adult patient to an internist. We must also reckon with the psychological inadequacy which is characteristic of these patients. They tend to be problem students in school, and undependable employees. There is more than average alcoholism and involvement with the drug scene. Comparatively few of them get married, although most of them are sexually potent. Some of them have reduced intelligence, but mostly they lack an indefinable element of aggressiveness and drive toward achievement. They are mostly likeable chaps, but totally lacking in achievement.

Under these circumstances, the physician is naturally stimulated to consider whether male hormone administration would be helpful, since these frustrating personality features are also characteristic of eunuchs. In practice, it often can be demonstrated that plasma testosterone levels are moderately diminished in these patients, and that some improvement is possible through systematic replacement therapy. However, I have had too many of them neglect their therapy to believe that it universally produces a miraculous result. Perhaps earlier treatment would be of value, since there is evidence that testosterone is active and necessary even in fetal life. It seems more likely that the chromosomal difficulty causes the personality problem through direct effects on aggressiveness centers in the brain (whatever they may be).

Klinefelter's (XXY) syndrome is just about the only non-traumatic cause of eunuchoidism for which we know the cause, but it is certain that there are other etiologies. At the moment, these can only be called idiopathic testicular atrophy or idiopathic absence of the testicle. Experimental embryology would suggest that testosterone must have been present in those patients during fetal life in order to cause them to be born phenotypic males. Whether because of this factor or for other reasons, such patients seldom have the same degree of personality impairment, and respond much more dramatically to male hormone therapy then the XXY patients do.

Even the marine sergeant can recognize that a twenty-year-old draft inductee with infantile genitalia is eunuchoid. It is much more difficult to be certain at age fifteen. And it is very difficult to recognize hypogonadism at any age when the secondary sex characters have been developed by therapy which was later discontinued, or if there has been spontaneous involution of the testis after the time of puberty. The ladies in the (unexpurgated) *Arabian Nights* were familiar with the persistence of sexual function for a considerable period after castration, and the deepened voice, beard growth and phallus size do not regress for many years. Thus, a brief "trial" of therapy when the diagnosis is easy can obscure the diagnosis semi-permanently. It is true that there are subtle secondary sex characters which can still be recognized by a shrewd observer, such as lack of facial oiliness, decreased general plethora and pigmentation, and diminished vascularity of the genitals. But it remains extremely probable that there are a great many untreated eunuchs who would greatly benefit from treatment, as well as uncertain numbers of insecure men receiving supplementation who have no deficiency.

References

Albert, A. L., et al.: Male hypogonadism: I, II, III, IV, V, VI, VII, Proc. Staff Meet. Mayo Clinic, *28*:409, 557, 698, 1953; *29*:131, 317, 368, 1954; *30*:31, 1955.

Federmann, D. D.: Abnormal Sexual Development. A Genetic and Endocrine Approach to Differential Diagnosis. Philadelphia, W. B. Saunders Co., 1967.

Klinefelter, H., Reifenstein, E., Jr., and Albright, F.: Klinefelter syndrome characterized by gynecomastia, aspermatogenesis without A-Leydigism, and increased excretion of follicle-stimulating hormone. J. Clin. Endocrinol., *2*:615, 1942.

22. Stein-Levinthal Syndrome

GEORGE ROSS FISHER, III

Cause: Polycystic ovaries.

Early Manifestations: Hirsutism. Other evidence of virilization may be questionable. Amenorrhea.

Treatment: Small doses of prednisone (30% success). Wedge resection of ovary.

Possible Dire Consequences without Treatment: Infertility, deficient estrogen effect.

All women make a certain amount of male hormone. Our present understanding is that the ovaries produce a small amount of testosterone (1/10 the amount produced in the male by the testicle) and that the female adrenal produces about the same amount of androsterone as the male. Androsterone is very weakly androgenic and does not cause much masculinization unless produced in gross excess.

A woman with beard growth thus raises three questions:

1. Are her hair follicles unusually sensitive to normal amounts of male hormone? That is, does she have hereditary hirsutism?
2. Is she producing excessive amounts of adrenal androsterone (*i.e.* urinary 17 ketosteroids)?
3. Are her ovaries producing excessive amounts of testosterone (as measured by plasma testosterone levels)?

It can be assumed that the history and physical examinations have eliminated syndromes of gross masculinization. If the virilizing condition has been present since early childhood, and if there are congenital malformations of the genitals, it is strongly suggested that the patient has the adrenogenital syndrome. If the condition has been of recent origin and progresses rapidly to enlarge the clitoris or deepen the voice, an androgen-secreting tumor is likely.

In the usual case, however, there is only questionable enlargement of the clitoris, little or no deepening of the voice, and a history of hirsutism over a period of years since the late teens. Both tumors and the adrenogenital syndrome can cause amenorrhea, but if the androgen production is too weak to enlarge the clitoris, it should also be too weak to cause amenorrhea. Therefore, the presence of amenorrhea with only mild masculinization suggests an ovarian rather than an adrenal origin—almost all such cases will be confirmed by the presence of a mildly elevated plasma testosterone level.

By this comparatively simple process, we can arrive at a reasonable defensible clinical diagnosis of the Stein-Levinthal syndrome. It may be fairly safely presumed that such a patient has polycystic ovaries, even though it may not be possible to palpate enlarged adnexae.

The therapeutic management varies with the situation. If the woman is complaining of infertility, the best approach may be to suggest laparotomy and wedge resection of the ovaries, possibly preceded by culdoscopy. If the patient is unmarried or does not contemplate children for some time, it probably is worthwhile to attempt a trial of several months of prednisone, 2.5 mg. twice daily. The rationale for this therapy is obscure, but it achieves rather prompt restoration of normal menses in about 30% of cases. This is the same therapy one would employ for the adrenogenital syndrome, and it seems likely that its empirical value in polycystic ovaries was merely stumbled upon.

The urge to employ clomiphene for the infertility should be met cautiously, since this drug may precipitate massive enlargement of the cysts. However, there may be a place for stilbestrol therapy to cause ovarian atrophy and hence some improvement in the hirsutism; obviously, the woman is infertile while she takes what amounts to a birth control pill.

As a matter of fact, the drug treatment of all varieties of hirsutism is discouraging. Electrolysis should be routinely advised, because even total cure of the androgen oversecretion will not cause the hair to fall out for many years. One can probably halt any further progression of the beard, but it is unwise to promise more. There was a time when testosterone was given to women with myopathies, and the resulting hirsutism persisted for years after the drug was discontinued From such experience we can probably generalize that relief of the masculinization cannot be measured by disappearance of the beard.

References

Lloyd C. W., et al.: Plasma testosterone and urinary 17-ketosteroids in women with hirsutism and polycystic ovaries. J. Clin. Endocr., *26*:314, 1966.

Neumann, F., et al.: Aspects of androgen dependent events as studied by antiandrogens. In Recent Progress in Hormone Research. Astwood, E. B. (ed.). New York, Academic Press, Inc., 1970, Vol. 26.

The Hormones and Sugar

The origin of the blood sugar is from liver and kidneys. There may be dissynergism between production and output, with interim storage in the form of glycogen and release by epinephrine and glucagon. Storage may be inadequate due to unavailability or malabsorption of food stuffs generally, with resultant hypoglycemia. Inadequate interconversions to carbohydrate from the amino acid pool may occur, due to inadequate cortisol, in pituitary and adrenocortical failure. Or this pathway may become unavailable in the alcoholic due to competitive reduction of NAD by alcohol dehydrogenases. In diseases primary to the liver, terminal involvement may occur without hypoglycemia, yet otherwise trivial disease may be attended chiefly by hypoglycemia. A huge liver may then be the principal other manifestation, including such importantly different conditions as primary hepatoma and the fatty infiltrations of alcoholism and of kwashiorkor. Primary renal disease is an even less common cause of spontaneous hypoglycemia, but it may be induced by an insulin tolerance test, analogous to measures sometimes taken to reduce a threateningly raised [K]s. Not only do the kidneys put out glucose; they normally extract about a third of the arterial insulin that perfuses them. Cohen and colleagues noted a slower recovery from identical initial hypoglycemia in uremics as compared to patients otherwise as ill from other conditions. A similar challenge is occasioned by the endogenous insulin provoked by hypertonic rinsing solutions in hemodialyzed uremic patients.

Most hypoglycemia is induced rather than spontaneous, usually by insulin. The insulin is endogenous in the prediabetic and in the patient receiving sulfonylureas. In other diabetic subjects it is exogenous. Hypoglycemia in these situations is considered in the two sections that follow.

References

Cohen, B. D., et al.: Hyperguanidinemia and hypoglycemia unresponsiveness in renal disease. Ann. Intern. Med., *54*:1062, 1961.

DeGroote, J.: Liver and brain. Postgrad. Med. J., *39*:224, 1963.

Madison, L. L.: Ethanol-induced hypoglycemia. Adv. Metab. Dis., *3*:85, 1968.

Mellinkoff, S. M., and Tumulty, P. A.: Hepatic Hypoglycemia. New Eng. J. Med., *247*:745, 1952.

Rabkin, R., and Colwell, J. A.: The renal uptake and excretion of insulin in the dog. J. Lab. Med., *73*:893, 1969.

Tomlinson, B. E.: Fatal hypoglycemia in early non-icteric infective hepatitis. Brit. Med. J., *1*:1300, 1955.

Zimmerman, H. J., Thomas, L. J., and Scherr, E. H.: Fasting blood sugar in hepatic disease with reference to infrequency of hypoglycemia. Arch. Intern. Med., *91*:577, 1953.

23. Functional Hypoglycemia

GUY LACY SCHLESS

Cause: Theorized to be a latent diabetic defect of the insulin-glucose transport-utilization mechanism at the peripheral cell membrane level.

Symptoms: Nonspecific: fatigue, weakness and tremors.
Neuroglycopenic: detachment, somnolence, near-syncope, abnormal behavior and negativism
Systemic: hunger, epigastric pain and neuropathies.
Adrenergic: tachycardia, palpitations, sweating, flushing and arterial insufficiency.

Signs: Obesity.

Treatment: Achievement of ideal weight with an isocaloric A.D.A. diet, including snacks two hours p.c. of 6 oz. unsweetened fruit juice or skimmed milk and 1 meat or 2 fat exchanges.
Phenformin timed-disintegration capsules, 50 mg. twice daily.
Avoidance of CATS: caffeine, alcohol, tobacco, stress and sweets.

Possible Dire Consequences without Treatment: Continued fatigue, weakness, tremors and development of frank diabetes.

The significance of functional hypoglycemia (FH) is that 80% of cases represent a latent stage of diabetes mellitus, which, if untreated, may progress to overt diabetes.

Symptoms of FH may vary greatly.

(1) Nonspecific feelings of weakness, fatigue, headache and tremors, worse in the postprandial period and helped by food.

(2) Neuroglycopenic symptoms of light-headedness, detachment from one's surroundings, sluggish mental responses and near-syncope but no true unconsciousness. Syncope does not occur in FH alone since the low sugar associated with this condition brings about a release of adrenalin, resulting in hepatic glycogenolysis, which should be an adequate compensatory mechanism to normalize the depressed blood sugar. In organic hypoglycemia, such as an insulinoma, there is complete loss of consciousness in the fasting state primarily. Should syncope happen postprandially and the glucose tolerance test (GTT) indicates FH, then one must consider the possibility of

TABLE XI–5.

| | Blood Sugar | | | | | |
	Fasting	Postprandial	Unconsciousness	Idiopathic Epilepsy	Latent Diabetes	Treatment
Functional hypoglycemia	Normal	Low	Absent	Absent	Common	Diet Phenformin
Organic hypoglycemia	Low	Low	Present	Absent	Rare	Removal of cause
Postprandial temporal lobe epilepsy	Normal	Low	Present	Present	Common	Diet Phenformin Anticonvulsants

postprandial temporal lobe epilepsy, a syndrome of FH transiently precipitating an underlying seizure disorder (Table XI–5). Just as the insulin-dependent diabetic, who having taken too much insulin, experiences hypoglycemia which causes emotional upset, abnormal behavior and negativism, so FH may present with psychiatric symptoms postprandially.

(3) Systemic symptoms, such as a hunger for sweets, may contribute towards a recent gain in weight. Since hypoglycemia is a strong stimulant for gastric acid production, some patients present with complaints suggesting a peptic ulcer. One case referred by a gastroenterologist experienced peptic ulcer symptoms but had a normal upper GI series. As her blood sugar fell to 22 mg.%. during a GTT, the gastric acid rose 13-fold, and her severe epigastric pain was reproduced. Attributed to latent diabetes are neuropathies, such as gastric atony, with delayed transient time of food demonstrated by upper GI series, producing epigastric fullness, bloating and dyspepsia.

(4) Secondary to the rapid fall of the blood sugar are adrenergic symptoms of tachycardia, palpitations, sweating and flushing. Vascular insufficiency and thrombosis has been attributed to the increased norepinephrine mobilizing more free fatty acids which in turn activate clotting factors XI and XII as well as increasing platelet aggregation.

(5) Especially in the early stages, the diagnosis is indicated objectively by an abnormal GTT and there are no symptoms.

Often indicative of this diabetic tendency is a family history of diabetes or gout, early arterial disease in immediate relatives, familial hyperlipoproteinemias, unexplained miscarriages, giving birth to a baby weighing over 9 pounds and the finding of asteroid hyalitis or Dupuytren's contracture.

Diagnosis is confirmed during a standard GTT by normal blood sugars in the first two hours followed by a fall below 50 mg.% between the second to fifth hours, after which the blood sugar spontaneously rises towards normal levels. In 44% of GTTs, the lowest blood sugar occurred at two and one-half, three and one-half and four and one-half hours and 57% of the hypoglycemic values were between the third to fifth hours (Fig. XI–4). Spontaneous adrenergic response returns the blood sugar towards normal in fifteen to twenty minutes. Thus, in order not to miss this tail-end genetic tag of latent diabetes, which the hypoglycemic fall represents, one should continue the GTT for four and preferably five hours, with blood sugars every half-hour. Under these conditions of testing, GTTs repeated over the years have shown a high degree of reproducibility in untreated cases. (See Fig. XI–2.)

Once the standard-GTT confirms the diagnosis of FH, a cortisone-GTT is performed to evaluate the latent diabetic status. Using the method of Fajans and Conn,* the upper limits of normal blood sugars at one, one and one-half and two hours of the cortisone-GTT are 180, 160 and 160 mg.%. Latent diabetes refers to 2 or more abnormal values and early latent diabetes to only one elevated blood sugar.

Treatment—*Diet.* In the earliest stages, weight and insulin levels of these patients are normal. The etiology of FH is theorized to be a latent diabetic defect of the insulin-glucose transport-utilization mechanism at the peripheral cell membrane, and so as time progresses, this defect probably results in a secondary hyperinsulinism which further inhibits the hydrolysis of triglycerides and so enhances obesity. However,

---

* Cortisone acetate PO, 50 or 62.5 mg., if weight below or above 160 pounds respectively, in two doses, eight and one-half and two hours prior to GTT.

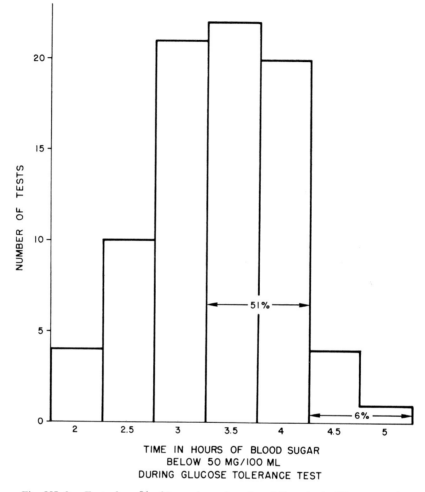

Fig. XI–2. Forty-four % of hypoglycemic values fell at the half-hour sample and 57% between hours three to five of the GTTs.

from the practical aspect the majority of patients also have poor eating habits, the exogenous intake of calories exceeding their physiological requirements. For these reasons, they are instructed in the American Diabetic Association diet and exchange systems with a limitation of 6 bread exchanges daily and omission of all sweets. If overweight, the daily total caloric intake is calculated as the isocaloric requirement minus 500 calories, which is 3500 calories less per week, or a reduction of 1 pound per week. Included are snacks between meals and at bedtime consisting of 4 to 6 ounces of fruit juice or skimmed milk and 1 meat or 2 (unsaturated) fat exchanges.

Medication is phenformin timed-disintegration capsules, 50 mg. twice daily. Should gastrointestinal symptoms occur, taking the drug after meals usually will prevent further complaints; rarely, the medication has to be reduced to once daily. Sulfonyl-ureas are poorly tolerated and may accentuate the hypoglycemic symptoms. Symptoms may improve with diet alone, but it is unusual for the abnormal cortisone-GTT to be normalized without medication. In contrast to Wilansky's reports of the beneficial effects of short term phenformin therapy in correcting abnormal cortisone-GTTs, we found an average of two years of 50 mg. twice daily gave the best results, although smaller doses for shorter periods of time were successful in some cases.

CATS. Patients with FH should avoid caffeine, alcohol, tobacco, stress and sweets. Alcohol inhibits the protective effect of adrenalin while the other factors enhance hyperglycemia.

Once the cortisone-GTT is normal, medication is stopped, diet continued and retesting is done annually. In our series, those who adhered to diet usually showed no recurrence of latent diabetes or symptoms of FH. In a separate four-year study of untreated latent diabetics, 50% progressed to overt disease and 10% reverted to a normal cortisone-GTT. The results in our three-year series of treated latent diabetics revealed that 48% of abnormal cortisone-GTTs were normalized and 34% significantly improved from latent to early latent diabetes, and less than 5% became overtly diabetic.

The importance of diagnosing FH is that most cases represent a latent stage of diabetes, which, with diet and medication, hopefully can prevent or delay the onset of overt diabetes with its many complications.

References

Kwaan, H. C.,, Colwell, J. A., and Suwanwela, N.: Disseminated Intravascular Coagulation in Diabetes. Diabetes, *21*:108, 1972.

Marks, V., and Rose, F. C.: Hypoglycemia. Philadelphia, F. A. Davis Co., 1971.

Schless, G. L.: Functional Hypoglycemia as an Early Manifestation of Diabetes Premellitus. Excerpta Medica International Congress Series. *140*:61, 1967, Stockholm.

Schless, G. L.: Functional Hypoglycemia: A Latent State of Diabetes. (*a*) Int. Med. Dig., *2*:23, 1967; (*b*) Brit. J. Hosp. Med., *3*:389, 1968.

Schless, G. L.: Postprandial Temporal Lobe Epilepsy. Diabetes, *20*:375, 1971.

Shochat, G., Kessler, J., and Wilansky, D. L.: Early Latent Diabetes. Metabolism, *15*:492, 1966.

Wilansky, D. L., and Shochat, G.: The Course of Latent Diabetes. Ann. N.Y. Acad. Sci., *148*:845, 1968.

24. Hypoglycemia from Insulin

Theodore G. Duncan

Cause: An excess of insulin can be caused by many factors. The most common are: (*a*) excessive dosage of exogenous insulin; (*b*) increased exercise; (*c*) decreased caloric intake; (*d*) islet cell tumor; (*e*) surreptitious administration.

Early Manifestations: The signs of hypoglycemia vary and may range from no symptoms to hypoglycemic coma. Others include temporary personality change, nervousness, sweating, tremors, tachycardia, hypothermia, decreased mental and manual dexterity, headache, restless sleep, nightmares and a variety of neurologic signs and symptoms.

Treatment: Prevention. Decrease the dosage or stop the offending hypoglycemic drug. Review the patient's other drug therapy to determine if this additional medication causes further hypoglycemic effect. Administer oral or intravenous glucose and when necessary glucagon and/or hydrocortisone hemisuccinate. Surgery.

Possible Dire Consequences without Treatment: Progression of symptoms.
Hormonal defense mechanisms may alleviate the hypoglycemia and the signs and symptoms clear without therapy.
Hypoglycemia usually does not cause permanent disability but if severe and prolonged can result in a permanent decreased mental acuity.
Hypoglycemia can cause stress to aggravate other existing diseases.

Hypoglycemia is defined in the medical dictionary as the "concentration of glucose in the blood below the normal limit." The direct translation from the Greek means "below sweet blood." The clinical and practical interpretation needs further definition since several essential factors help us in determining when the patient is having impaired function due to low sugar. The patient can have definite impaired mental acuity and mechanical dexterity from a high value to a lower value in a short period of time. The rate of drop of the blood sugar or the absolute number of units decrease seems to be of more value in producing recognizable signs and symptoms than the absolute blood sugar value at the time of the hypoglycemic reaction.

For example, characteristically, a patient having symptoms of hypoglycemia with associated blood sugar below 40 mg.% usually is accepted by the physician as definite proof for the patient's difficulty. On the other hand, coma with all the associated signs and symptoms of hypoglycemia has been well documented in patients having a blood sugar in excess of 150 mg.%. Conversely, the patient may be conscious, alert, cooperative and no evidence of hypoglycemia but have blood sugar levels below 30 mg.%.

Doctor W. J. H. Butterfield recorded in the literature, a case record of a twenty-three-year-old diabetic, taking insulin, who on one occasion had hypoglycemic coma and convulsions with a blood sugar value, prior to treatment, of 159 mg.%. On three other occasions, he was cooperative, alert and conscious with values of 25, 27 and 30 mg.% and a few months later he again developed coma, convulsions with abnormal EEG changes, with a blood sugar of 150 mg.%. On other occasions, frank hypoglycemia occurred with blood sugars below 40 mg.%. This case demonstrates three important features of hypoglycemia. (1) Symptoms and coma of hypoglycemia can occur in patients with blood sugar values considered in the normal range. (2) No obvious symptoms need exist in patients having definite hypoglycemia with blood sugar values below 40 mg.%. (3) The response to hypoglycemia can vary in one individual and indeed, varies among individuals.

Studies using the Phystester, developed by Delco Electronics, a division of General Motors, better known as "the drunkometer," can definitely detect impaired mental process when an excess of alcohol is imbibed or when symptomatic or asymptomatic hypoglycemia exists. It became quite evident, when using this instrument to detect impaired function, that the patient having hypoglycemia usually is not aware of his difficulty, resists help when orange juice was offered and completely denied, frequently in a hostile fashion, that he was having any difficulty whatsoever. Sixty % of the patients who had functional impairment to the degree that would cause hazardous driving had no idea that their mental acuity and dexterity was markedly impaired due to hypoglycemia. Literature documents frequent occurrence of asymptomatic hypoglycemia but does not stress the undetected impairment of function during this hazardous period of a diabetic's routine. One explanation for asymptomatic hypoglycemia is the lack of epinephrine effect due to a gradual lowering of the blood sugar to hypoglycemic ranges—for example, a slow decrease in blood sugar from 70 to 20 mg.%. Epinephrine effect can cause nervousness, sweating and palpitations.

With this information physicians are frequently presented with a perplexing situation of not knowing what to do and in fact, sometimes having difficulty not knowing whether the patient is having low sugar reactions. Patients have been accused of having symptoms due to mental stress or neurosis, as the blood sugar values during their difficulty do not represent the typical hypoglycemic range. The juvenile diabetic, well controlled, when monitored by frequent blood sugar values will quite characteristically have blood sugars peaking to an excess of 300 mg.% and to a level below 50 mg., which can occur several times daily. Therefore, patients receiving insulin will invariably approach the hazards of hypoglycemia several times daily and will not be able to recognize the potential danger, for the majority have no symptoms associated with hypoglycemia.

When symptoms do exist, a multitude of changes may occur in the diabetic which makes it somewhat difficult to render a clear-cut diagnosis.

Patients receiving insulin and oral drugs for the treatment of diabetes are more prone to have hypoglycemic reactions or "shock" after a period of fasting. These exist prior to lunch, supper and breakfast times. The number of abnormal changes that may be detected is great and may vary from one noticeable sign or symptom to a variety of detectable abnormalities. A normally good-natured individual may show marked hostility and refuse help and on occasion, a patient has taken the orange juice that has been offered and thrown it across the room, shouting, "I do not need your help, there is nothing the matter with me." Hostility is a common personality change that is seen associated with hypoglycemia. On the other hand, he may become withdrawn and show marked fatigue and frequently a relative will notice that he has become "glassy eyed." Nervousness, sweating and tremors associated with tachycardia are caused by an increased release of epinephrine which have been characteristically outlined in all texts describing hypoglycemia but their occurrence is not as frequent as one would think. In addition, a quiet person may become talkative, sometimes incoherent and irrational and his speech may be slurred and stuttering can occur. The patient may notice a decrease in his thinking ability and also note poor coordination. A frequent first sign in one of our patients who does figure skating is the inability to perform intricate coordinated skating patterns with normal ease. A glass of orange juice usually clears the difficulty. Amnesia for events during hypoglycemia is not unusual for not only will the existence of low sugar be denied during the actual episode but afterwards he will have no recall for the incident. One of our patients did drive from Philadelphia to Atlantic City without recalling the event. The blood sugar prior to this trip showed definite hypoglycemia.

Headaches are quite common. They are usually bilateral, frontal and occipital. The patients complain about pain behind the eyes. This may be the only symptom of hypoglycemia and when food is taken, the difficulty clears. Headache can occur with many of the other symptoms mentioned and it can persist for a day after the hypoglycemia has been treated. Headache prior to breakfast may denote low sugar during the night and other evidence of nocturnal hypoglycemia is a restless night's sleep, nightmares, and awakening with the bed clothes drenching from "cold sweat." It is not unusual for a patient to sleep through a hypoglycemic reaction and then awaken after difficulty has cleared.

Hypothermia exists and frequently the patient will feel cold and perspiration may or may not be present. Mothers will frequently check their diabetic children during the night and assume that they are all right with no hypoglycemia if the skin temperature is normal. Rectal temperatures have decreased to 95° or 92° F. in patients with coma due to hypoglycemia.

Neurological symptoms in the conscious or unresponsive patient are quite common and include paresthesias, ataxia, diplopia, headache and sometimes localizing neurological signs. Hypoglycemia can trigger a seizure in an epileptic, migraine headache or signs and symptoms of a brain tumor or a stroke if primary sub-clinical cerebral ischemia exists prior to the hypoglycemic episode.

The symptoms of children and adults receiving insulin for the treatment of juvenile diabetes may vary. A child rarely complains about paresthesias, double vision or unstable gait and tremors are rare. A youngster will show a pallor, staring gaze and sweating. Blurred vision is common. Convulsions are more common in children than in adults. A teacher or a parent may notice a loss of attention and concentration or other changes in behavior, such as irritability in the period prior to lunch or supper, which are due to a low blood sugar level. If these are not recognized and treated, undeserved punishment might ensue.

Unconsciousness due to hypoglycemia is associated with a variety of signs and symptoms. These include perspiration, hypotonia, primitive movements such as grimacing, grasping, sucking, restlessness, chronic spasms, hyperresponsiveness to pain, tachycardia and mydriasis. Ocular deviation can exist and abnormal neurologic signs such as a Babinski have been noted. Deep coma has been associated with shallow respiration, bradycardia, miosis, no pupillary reaction to light, hypothermia, atonia, hyporeflexia, reflexia and absent reflex.

In review, it is evident that hypoglycemia is frequently asymptomatic and when symptoms do occur a bizarre variety of mental and physical changes are elicited. Decreased mental acuity definitely exists in almost all episodes of hypoglycemia even when obvious signs and symptoms are absent.

References

Bleicher, S. J.: Hypoglycemia. Ellenberg, M. and Rifkin, H. (eds.): Diabetes Mellitus: Theory and Practice. New York, McGraw-Hill Book Co., 1970, pp. 958–989.

Gastineau, C. F.: Hypoglycemia Secondary to Therapy. Fajans, S. S., Sussman, K. (eds.): Diabetes Mellitus: Diagnosis and Treatment, Vol. III. New York, American Diabetes Association, Inc., 1971, pp. 261–268.

Marks, V., and Rose, F. C.: Hypoglycemia. Philadelphia: F. A. Davis Co., 1965.

Hormonal and Other Controls of Water and Salt

The body's mechanism for governing water intake seems to need and actually to have a sensing element for substances dissolved in the circulating fluids. The prevailing hydration state then is ascertained much as an experimenter might do, when he needs to know the water content of some heterogeneous volume. He might, for example, determine the equilibrium count rate after administering a radiosodium salt, count rate ranges being known for established doses and conditions. A given

TABLE XI-6.

Dilute Polyurias (Water Diuresis)

1. Vasopressin Deficient
    (*a.*) Idiopathic nuclear atrophy
    (*b.*) Hypophyseal surgery or irradiation
    (*c.*) Sellar or parasellar tumor
    (*d.*) Granulomatous disease
    (*e.*) Hereditary pituitary diabetes insipidus
2. Vasopressin Suppression
    (*a.*) Physiologic (Hydration, positive pressure respiration, immersion, tachycardia)
    (*b.*) Pharmacologic (Alcohol)
    (*c.*) Psychologic (Hypnotism, conditioned reflex)
3. Vasopressin Resistance
    (*a.*) Inherited trait
    (*b.*) Functional (Prolonged psychogenic water drinking)
    (*c.*) Structural (Filtrable proteins, hypokalemia, hypercalciuria, medullary sickling, pyelonephritis, raised intratubular pressures)

Load Polyurias (Solute Diuresis)

1. Decreased reabsorption of endogenous solute
    (*a.*) Glucose: Phlorizin
    (*b.*) $NaHCO_3$: Carbonic anhydrase inhibitors
    (*c.*) NaCl: Chloruretic agents
2. Increased filtration of endogenous solute
    (*a.*) Urea, glucose
3. Increased filtration of exogenous solute
    (*a.*) Sucrose, hexoses, hexitols
    (*b.*) Na_2SO_4, NH_4NO_3, NH_4Cl, $CaCl_2$, KCl

Load Polyurias (Filtration Diuresis)

1. Increased renal blood flow
    (*a.*) Adequate circulation with plethora
    (*b.*) Failing circulation treated by digitalis, rest and recumbency
    (*c.*) Adequate circulation with renal vasodilation (Cholinergic, B-adrenergic, dopaminergic vasodilators) (Direct vasodilators: Pyrogens, hydralazine, diazoxide).

count rate would bespeak a certain water volume. No such injection is necessary in biology where nature already has provided a suitable indicator in the form of the native sodium salts. The fact that these are present in much more than indicator quantities, which of course assures the retention extraprotoplasmically of sufficient water for their own best circulation from portal to portal, in no way vitiates their fortuitous utility in this regard. Hence raised sodium salt concentrations in circulating fluids occasion thirst in responsive subjects, and in therapy are the warrant for allocating more water to replenish body stores.

The deficiency of water may have arisen through insufficient intake or through losses by extrarenal and renal routes. The principal agencies for the losses of hypotonic fluids are the sweat glands and the kidneys. Urine formation according to current concepts is the resultant of large proportionate transfers of solutes, with solvent, across glomerular capillaries (in the cortical labyrinth of Fig. XI–5), followed by nearly as large a reabsorption across peritubular capillaries in proportions modified by properties of the tubular epithelium. The propensity for copious polyurias in such a scheme are so obvious that it is unsurprising to encounter them under occasional and diverse circumstances of clinical medicine. Early appreciation of a distinction between the dilute polyuria of diabetes insipidus and the solute-coupled polyuria of diabetes mellitus anticipated modern classifications of diuresis. An example is given in Table XI–6.

The kidney is functionally hybrid, so dominated by a vascular supply specialized as an enormous filtration system that perfusion tends to dictate metabolic activity, rather than the reverse. There is a notorious proneness to vascular injury, an aspect

TABLE XI–7.

	WATER	SOLUTE		FILTRATION
		Reabsorption	Filtered	
		Decrease	Increase	
	DIURESIS	DIURESIS		DIURESIS
Solute Partition	2/3 Electrolyte		1/3 Electrolyte	
Solute Rejection Fraction	1–3%	10–50%	10–30%	Up to 12.5%
Water Rejection Fraction	Up to 12.5%	10–50%	10–30%	Up to 12.5%
Urine	Hypotonic	Isotonic		Isotonic
Flow Increase	Distal Tubular and Ductular	Tubular		Glomerular
Urea Rejection Fraction	60%	80%		60%
Potassium Rejection Fraction	10%	50–125%		10%

that was considered in Chapter VIII; failure of the tubules as conduits was considered in Chapter X.   Here we consider the kidneys as glands.

Figure XI–3 shows that the kidney tubules which, in panel 2, are highly permeable to water, subsequently become waterproof as indicated in panel 3.   The inset over panel 3 shows that the diluting system arises as the straight distal tubular segments emerge from each of 6 to 10 medullary (Malpighian) pyramids of human kidneys. These course toward their glomeruli of origin in the cortical labyrinth.   An eighth of them, returning to juxtamedullary glomeruli, drain long thin loops extending into the inner (papillary) medulla, their points of emergence delineating the region's border with the outer (boundary) medulla more or less sharply in all species. Those segments with origin from more superficial glomeruli begin their outward turns at varying higher levels within the outer medulla, so that diluting (distal) and proximal straight segments with their vasculature run parallel to collecting ducts in the medullary rays.   Uniform inner medullary descent of proximal segments gives it a two-striped appearance in some species.   Passing from the diluting system, the tubules in panels 4, 5, and 6 remain waterproof and, insofar as solute is removed, permit still further dilution except as modified by the presence of vasopressin.

At usual hydration, the pituitary releases vasopressin at a rate resembling administration of about 7.5 to 50 milliunits commercial pitressin hourly.   Inactivation takes about thirty to seventy-five minutes and at this interval after a forced water load of 20 ml./kg., a physiologic diabetes normally ensues.   Ingestion of far less fluid in the form of beer induces a pharmacologic diabetes insipidus.   Another similar effect is obtained by maneuvers which displace blood into the thorax, distending both pulmonary vascular bed and left atrium.   Two such maneuvers are sitting in a tank of water (Ba gett) and negative pressure breathing (Henry and Gauer).   To a certain extent lying recumbent does the same thing.   Left atrial distension is believed to signal to a central mechanism, capable of shutting off vasopressin, that the circulation is overfilled.

The diuresis occasioned by the absence of vasopressin is dilute.   It requires narrow operant conditions of filtration.   It is not seen in the hypoperfused mate of a normal kidney because of insufficient solute filtration per nephron, nor in bilateral renal disease because of excessive solute filtration per nephron.   In both circumstances coupling of solute and solvent reabsorption in the diluting segment approaches identity with filtrate proportions as an asymptote.   Under certain circumstances of increased filtration without similarly augmented reabsorption there may be a "filtration diuresis."   Such may occur in the cardiac patient whose cardiac output improves when he goes to bed, and this may be the chief mechanism by which diuresis is induced with aminophyllin or with coffee.   Furthermore, there is reason to believe that the observed augmentation of urine flow may reflect primarily the activity of juxtamedullary glomeruli, in which case measurements of total filtration rate will underestimate the actual change in load involved in the flow rate change.   The exaggerated natriuresis in response to fluid overload that characterizes most hypertensive states, and a marked tendency to nocturnal diuresis in a few patients with unilateral renal ischemia, may be additional manifestations of a lesser autoregulation of flow, in the face of perfusion pressure changes, on the part of these glomeruli.

Any variety of polyuria is imminently desiccating unless great exactitude of water intake can be maintained.   In water diuresis, increased loss of "free" water alone causes the increased urine flow.   Solute-borne or osmotic diureses bring out water obligated by increased solute loss as well.   If you give hypertonic mannitol, which

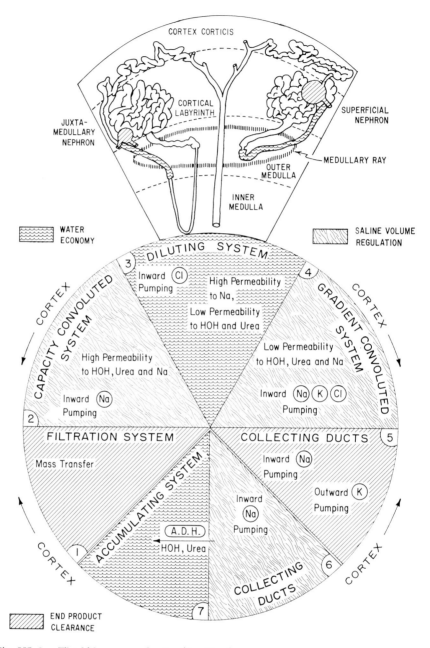

Fig. XI–3. The kidney as a gland. (See Text).

One of the more recently discovered glandular functions of the kidney is the transformation of monohydroxy vitamin D into dihydroxy vitamin D in one of two forms. The 24–25 dihydroxy product seems to be largely inactive, while the 1–25 dihydroxy product is extremely active in calcium and phosphorus mobilization. The autoregulation of choice between these two products seems to be internally responsive to parathyroid hormone levels and circulatory ion concentrations. The characteristic hypocalcemia of uremia may be entirely due to lack of available enzymes to produce the 1–25 product, and the treatment of renal bone diseases may be greatly modified when suitable commercial preparations (or analogs) of 1–25 dihydroxy vitamin D become available.

the tubules cannot reabsorb, and bring out a urine that is largely isotonic mannitol, this occasions net water removal from the body, despite the fact that the urine is not dilute. A distinctive added hazard of the solute-borne polyurias is their disproportionate withdrawal of protoplasmic as compared to circulating water. Ameliorating this disparity at the momentary expense of the circulation, but possibly enhancing immediate survival is a regular renal response whereby saluresis is added to the effects of the original loading solute. Actually in mannitol diuresis about two-thirds of the increased volume is due to the loading solute and about one-third to sodium and its anions. Wesson and Anslow gave a possible explanation of this in terms of the energetics of salt transfer. The unreabsorbable mannitol dilutes the contents of the proximal tubule by means of the water that it draws in, increasing the gradient against which sodium is reabsorbed.

However, the same thing appears to occur to a lesser degree in uncomplicated water deprivation. This was studied by McCance and Young in such a way as to engender vasopressinism but not an adrenocortical stress response, sodium losses being about 200 mM/L (100 mM/day) and potassium losses half this. Water restitution did not immediately augment urine flow rate. Instead there was a prompt change in urine solute partition, with increased urea excretion matching a reciprocally decreased electrolyte excretion. A renal response which dumps electrolyte to match shrinking water stores, is able to regain it when they are replenished, and does so within the compass of a relatively brief time constant has the hallmarks of an autoregulation. A degree of gain permitting a still raised sodium concentration is itself serviceable if it induces the patient to take water.

If instead of replenishing water, a surfeit of some solute is introduced, excretion of urea and electrolyte increase simultaneously, and urine flow rate then increases irrespective of the loading solute (urea, NaCl, KCl). This is an osmotic diuresis with the consequence that despite continued vasopressinism, not as much water can be conserved. Despite more electrolye in urine, its ratio to water in a lessened reabsorbate may rise, enhancing the tendency to hypernatremia. This has been noted after gastrointestinal hemorrhage, where the solute is endogenous, and after protein tube feedings where it is exogenous. It is not abolished if the kidney is denervated (newly transplanted).

The minimum conditions necessary for concentrating the urine include (1) generation of medullary hypertoxicity, and (2) permeability of the pyramidal collecting ducts to water. The former is attained via pumping solute without water out of the loops of Henle as the ascent from the medulla and to some extent from the ducts themselves. Escape of the pumped solute is prevented by a parallel arrangement of the medullary vessels (vasa rectas); since solute escapes from outgoing and into incoming vessels they function as "counter-current exchangers." The pumping requirement upon the tubular structures that must generate the hypertoxicity is decreased by a second parallel arrangement of the tubules themselves. If sodium is pumped out of waterproof ascending limbs against a gradient, the gradient is decreased insofar as solute diffuses into descending limbs, and intraluminal concentrations coming around the bends in each loop progressively increase. This arrangement of the tubules constitutes a "counter-current multiplier," the attainable hypertoxicity depending upon (1) length of the loops, (2) the gradient between adjacent portions of the loops, and (3) velocity of flow out of the system into the distal convoluted segments.

Once medullary hypertoxicity is established, a concentrated urine results providing collecting duct epithelium is made permeable to water or flow through the ducts is extremely limited. Ordinarily the presence of vasopressin ensues sufficient permeability. In the conditions of hypercalcemia and hypokalemia, sufficient permeability may not be attained despite normal or high vasopressin levels. If all of these factors do not suggest a reason, inability to concentrate the urine implies medullary destruction or disorganization, a high osmotic load per nephron, or both. Both impair the attainment of maximal dilution as well. Were this not so, extreme polyuria would be seen more often in primary renal disease than it is.

References

Burg, M., and Stoner, L.: Sodium transport in the distal nephron. Fed. Proc., *33*:31, 1974.
Elkinton, J. R., and Taffel, M.: Prolonged water deprivation in the dog. J. Clin. Invest., *21*:787, 1942.
McCance, R. A., and Young, W. F.: The secretion of urine during dehydration and rehydration. J. Physiol., *102*:415, 1944.
Schreiner, G. E.: The use of diuretics in edema of renal origin. In Edema, Mechanisms and Management. J. H. Moyer and M. Fuchs (eds.). Philadelphia, W. B. Saunders Co., 1960.
Wesson, L. G., Jr., and Anslow, W. P., Jr.: Excretion of sodium and water during osmotic diuresis in the dog. Am. J. Physiol., *153*:465, 1948.

25. Diabetes Insipidus

Joseph H. Magee

Cause: Idiopathic atrophy of supraoptic, paraventricular and filiform nuclei. Posthypophysectomy or irradiation. Neoplasia. Granulomatous disease. Hereditary pituitary diabetes insipidus. The condition does not appear if the anterior pituitary gland is also destroyed, although cortisone therapy will bring it forth.

Early Manifestations: Dilute polyuria (S.G. <1.005, cryoscopy <100 mOsm/kg. water); nocturia. Thirst. Afternoon fever. Weight loss. Constipation. Amelioration by self-selected diet low in salt and protein, amelioration by increased tobacco smoking. Amelioration by aqueous vasopressin or vasopressin tannate. The patient may be quite unaware of his polyuria until it is measured.

Late Manifestations: Hypernatremia. Low arterial and venous pressure. Anorexia, nausea, vomiting, convulsions.

Treatment: Chlorpropamide 250 to 750 mg./day. Chlorothiazide 500 mg./day, primarily to antagonize insulin release by chlorpropamide. Synthetic lysine vasopressin nasal spray. Pitressin tannate 5 units (1 ml.)/day.

Possible Dire Consequences without Treatment: Severe and conceivably fatal dehydration, especially in patients subjected to surgery or severe trauma.

References

Crawford, J. D., and Kennedy, G. C.: Chlorothiazide in diabetes insipidus. Nature, *183*:891, 1959.

Forssman, H.: On hereditary diabetes insipidus. Acta Med. Scand., *121*:Suppl 159:1, 1956.

Harard, C. W. H., and Wood, P. H. N.: Antidiuretic properties of hydrochlorothiazide in diabetes insipidus. Brit. Med. J., *1*:1306, 1960.

Webster, B., and Bain, J.: Antidiuretic effect and complications of chlorpropamide therapy in diabetes insipidus. J.C.E.M., *30*:215, 1970.

26. Nephrogenic Diabetes Insipidus

Joseph H. Magee

Cause: X-linked genetic trait expressed as endorgan (distal convolution, collecting duct) unresponsiveness to endogenous and exogenous vasopressin, fully in hemizygous males, variably in heterozygous females). Acquired hypercalciuria. Acquired hypokalemia.

Early Manifestations: Dilute polyuria (SG < 1.005, cryoscopy < 100 m Osm/kg. water), nocturia. Thirst. Afternoon fever. Weight loss. Constipation. Amelioration by decreased dietary salt and protein (decreased urine solute). Not ameliorated by aqueous vasopressin or vasopressin tannate.

Late Manifestations: Hypernatremia. Low arterial and venous pressure. Anorexia, nausea, vomiting, convulsions.

Treatment: Constant availability of water.
Chlorothiazide 10 mg./kg./day.
Salt restriction and potassium supplementation.
Intravenous fluid therapy. "5 percent dextrose in water, although the fluid of choice in other instances of dehydration, may aggravate the hypertonicity . . . it is virtually impossible to maintain positive water balance if 5 percent dextrose is administered to patients with this disorder. Successful correction . . . may be accomplished by administering $2\frac{1}{2}$ to 3 percent dextrose in water . . . it is advisable to administer water without solute orally as soon as is clinically feasible."

Possible Dire Consequences without Treatment: Severe and conceivably fatal dehydration, especially in patients subjected to surgery or severe trauma.

Reference

Orloff, J., and Burg, M. B.: Vasopressin-resistant diabetes insipidus. In Metabolic Bases of Inherited Diseases, Wyngaarden, J. B., Stanbury, J. B., and Fredrickson, D. S. (eds.). New York, The Blakiston Co., 1970.

27. Water Loss due to Load

Joseph H. Magee

Synonyms: Load polyuria. Solute diuresis. Osmotic diuresis.

Result: Renal water loss. Hypernatremia.

Causes: Urea diuresis: Diuretic phase of acute renal failure.
Urea diuresis: Due to gut bleeding, concealed bleeding, catabolism.
Urea diuresis: Due to tube feedings.
Urea diuresis: Feeding fluid cow's milk (2.5 times the protein content and 4 times the salt content of human milk) to babies with insufficient additional water.
Urea diuresis: Feeding powdered cow's milk to babies with insufficient dilution.
Urea diuresis: Hypertonic intravenous urea solutions to lower intracranial pressure.
Mannitol diuresis: Hypertonic intravenous mannitol solutions for same purpose.
Glucose diuresis with insufficient water repletion during therapy of ketotic and non-ketotic diabetic coma.

Early Manifestations: Non-dilute polyuria. Thirst. Glycosuria may be present. Azotemia may be present. Azotemia disproportionate to creatininemia.

Late Manifestations: Fever. Hypernatremia. Worsening neurologic status (obtundity, behavioral change, vomiting, convulsions).

Treatment: Plain water by ingestion or tube.
If insufficient water can be given internally, dextrose in water, with appropriate insulin in diabetics.
Where both water and insulin are given, to subjects in whom water originally is sequestered outside cells, by glucose, progression may be from hypernatremia to pseudohyponatremia to normal [Na]s.
Appropriate dilution of tube feedings in adults.
Appropriate dilution of cow's milk in infants.
Substitution of carbohydrate and fat calories in tube feedings, depending upon condition causing incapacity, and associated conditions.

Possible Dire Consequences without Treatment: Where [Na]s exceeds 158, incidence of convulsions is 71%.

References

Borst, J. G. G.: The cause of hyperchloremia and hyperazotemia in patients with recurrent massive hemorrhage with peptic ulcer. Acta Med. Scand., 97:68, 1938.

Doolan, P. D., et al.: Post-traumatic acute renal insufficiency complicated by hypernatremia. Ann. Intern. Med., 42:1101, 1955.

Engel, F. L., and Jaeger, C.: Dehydration with hypernatremia, hyperchloremia and azotemia complicating nasogastric tube feeding. Am. J. Med., 17:196, 1954.

Gault, M. H., et al.: Hypernatremia, azotemia and dehydration due to high-protein tube feeding. Ann. Intern. Med., 68:778, 1958.

Morris-Jones, P. H., Houston, I. B., and Evans, R. C.: Prognosis of the neurological complications of acute hypernatremia. Lancet, 2:1385, 1967.

Parc, C.: Hypernatremia in a premature infant associated with feeding a concentrated formula. Canad. M. A. J., 82:85, 1960.

Skinner, A. L.: Water depletion associated with improperly constituted powdered milk formulas. Am. J. Dis. Child., 39:625, 1967.

Welt, L. G., et al.: Role of the central nervous system in metabolism of electrolyte and water. Arch. Intern. Med., 90:355, 1952.

Wise, B. L.: Hyperosmolality (hypernatremia) and azotemia induced by administration of urea. Arch. Neurol., *2*:160, 1960.

Zierler, K. L.: Hyperosmolality in adults. J. Chron. Dis., *7*:1, 1958.

28. Salt-Poisoning

JOSEPH H. MAGEE

Causes: Inadvertent addition of NaCl to infant formulas.

Self-ingestion of NaCl by older infants.

Addition of NaCl to milk for treatment of infantile gastroenteritis.

Use of electrolyte powders (Lytren) for infantile gastroenteritis.

NaCl as home remedy for menstrual cramps.

Suicidal ingestion of NaCl.

Ingestion of sea water (1200 mOsm./kg.).

Chinese restaurant syndrome (NaCl, Na Glutamate).

Massive sodium penicillin therapy.

Early Manifestations: Infant irritability, later lethargy. Anorexia, vomiting. Tachypnea, hyperpnea.

Late Manifestations: Convulsions. Death.

Treatment: Plain water in conscious adults. Dextrose 5% in water intravenously 0.5–2.5 ml./kg./minute for two hours. Peritoneal dialysis where [Na]s is >180 mM/l.

Possible Dire Consequences without Treatment: Convulsions, death.

References

Brunner, F. P., and Frick, F. G.: Hypokalemia, metabolic alkalosis and hypernatremia due to "massive" sodium penicillin therapy. Brit. Med. J., *4*:550, 1968.

Calvin, M. E., Knepper, R., and Robertson, W. O.: Hazards to health. Salt poisoning. New Eng. J. Med., *270*:625, 1964.

Colle, E., Ayout, E., and Raile, R.: Hypertonic dehydration. Pediatrics, *22*:5, 1958.

Daves, N. E.: Chinese restaurant syndrome. New Eng. J. Med., *278*:1124, 1968.

Finberg, L.: Pathogenesis of lesions in the nervous system in hypernatremic states. Pediatrics, *23*:40, 1959.

Finberg, L., and Harrison, H. E.: Hypernatremia in infants. Pediatrics, *16*:1, 1955.

Finberg, L., Kiley, J., and Luttrell, C. N.: Mass accidental salt poisoning in infancy. J.A.M.A., *184*:187, 1963.

Franz, M. N., and Segar, W. E.: The association of various factors and hypernatremic diarrhea dehydration. Am. J. Dis. Child., *97*:298, 1959.

Kivok, R. H. M.: Chinese restaurant syndrome. New Eng. J. Med., *278*:796, 1968.

Schatz, W. J.: Treatment based on physical principles followed by recovery in sodium chloride poisoning. Med. Rec. Ann., *145*:487, 1937.

Schaumburg, H. M., and Byck, R.: Sin Cib-Syn. Accent on glutamate. New Eng. J. Med., *279*:105, 1968.

Weil, W. B., and Wallace, W. M.: Hypertonic dehydration in infancy. Pediatrics, *17*:171, 1956.

29. Neurogenic Hypernatremia

Joseph H. Magee

Causes: Primary atrophy of thirst center(s) and/or osmoreceptor nuclei. Postoperative or posttraumatic. Neoplasia including pinealoma. Granulomatous disease. Angiomata, aneurysms, subarachnoid hemorrhage.

Result: Primary hypodipsia (thirst center lesions). Reset hypodipsia (Osmoreceptor lesions).

Early Manifestations: Presentation may be as periodic paralysis.
Serum drawn for electrolytes may reveal normal [K]s, but [Na]s in the vicinity of 170 to 180 mM/l. without thirst.
Paresthesias and objective muscle tenderness may accompany weakness.
Arterial and venous pressures and measured plasma volumes are normal.
Muscle strength improves and [Na]s falls to high normal values with Na restriction. Thirst is present on arising (and if usual daily intake of $1\frac{1}{2}$ to 2 liters is further restricted) in patients with osmoreceptor lesions.
Urine is usually concentrated, but dilutes appropriately with water-loading tests.

Treatment: Diet free of added salt and using salt-poor bread and milk, aimed at about 35 mM/day intake.
High potassium food items and supplementation with liquid KCl supplementation to attain 250 mM/day intake.
Ad libitum fluid intake.
Spironolactone 100 mg. daily if [K]s is low or low normal.

Possible Dire Consequences without Treatment: Periodic paralysis.

References

Allot, E. N.: Hypernatraemia and hyperchloremia in bulbar poliomyelitis. Lancet, *1*:246, 1957.
DeRubertis, F. R., et al.: Essential hypernatremia due to ineffective osmotic and intact volume regulation of vasopressin secretion. J. Clin. Invest., *50*:97, 1971.
Goldberg, M., et al.: Asymptomatic hypovolemic hypernatremia. Am. J. Med., *43*:804, 1967.
Golonka, J. E., and Richardson, J. A.: Postconcussive hyperosmolality and deficient thirst. Am. J. Med., *48*:261, 1970.
Kastin, A. J.: Asymptomatic hypernatremia. Am. J. Med., *38*:306, 1965.
Katzman, R., and Pappius, H. M.: Brain Electrolytes and Fluid Metabolism. Baltimore, The Williams & Wilkins Co., 1972.
Mahoney, J., and Goodman, A. D.: Hypernatremia due to hypodipsia and elevated threshold for vasopressin release. New Eng. J. Med., *279*:1191, 1968.
Pleasure, D., and Goldberg, M.: Neurogenic hypernatremia. Arch. Neurol., *15*:78, 1966.
Sweet, W. H., et al.: Gastrointestinal hemorrhage, hyperglycemia, azotemia, hyperchloremia and hypernatremia following lesions of the frontal lobe in man. Proc. Assn. Res. Nerv. Ment. Dis., *27*:795, 1948.
Welt, L. G.: Hypo and hypernatremia. Ann. Intern. Med., *56*:161, 1962.

30. Primary Hyponatremia

Joseph H. Magee

Cause: Non-osmotic vasopressinism due to alarm reaction or drugs.

Pain, trauma, surgery, heat stress, fright, noise, excitement, exercise, coitus, suckling, hypnosis, conditioned reflexes.

Ether, cyclopropane, nitrous oxide.

Opiates, barbiturates.

Procaine and congeners.

Acetyl choline, nicotine, lobeline, neostigmine.

Histamine, bradykinin, serotonin.

Ferritin, angiotensin, norepinephrine, large doses of epinephrine.

Result: Non-osmotic vasopressinism.

Early Manifestations: Body fluid dilution. Paradoxical (inappropriate) antidiuresis despite continued fluid intake.

Treatment:

Monitor $\left\{ \begin{array}{l} \text{Urine solute concentration} \\ \text{Serum sodium concentration} \end{array} \right\}$ as guide to fluid administration

Possible Dire Consequences without Treatment: Encephalopathy ("Water intoxication").

Hyponatremia is a leading sign of water retention. It is highly sensitive though slightly non-specific for this purpose, as among several physical indicators of water gain by biological solutions. Increased presence of solvent is most directly detected as decreased activity of solutes in toto in an external osmometer. Although invariably called osmometers, instruments for this purpose variously detect the lowered osmotic pressure or boiling point of a solution, compared to pure solvent, or its raised vapor pressure or freezing point. Available devices usually evaluate one of the latter two properties, most often the latter.

It would be helpful to use an internal osmometer such as might be afforded by mean corpuscular volume (MCV) of red cells, that we already obtain routinely. To serve, indirectly, as an osmometer, MCV would have to increase reciprocally as external solute concentration [S] decreases, the constant product being N, the osmotic value of red cell internal solutes. The trouble with MCV is that the value of N fails to hold constant as it should when the red cells gain volume. However, this deviation from ideal behavior may not be critical if we presuppose, operationally, that hemoglobin is a relatively dilute solute in red cell water, and use it as an alternative to N. Instead of taking an assumed value for hemoglobin we measure hemoglobin concentration (MCH), saying that insofar as the amount of hemoglobin in the red cell is unchanged there will be a dependable relationship between falling concentration, MCH, and expanding volume, MCV. For every value of MCH, as was postulated for N, there is a constant product of MCV times a varying [S] so that $MCV[S] = MCH$. The solution for [S] is MCH/MCV which is the remaining and here preferable hematologic index, MCHC. This was found to be satisfactory for quantitating the dilution incident to a standard 20 ml./kg. water load. The requirements are that hematologic disease, if present, be in a steady state, and that recalibrated hematocrit tubes be used. Where automated techniques have been adopted for hematologic determinations, hematocrit is now a derived quantity obtained from Coulter red cell counts and from MCV estimations that are obtained directly; MCHC is obtained then from the hematocrit, thus derived, and from an independent hemoglobin determination.

A third indicator of water gain is the serum protein concentration [Pr]s. Exceptionally it might be preferable to [Na]s, the chief reason being thrift, in which case another advantage might creep in. The thriftiest way to do serum protein is by the specific gravity method with graduated copper sulfate solutions. Here it is always desirable to institute a check for spuriously low specific gravities, accomplished by observing a chilled tube of serum for lactescence. If this is present both [Pr]s and [Na]s will be spuriously low, when done by conventional techniques as well, because normal values will have assumed a 10% displacement of serum water by hydrophobic molecules, which may now have risen to 20%. A [Na]s which would have been 140 mM/l. in non-lactescent serum will be reported as 124mM/l.

A different variety of pseudohyponatremia occurs when protoplasmic water is displaced, into the interstitial spaces and into plasma, by raised glucose levels. This will be undetected with [Na]s, [Pr]s, or cryoscopic methods, unless the blood glucose value becomes known. Since glucose enters the red cell, its volume changes will retain a reciprocal relationship to dilution of the other plasma solutes, and hence may be of value in replacement therapy while the value of [Na]s as an indicator is still impaired.

References

Katz, M. A.: Hyperglycemia-induced hyponatremia. New Eng. J. Med., *290*:19, 1974.
Streeten, D. H. P., and Thorn, G. W.: Use of the mean corpuscular hemoglobin concentration as an index of erythrocyte hydration. J. Lab. & Clin. Med., *49*:661, 1957.

31. Inappropriate ADH (Primary Hyponatremia) (Syndrome of Inappropriate Secretion of Antidiuretic Hormone)

JOSEPH H. MAGEE

Causes: Non-osmotic vasopressinism of aberrant origin or of neurohypophyseal origin in the absence of alarm reaction and drugs.
1. Malignant Tumors:
   Carcinoma of lung. Carcinoma of duodenum. Carcinoma of pancreas. Thymoma.
2. Central nervous system disorders:
   Myelitis (Guillain-Barré). Meningitis. Encephalitis. Brain Abscess. Brain Tumor. Brain Injury. Subarachnoid Hemorrhage. Encephalopathy (Porphyria).
3. Lung Disorders:
   Pneumonia. Tuberculosis. Cavitation (Aspergillosis).

Early Manifestations: Body fluid dilution.
Paradoxical (inappropriate) antidiuresis: urine may be transiently, but never maximally, dilute accompanying variations (expansion or contraction) of body fluid volume rather than osmolality.
Adrenal function is normal. Circulatory function is normal.

Treatment: Water restriction. This must be stringent enough to attain a 2 to 4 kg. negative balance, frequently requiring limitation to 500 to 700 ml. fluid/day.

Possible Dire Consequences without Treatment: Encephalopathy ("Water Intoxication").

Reference

Bartter, F. C., and Schwartz, W. B.: The syndrome of inappropriate secretion of antidiuretic hormone. Am. J. Med., *42*:790, 1967.

32. Primary Hyponatremia (Cortisol Lack)

JOSEPH H. MAGEE

Cause: Cortisol lack, without associated mineralocorticoid lack, due to failure of pituitary stimulation.

Extrasellar cysts and craniopharyngiomas causing pituitary failure in childhood.

Intrasellar cysts, metastatic carcinoma.

Enlarging pituitary adenoma following degeneration or hemorrhage.

Hemorrhagic necrosis (postpartum) (Sheehan's syndrome).

Ischemic necrosis (basilar skull fracture, primary infection especially in diabetics, cavernous sinus thrombosis).

Granuloma (syphilis, tuberculosis, fungal, sarcoidosis, idiopathic).

Hemochromatosis.

Early Manifestations: Hyponatremia.

Normal [urea]s.

Sensitivity to forced fluids manifested by headache, blurred vision, muscle cramps, changes in sensorium.

Impaired water diuresis with standard 20 ml./kg. load.

Antidiuresis or curtailed diuresis following water load reversible by ethanol, especially if there has been pretreatment with submaximal doses of cortisone, unlike sustained vasopressinism in Schwartz-Bartter syndrome.

Sensitivity to narcotics, hypnotics, anesthetic agents, thyroid hormone, and operative stress.

Episodes of hypoglycemia, occasioned by anorexia and insufficient gluconeogenesis, must be differentiated from water intoxication.

Late Manifestations: Even in selective ACTH deficiency there may be amenorrhea, anorexia, lassitude, muscular weakness and postural hypotension, all reversed by cortisol replacement alone.

Evidence of hypogonadism (failure to lactate, amenorrhea, loss of pigmentation, body hair and libido) may antedate overt adrenal and thyroid deficiency by years.

Retarded growth rate and delayed puberty due to growth hormone deficiency.

Pituitary myxedema.

Reduced visual acuity, bitemporal hemianopia.

Treatment: Cortisol replacement: As much as 50 mg./day cortisone (10 mg. prednisone) may be required to restore response to water load. Hypopituitary patients appear to be unusually susceptible to iatrogenic cortisolism and the smallest doses affording freedom from hyponatremia, hypoglycemia and postural hypotension should be sought.

Precede elective surgery by 100 mg. cortisone acetate I.M. the night before and by 100 mg. hydrocortisone hemisuccinate I.V. on the morning of surgery.

Thyroid replacement, which potentially may precipitate adrenal crisis, angina, and cardiac circulatory failure, should follow adrenal replacement; beginning with gr. 1/8 (8 mg.) thyroid extract or 0.1 mg. 1-thyroxine, daily; and taking about six weeks to attain full dosage of up to gr. 3 (180 mg.).

Cyclic estrogen (0.5 to 3 mg. stilbestrol daily for twenty-one days) for female hypogonadism and breast atrophy; testosterone evanthate 300 mg. per month in males.

Surgery or radiotherapy of pituitary adenoma depending upon threat to vision. Since aldosterone secretion is partly independent of ACTH secretion, since nearly 98% of the anterior pituitary must be destroyed before panhypopituitarism appears, since the secretion of some pituitary hormones may be more affected than others, since diabetes insipidus may or may not be present, and since the dietary solute load is a significant factor—the development of this condition is quite variable; and the treatment must be highly individualized.

Possible Dire Consequences without Treatment: Water intoxication. Hypoglycemia. Adverse reactions to drugs. Postural hypotension. Adverse reactions to trauma, operative stress.

References

Agus, Z., and Goldberg, M.: Role of antidiuretic hormone in the abnormal water diuresis of anterior hypopituitarism in man. J. Clin. Invest., *50*:1478, 1971.

Garrod, O., and Burston, R. A.: The diuretic response to ingested water in Addison's disease and panhypopituitarism and the effect of cortisone thereon. Clin. Sci., *11*:113, 1952.

Goldberg, M., and Elkinton, J. R.: The role of vasopressin in the antidiuresis of anterior pituitary insufficiency. Jr. Am. Ass. Phys., *75*:129, 1962.

Rose, E. J., et al.: Aldosterone excretion in hypopituitarism and after hypophysectomy in man. Am. J. Med., *28*:229, 1960.

Wynn, V., and Garrod, O.: Spontaneous and induced water intoxication in two cases of hypopituitarism. Brit. Med. J., *1*:505, 1955.

33. Secondary Hyponatremia without Edema

Joseph H. Magee

Causes: Non-edematous salt-retaining states (oligemic reaction).
Blood sequestration by gravity, exercise, positive pressure breathing.
Relief of atrial distention.
Circulating protein loss.
(*a.*) External hemorrhage.
(*b.*) Concealed hemorrhage, hemolysis.
(*c.*) Inadequate synthesis.
(*d.*) Gut loss. (Constrictive pericarditis may produce this.)
(*e.*) Kidney loss.
Non-renal saline volume loss.
(*a.*) Skin: Heat exhaustion, burns.
(*b.*) Gut: vomiting, suctioning, external fistulae, enteritis (salmonella, shigella, cholera), internal fistulae, pancreatic cholera (pancreatic adenoma), villous, adenoma (colon).
(*c.*) Peritoneal: Paracenteses, dialyses.
(*d.*) Third space losses: Hepatic or portal venous hypertension, peritonitis, burns, hypodermolyses, toxic megacolon, idiopathic edema.
(*e.*) Surreptitious self-administration of diuretics.

Result: Hypoperfusion of organs generally including the kidney. Reflex by increased baroceptor vasomotor center and sympathetic activity, sympathetic dependent salt retention. Aldosteronism. Non-osmotic vasopressinism. Non-osmotic thirst.

Early Manifestations: Body fluid dilution, dilutional hyponatremia.
Underfilled circulation with valveless vein hypotension.
Arterial hypotension may be present.
Normal arterial pressure and edema may be present in nephrotic syndrome, enteropathy, and cirrhotic syndrome despite decreased plasma volume.
Prerenal (appropriate) oliguria with urine flow rate less than 480 ml./day (20 ml./hr., or 1/3 ml./min.).
Antinatriuresis with [Na]u usually under the [K]u usually over 20 mM/l.; and with [Cl]u usually under 50 mM/l. Approximately the reverse findings occur in oliguria due to intrinsic renal damage.

Treatment:

Monitor $\left\{ \begin{array}{l} \text{Urine sodium concentration} \\ \text{Serum sodium concentration} \end{array} \right\}$ as guide to fluid administration

Monitor $\left\{ \begin{array}{l} \text{Arterial pressure} \\ \text{Venous filling} \end{array} \right\}$ as guide to colloid administration

Possible Dire Consequences without Treatment: Inadequancy of circulation despite compensating mechanisms.

Reference

Greenberger, N. J., Tennenbaum, J. T., and Ruppert, R. D.: Protein-losing enteropathy associated with gastrointestinal allergy. Am. J. Med., *43*:777, 1967.

Pituitary Dysfunctions

34. Secondary Hyponatremia with Edema

JOSEPH H. MAGEE

Cause: Edematous salt-retaining states (non-cardiac circulatory congestion).

Result: Dilutional hyponatremia, due to continued intake of fluids and sodium salts; in oliguric acute renal failure, especially acute glomerular nephritis.

Early Manifestations: Body fluid dilution. Circulation overfilled (valveless vein hypertension) with retinal and facial edema and serous effusions preceding exertional dyspnea and orthopnea. Arterial pressure raised, initially in systole by preload (volume overload) with increased pulse pressure and stroke volume. Circulation time normal. Arteriovenous oxygen difference normal. Plasma volume increased with or without RBC volume increase.

Treatment: Water restriction. Peritoneal dialyses.

Possible Dire Consequences without Treatment: Hypertensive encephalopathy.. Ventricular dilatation, presaged by ventricular gallop with fatal pulmonary edema.

References

Davies, C. E.: Heart failure in acute nephritis. Quart. J. Med., *20*:163, 1951.
DeFagro, V., et al.: Circulatory changes in acute glomerulonephritis. Circulation, *20*:190, 1959.
Eichna, L. W., et al.: Non-cardiac circulatory congestion simulating congestive heart failure. J. Am. Assoc. Phys., *67*:72, 1954.
Peters, J. P.: Edema of acute nephritis. Am. J. Med., *14*:448, 1953.
Swan, R. C., and Merrill, J. P.: Clinical course of acute renal failure. Medicine, *32*:215, 1953.

35. Acromegaly

George Ross Fisher, III

Cause: Hypersecretion of eosinophil cells of the anterior pituitary.

Early Manifestations: Disease is well named. The hormone incites growth in all osseous organs where there is room to grow. This necessarily includes only the bones of extremities including the skull and jaw. The cartilages enlarge before the bones. Patient may present with arthritis, diabetes, peptic ulcer, goiter, hypertension, dental problems, or visual loss.

Treatment: Surgical excision or roentgen ray to the eosinophilic cells.

Possible Dire Consequences without Treatment: Disfigurement, loss of vision, compression of the hypothalamus, compression of the normal pituitary, sudden hemorrhage, death.

Acromegaly is a disfiguring disease. Treatment by surgery or radiation is effective, but the disfigurement is only partly improved. For this reason, it is important to discover and treat the condition as early as possible, rather than to wait until the condition has advanced to produce the facial appearance which is so commonly portrayed in textbook photographs, and described as "classical."

An acropolis is a city on a mountain peak, acromegaly is enlargement of the "peaks" of the body. That is, big feet, big hands, big nose, big ears. The soft tissues enlarge first, then cartilage, then bone. Only the soft tissue enlargement reliably improves with therapy. Such enlargement is perceived as enlarged finger and toe tips, with the distinguishing characteristic that the fingernails and toe nails (which do not enlarge) appear to be disproportionately small. The return of proper proportionality between nail and digit is a favorable sign that therapy is effective.

There are a great many normal people with large jaws, heavy frontal bossae, big feet and big hands. While the idea of acromegaly is properly considered briefly in such persons, it need not be considered seriously if the nose and ears are reasonably small or in proportion. The reasoning would be that the cartilaginous structures should enlarge before the bone structures, since growth is more rapid.

The creases of the forehead and the nasolabial folds are characteristically deepened into an appearance usually called lion-like. These creases are surprisingly resistant to therapy, and may be a clinical parallel to the usual experience that serum growth hormone levels do not universally return to completely normal values even when therapy seems otherwise to be quite satisfactory. This last disappointing fact has caused considerable uncertainty about which form of surgery or irradiation is best, and there is room for the argument that therapy has not improved much in fifty years.

The cartilages of the joints are affected early, and the irregular-hinge effect causes the patients to complain of, and be treated for, osteoarthritis. The ankles and the neck are usually most bothersome. This, too, may not completely improve with otherwise satisfactory therapy.

Although the incidence is only about 30%, there are a fair number of patients who present for treatment of peptic ulcer, hypertension, goiter, or diabetes. In a rare case, the diabetes may be extraordinarily insulin-resistant, requiring thousands of units daily.

The patients develop spreading and protrusion of the teeth, which contributes to the appearance of grossness about the lips and mouth. The teeth may be removed before the diagnosis is made, but the appearance can be quite typical. A perceptive patient will complain that he can no longer chew lettuce.

The diagnostic measure which should be employed first is a lateral roentgenogram of the skull, since 80% of patients will have enlargement of the sella turcica at the earliest time the disease is suspected. Enlargement of the nasal sinuses is usually also noted. Carefully measured, the thickening of heel pad is also often helpful, and roentgenograms of the heel have value in the assessment of therapy.

There is confirmatory value to a glucose tolerance or thyroid function studies, but when normal they do not exclude the disease. The chemical test of most value is the serum growth hormone level, which may be elevated or normal, but which characteristically does not respond to sleep, the administration of glucose, or insulin.

Once the diagnosis of acromegaly is made, there are several complications which may be present or may develop later. The pituitary tumor may compress the other contents of the sella turcica, causing simultaneous hypopituitarism. The tumor may expand upward against the optic chiasm, causing bitemporal hemianopsia. The tumor may rarely undergo hemorrhage causing either sudden neurological signs, or bloody spinal fluid. And the tumor may continue to grow in size, even though it does not produce growth hormone. There is general reluctance to perform pneumoencephalograms because of the morbidity of the procedure, but this should always be considered when a person with acromegaly is not doing well, since arteriograms and scans are of little value in midline lesions.

Reference

Roth, J., et al.: Acromegaly and other disorders of growth hormone secretion. Ann. Intern. Med., *66*:760, 1967.

36. Hypopituitarism, Sheehan's Syndrome

GEORGE ROSS FISHER, III

Cause: Loss of more than 90% of pituitary cells, congenital or from tumor. Necrosis secondary to shock at the time of obstetrical delivery.

Early Manifestations: Vague, not feeling right, later amenorrhea, and others. Loss of axillary and pubic hair. Hypoglycemia. Decrease of general skin pigmentation.

Treatment: Correction of secondary hypothyroidism, hypogonadism or hypoadrenocorticism— In children, administration of human growth hormone will induce some linear growth. If pregnancy can be induced, it may be curative.

Possible Dire Consequences without Treatment: Lack of proper growth, diabetes, hypogonadism, Addison's disease, death.

Textbooks have finally stopped including a picture of an emaciated victim of what was called Simmond's disease, but it may be another generation before the concept dies out. Patients with hypopituitarism are, in fact, usually slightly overweight.

The concept of emaciated hypopituitarism has persisted as long as it has because starvation will frequently cause cessation of menstruation, and occasionally the amenorrhea will persist after the patient regains weight. The emotional disturbance which is behind anorexia nervosa is usually severe enough to be obvious, particularly when the patients begin to resist feeding efforts by deviousness or even outright deceit. The important issue to recognize in anorexia nervosa is not the endocrine one, but the startlingly high mortality and suicide rate.

Sheehan was the first to clarify the clinical features of hypopituitarism, which include loss of axillary and pubic hair, as well as loss of skin pigmentation. Sheehan also identified the usual cause, which is hemorrhage in the course of a stormy obstetrical delivery. The patient with Sheehan's syndrome will state that she has had no menstrual periods since a stormy delivery, and that she was unable to nurse the baby. The hair loss is reported in terms like "they shaved me for the delivery, and the hair never grew back."

To develop hypopituitarism, the patient must lose 90% of the functioning pituitary cells. This degree of reserve in the gland makes it possible to have states of borderline or incomplete hypopituitarism which may be difficult to recognize. Since the best hope for cure is renewed pituitary hyperplasia of pregnancy, the diagnosis of borderline Sheehan's syndrome is an important one. These patients recognize that they have "never been right" since a delivery, and their natural reaction is to fear further pregnancies. For his part, the physician may have the misconception that further pregnancy would be impossible, and thus considers neither the diagnosis nor its remedy.

Disregarding congenital defects in the anterior pituitary (which quite often prove to be defects in the hypothalamus), the usual cause of hypopituitarism in regions of good obstetrical practice is tumor-compression of the gland within the tight sella turcica. In children, the usual tumor is a suprasellar cyst, in adults it is usually a chromophobe adenoma. A lateral roentgenogram of the skull will demonstrate expansion of the sella in more than 80% of such cases. It is important to extend the investigation to a pneumoencephalogram, since the size and location of the tumor is quite unpredictable. The patient may lose any or all of the pituitary hormones, and so may be dwarfed (in children), myxedematous, eunuchoid, amenorrheic or addisonian. It is curious that they do not develop diabetes insipidus unless cortisone is given, and then the polyuria may be astonishing within forty-eight hours.

The pituitary may be compressed through damming and dissection by the "subarachnoid" fluid. This situation is called the "empty sella syndrome," and its recognition through pneumoencephalography is important. It is quite unsatisfactory to decide upon either radiotherapy or neurosurgery until this point is clarified. Ever since Harvey Cushing interested himself in pituitary tumors, there has been a doctrine that neurosurgery is mandatory if visual field cuts imply that there is pressure on the optic chiasm. By implication, radiotherapy is indicated for the smaller adenomas. However, transnasal approaches are now so simplified that the recommendation of surgery is easier in all cases. In fact, biopsy of the pituitary may be desirable in many cases, even if they are treated by radiotherapy.

The laboratory tests for hypopituitarism are numerous, and satisfying in their demonstration of physiologic principles. But they are all somewhat invalidated by the generalized effects of myxedema. Almost any myxedematous patient will have some impairment in production of urinary hormones after ACTH administration. If possible, hypothyroidism should be corrected before the tests are run. The administration of metyrapone blocks the adrenal production of hydrocortisone, hence stimulating ACTH production. The plasma corticoids are best measured before and after metyrapone administration in children. The twenty-four-hour urinary corticoids are less equivocal in adult patients. If the patient fails to respond to metyrapone, it must be demonstrated that his adrenal can respond to ACTH administration. This test, of course, continues to leave uncertainty about the hypothalamic corticotrophin-releasing factor.

A similar maneuver can be employed using plasma prolactin values before and after thorazine or L-dopa administration. This test has not yet had the test of time, and prolactin determinations are difficult to obtain. However, normal response requires an intact hypothalamus, and there are thus advantages which may be useful.

The administration of hypothalamic TSH-releasing factor (measuring plasma TSH, thyroxin or both) may well become a useful measure of all three components of the system. However, it should be remembered that the thyroid system may be spared by a tumor, or on the contrary it may be the only pituitary function impaired.

Hypothalamic TRH (thyrotropin releasing factor) is available in the United States, but gonadotropin releasing hormones are not. Presumably they will be useful for testing when they are released by the Food and Drug Administration.

The administration of cortisone to precipitate diabetes insipidus is a useful test when the posterior pituitary is involved, since the drug is easily available, and urine volume is simple to measure.

Plasma testosterone may be measured before and after gonadotropin administration. Obviously, this test is of value only when the testosterone level is low, and has only negative implications.

Plasma growth hormone may be measured, before and after the patient falls asleep (sleep is a stimulus to secretion). The value may be measured in the fasting state (when it is high) and again after administering glucose (when it should fall).

In the special case of a post-menopausal woman, a fairly easy test of pituitary function is available. The menopause appears to be a failure of the ovaries, and consequently the unopposed pituitary produces excessive amounts of gonadotrophin. Therefore, a low gonadotrophin titer in the urine of a menopausal woman may be taken as a sign of underfunction of the pituitary.

The pituitary appears to produce its hormones in spurts, some of which fluctuate in a diurnal manner and some of which are triggered by falling asleep (growth), fasting (growth), stress (ACTH), and other undetermined forces such as the monthly spike of LH production in fertile women. This characteristically irregular production of hormone means that a single determination of any hormone is of doubtful significance. It is necessary to test the pituitary under circumstances which are known to trigger secretion of a particular hormone, and to compare that value with a baseline value under circumstances when minimal secretion is expected. If the target gland reacts promptly, as the adrenal cortex does, one can measure the blood level of target hormone. Therefore, a plasma corticoid level is normally high in the morning, and low in the evening. Disruption of the diurnal pattern is therefore a good clue to pituitary dysfunction.

The plasma thyroxin value will not serve for this type of approach, because thyroxin remains in the blood for too long after secretion.

Obviously, the assessment of pituitary function is difficult, expensive, and subject to error. It probably is not practical to evaluate every pituitary hormone, but better to concentrate on a few which are easy to measure. Our limited goals should be:

1. To confirm the diagnosis of pituitary tumor, which can be strongly suspected from enlargement of the sella or visual field cuts.

2. To confirm a history of difficulties dating from an obstetrical delivery.

3. To establish whether end-organ failure (amenorrhea, eunuchoidism, hypo-adrenalism, or myxedema) is pituitary in origin. The absence of urinary gonado-tropin, or the inability to respond to metyrapone, or TSH, should serve for this purpose.

4. To evaluate dwarfism. In this case, the measurement of growth hormone before and after falling asleep is a direct approach. It must be admitted that our understanding of the pathogenesis of growth failure is limited, at present. The early reports of good growth following growth hormone administration are now somewhat tempered.

5. To evaluate the degree of underfunction which may accompany the "empty" sella syndrome. For the most part, these cases are discovered on routine roentgeno-grams of the skull taken for other purposes. The pneumoencephalogram shows that the enlarged sella is not due to a tumor, but it is an exaggeration to say that the sella is empty. Rather, the incompetent diaphragm sellae allows the pulsatile subarach-noid fluid to balloon the walls of the sella. Recalling the fact that 80 to 90% of the pituitary can be destroyed before hypofunction appears, it would appear that this type of compression is less destructive than tumor growth. In any event, most patients with the "empty" sella syndrome have no demonstrable degree of functional impairment. If growth is complete and menstrual function is normal, it is enough to be satisfied with a normal PBI or T-4, as well as a good response to metyrapone. Even the adrenal studies are superfluous if the patient is hypertensive. For some reason, most empty sella patients are obese, hypertensive, middle-aged women.

It would be very helpful if the components of pituitary failure made their appear-ance in a regular sequence. But they do not. Any combination of hormones may be missing or normal. Growth and prolactin are the hormones most commonly lost. TSH and ACTH are the hormones whose loss may give greatest clinical danger. Since it may be unpractical to measure all hormones, before and after a particular stimulus, it may be better to concentrate on the ones which matter. A child who is growing normally has enough growth hormone, and an adult does not need it. A fertile person need not worry about gonadotropin function, nor a postmenopausal woman, either.

Therefore, a metyrapone test will establish adrenal function and reserve. Any of several thyroid tests will establish the condition of TSH. Other tests are not to be discouraged, but typically they do not alter the clinical management.

Reference

Brasel, J. A., et al.: An evaluation of seventy-five patients with hypopituitarism beginning in childhood. Am. J. Med., *38*:484, 1965.

Chapter XII

Adrenal and Pseudoadrenal Disorders

Introduction

Francis H. Sterling

The syndromes of adrenocortical excess and deficiency are numerous. At two extremes are Addison's disease, with total deficiency of glucocorticoids, mineralocorticoids and adrenal androgens, and Cushing's disease with excesses of all these. Far more complex (the adrenogenital syndromes) are instances where excesses of certain hormones are combined with deficiencies of others. Few physicians have occasion to memorize the arcane details of steroid nomenclature and metabolic pathways. Use of the accompanying color-coded "road ways" in the discussions that follow is, however, recommended because:

(1) When visualized in this way an account of the clinical presentation diagnosis and treatment of the several adrenogenital syndromes is readily followed.
(2) The laboratory aspects of the diagnosis of adrenal and pituitary diseases depend upon understanding the relationships depicted in the diagram.
(3) Many features of testicular and ovarian diseases can also be understood in terms of the same biosynthetic pathways (Fig. XII–1).

To use Figure XII–1 first look at its upper left corner, and note cholesterol. Cholesterol is included for two reasons: It is a precursor of the steroids (although most steroids can be synthesized from acetate) and it shows the numbering of steroid compounds. Certain positions are of special interest and will be discussed. These include the 3 position in the A ring, the 11 position in the C ring and the 17 position in the D ring. One would think that the carbon coming off the top from 17 would be 18, but the 18 and 19 carbons are represented by little sticks which are methyl groups between the C and D rings and between the A and B rings respectively. The carbon arising from the top of the 17 position is 20 and the next carbon is 21. The 17, 20, 21 side chain configuration is important in clinical testing as will be shown below. Many of the steroids on this chart have 21 carbons while others have the 20, 21 carbon side chain removed, leaving 19 carbons. C-21 compounds include glucocorticoids, mineralocorticoids and progestational hormones. C-19 compounds include the androgens, and C-18 compounds (not shown) include the estrogens.

Figure XII–1 as labeled in its upper right-hand corner, is divided into two sections. Inside the square are steroids in the adrenal cortex or plasma, those outside are their urinary metabolites. Colors indicate the several varieties of urinary metabolites as follows:

GREEN (17-KS)	17-Keto-Steroids	Zimmerman Reaction	10–20 mg./day ♂ 5–15 mg./day ♀
RED (17-OHCS)	17-Hydroxy-Steroids	Porter-Silber Reaction	2–10 mg./day
BLUE & RED (17-KGS)	17-Ketogenic Steroids	Norymbersky Reaction	8–25 mg./day

The compounds which are colored *green* are the principal neutral 17-ketosteroids (17-KS) and are measured by the Zimmerman reaction. These compounds have a ketone at the 17 position and referred to, unfortunately, as the adrenal androgens. Only the compound at the top, dehydroepiandrosterone, has any androgenic activity and therefore, these compounds are better thought of as by-products of the synthesis of hydrocortisone. There are other 17-ketosteroids such as estrone which are not measured because they are phenolic rather than neutral. The normal values for the urinary neutral 17-ketosteroids in most laboratories are 10 to 20 mg. per twenty-four hours in males and 5 to 15 mg. per twenty-four hours in females. The values are higher in males for two reasons: (1) men are bigger than women and the amount of steroids produced during a twenty-four hour period is proportional to body weight (large or fat people produce more steroids than small or thin people). (2) One-third of the 17-ketosteroids in the male are of testicular origin. Testosterone is not a 17-ketosteroid. The testicle produces 17-ketosteroids in the process of making testosterone.

The *red* compounds are the Porter-Silber chromogens (17-OHCS). The essential feature of a Porter-Silber chromogen is the presence of a 17-hydroxy, 20-keto, 21-hydroxy side chain. Note that all red compounds have this dihydroxy-acetone configuration. In normal individuals, the Porter-Silber chromogens in the urine are for the most part tetrahydro E and F with small amounts of other compounds. The normal values for the Porter-Silber chromogens vary with the laboratory but are generally in the neighborhood of 2 to 10 mg. per twenty-four hours. In many laboratories when a plasma cortisol is ordered, this same colorimetric reaction is performed on plasma. In normal individuals, the only plasma Porter-Silber chromogen present in significant amounts is cortisol (compound F). However, in certain disease states, the immediate precursor 11-desoxy cortisol (compound S) may also be present and will be measured. A small fraction of cortisol is excreted as urinary free cortisol. Presently it is preferable to the other urine tests in the diagnosis of Cushing's disease. Normal values are less than 120 micrograms per twenty-four hours with some variation depending on the laboratory.

The *red* plus the *blue* compounds are the 17-ketogenic steroids (17-KGS) and are measured by the Norymbersky reaction. Do not confuse 17-keto-steroids with 17-ketogenic steroids. In order to be ketogenic, the compound must have a 17-hydroxyl and at the 20 position either a ketone or hydroxyl group. The term "17-ketogenic steroid" is derived from the method of the test. Very simply, the procedure is as follows: an aliquot for the twenty-four-hour urine is assayed for the green compounds, the neutral 17-ketoste-roids (Zimmerman reaction). Subsequently, another aliquot of the same urine is oxidized and the Zimmerman reaction repeated. The red and blue compounds are readily oxidized by splitting off the side chain and are con-verted into new 17-ketosteroids. The first value is subtracted from the second and the difference is reported as the 17-ketogenic steroids.

Example:

Zimmerman reaction after oxidation	35 mg.	(total steroids)
Initial Zimmerman reaction	15 mg.	(ketosteroids)
	20 mg.	(ketogenic steroids)

In normal individuals, the principal 17-ketogenic steroids are tetrahydro E and F plus cortol and cortolone. The normal values are about 8 to 25 mg. per twenty-four hours (double the Porter-Silber chromogens). What is measured when urinary 17-hydroxysteroids are requested? Certain labora-tories measure the Porter-Silber chromogens and others the ketogenic steroids. It is important to know which test is used if a patient is being evaluated for virilization. In a patient with 21-hydroxylase deficiency, the "17-hydroxy-steroids" would be low if the Porter-Silber reaction were used but high if 17-ketogenic steroids were measured (see below). Hopefully, in the near future these difficulties can be obviated by measuring the individual com-pounds.

Let us now look at the urinary metabolites along the bottom of the chart. Each compound is identical to the parent compound above, except for the fact that the double bonds are now broken (reduced). If the double bond in the A ring is reduced, two hydrogens are added and the compound is re-ferred to as dihydro. If, in addition, the double bond at the 3 position is reduced, two more hydrogens are added and the compound is referred to as tetrahydro (*e.g.* tetrahydro E and F). Finally, by reducing the double bond at the 20 position, a hexahydro compound results. The hexahydro com-pounds have special names such as pregnanediol, pregnanetriol, cortolone and cortol.

Cortisone (compound E) is shown outside the square because only minimal amounts of cortisone are secreted as such and most is a metabolite of the liver. The only difference between corti*sol* and corti*sone* is the presence of a hydroxyl group on the former and a ketone in the latter at the 11 position. (Note tetrahydro E and F and their metabolites cortolone and cortol.)

Now locate progesterone at the center of the chart. Let us consider how the adrenal cortex transforms progesterone to cortisol (hydrocortisone). This involves three enzymatic steps. The first is the addition of a hydroxyl group at the 17 position. The enzyme 17-alpha hydroxylase is indicated by the *yellow* X-s. If this enzyme is missing, the Biglieri (hypertensive hypogonadal) syndrome results. The clinical features are discussed below. It is easy to

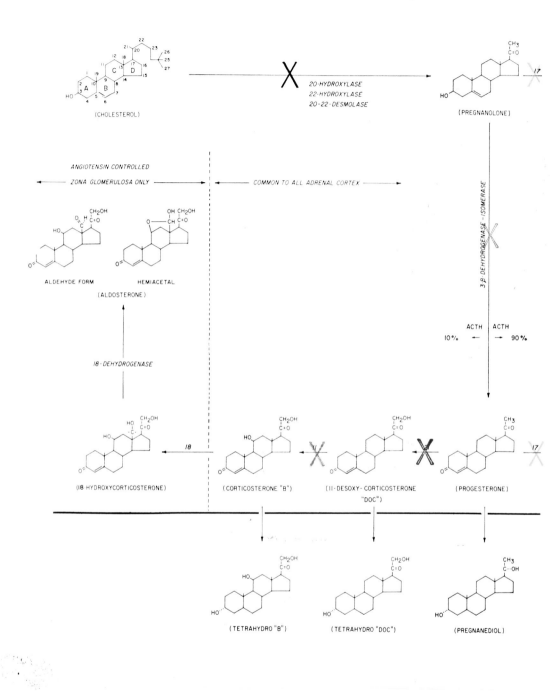

Fig. XII-I.

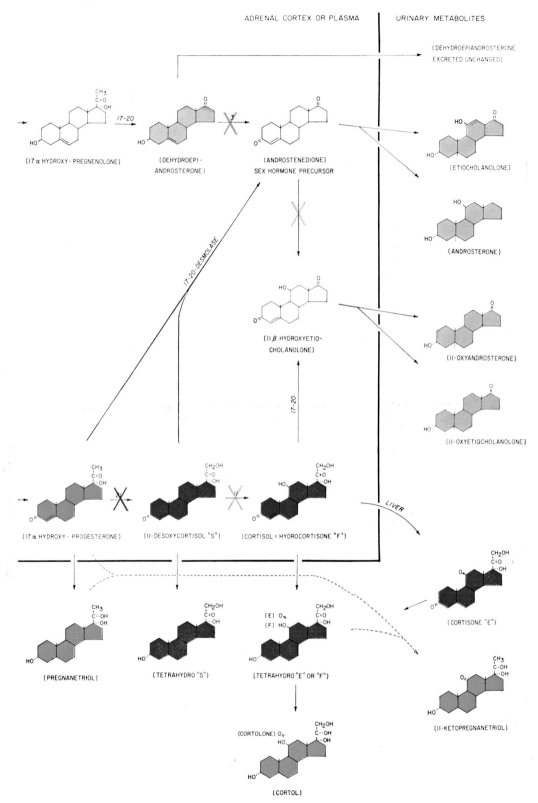

ADRENAL CORTEX OR PLASMA   URINARY METABOLITES

(DEHYDROEPIANDROSTERONE
EXCRETED UNCHANGED)

(17 α HYDROXY- PREGNENOLONE)

17-20

(DEHYDROEPI-
ANDROSTERONE)

3

(ANDROSTENEDIONE)
SEX HORMONE PRECURSOR

(ETIOCHOLANOLONE)

(ANDROSTERONE)

17-20-DESMOLASE

(11 β HYDROXYETIO-
CHOLANOLONE)

17-20

(11-OXYANDROSTERONE)

(11-OXYETIOCHOLANOLONE)

(17 α HYDROXY- PROGESTERONE)

(11-DESOXYCORTISOL "S")

U

(CORTISOL = HYDROCORTISONE "F")

LIVER

(CORTISONE "E")

(PREGNANETRIOL)

(TETRAHYDRO "S")

(E) O
(F) HO

(TETRAHYDRO "E" OR "F")

(11-KETOPREGNANETRIOL)

(CORTOLONE) O

(CORTOL)

Fig. XII-I (*Continued*).

see that in this syndrome, the excretion of Porter-Silber chromogens, 17-keto-steroids and ketogenic steroids will all be low since no compounds to the right of the yellow X's can be synthesized. The compound resulting, 17-hydroxy-progesterone, is physiologically inert. The next step involves the addition of hydroxyl group at the 21 position. Red X's mark the site of action of 21-hydroxylase, a deficiency of which results in the common adrenogenital syndrome which may be partial or complete. Partial deficiency results in virilization. Complete deficiency results in virilization plus salt wasting since all mineralocorticoids require 21-hydroxylation. It can be seen that a block in 21-hydroxylase would result in low Porter-Silber chromogens but elevated 17-ketogenic steroids due to the accumulation of large amounts of 17-hydroxyprogesterone. The reason for virilization is as follows: Since the cortisol levels are low, the ACTH secretion is not inhibited. Excessive ACTH results in hyperplastic adrenals which produce large quantities of 17-hydroxyprogesterone. This steroid is metabolized in two ways; it can be reduced (arrow down) to pregnanetriol, or via side chain cleavage (arrow up), changed to androstenedione. Special attention should be paid to andro-stenedione. This compound is the precursor of testosterone and all natural estrogens. It is a 17-ketosteroid but is not colored green because it does not contribute significantly to the urinary 17-ketosteroids. The only difference between androstenedione and testosterone is that testosterone has a hydroxyl group rather than a ketone on the 17 position. The conversion of androste-nedione to testosterone is a relatively simple reaction and readily occurs in the liver and elsewhere. The secretion of androstenedione is, therefore, tantamount to the secretion of testosterone, hence the virilization in this syndrome. The steroid to the right of 17-hydroxyprogesterone is called compound S or 11-desoxycortisol. It is a weak mineralocorticoid.

The final step in the synthesis of hydrocortisone involves the addition of the hydroxyl at the 11 position. The green X's on the chart mark the site of action of 11-beta hydroxylase. If this enzyme is missing, the hypertensive adreno-genital syndrome results due to the accumulation of mineralocorticoid (specifically 11-desoxycorticosterone, DOC). The principal steroid produced by the adrenal in this disease is compound S which is metabolized to the virilizing androstenedione. The clinical manifestations of this syndrome are discussed below. It can be noted at a glance that Porter-Silber chromogens, 17-ketogenic steroids and 17-ketosteroids will all be elevated.

Let us now direct our attention to the left-hand side of the chart and to those adrenal steroids (in man only 10%) in which the 11-hydroxylase stop, indi-cated by yellow X's is skipped. As before, locate progesterone in the center of the chart. Moving left (red arrow) its first hydroxylation is in the 21 position. The resulting compound 21-hydroxyprogesterone, also known as 11-desoxycorticosterone or DOC is a potent mineralocorticoid. The next step, involving addition (green arrow) of a hydroxyl group in the 11-position, forms corticosterone, the principal glucocorticoid in some species, including the rat. In man this compound has little physiologic action and is a poor inhibitor of the pituitary (the ability of a steroid to inhibit the pituitary is directly proportional to its glucocorticoid activity). The principal reason for portraying this pathway to the left is that it leads to the production of aldos-terone. The conversion of corticosterone to aldosterone involves enzymes uniquely present in the part of the adrenal (zona glomerulosa) regulated primarily by angiotensin II rather than by ACTH. The first step (18-hydroxylation) produces 18-hydroxycorticosterone; removal of two hydrogen atoms by the enzyme 18-dehydrogenase yields an aldehyde group in the 18 position, hence the designation aldosterone. A hemiacetal configuration between the 11 and 18 positions is assumed in body fluids.

1. Addison's Disease

FRANCIS H. STERLING

Cause: Tuberculosis   Hemorrhagic necrosis
Histoplasmosis   Idiopathic atrophy
Autoimmune disease   Congenital absence
Amyloidosis   Therapeutic adrenalectomy
Metastatic carcinoma   o,p' – DDD

Early Manifestations: Plasma cortisol very low or zero. Plasma ACTH very high (normal 0.1 to 0.4 mμ/100 ml.). Plasma cortisol very low after ACTH. Low [Na]s; high [K]s, [Ca]s; azotemia. Renal salt loss. Fatigue, weakness, postural hypotension, low venous and arterial pressures, exaggerated decreased circulation reflexes. Anorexia, salt craving, hypoglycemia. Weight loss. Vitiligo. Pigmentation of skin, mucous membranes, hair. Eosinophilia. Delayed excretion of standard water load.

Treatment: Hydrocortisone 30 mg./day. 9α—fluorohydrocortisone 0.05 to 0.1 mg./day.

Possible Dire Consequences without Treatment: Fatal adrenal crisis with trauma, anesthesia, parturition, surgery, infection.

In Addison's disease all measurements of adrenocortical steroids are low. When suspected, the diagnosis is established by demonstrating that there is no rise in adrenal steroid production following the administration of 0.25 mg./25 units of synthetic ACTH intramuscularly or intravenously. In the screening version of the test, plasma cortisol is measured prior to administration of ACTH and again thirty to sixty minutes later. If the patient does not have a significant increase in plasma cortisol following ACTH, it may indicate Addison's disease or adrenal atrophy due to long standing hypopituitarism or even chronic illness. It is then necessary to give 0.25 mg. ACTH by intravenous drip over an eight-hour period on each at least two days. Plasma cortisol is remeasured at the end of the second infusion; failure to increase proves the diagnosis of Addison's disease.

References

Addison, T.: On the Constitutional and Local Effects of Disease of the Suprarenal Capsules. London, Highley, 1855.

Blijjard, R. M., et al.: Adrenal antibodies in Addison's disease. Lancet, *2*:901, 1962.

Crispell, K. R., et al.: Addison's disease associated with histoplasmosis. Am. J. Med., *20*:23, 1956.

Forsyth, C. C., Forbes, M., and Curnings, J. N.: Adrenocortical atrophy and diffuse cerebral sclerosis. Arch. Dis. Child., *46*:273, 1971.

Migeon, C. J., et al.: Study of adrenal function in children with meningitis. Pediatrics, *40*:163, 1967.

Migeon, C. J., et al.: The syndrome of congenital adrenogenital unresponsiveness to ACTH. Pediatrics Research, *2*:501, 1968.

Rowntree, L. G., and Snell, A. M.: A Clinical Study of Addison's Disease. Philadelphia, W. B. Saunders Co., 1931.

2. Lipoid Adrenal Hyperplasia

FRANCIS H. STERLING

Cause: Congenitally deficient adrenal and gonadal steroidogenesis due to enzymatic block in cleaving cholesterol side chain, located by black "x" in Figure XII–1.

Result: Combined hypoadrenal and hypogonadal syndrome:
Inability to synthesize pregnenolone, precursor of gonadal steroids and of adrenal androgens, cortisol and aldosterone.
Accumulation of cholesterol and lipid in adrenal cortex, gonads, male genital tract.
Congenital adrenal and gonadal hyperplasia due to pituitary stimulation.
Incomplete masculinization of genotypic males due to androgen deficiency *in utero* (male pseudohermaphroditism).

Early Manifestations: Failure to thrive. Salt-wasting. 17 KS and 17 OHCS absent from urine. Ambiguous external genitalia with cryptorchidism, hypospadias and incomplete labial fusion in genetic males.

Treatment: Glucocorticoid and mineralocorticoid hormone replacement.

Possible Dire Consequences without Treatment: Addisonian crisis.

This disease is probably due to a deficiency of 20-hydroxylation in both adrenal and gonadal tissue. Since no androgen is made *in utero*, failure of labial fusion causes genotypic males to have the external genitalia of a female. However, the fetal testicle has been able to make the protein known as "organizing substance," with regression of the Müllerian system, so that the vagina is short and without a uterus and fallopian tubes. The syndrome is extremely rare, usually fatal and is included here for the sake of completeness.

References

Camacho, A. M., et al.: Congenital adrenogenital hyperplasia due to a deficiency of one of the enzymes involved in the biosynthesis of pregnenolone. J. Clin. End. Metab., *28*:153, 1968.

Prader, A., and Gustner, H. P.: Das syndrom des pseudohermaphroditismus masculinus bei kongenitaler nebenniere winden hyperplasie ohne and regeniiber production. Helvet. Ped Acta, *10*:397, 1955.

3. 3-Beta-"ol" Syndrome

Francis H. Sterling

Cause: Congenitally deficient adrenal and gonadal steroidogenesis due to enzymatic block (3-beta-hydroxysteroid dehydrogenase-isomerase) located by the blue "x's" in Figure XII–1.

Result: Combined hypo- and hyperadrenal syndrome. Hypogonadal syndrome. Inability to synthesize progesterone, precursor of gonadal steroids, and of adrenal △ 4,3 keto androgens, cortisol and aldosterone.
Accumulation of △ 5,3 hydroxy adrenal androgens and metabolites.
Congenital adrenal and gonadal hyperplasia due to pituitary stimulation.
Virilization of genotypic females *in utero* by adrenal androgen; incomplete masculinization *in utero* of genotypic males (female and male pseudohermaphroditism).

Early Manifestations: Failure to thrive. Salt-wasting. 17-KS and 17-OHCS low in urine. 17-KS entirely due to △ 5,3 hydroxy metabolites, 25% being dehydroepiandrosterone. Ambiguous external genitalia.

Treatment: Glucocorticoid and mineralocorticoid hormone replacement.

Possible Dire Consequences without Treatment: Addisonian crisis. Continued mild virilization in absence of replacement doses of cortisol or equivalent.

A block in steroidogenesis at this point was first described by Bongiovanni and colleagues. As can be seen in Figure XII–1, inability to make androstenedione, the essential precursor of testosterone and the estrogens can result from a block at the site of *either* the blue or the black "x's". With a block at the blue "x's" as in the present instance, the adrenal can and does make large quantities of dehydroepiandrosterone, which is a weak androgen. This results in some labial fusion and slight development of the phallus in both sexes. The syndrome is named, not according to the enzyme that is missing, but rather according to the steroids which occur in the urine. With block at the two blue "x's", it can be seen that three compounds will accumulate: pregnenolone, 17-hydroxypregnenolone, and dehydroepiandrosterone. All of these compounds have a hydroxyl group at the 3 position; hence, the designation as the 3-beta-"ol" adrenogenital syndrome.

References

Bongiovanni, A. M., et al.: Disorders of steroid hormone biogenesis. Recent Prog. Hormone Res., *23*:375, 1967.
Bongiovanni, A. M., and Root, A. W.: The adrenogenital syndrome. New Eng. J. Med., *268*:1283, 1342, 1391, 1963.
Janne, O., Perheentupee, J., and Vikho, R.: Plasma and urinary steroids in an eight year old boy with 3B-hydroxysteroid dehydrogenase deficiency. J. Clin. End. Metab., *31*:162, 1970.

4. Hypertensive Hypogonadal Syndrome

Francis H. Sterling

Cause: Congenitally deficient adrenal and gonadal steroidogenesis due to enzymatic block (17-hydroxylase) located by yellow "x's" in Figure XII-1.

Synonym: Biglieri's syndrome.

Results: Combined hypo- and hyperadrenal syndrome.
Inability to hydroxylate 17 positions of pregnenolone and progesterone, precursor compounds of gonadal steroids, of adrenal androgens and of cortisol.
Unblocked C21 steroidogenesis with accumulation of DOC and corticosterone.
Congenital adrenal and gonadal hyperplasia due to pituitary stimulation.
Incomplete masculinization *in utero* of genotypic males (male pseudohermaphroditism).
Reversible renin and aldosterone suppression due to mineralocorticoid (DOC) excess.

Early Manifestations: Hypertension due to mineralocorticoid excess.
Hypokalemic alkalosis due to mineralocorticoid excess.
Low urine 17-KS, 17-KGS, 17-OHCS and aldosterone levels.
Raised urine pregnanediol, tetrahydro DOC and tetrahydrocorticosterone levels.
Sexual infantilism with absence of menarche, breast development, axillary and pubic hair in females.
Female external genitalia, short vagina, absent uterus in genetic males.

Treatment: Adults: Hydrocortisone 30 mg. per day.
Children: Hydrocortisone 10 to 20 mg. per day.
Adults: Cyclic or combined estrogen and progesterone to induce menses (in genotypic females) and small amount of androgen to induce secondary sexual characteristics.

Possible Dire Consequences without Treatment: Hypertension. Periodic paralyses, ventricular escape rhythms, kaliopenic nephropathy.

Since no androgen can be made in this syndrome, all individuals both male and female will have female external genitalia. The disease is not life-threatening due to the production of excess mineralocorticoid. Since the enzyme is missing from the testicle and ovary as well as the adrenal, the patient will be unable to make sex hormones and will not enter puberty. The usual clinical presentation is that of a "girl" with primary amenorrhea, absence of breast development and absence of pubic and axillary hair, who on physical examination has hypertension. Sodium retention and potassium wasting are, however, not due to excess aldosterone but rather due to excess DOC. The aldosterone levels are low for the following reasons:

(*a.*) Since hydrocortisone cannot be adequately synthesized, there is no inhibition of ACTH.

(*b.*) Excess ACTH secretion results in hyperplasia of the adrenal cortex.

(*c.*) Large amounts of DOC are secreted as well as corticosterone.

(*d.*) DOC causes renal retention of sodium and potassium wasting.

(*e.*) Sodium retention results in expanded plasma volume, increased renal profusion and suppression of renin production.

(*f.*) Suppressed renin production results in decreased conversion of angiotensinogen to angiotensin I and angiotensin II.

(*g.*) The enzymatic pathways culminating in the conversion of corticosterone to aldosterone, present only in the zona glomerulosa are regulated by angiotensin II.

The treatment of the 17-hydroxylase deficiency is replacement doses of hydrocortisone. This is effective in correcting hypertension because it inhibits ACTH secretion and results in decreased production of DOC. In order to get secondary sex characteristics, however, estrogens must also be administered. If the patient is a genotypic male (XY), the individual must be continued to be regarded as a female.

The diagnosis of the 17-hydroxylase deficiency is established when patients with the above syndrome are found to have low 17-OHCS, 17-KGS and 17-KS, and elevated pregnanediol levels. Special techniques are necessary to measure tetrahydrocorticosterone and tetrahydro DOC, the metabolites of corticosterone and DOC respectively.

References

Biglieri, E. G., Herron, M. A., and Brust, N.: 17-hydroxylase deficiency in man. J. Clin. Invest., *45*:1946, 1966.

Goldsmith, O., Solomon, D. H., and Horton, R.: Hypogonadism and mineralocorticoid excess: The 17-hydroxylase deficiency syndrome. New Eng. J. Med., *277*:673, 1967.

Mallin, S. R.: Congenital adrenal hyperplasia secondary to 17-hydroxylase deficiency. Ann. Intern. Med., *70*:69, 1969.

New, M.: Male pseudohermaphroditism due to 17α-hydroxylase deficiency. J. Clin. Invest., *49*:1930, 1970.

5. Common Adrenogenital Syndrome

Francis H. Sterling

Cause: Congenitally deficient steroidogenesis due to enzymatic block (^{21}-hydroxylase) located by red "x's" in Figure XII–1.

Result: Combined hypo- and hyperadrenal syndrome.

Inability to synthesize precursor compounds (11-deoxycortisol, substance S) of cortisol and (DOC) of corticosterone and aldosterone.

Unblocked C17 steroidogenesis with excess adrenal androgen formation.

Virilization of genotypic females *in utero* by adrenal androgen (female pseudo-hermaphroditism).

Congenital adrenal hyperplasia due to excess ACTH (deficient cortisol feedback).

Reversible gonadal hypoplasia due to inhibition of pituitary by adrenal androgens.

Early Manifestations: Low cortisol:
  (a.) Insulin sensitivity.
  (b.) Impaired stress tolerance, Addisonian crises.
  (c.) Increased C-17 steroidogenesis (high excess ACTH).
High androgens, congenital virilization:
  (a.) Pseudoprecocious puberty in males.
  (b.) Hirsutism, absent menarche and breast development in females.
  (c.) Muscularity, acne, seborrhea, voice changes, temporal baldness, accelerated linear growth, premature epiphyseal closure, shortened adult stature in both sexes.
Low aldosterone depending upon completeness of C21 block:
  Salt-wasting, episodic weakness and syncope.
  Raised 17KS, 17KGS, pregnanetriol in urine.
  Low 17OHCS and free cortisol in urine.
  Raised plasma testosterone and androstenedione levels.
  Low plasma cortisol and compound S levels.

Treatment: Adults: Hydrocortisone, 30 mg./day. Children: Hydrocortisone, 15 to 20 mg./day. Salt-wasting children, 0.5 to 1.0 mg. 9α-fluorohydrocortisone/day.

Possible Dire Consequences without Treatment: Fatal salt-wasting in childhood. Subsequent fatal adrenal crisis subsequently precipitated by trauma, surgery, infection in adults not receiving supportable glucocorticoid. Suppression of true puberty. Premature epiphyseal closure.

Figure XII–2 shows a patient who was diagnosed at the age of thirty-seven as having a deficiency of 21-hydroxylase. This patient related that she was very large as a child but stopped growing early, reaching a height of 5 feet. This is characteristic of the adrenogenital syndromes and is due to the fact that there is an early growth spurt from the excess androgen production but early closure of the epiphyses. At the age of seventeen the patient had a D & C and was treated with cyclic estrogen therapy, following which there was some withdrawal bleeding on several occasions. At the time she was studied little was known of the adrenogenital syndromes and she was advised to buy a wig, a padded brassiere and a sharp razor. Also significant in the history was the fact that the patient had frequent fainting spells, hypotension and marked weakness. A glance at the chart will show in patients with a deficiency of 21-hydroxylase (red X), no mineralocorticoid (*i.e.*, D.O.C. and aldosterone) can be made. If this deficiency is complete, patients usually die in the first weeks of life. However, those with partial defects are able to survive because the hypertrophied adrenal glands can make the minimum requirement of steroids.

374

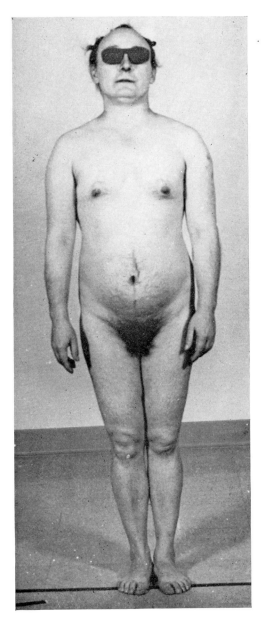

Fig. XII–2. A thirty-seven-year-old patient diagnosed as having 21-hydroxylase deficiency.

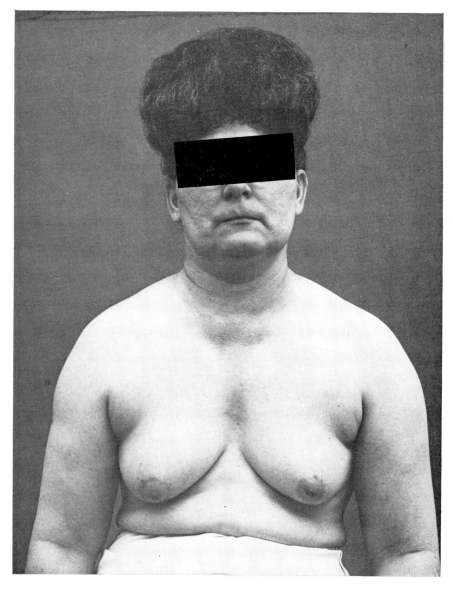

Fig. XII–3. Same thirty-seven-year-old patient following replacement
therapy with hydrocortisone.

Since this patient has ovaries, why did she not enter normal puberty? In order to understand the syndrome it is necessary to remember that there is a double feed-back on the pituitary gland. (1) Since hydrocortisone cannot be made, excess ACTH is produced resulting in adrenal hyperplasia with increased androgen production. (2) The excess androgen results in inhibition of gonadotropin secretion. (3) Therefore, the ovary is not stimulated. If hydrocortisone is administered in replacement doses, this process is reversed; androgen production diminishes and gonadotropins are produced. Figure XII–3 shows the patient following treatment with replacement doses of hydrocortisone. No estrogens were administered and puberty was initiated at the age of thirty-seven. Figure XII–4 shows the external genitalia of this patient. There is striking clitoral hypertrophy although the modest degree of labial fusion is not readily apparent in the photograph. If the labial fusion were complete, the patient would have been diagnosed as a boy with undescended testicles and hypospadias (female pseudohermaphroditism). Patients who are raised as boys could readily be converted to normal females capable of reproducing by severing the labial fusion and administering hydrocortisone. Such therapy is rarely possible, however, because once past the age of two or three years, the patients are psychologically oriented to being male and in this country at least, are usually treated with a hysterectomy and bilateral salpingo-oophorectomy. Following this, they are treated with hydrocortisone plus testosterone. The diagnosis is proven by demonstrating low Porter-Silber chromogens, elevated pregnanediol and elevated 17-ketosteroid levels.

Figure XII–5 shows a three and a half year old boy with pseudoprecocious puberty (virilization without testicular stimulation by gonadotropins) due to a deficiency of 21-hydroxylase. The bone age in this child was twelve years at the time of the initial diagnosis. Such an advanced bone age makes it virtually certain that he will be a short adult in spite of treatment. The earlier therapy is instituted, the more likely the patient is to achieve his full height. Treatment consists of replacing hydrocortisone. The dose for adults is generally about 30 mg. per day with 15 or 20 mg. generally being required in children. The smallest dose necessary to suppress androgen production should be used since larger doses will impair growth in children, in addition to causing the well known steroid side effects. It is possible to minimize the total amount of steroid required by giving two-thirds of the daily requirement at bed time. Since ACTH production is highest during sleep, a lower total steroid dose is necessary with this

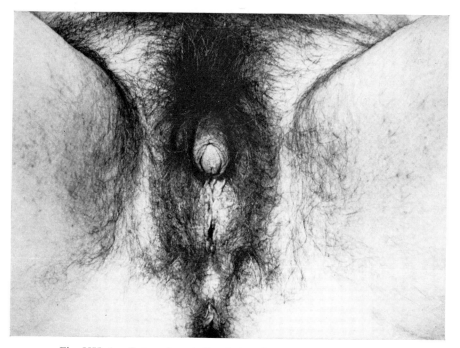

Fig. XII–4.   External genitalia of the thirty-seven-year-old patient.

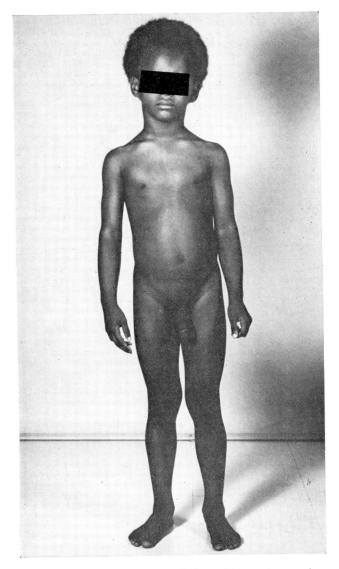

Fig. XII–5. A three and one-half year-old boy with pseudoprecocious puberty.

regimen. Children with complete defects of 21-hydroxylase (salt losing) require the addition of mineralocorticoid, usually 9-alpha fluoro-hydrocortisone in doses of .05 to .1 mg. per day.

The 21-hydroxylase deficiency is inherited as an autosomal recessive. If one child has the syndrome, each sibling has a one in four chance of showing the defect and in the same degree of severity. Patients should be treated for life. Adult males with this syndrome are likely to be infertile unless treated with hydrocortisone since their androgen production is of adrenal rather than testicular origin and the gonadotropins are generally suppressed.

References

Bongiovanni, A. M., and Root, A. W.: The adrenogenital syndrome. New Eng. J. Med., *268*:1383, 1342, 1391, 1963.

Fleischer, N., Brown, H., and Graham, D. Y.: The juxtaglomerular cells of the kidney and the zona glomerulosa in sodium losing and the hypertensive forms of virilizing adrenal hyperplasia. Pediatrics, *32*:825, 1963.

Gardner, L. I., and Migeon, C. J.: Unusual plasma 17-ketosteroid pattern in boy with congenital adrenal hyperplasia and periodic fever. J. Pediat., *57*:461, 1960.

Perloff, W. H., and Hadd, H. E.: Adrenogenital syndrome "virilizing type" in adult male. J. Clin. End., *19*:506, 1957.

6. Hypertensive Adrenogenital Syndrome

Francis H. Sterling

Cause: Congenitally deficient adrenal steroidogenesis due to enzymatic block (11-beta hydroxylase) located by green "x's" in Figure XII–1.

Synonym: Virilizing adrenal hypertension.

Result: Combined hypo- and hyperadrenal syndrome.
Inability to synthesize cortisol, corticosterone and aldosterone.
Unblocked C17 steroidogenesis with excess adrenal androgen formation.
Virilization of genotypic females *in utero* by adrenal androgen (female pseudohermaphroditism).
Unblocked C21 steroidogenesis with accumulation of DOC and 11-deoxycortisol (substance S) (17OH-DOC).
Congenital adrenal hyperplasia due to pituitary stimulation (absent cortisol feedback).
Reversible gonadal hypoplasia due to pituitary inhibition.
Reversible renin and aldosterone suppression due to mineralocorticoid (DOC) excess.

Early Manifestations: Hypertension due to mineralocorticoid excess.
Hypokalemic alkalosis due to mineralocorticoid excess.
Low cortisol.
(*a.*) Insulin sensitivity.
(*b.*) Impaired tolerance of infectious and traumatic stress.
(*c.*) Increased C-17 and C-21 steroidogenesis (increased ACTH).
High androgens, congenital virilization.
(*a.*) Pseudoprecocious puberty in males.
(*b.*) Hirsutism, absent menarche and breast development in females.
(*c.*) Muscularity, acne, seborrhea, voice changes, temporal baldness, accelerated linear growth, premature epiphyseal closure, shortened adult stature in both sexes.
Raised urine 17-KS, 17-KGS, 17-OHCS, tetrahydro DOC and tetrahydro 5 levels; decreased tetrahydrocortisol metabolites, free cortisol and aldosterone.
Raised plasma ACTH levels; decreased cortisol and compound 5 levels.

Treatment: Adults: Hydrocortisone 30 mg./day. Children: Hydrocortisone 15 to 20 mg./day.

Possible Dire Consequences without Treatment: Accelerated hypertension, precocious stroke. Periodic paralyses, ventricular escape rhythms, kaliopenic nephropathy.

The clinical picture in patients with a deficiency in 11-beta hydroxylase resembles that of the classical adrenogenital syndrome; however, no defect of mineralocorticoid is present. Both DOC and compound S may accumulate as may be realized from Figure XII–1. The principal C21 compound secreted is compound S, on the right side of the diagram; however, DOC, on the left side oₗ the diagram, is a much more potent mineralocorticoid. Aldosterone production is suppressed by the same mechanism discussed in connection with 17-hydroxylase deficiency. This deficiency is much more rare than the classical adrenogenital syndrome; since it may not be recognized until adult life, it may be confused with Cushing's disease, despite the fact that here the efficacious treatment is to *give* hydrocortisone. It is of interest that the metabolic block induced by the drug Metopirone is at the 11-beta hydroxylase step responsible for this syndrome.

Reference

Eberlein, W. R., and Bongiovanni, A. M.: Plasma and urine corticosteroids in hypertensive form of congenital adrenal hyperplasia. J. Biol. Chem., *223*:85, 1956.

7. Cushing's Syndrome

Francis H. Sterling

Cause: Bilateral adrenal cortical hyperplasia due to ACTH of pituitary origin or adrenal tumor.

Early Manifestations:

	Literature Survey n = 189	Presbyterian Hospital n = 33	Brigham Hospital n = 52	Utah-Vanderbilt n = 52	Utah-Vanderbilt n = 59
					Not Cushing's Disease
		Cushing's	Disease		
Osteoporosis	72%	—	—	64%	3%
Weakness	50	83%	87%	65	7
Bruising	23	60	65	53	6
Hypokalemia	—	—	—	25	4
Trunk Obesity	97	97	97	90	29
Florid Facies	50	89	97	82	31
Hypertension	85	84	82*	39**	17
Acne	26	82	—	52	24
Purple Striae	71	60	67	46	22
Edema	28	60	62	38	17
Leukocytosis	—	48†	—	58††	30
Hirsutism	69	73	80	50	29

  * Diastolic arterial pressure 90 mm.Hg or more.
 ** Diastolic arterial pressure 105 mm. Hg or more.
  † WBC 10,000 mm.^{3} or more.
 †† WBC 11,000 mm.^{3} or more.

Glucocorticoid Effects: Centripetal redistribution of fat. Gluconeogenesis, diabetes, polyuria, polydipsia. Osteoporosis, weakness, bruising, florid facies, striae, peptic ulceration. Alterations of mood. Eosinopenia.

Androgen Effects: Acne, hirsutism, diminished menses. Leukocytosis.

Treatment: Usually bilateral adrenal extirpation.

Possible Dire Consequences without Treatment: Accelerated atherogenesis, hepatic steatosis, fat emboli.
Diabetes mellitus, diabetic neuropathy and nephropathy.
Compression fracture, femoral neck fracture, tendon ruptures, poor wound healing, peptic ulceration.
Hypertensive cardiovascular disease, accelerated hypertension, cardiac failure, cerebrovascular disease.
Psychosis

Generalized Increase in Adrenocortical Production. Cushing's syndrome is characterized by the well-known effects of excess glucocorticoid, mineralocorticoid and androgen production. The syndrome can be produced by the administration of steroids, by tumors of the adrenal cortex (benign or malignant) which secrete these steroids or by generalized hyperplasia of the adrenal cortex due to ACTH of pituitary or non-endocrine tumor origin, such as bronchogenic carcinoma. Cushing's disease is bilateral adrenal hyperplasia due to ACTH of pituitary origin. In Cushing's disease, the abnormality is not in the adrenal. It is either in the pituitary or in the hypothalmus or elsewhere in the central nervous system. This concept of disturbed neural regulation of ACTH secretion is indispensable for an understanding of the diagnostic procedures in Cushing's disease.

A normal person who is given the equivalent of a daily replacement dose of hydrocortisone (1.2 mg. dexamethasone) will cease to secrete ACTH and adrenal steroidogenesis will diminish rapidly. A patient with Cushing's diseae (bilateral adrenal hyperplasia) requires much larger doses of hydrocortisone or dexamethasone to suppress ACTH secretions. Nevertheless, it can be suppressed. A patient with a tumor in the adrenal gland, either benign or malignant with excess production of glucocorticoid *already* has suppressed ACTH. Further administration of steroids will not likely diminish the production of steroids by the tumor. Therefore, the following procedures are recommended in diagnosis:

(*a*.) As a screening test, a 1 mg. dexamethasone suppression test is useful. The patient is instructed to take 1 mg. dexamethasone p. o. at midnight, and blood for a plasma cortisol determination is drawn at 8 a.m. Normally, this value should be less than the lower limit of normal. If the a.m. plasma cortisol is still within normal limits, then further testing must be performed. It is extremely important that all barbiturates, phenothiazines, and sedatives as well as any unnecessary medication be eliminated for several days prior to testing. The specific drugs which are known to interfere with the colorimetric (Porter-Silber) or fluorometric methods of measurement of plasmacortisol, are too numerous to mention.

(*b*.) If the patient did not suppress with 1 mg. of dexamethasone at midnight, then 0.5 mg. is administered p. o., q 6h. for two days. During the second day, urine is collected for urinary cortisol and blood is drawn for plasma cortisol determination at 8 a.m. following the second day of dexamethasone administration. If urinary cortisol measurements are not available, 17-OHCS, 17-KGS, or 17-KS can be measured. These should all be below the normal range. If suppression does not occur, it is likely that the patient has Cushing's syndrome. Additional studies which are useful include a skull roentgenogram for enlargement of the sella turcica and an intravenous pyelogram with tomography to look for enlargement of the adrenals. The next question which arises is whether the excess steroid production is due to ACTH stimulation of the adrenal glands (Cushing's disease), or due to tumor of the adrenals. Therefore, the dose of dexamethasone is quadrupled and 2 mg. administered every six hours for two days. Again urine is collected on the second day and blood drawn for plasma cortisol at 8 a.m. following the second day of dexamethasone administration. If steroid synthesis is not suppressed following the larger dose of dexamethasone, it is likely that the patient has an adrenal tumor or the ectopic ACTH syndrome. However, there are occasional patients with Cushing's disease whose ACTH secretory regulation is so altered that even larger doses of dexamethasone will be required. Such patients often have increased pigmentation of the skin due to the excess ACTH and MSH production. Contrast radiography such as arteriography, venography and retroperitoneal carbon dioxide insufflation are rarely of more help than simple tomograms during intravenous pyelography. Ideally, ACTH should be measured but this is technically not possible at the present time in most hospitals. Treatment of Cushing's disease is bilateral adrenal extirpation. If the syndrome is due to an adrenal tumor, obviously only the involved gland should be removed.

References

Fucci, J. R., et al.: Rapid dexamethasone suppression test for Cushing's syndrome. J.A.M.A., *199*:379, 1967.

Hellman, L., et al.: Cortisol is secreted episodically in Cushing's syndrome. J. Clin. Endo., *30*:686, 1970.

Lanker, D. P., Williams, G. H., and Thorn, G. W.: Diseases of the adrenal cortex in Principles of Internal Medicine, 6th Ed., Wintrobe, M. M., et al. (eds.). New York, McGraw-Hill Book Co., 1970, pp. 477–518.

Levine, R., and Weisberg, H. F.: Cushing's syndrome in Progress in Endocrinology, Soskin, S. (ed.). New York, Grune and Stratton, 1951, pp. 160–167.

Nugent, C. A., et al.: Probability theory in the diagnosis of Cushing's syndrome. J. Clin. End. and Metab., *24*:621, 1964.

Orth, D. N., and Liddle, G. W.: Results of treatment in 108 patients with Cushing's syndrome. New Eng. J. Med., *285*:243, 1971.

Plotz, C. M., Knowlton, A. I., and Ragan, C.: The natural history of Cushing's syndrome. Am. J. Med., *13*:597, 1952.

8. Ectopic ACTH Syndrome

FRANCIS H. STERLING and JOSEPH H. MAGEE

Cause: Bilateral adrenal cortical hyperplasia due to ACTH of non-pituitary origin.

Source:		
Bronchus	— oat cell carcinoma	62
Bronchus	— malignant carcinoid	5
Mediastinum	— carcinoma	11
Thymoma		14
Thyroid	— carcinoma	3
Parotid tumor		2
Pancreas	— islet cell carcinoma	11
Ovarian tumor		2
		110

Rare Sources: Carcinomas of breast, esophagus, gallbladder, colon, kidney, prostate, testes, uterus.

Early Manifestations: Glucocorticoid Effects:

Weight loss common; truncal obesity absent; non-ketotic hyperglycemia frequent; striae uncommon. Objective wasting in addition to weak muscles.

Mineralocorticoid Effects:

Marked hypokalemic alkalosis, hypertension, edema (may accompany ascites, pulmonary congestion, superior vena caval syndrome, with mediastinal, hilar, supraclavicular lymphadenopathy and/or tumor masses).

ACTH or MSH Effects. Hyperpigmentation.

Laboratory Study:

Plasma cortisol and urine steroids elevated before and after high dose dexamethasone, 2.0 gm. every six hours.

No urine steroid response to ACTH or metopirone; plasma cortisol may be hypersuppressible, though showing no baseline diurnal variation.

Treatment: Sodium restriction and potassium repletion. Spironolactone 400 to 600 mg./day. Metopirone. Dexamethasone may potentiate the action of metopirone. Bilateral adrenalectomy if expectation of survival warrants.

Possible Dire Consequences without Treatment: Inanition from primary malignancy. Muscle weakness, neuromuscular irritability, polyuria, ileus, from potassium depletion and alkalosis.

References

Bagshawe, K. D.: Hypokalemia, carcinoma and Cushing's syndrome. Lancet, *2*:284, 1960.

Brickner, P. W., Lyons, M., and Landau, S. J.: Cushing's syndrome associated with non-endocrine neoplasms. Am. J. Med., *31*:632, 1961.

Brown, W. H.: A case of pluriglandular syndrome. Lancet, *2*:1022, 1928.

Liddle, G. W.: Nonpituitary neoplasms and Cushing's syndrome. Arch. Intern. Med., *111*:471, 1963.

Liddle, G. W., et al.: The ectopic ACTH syndrome. Cancer Res., *25*:1057, 1965.

O'Riodan, J. L. H., et al.: Corticotropin-secreting carcinomas. Quart. J. Med., *35*:137, 1966.

Schambelen, M., Slaton, P. E., and Biglieri, E. G.: Mineralocorticoid production in hyperadrenocorticism: Role in pathogenesis of hypokalemic alkalosis. Am. J. Med., *51*:299, 1971.

Stott, C. A., Nugent, C. A., and Tyler, F. H.: Cushing's syndrome caused by bronchial adenoma. Am. J. Med., *44*:97, 1968.

Thorne, M. G.: Cushing's syndrome associated with bronchial carcinoma. Guy's Hospital Reports, *101*:251, 1952.

Introduction: Bystanding Corticotrophs

In the derangements so far considered adrenal control by corticotrophin (ACTH) has been maximally exerted upon a gland variably able to respond. Seemingly normal ACTH levels encountered in pituitary Cushing's disease are seen in actuality to be high; occurring as they do in setting of higher than normal cortisol levels, indicating an upward resetting of the pituitary control mechanism. ACTH is a peptide hormone variably present in blood due to the nature of its release, in about 8 bursts per day, and to its rapid decay time. There is a further rapid inactivation in shed blood so that facilities for refrigerated centrifugation and subsequent freezing are necessary in order to use plasma ACTH levels as diagnostic aids. High ACTH levels, as seen in the Ectopic ACTH syndrome, reveal a like response to antibodies, raised against the N-terminal 24 amino acids of the molecule used in radioimmunoassay, by tumor and pituitary ACTH. Despite the high assayed levels, ACTH genuinely of pituitary origin is probably absent in this syndrome, being reflexly suppressed by high levels of cortisol.

Subsequently, to be considered are conditions in which cortisol levels are autonomously or iatrogenically high, and ACTH is both reflexly suppressed and low as measured in plasma. The suppression of ACTH is brought about by external or long-loop negative feedback which may be multistage. The principal feedback point is at the corticotroph or ACTH secretory cell, with others at higher levels of control. This may be reinforced by internal or short-loop feedback in which ACTH itself prevents release of its hypophysiotrophic hormone, or corticotrophin releasing factor (CRF), from transducer neurons, into the portal venous plexus which runs through the pituitary stalk from the median eminence to the pituitary secretory cell.

Electron microscopy discloses six classes of secretory cells when peroxidase labels are added to antibodies against the adenohypophyseal hormones. Their stained analogs in light microscopy include intermediate lobe melanotrophs which secrete melanocyte stimulating hormone (MSH), and, in the anterior lobe the mammotrophs (red acidophils) which produce prolactin and somatotrophs (orange acidophils) which produce growth hormone. All of these are hormones which regulate target organs more or less directly, without the intermediary of another endocrine gland. However, they are themselves under dual hypophysiotrophic hormone control in having both releasing and inhibiting factor by which their own secretion is regulated.

Gonadotrophs (purple basophils) secrete follicle stimulating hormone (FSH) and luteinizing hormone (LH), controlled by a hypophysiotrophic releasing factor, peptide in nature and produced in transducer neurons under feedback control to this stage, plus higher stage control by monoaminergic neurons. Thyrotrophs (blue basophils) are similarly controlled by a tripeptide (thyrotrophin releasing factor, TRF), which has been prepared synthetically. CRF, which regulates secretion by the corticotrophs (pale basophils, chromophobes), is or closely resembles vasopressin, which has composite CRF, antidiuretic and pressor potencies. Secretion into a portal system achieves predominance of local over distant effects. The physiologic CRF may be one of several analogs having higher CRF/pressor activity ratios than does lysine vasopressin.

It is believed that the elevated ACTH seen in Addison's disease and following adrenalectomy comes about through an increase in CRF. This takes about two weeks to occur but during this time stress induced rises in ACTH may occur. Nelson refers to the first or slow rising ACTH increase as due to CRF-D (for diurnal), and

14

to the acute rises as CRF-S (for stress). Separate nervous pathways to the hypothalamic area secreting CRF may explain the differences.

Reference

Nelson, D. N.: Regulation of glucocorticoid release. Am. J. Med., *53*:590, 1972.

9. Functioning Adrenal Carcinoma

Joseph H. Magee

Cause: Functioning endocrine neoplasm. (Many adrenal malignancies are non-functional.) Reflex suppression of ACTH. Atrophy of non-neoplastic adrenal cortex.

Early Manifestations: Females 2:1, ages $\frac{1}{2}$–72 years (average 36).

Cushing's Syndrome (including hirsutism)	52%
Cushing's Syndrome plus virilism	12%
Virilism only	35%
Feminization	11%
Mineralocorticoid effects only	4%
No endocrine manifestations	6%
Metastases, kidney and local	65%
Lung	53%
Liver	44%
Bone	7%
Brain	4%
Palpable abdominal mass	40%
Pain	50%

Laboratory Study:
Plasma ACTH low (Normal 0.1–0.4 mμ/100 ml.).

Elevated 17-KS excretion	76%
Elevated 17-OHCS and 17-KS excretion	54%
Elevated 17-OHCS excretion only	5%
Neither elevated	19%

Failure of plasma cortisol levels, or of urine cortisol 17-OHCS and 17-KS excretions, to fall with high dose dexamethasone.

Treatment: Adrenal extirpation. Maintenance corticosteroid therapy. Palliative excision of recurrent intra-abdominal masses. Chemotherapy: o'p'–DDD.

Possible Dire Consequences without Treatment: Untreated maximum survival rate from time of diagnosis is eight months, mean 2.9 months. Surgical four-year survivals after diagnosis are 52% for females, 38% for males.

References

Hutter, A. M., Jr., and Kayhoe, D. E.: Adrenal cortical carcinoma. Clinical feature of 138 patients. Am. J. Med., *41*:572, 1966.

Hutter, A. M., Jr., and Kayhoe, D. E.: Adrenal cortical carcinoma. Results of treatment with o, p'DDD in 138 patients. Am. J. Med., *41*:581, 1958.

Mac Farlane, D. A.: Cancer of the adrenal cortex. Roy. Coll. Surg. Eng., *23*:155, 1958.

10. Functioning Adrenal Adenoma

Joseph H. Magee

Cause: Functioning endocrine neoplasm. Reflex suppression of ACTH. Atrophy of non-neoplastic adrenal cortex.

Early Manifestations:

Females 4:1, ages one-half to sixty-three years.

Glucocorticoid effects.

	Effect/ Total Cases
Osteoporosis	8/15
Weakness	8/13
Bruising	7/15
Trunk obesity	14/15
Striae	4/15

Mineralocorticoid effects.

Hypertension	13/15
Edema	7/15

Androgen effects.

Hirsutism	9/15

Laboratory Studies:

Plasma ACTH low (normal 0.1–0.4 mμ/100 ml.)

Elevated 17–KS excretion	10/15
Elevated 17-OHCS excretion	15/15
Failure of plasma cortisol levels or if urine cortisol, 17-OHCS and 17-KS excretions to fall with high dose dexamethasone	15/15

Treatment: Bilateral adrenal exploration. Removal of involved gland(s). Bilateral extirpation if adenoma not identifiable.

Possible Dire Consequences without Treatment: Continuation and exaggeration of above symptoms and ultimate death.

Reference

Scott, H. W., Jr., et al.: Cushing's syndrome due to adrenal tumor. Ann. Surg. *162*:507, 1964.

11. Iatrogenic Cortisolism

Joseph H. Magee

Cause: Glucocorticoid therapy. ACTH therapy.

Oral Glucocorticoid Agents		Mg. Equiv. to 25 mg. Cortisone Acetate	Other Available Strengths (mg.)
Betamethasone	(Celestone)	0.6	——
Dexamethasone	(Decadron, Decagenic, Dronactin)	0.75	0.25 0.5
	(Gammacorten, Hexadrol)		15
Paramethasone	(Haldrone)	2	1
Triamcinolone	(Aristocort, Aristogesic)	4	2 8
	(Aristomin, Kenacort)		16
Methylprednisolone	(Medrol, Medaprin)	4	2, 16
Prednisolone	(Atataxoid, Delta-Cortef)	5	——
Prednisone	(Arthralgen, Betapar, Delta-Dome) (Deltasmye, Deltasone, Sterazolidin)	5	2.5
Hydrocortisone	(Cortef)	20	5, 10
Cortisone	(Cortone)	25	5, 10

Result: Chronic suppression of pituitary ACTH.
  Hypoplasia (with glucocorticoid therapy), or hyperplasia (with ACTH therapy) of adrenal cortex.
Inadequate pituitary ACTH response to surgical, traumatic or infectious stress.
Antianabolic effect.
Impaired cell mediated (delayed) immunity

Early Manifestations: Cushingoid habitus. Salt intolerance, hypertension and edema. Potassium depletion and carbohydrate intolerance. Skeletal muscle weakness, striae. Delayed epiphyseal growth, osteoporosis. Peptic ulceration.

Treatment: Unless the condition requiring corticoid therapy flares up as corticoids are removed, comparatively few symptoms appear, until the patient is stressed. Usually, a physiological dose (one tablet a day) will protect against most moderate stresses and symptoms of adrenal insufficiency. However, in the face of severe illness or major surgery, there should be no hesitation in going to high doses.
  Precede elective surgery by 100 mg. cortisone acetate I.M. night before surgery and 100 mg. hydrocortisone hemisuccinate IV on morning of surgery.
  Replace preparations of glucocorticoid in combination with other drugs, such as salicylates that require divided daily doses.
  Transfer patient to alternate day glucocorticoid therapy using short acting preparations such as prednisolone, prednisone, hydrocortisone or cortisone if possible.

Possible Dire Consequences without Treatment: Inadequate pituitary ACTH response to surgical, traumatic or infections stress: Irreversible oligemic, neurogenic or endotoxic shock.
Glucocorticoid excess.

388

(*a.*) Disseminated infection from tuberculoma, histoplasmoma.
(*b.*) Superinfections with antimicrobial therapy (esp. pulmonary).
(*c.*) Opportunistic infections with candida, aspergillus, nocardia, pneumocystis, megalovirus, other herpes viruses.
(*d.*) Tendon rupture.
(*e.*) Compression fractures.
(*f.*) Anemia, hematemesis, melena, exsanguination.
(*g.*) Overt diabetes.
Rapid dose reduction.
(*a.*) Period of adrenal insufficiency.
(*b.*) Pseudotumor cerebri.
(*c.*) Exacerbations of arthritis, asthma, allergies.

References

Graber, A. C., et al.: Natural history of pituitary-adrenal recovery following long-term suppression with corticosteroids. J. Clin. Endocr., *25*:11, 1965.

Nelson, D. H.: Present status of the problem of iatrogenic adrenal cortical insufficiency. Anesthesiology, *24*:457, 1963.

Introduction: Mineralocortex

"Control of aldosterone secretion by the integrative center presumably involves one or more of the following mechanisms:

(*a.*) Impulses delivered over the hypothalamic-hypophyseal tracts cause the liberation of antidiuretic hormone (ADH) from the median eminence, ADH passes into the portal system supplying the adenohypophysis and stimulates the secretion of ACTH. The latter hormone, in turn, activates the zona glomerulosa of the adrenal and increases the output of aldosterone.

(*b.*) ADH (arginine vasopressin), acting directly on the adrenal glands, stimulates the secretion of both hydrocortisone and aldosterone.

(*c.*) Impulses to a presumed diencephalic or pineal neurosecretory system liberate adrenoglomerulotropin, which stimulates the secretion of aldosterone.

(*d.*) Impulses to sympathetic centers of vascular control are relayed to the kidney and cause vasoconstriction of afferent arterioles. Renin is liberated, and the angiotensin formed in peripheral blood stimulates the secretion of aldosterone.

(*e.*) Sympathomimetic hormones, liberated from the adrenal medulla, cause the release of ACTH and the stimulation of aldosterone secretion. The relative significance, or even the existence of some of these mechanisms, has not been definitely established. However, the fact remains that secretion of aldosterone is increased by volume depletion and reduced by volume expansion."

Cells of mineralocortex occupy the outermost reaches (zona glomerulosa) of the adrenal cortex. Since the glomerulosa widens under conditions in which aldosterone does not increase and vice versa, the mineralocortex is primarily a physiologic entity. Unlike the underlying glucocortex, its secretion is not regulated exclusively nor even primarily by ACTH. Instead there are a number of AGTHs (adrenoglomerulo-tropins) of which ACTH is but one. ACTH itself conforms to our idea that hormones, including trophic ones, tend to be peptides when not themselves steroids, and that they are prone to enlist a second messenger (cyclic adenosine monophosphate) to complete their definitive mission within the target cell. Its effect upon the mineralocortex appears to be transient in comparison with other AGTHs, which include potassium ions, angiotensin II and serotonin. These latter substances conform more to the concept of autocoids, substances more immediate in their action and originating in more immediate proximity to their sites of ultimate action than hormones as strictly defined. Within mineralocorticoid cells all of the AGTHs appear to exert their effect at the point (Fig. XII–6) where the isocaproaldehyde side chain of cholesterol is split off by successive hydroxylations at C20 and C22 and the action of a 20,22 desmolase, yielding pregnenolone. This subsequently becomes progesterone by transfer of a double bond from $\triangle^5$ to $\triangle^4$ position and adding the 3 B-ol group. At this point the synthetic pathways in the mineralocortex begin to diverge from those in the glucocortex.

Since the mineralocortex lacks a system for the 17-hydroxylation of either pregnenolone or progesterone, neither cortisol nor the adrenal androgens are synthesized and further transformation of progesterone follows the route of 21-hydroxylation exclusively. The next compound formed is 11-deoxycorticosterone, which as implied by its name requires a further 11-hydroxylation to form corticosterone.

As in the glucocortex, this hydroxylation can be blocked by metopirone, and it is congenitally blocked in the hypertensive variety of the adrenogenital syndrome. Corticosterone stands at the end of this synthetic pathway in the glucocortex; in man it is a glucocorticoid about a fifth as abundant and about half as potent as cortisol.

MINERALOCORTEX AND ANALDOSTERONISM

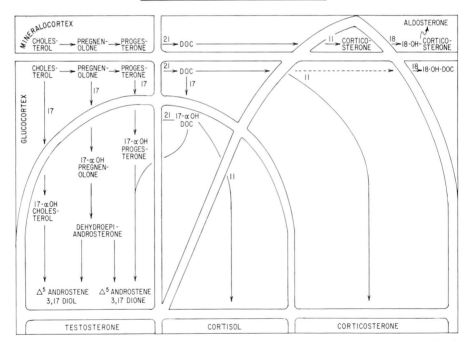

Fig. XII–6. Synthetic blocks resulting in isolated analdosteronism do not produce the spectacular clinical features of combined adrenal excess and deficiency seen in the adrenogenital syndromes. Because 17 and 21 hydroxylations proceed normally, drive to ACTH by deficient cortisol production does not occur. Corticosterone excretion increases somewhat in the inborn, and 18-OH corticosterone in the heparin-induced, forms of analdosteronism, indicating increased drive of AGTHs (see text) other than ACTH, one of which is raised [K]s.

Uniquely in the mineralocortex the sequence goes further; by an 18-hydroxylation and subsequent hydroxydehydrogenation, aldosterone is formed. Metopirone has another blocking action at the first and possibly both of these steps which is even more pronounced than its 11-B-hydroxylase blocking action.

Hence the first and probably rate limiting intra-adrenal step in ultimate aldosterone formation is the interconversion of cholesterol to pregnenolone. Since more than one AGTH can enhance the reaction rate at this step, there is redundance of potential command without there necessarily being an additive effect. Pituitary ACTH is most prominent in general neurogenic stress and angiotensin II in such cardiovascular stresses as orthostasis and hemorrhage. In a setting of potassium depletion, potassium repletion increases aldosterone secretion, unaided, without demonstrable increase in angiotensin II. The latter is absent despite continued aldosterone secretion in bilaterally nephrectomized men, dogs and sheep. When autonomous (adenoma) tissue, in Conn's syndrome, turns off secretion in the remaining mineralocortex, withdrawn support by angiotensin II and the other mineralotroph system may explain the absent function.

The last element of glucocortex control was ACTH, a long polypeptide which becomes blood-borne from discrete cells, the pituitary corticotrophs. In mineralocortex control, several of the final elements (AGTHs other than ACTH itself) are themselves systems. Angiotensin II is assembled piecemeal, with a proteolytic enzyme from renal lysosomes splitting leucyl-leucyl bonds of an hepatic substrate, repeated in pulmonary capillaries with splitting of a phenylalanyl-leucyl bond, to form an active hormone which survives according to the action of blood aminopeptidases upon its other end, and to such binding as occurs by tissues. Potassium ions emerge from protoplasm generally, importantly conditioned by ambient hydrion gradients between protoplasm and surrounding fluids, and by growth, glycogenolysis, and external balances. Serotonin is an important AGTH *in vitro* for cow, guinea pig, human, rabbit, and rat, but not for sheep or dog, adrenals. The sequestration of serotonin by platelets has so far proved an insuperable obstacle to confirming the reality of its role as an AGTH *in vivo* in man. A common denominator of the AGTHs is that their stimulation has a short time constant so that responses may be effected within minutes.

The final critical steps whereby the angular aldehyde group of aldosterone is added to the molecule appears, however, to respond to stimuli having a far longer time constant of perhaps days. Most influential are a raised [K]s or a lowered [Na]s, either independently or divergently so that the ratio [Na/K]s falls, departing from a normal of 30 or greater. If there is an impaired reaction to stimulus at this point, analdosterone may occur as a consequence despite adequate drive to earlier synthetic steps in the sequence by action of the mineralotrophs.

Discussion of 12 vagaries of aldosterone secretion follows. Secretion is deficient despite adequate stimulation of the target cortex in the first 3; in the others it is raised, secondary to these same controlling mechanisms. The patient here may attract attention because of hypertension or edema, or because [K]s is low.

References

Davis, J. O.: A critical evaluation of the role of receptors in the control of aldosterone secretion and sodium excretion. Prog. Cardiovasc. Dis., *4*:27, 1961.
Farrell, G.: Adrenoglomerulotropin. Circulation, *27*:1009, 1960.

Hilton, J. G.: Adrenocorticotropic action of antidiuretic hormone. Circulation, *21*:1038, 1960.

Pitts, R. F.: Physiology of the Kidney and Body Fluids. 2nd Ed. Chicago, Year Book Medical Publishers, Inc., 1968, p. 219.

Sawyer, W. H., Munsick, R. A., and Van Dyke, H. B.: Antidiuretic hormones. Circulation, *21*:1027, 1960.

Shafer, E. A.: The Endocrine Organs, New York, Longmans, Green, 1916; cited by W. W. Douglas, Autacoids, in the Pharmacologic Basis of Medical Practice. Goodman, L. S. and Gilman, A. (Eds.), New York, Macmillan, 1970.

Veyrat, R., et al.: Inhibition of renin by potassium in man. Acta Endocrin. Suppl., *119*:86, 1967.

12. Isolated (Inborn) Analdosteronism

JOSEPH H. MAGEE

Cause: Defective 18-hydroxylation of corticosterone. Defective hydroxydehydrogenation of 18-hydroxycorticosterone.

Early Manifestations: Nausea, vomiting, failure to thrive in newborns.
Intolerance to salt deprivation in adults with partial deficiency.
Improvement with salt.
Salt-craving in older children and adults.
Hyperkalemia and hyponatremia.
Renal salt loss and potassium retention.
Aldosterone absent from urine.
Corticosterone high in defect.
Corticosterone and 18-hydroxycorticosterone high in defect.
Renin activity and concentration normal or high.
Adams-Stokes attacks.
Periodic paralysis.
Postural hypotension.

Treatment: 9α Fluorohydrocortisone, 0.1 to 0.3 mg./day in infants and young children, 0.5 to 1.0 mg./day in adults. The condition may be transient in infants and lifelong treatment is not inevitable.

Possible Dire Consequences without Treatment: Fatal asystole or ventricular escape rhythm.

References

David, R., Golan, S., and Doucker, W.: Familial aldosterone deficiency, enzyme defect, diagnosis and clinical course. Pediatrics, *41*:403, 1968.

Mc Giff, J. C., et al.: Interrelationship of renin and aldosterone in a patient with hypoaldosteronism. Am. J. Med., *48*:247, 1970.

Ulick, S., et al.: An aldosterone biosynthetic defect in a salt-losing disorder. J.C.E.M., *24*:669, 1964.

Visser, H. K., and Cost, W. S.: A new hereditary defect in the synthesis of aldosterone: Urinary C21-corticosterone in three related patients with a salt-losing syndrome and an 18-oxidation defect. Acta Endocrinologic, *89*:31, 1964.

13. Isolated (Pharmacologic) Analdosteronism

Joseph H. Magee

Cause: Selective atrophy of mineralocortex (zona glomerulosa) during prolonged administration of heparin or natriuretic heparinoid Rol-8307.

Early Manifestations: Decreased aldosterone and 18-OH-corticosterone secretion. Renal salt loss and potassium retention. Salt-craving, anorexia, vomiting. Periodic paralysis and/or Adams-Stokes attack.

Treatment: Heparin withdrawal. Salt repletion. 1 mg. 9α fluorohydrocortisone/day if necessary.

Possible Dire Consequences without Treatment: Fatal asystole or ventricular escape rhythm. Both heparin and heparinoids have been used therapeutically to decrease aldosterone secretion in primary aldosteronism.

References

Abbott, E. C., et al.: The influence of a heparin-like compound on hypertension, electrolyte and aldosterone in man. Canad. Med. Ass. J., *94*:1155, 1966.

Abbott, E. C., et al.: Effect of a sulfated polysaccharide (Rol-8307) on the zona glomerulosa of the rat adrenal gland. Endocrinology, *78*:651, 1966.

Cejka, V., et al.: Effect of heparinoid and spironolactone on the renal excretion of sodium and aldosterone. Lancet, *1*:317, 1960.

Conn, J. E., Cohen, E. L., and Anderson, J. E., Jr.: Inhibition by heparinoid of aldosterone biosynthesis in man. J.C.E.M., *26*:527, 1966.

Ehrlich, E. N.: Heparinoid-induced inhibition of aldosterone secretion in pregnant women. Am. J. Obstet. Gyn., *109*:963, 1967.

Ford, H. E., and Bailey, R. E.: The effect of heparin on aldosterone secretion and metabolism in primary aldosteronism. Steroids, 7:30, 1966.

Glay, E., and Sugar, K.: Effect of heparin and heparinoids on the systems of aldosterone and corticosterone by the rat adrenal gland. Endocrinology, *74*:159, 1964.

Schlatman, R. J.: The natriuretic and aldosterone-suppressive action of heparin and some related polysulfated polysaccharides. J.C.E.M., *24*:35, 1964.

Veyrat, R., et al.: Mesura de la secretion de l'aldosterone sons administration d'un adrenostatique semi-synthetique, l'heparinoide Rol-8307. Res. Franc. Eterol Clin. Biol., *8*:677, 1963.

Wilson, I. D., and Goetz, F. C.: Selective aldosteronism and prolonged heparin administration. Am. J. Med., *36*:635, 1964.

14. Isolated Analdosteronism: Unheeded Signals

Joseph H. Magee

Cause: Mineralocortex unresponsive, despite stimulation by oligemia or potassium excess, following resection of aldosterone-producing adenoma.

Mineralocortex unresponsive despite like stimulation, with a preceding history of prolonged chronic volume overload, usually due to cardiac circulatory failure.

Early Manifestations: Raised [K]s.

Episodes of periodic paralysis or Adams-Stokes syncope.

Intolerant of salt restriction beyond 4 gm./day (78 mM), but edema readily accumulates with small doses of desoxycorticosterone acetate or of alpha-fluoro-hydrocortisone.

Low aldosterone secretion and excretion.

Normal renin activity and concentration.

Treatment: Fluorohydrocortisone 1 mg./day, reduced to once every two to three days if edema occurs.

Possible Dire Consequences without Treatment: Ventricular escape rhythm or asystole.

References

Bigheri, A. H., et al.: Post-operative studies of adrenal function in primary aldosteronism. J. Clin. Endocrin., *26*:553, 1966.

Hill, S. R., et al.: Studies in man on hypo and hyperaldosteronism. Arch. Intern. Med., *104*:982, 1959.

Hudson, J. B., Chobamian, A. V., and Relman, A. S.: Hypoaldosteronism. A clinical study of a patient with an isolated adrenal mineralocorticoid deficiency, resulting in hyper-kalemia and Stokes-Adams attacks. New Eng. J. Med., *257*:529, 1957.

Mc Giff, J. C., et al.: Interrelationship of renin and aldosterone in a patient with hypo-aldosteronism. Am. J. Med., *48*:247, 1970.

Molnar, G. D., Mason, H. L., and Power, M. H.: Chronic adrenocortical dysfunction, including aldosterone deficiency. Studies of steroid and electrolyte metabolism. J.C.E.M., *19*:1023, 1959.

Vagnucci, A. H.: Selective aldosterone deficiency. J. Clin. Endocrin., *29*:279, 1969.

15. Hypertensive Aldosteronism: Renal or Renal Artery Hypertension

Joseph H. Magee

Cause: Renal secreting tumors or renin release reflexly increased bilaterally or renin release increased ipsilaterally, and reflexly decreased contralaterally and net increased mineralocortex stimulation.

Early Manifestations: Compared to Conn's adenoma.
(a.) Renin high rather than low.
(b.) Hypertension may be more severe.
(c.) Serum sodium low rather than high.
(d.) Circulatory reflexes normal.
Hypokalemic alkalosis worsened by saluretics.
(a.) Glucose intolerance reversible by potassium repletion.
(b.) Polyuria, nocturia, weakness, paresthesias.
(c.) Urine pH 6–7 in alkalosis with low titratable acid but reciprocally increased ammoniation.

Treatment: Renal revascularization if possible. Resection for contracted kidney, revascularization failure, or renal cell carcinoma. Spironolactone, adjunctive to preoperative potassium repletion.

Possible Dire Consequences without Treatment: Accelerated hypertension. Perpetuation of hypertension by arteriolar sclerosis in contralateral unprotected kidney if revascularization delayed.

References

Barraclough, M. A., et al.: Plasma-renin and aldosterone secretion in hypertensive patients with renal or renal-artery lesion. Lancet, 2:1310, 1965.

Conn, J. W., and Cohen, E. L.: Primary aldosteronism versus hypertension disease with secondary aldosteronism. Recent Prog. Hormone Res., 17:389, 1961.

Cope, C. L., Harwood, M., and Pearson, J.: Aldosterone secretion in hypertensive disease. Brit. Med. J., 1:659, 1962.

Derot, M., et al.: Hypertension arterielle seven et depletion potassique. J. Urol., 67:57, 1961.

Dollery, C. T., Shackman, R., and Shillingford, J.: Malignant hypertension and hypokalemia cured by nephrectomy. Brit. Med. J., 2:1367, 1959.

Foster, J. H., et al.: Malignant hypertension secondary to renal artery stenosis in children. Ann. Surg., 164:700, 1966.

Goldberg, M., and Mc Curdy, D. K.: Hyperaldosteronism and hypergranularity of the adrenal cortex in renal hypertension. Ann. Intern. Med., 59:24, 1963.

Laidlaw, J. C., Cohen, M., and Gornall, A. G.: Hypertension caused by renal artery occlusion simulating primary aldosteronism. Metabolism, 9:612, 1960.

Ledingham, J. G. G., Bull, M. B., and Laragh, J. H.: The meaning of aldosteronism in hypertensive disease. Circulation Res., 10, 11:Suppl. 1:177, 1967.

Maxwell, M. H., Lupu, A. N., and Franklin, S. S.: Clinical and physiological factors determining diagnosis and choice of treatment in hypertension. Circulation Res., 10, 11:Suppl. 1:201, 1967.

Robertson, P. W., Kliduian, A., and Harding, L. K.: Hypertension due to a renin-secreting renal tumor. Am. J. Med., 43:973, 1967.

Sambhi, M. P., et al.:   The rate of aldosterone secretion in hypertensive patients with demonstrable renal artery stenosis.   Metabolism, *12*:498, 1963.

Sharpe, A. R., Jr., Magee, J. H., and Richardson, D. W.:   Unilateral renal disease and hypertension.   Arch. Intern. Med., *118*:546, 1966.

Slaton, P. E., and Biglieri, E. G.:   Hypertension and hyperaldosteronism of renal and adrenal origin.   Am. J. Med., *38*, 323, 1965.

Timmis, G. C., and Gordon, S.:   A renal factor in hypertension due to coarctation of the aorta.   New Eng. J. Med., *270*:814, 1964.

Wrong, O.:   Hyperaldosteronism caused by renal artery occlusion.   Quart. J. Med., *26*:586, 1957.

16. Hypertensive Aldosteronism: Vasoconstricted Kidneys

Joseph H. Magee

Cause: "Malignant" (accelerated) hypertension, de novo or as event (vascular crisis) in the course of established hypertension of non-adrenal origin.
Vasoconstricted kidneys.
Renin release reflexly increased bilaterally.
Net increased mineralocortex stimulation.

Early Manifestations: Compared to lateralized renal or renal artery hypertension.
  (*a.*) Male predominance is similar; onset is typically at age forty-four in men, thirty-six in women; either extreme of age favors lateralized disease.
  (*b.*) Creatininemia is evidence of bilateral involvement.
  (*c.*) Tomography may give evidence of symmetrical involvement.
Compared to Conn's adenoma.
  (*a.*) Males predominate rather than females.
  (*b.*) Renin high rather than low.
  (*c.*) Serum sodium low rather than high.
  (*d.*) Edema may be present.
  (*e.*) Papilledema common (75%) rather than rare.
  (*f.*) Hypertension severe by definition.
Compared to accelerated hypertension in Cushing's syndrome.
  (*a.*) Males predominate.
  (*b.*) Changes in appearance absent.
  (*c.*) Urine aldosterone, but not cortisol, 17-OHCS and 17-KS excretion is raised.
Compared to above.
  (*a.*) Average duration of preceding moderate hypertension is six years.
  (*b.*) History of unexplained weight loss over preceding six months is common.
Hypokalemic alkalosis worsened by saluretics.
  (*a.*) Glucose intolerance reversible by potassium repletion.
  (*b.*) Polyuria, nocturia, weakness, paresthesia.
  (*c.*) Urine pH 6 to 7 in alkalosis with low titratable acid but reciprocally increased ammoniation.

Treatment: Spironolactone as adjunct to potassium repletion.
  Discontinue spironolactone in creatininemia.
  Other saluretics may be used in creatininemia.
  Direct vasodilators, ganglionic and adrenergic neuron blocks.

Possible Dire Consequences without Treatment: 99% deaths in 5 years (untreated). 95% deaths in 3 years (untreated). 67% deaths in 1 year (untreated). Mode of death: (a.) Uremia 60%. (b.) Stroke 20%. (c.) Myocardial infarction 10%. (d.) Circulatory congestion 10%.

References

Castleman, B. E.: Case records of the Massachusetts General Hospital 38092. Malignant nephrosclerosis (Uremia with base-losing nephropathy). New Eng. J. Med., *246*:347, 1952.

Chalmers, T. M., et al.: Conn's Syndrome with severe hypertension. Lancet, *1*:127, 1956.

Fitzgerald, M. G., et al.: Malignant hypertension; adrenal hyperplasia and depletion of potassium. Scottish Med. J., *2*:473, 1957.

Holten, C., and Peterson, V. P.: Malignant hypertension with increased secretion of aldosterone and depletion of potassium. Lancet, *2*:918, 1956.

Jackson, P. E., and Oakley, C. M.: Potassium and paralysis. Brit. Med. J., *2*:881, 1955.

Kaplan, N. M.: Primary aldosteronism with malignant hypertension. New Eng. J. Med., *269*:1282, 1963.

Laragh, J. H., et al.: Aldosterone excretion and primary and malignant hypertension. J. Clin. Invest., *39*:1091, 1960.

Wyngaarden, J. B., Keitel, H. G., and Isselbacher, K.: Potassium depletion and alkalosis. Their association with hypertension and renal insufficiency. New Eng. J. Med., *250*:597, 1954.

17. Edematous Aldosteronism: Pump Failure

JOSEPH H. MAGEE

Causes: Decreased filling of right heart.
  (*a.*) Pericardial tamponade.
  (*b.*) Pulmonary artery obstruction.
  (*c.*) Rightward shunting of aortic or left chamber blood.
  (*d.*) Rapid arrhythmias.
Decreased filling of left heart.
  (*a.*) Atrial myxoma thrombus on pedicle.
  (*b.*) Valvular mitral stenosis.
Decreased emptying of heart.
  (*a.*) Conduction failure.
  (*b.*) Contraction failure (toxic, ischemic, intrinsic, endocrine).
  (*c.*) Valvular failure.

Results: Cardiac circulatory failure. Reflex by increased baroceptor, vasomotor center, and sympathetic activity.
Sympathetic dependent salt retention.
Normal or increased aldosterone levels (secondary aldosteronism); non-osmotic vasopressinism.
Steroid escape does not occur.
Positive salt balance, weight gain, edema.

Early Manifestations: Dependent edema.
May be aggravated in women in week before menses.
Heart disease may be occult with edema occurring before breathlessness and orthopnea.
Venous pressure slightly raised at rest.
Loss of arterial pressure overshoot (with bradycardia) following Valsalva maneuver.
End diastolic pressure of right ventricle raised without increased stroke work (mean minus end-diastolic pressure, times stroke volume).
Positive salt balance, weight gain, and venous pressure elevation; increased by exogenous mineralocorticoid, or sympathetic blockade (guanethidine).
Potassium and magnesium wasting, hypokalemic alkalosis.

Treatment: Same as Chapter XII. Section 16.

Possible Dire Consequences without Treatment: Passive circulatory congestion, thromboembolic complications.

References

Gill, J. R., Mason, D. T., and Barttes, F. C.: "Idiopathic" edema resulting from occult cardiomyopathy. Am. J. Med., *38*:475, 1965.
Gill, J. R., Mason, D. T., and Butler, F. C.: Adrenergic nervous system in sodium metabolism. J. Clin. Invest., *43*:177, 1964.
Luetscher, J. A., and Lieberman, A. H.: Idiopathic edema with increased aldosterone output. J. Am. Assoc. Phys., *70*:158, 1957.
Streeten, D. H. P., and Conn, J. W.: Studies on the pathogenesis of idiopathic edema. J. Lab. & Clin. Med., *54*:949, 1959.

18. Edematous Aldosteronism: Third Spaces

Joseph H. Magee

Cause: Portal obstruction usually due to hepatic cirrhosis. (Other causes of fluid sequestration, which may be less persistent, include caval obstructions by tumor, thrombosis, plication, or ligation; burns; toxic megacolon; peritonitis; and *hypodermoclyses*).

Result: Oligemic reaction due to fluid sequestration; altered peripheral dynamics in cirrhosis, with hypoperfusion of organs generally, despite normal or increased cardiac output and skin and muscle flows.
Increased sympathetic activity.
Sympathetic dependent salt retention.
Secondary aldosteronism.
Decreased hepatic catabolism of aldosterone.
Non-osmotic vasopressinism.

Early Manifestations: Plasma renin and angiotensin may be elevated.
(*a.*) Decreased pressor response to infused angiotensin.
(*b.*) Natriuretic response to infused angiotensin.
(*c.*) Increased aldosterone excretion due both to increased secretory rate and decreased inactivation.
Sodium retention.
(*a.*) Ratios Na_e/K_e and $[Na]s/[K]s$ are *increased.*
(*b.*) Ratios Na/K in urine, sweat, saliva and gut fluids are *decreased*
Potassium and magnesium wasting. This is of particular import in the cirrhotic who may have increased K loss via gut due to soft stools, and increased intracellular K transfer due to hypoventilation and respiratory alkalosis, and the adverse effects of alkalosis upon the renal vein output and the nervous tissue uptake of ammonia.

Treatment: Spironolactone, triamterene, amiloride, organomercurial diuretics (rather than equipotent doses of thiazide and other sulfonamide diuretics, and of ethacrynic acid), because of potassium sparing action.
Potassium repletion; dietary salt restriction.

Possible Dire Consequences without Treatment: Rapid ascites. Umbilical hernia. Hepatic coma.

References

As in Chapter XII, Section 17.

19. Edematous Aldosteronism: Protein Loss

JOSEPH H. MAGEE

Cause: Inadequate Synthesis. Gut Losses. Kidney Losses. External Hemorrhage. Concealed Hemorrhage.

Results: Oligemic reaction. Increased sympathetic activity. Sympathetic dependent salt retention. Secondary aldosteronism. Non-osmotic vasopressinism.

Early Manifestations: Hypoproteinemia with low serum albumin, raised serum beta-lipoprotein and cholesterol levels.
Hypoproteinemia may be inverse of proteinuria, or in exudative enteropathy with gut losses, urinary losses may be absent.
Raised plasma renin and angiotensin; aldosterone excretion.
Sodium retention and edema with or without serous effusions.
(*a.*) Ratios Na_e/K_e and $[Na]s/[K]s$ are *increased.*
(*b.*) Ratios Na/K in urine, sweat, saliva and gut fluids are decreased.
Potassium and magnesium wasting.

Treatment: Potassium-sparing saluretics. Corticosteroid and cyclophosphamide therapy of classic nephrotic syndrome.

Possible Dire Consequences without Treatment: Protein malnutrition. Susceptibility to infection.

References

As in Chapter XII, Section 17.

20. Normotensive Aldosteronism: Pregnancy and the Pill

Joseph H. Magee

Cause: Pills containing 0.05 to 0.1 mg. mestranol or ethinyl estradiol, plus 10 to 25 times as much progestogen simultaneously or sequentially.

Normal pregnancy.

Early Manifestations:
Increased renin substrate
Decreased renin concentration
Increased renin activity
Increased plasma aldosterone
Edema
"The striking activation of the renin/angiotensin/aldosterone system during contraceptive therapy is usually well compensated but may accentuate or precipitate the development of hypertension in susceptible women."

Treatment: Edema is an indication for alternative forms of contraception.

Possible Dire Consequences without Treatment: Usually none as far as we know presently.

References

Beekerhoff, R., et al.: Plasma-aldosterone during oral contraceptive therapy. Lancet, *1*:1218, 1973.

Laragh, J. H., et al.: Renin, angiotensin, and aldosterone system in pathogenesis and management of hypertensive vascular disease. Am. J. Med. *52*:633, 1972.

Watanabe, M., et al.: Secretion rate of aldosterone in normal pregnancy. J. Clin. Invest., *42*:1916, 1963.

21. Normotensive Aldosteronism: Bartter's Syndrome

Joseph H. Magee

Cause: Decreased pressor response to angiotensin II. Compensatory hyperreninism. Hyperaldosteronism. Hypokalemic alkalosis. Normotension.

Early Manifestations: Associated features include dwarfism and mental retardation with frequent occurrence in siblings.
High plasma renin activity.
Raised aldosterone secretion and excretion.
Hypokalemic alkalosis.
Resistance to infused angiotensin (8 to 25 times usual rate in mg./kg./min. to produce a standard pressor response).

Treatment: Spironolactone 100 mg./day, triamterene 100 mg./day singly or in combination.

Possible Dire Consequences without Treatment: Hypokalemia, weakness, periodic paralysis, postural hypotension. Kalipenic nephropathy.

References

Bartter, F. C.: So-called Bartter's syndrome. New Eng. J. Med., *281*:1483, 1969.
Bartter, F. C., et al.: Hyperplasia of the juxtaglomerular complex with hyperaldosteronism and hypokalemia alkalosis. Am. J. Med., *33*:811, 1962.
Brackett, N. C., Jr., et al.: Hyperplasia of the juxtaglomerular complex with secondary aldosteronism without hypertension (Bartter's syndrome). Am. J. Med., *44*:803, 1968.
Bryan, G. T., et al.: Effect of human renin in aldosterone secretory rate in normal man and in patients with the syndrome of hyperaldosteronism, juxtaglomerular hyperplasia and normal blood pressure. J. Clin. End., *24*:729, 1964.
Bryan, G. T., MacCardle, R. C., and Bartter, F. C.: Hyperaldosteronism, hyperplasia of the juxtaglomerular complex, normal blood pressure and dwarfism. Pediatrics, *37*:43, 1966.
Cannon, P. J., Leeming, J. M., and Sommers, S. C.: Juxtaglomerular cell hyperplasia and secondary hyperaldosteronism (Bartter's syndrome). Med., *47*:107, 1968.
Fleischer, D. S.: Prolonged hypokalemic alkalosis: A specific disorder associated with elevated level of unidentified anions. Am. J. Dis. Child., *102*:705, 1961.
Goodman, A. D., Vagnucci, A. H. and Hartroft, P. M.: Pathogenesis of Bartter's syndrome. New Eng. J. Med., *281*:1435, 1969.
Greenberg, A. J., et al.: Normotensive secondary aldosteronism. J. Pediat., *69*:719, 1966.
Kelsch, R. C., Gulhoed, G. W., and Vander, A. J.: Plasma renin in Bartter's syndrome. J. Pediatrics, *74*:821, 1969.
Trygstad, C. W., Mangos, J. A., and Bloodworth, J. M. B., Jr.: A sibship with Bartter's syndrome. Pediatrics, *44*:234, 1969.

22. Normotensive Aldosteronism: Desalting Therapy

Joseph H. Magee

Cause: Salt restriction. Saluretic agents, sometimes surreptitiously self-administered.

Result: Oligemia; preceding congestive state, usually cardiac. Hypoperfusion of organs. Increased sympathetic activity. Sympathetic dependent salt retention. Secondary aldosteronism. Non-osmotic vasopressinism.

Early Manifestations: Low [Na]s, [Cl]s. Raised serum urea N and creatinine. Anorexia, nausea, vomiting. Abdominal or peripheral cramps. Drowsiness, disorientation. Hypokalemic alkalosis.

Treatment: Potassium repletion postoliguria. Spironolactone, as saluretic therapy if resumed, adding second saluretic agent after one to three weeks spironolactone.

Possible Dire Consequences without Treatment: Aggravated azotemia from anorexia and vomiting. Oliguria or non-oliguria acute renal/failure. Weakness; periodic paralyses; asystole or ventricular escape rhythms.

References

Crabbe, J., Ross, E. J., and Thorn, G. W.: The significance of the secretion of aldosterone during dietary sodium deprivation in normal subjects. J. Clin. End., *18*:1159, 1958.
Schroeder, H. A.: Low salt diets and arterial hypertension. Am. J. Med., *4*:578, 1948.

23. Normotensive Aldosteronism: Extrarenal Salt Loss

Joseph H. Magee

Cause: Skin loss: Heat exhaustion, burns.
Gut loss: Vomiting, suctioning, internal fistulae.
Gut loss: Enteritis (salmonella, shigella, cholera).
Gut loss: Pancreatic cholera (pancreatic adenoma).
Gut loss: Villous adenoma (colon).
Peritoneal loss: Paracenteses, dialyses.

Early Manifestations: Low [Ks] and high [Na/K]s, with urine K loss less than 25 mm./ day initially.
Ratio [Na/K] not decreased initially in urine, sweat and saliva.
With oligemic stimulus, secondary aldosteronism occurs, and ratio [Na/K] is decreased in these fluids, added to initial extrarenal source of K loss.

Treatment: Saline volume replacement. Potassium replacement.

Possible Dire Consequences without Treatment: Weakness, postural hypotension, periodic paralyses, asystole or ventricular escape rhythms.

References

Fleischer, N., Brown, H., and Graham, D. Y.: Chronic laxative induced hyperaldosteronism and hypokalemia simulating Bartter's syndrome. Ann. Intern. Med., 70:791, 1969.
Schwartz, W. B., and Relman, A. S.: Metabolic and renal studies in chronic potassium depletion resulting from overuse of laxatives. J. Clin. Invest., 32:258, 1953.

Introduction: Unyielding Tubules

Lack of salt evokes distinctive responses depending upon the adequacy of renal function; the response of normal kidneys to salt scarcity is to save it. The response, centrally coordinated, is initiated by a drop in renal (glomerular) filtration rate (GFR), which occurs identically in normals and in hypoadrenal patients maintained solely on cortisol. A rise in aldosterone follows, in normals, two days later, at which time the Na/K ratios in urine, sweat, saliva and gut fluids fall. As salt is repleted, the reverse sequence ensues, with aldosterone secretion declining earliest, and with GFR subsequently returning to normal values. If the deprivation has been sufficiently severe, there will have been prerenal azotemia, but no indicators of renal disease will persist after correction is effected. We have seen that such a response occurs in Addison's disease, the result of endocrine fault. In the entities to follow, endorgan (tubular) fault simulates endocrine disease more or less closely; the degree of reversibility varies considerably.

24. Transient Tubular Acidosis (Lightwood's Syndrome)

Joseph H. Magee

Cause: Unknown.

Early Manifestations: Onset is from one to eighteen months following birth, usually six to nine months without history of renal disease in previous generations, and with recovery at about twenty-four months of age.

Sodium-wasting syndrome.

(*a.*) Low arterial and venous pressure.

(*b.*) Pre-renal azotemia.

(*c.*) Anorexia, vomiting, constipation, weight loss.

(*d.*) Irritability, thirst, polyuria, fever, apathy, marasmus.

(*e.*) High aldosterone secretion and excretion.

(*f.*) High renin activity and concentration.

Hyperchloremic acidosis.

(*a.*) Blood: Acidemia with $[HCO_3]$s 5 to 25 mM/l. and $[Cl]$s 105 to 135 mM/l.

(*b.*) Urine: Inappropriate (paradoxic) alkaluria with urine pH seldom below 6.1 to 7.1 at $[HCO_3]$s 18 to 22 mM/l.

(*c.*) Hyperpnea.

(*d.*) Effect of treatment: exclusive NaCl treatment worsens acidosis; treatment with $NaHCO_3$ or metabolizable salts to maintain urine pH at greater than 7.4 corrects both sodium-wasting syndrome and hyperchloremic acidosis.

Nephrocalcinosis and nephrolithiasis.

(*a.*) $[Ca]$s and filtered load of Ca usually are normal.

(*b.*) $[Ca]$u also usually is normal but its solubility is decreased by decreased $[citrate]$u, a consequence of systemic acidosis.

(*c.*) Nephrocalcinosis is demonstrable at postmortem in fatal cases but is seldom demonstrable by roentgenogram.

(*d.*) Bone lesions usually are absent.

Hypokalemia, weakness and polyuria usually are not prominent features following volume restoration and resumption of feeding but Shohl's and Harrison's solutions provide potassium supplementation during therapy.

Treatment: 3mM. (250 mg.) sodium bicarbonate, per kg., t.i.d., or

3mM. (3 ml.) 10% sodium citrate, per kg., t.i.d. or

3mM. (3 ml.) Shohl's solution* per kg., t.i.d., or

3mM. (1 ml.) Harrison's solution,† per kg., t.i.d.

Indices of adequacy are resumption of growth, healing of bone lesions if any, normal blood pH and $[HCO_3]$s levels and urine pH 7.4 or more. Urine calcium excretion should be less than 2 mg./kg./24 hours. Urine Sulkowitch tests,‡ which can be used for interim monitoring, should be 2 plus or less. Use of Shohl's or Harrison's solution doubles citrate excretion and enhances solubilization of urine calcium. Usual intakes of vitamin D may be employed following correction of acidosis.

Possible Dire Consequences without Treatment: Oligemia circulatory failure. Nephrocalcinosis.

---

* Citric acid monohydrate 140 gm. and trisodium citrate dihydrate 98 gm./l.

† Citric acid monohydrate 70 gm. trisodium citrate dihydrate and tripotassium citrate monohydrate 108 gm./l. in non-alcoholic fruit-flavored syrup base.

‡ 5 ml. reagent is added to 5 ml. urine in a test tube and rapidity and density of precipitate formation are empirically graded zero to four plus. The reagent is:

Oxalic acid	2.5 gm.
Ammonium oxalate	2.5 gm.
Glacial acetic acid	5.0 gm.
Distilled water q.s. ad.	150 ml.

Lightwood's syndrome presents as abrupt failure to thrive of a heretofore healthy infant. Lightwood elicited this information from chart review, when he found 6 instances of unexplained nephrocalcinosis in five to eleven month old babies, among 850 pediatric autopsies surveyed in 1935, and it was not at first realized that an acid-base disturbance was responsible. Indeed, as then suspected, infantile hypercalcemia may produce an identical picture, confirmed in a prospective study in 1952. However, Butler in 1936 had reported 4 more infants with the same fatal sequence, in whom antemortem studies had documented severe acidemia, yet with nephrocalcinosis identical to that seen in hyperparathyroid hypercalcemia. Serendipitously, it was later found that a research laboratory had documented an [HCO_3]s of 3.2 and [Cl]s 122 mM/l. in one of Lightwood's cases. Hartman then encountered a similar case, in which he pointed out the inappropriate alkalinity of the urine, and demonstrated both the efficacy of alkali therapy and the fact that it could ultimately be dispensed with. Following World War II, Lightwood began his prospective study of infantile failure to thrive, which then seemed typically to begin at four to six months. Ten infants studied had hypercalcemia alone, 29 had hyperchloremic acidosis only, and 2 had both. The condition, it now is known, was then at its apogee; 122 cases being reported from a group of British hospitals from 1950 to 1954, while from 1955 to 1959 only 21 were seen. There is considerable likelihood that both infantile syndromes elucidated by Lightwood and confreres—idiopathic hypercalcemia and transient tubular acidosis—had to do with the nature of vitamin D supplementation practices during their years of high incidence.

In a footnote to Butler's paper, mention was made of a case of the persistently acidotic syndrome suffered by a patient whom Albright again reported, along with a second case, in 1940. A salient feature of these cases was their bone disease, which Albright found to be true rickets, not the osteitis fibrosa of azotemic renal disease. Their maintenance requirement for alkali was modest, the acidification defect distal, and instances of familial occurrence emerged.

Edelmann and Rodriguez-Soriano have in recent years established the proximal location of the defect in cases studied by them, exclusively male, with high requirements for alkali and ultimate complete recovery, which appear to be identical to the cases encountered by Lightwood and contemporaries. No noxious agent such as vitamin D, mercury, or sulfonamides appears responsible for these cases, so they are to date designated as idiopathic or primary in nature. A case with adult onset, reported by York and Yendt, required high dose bicarbonate therapy throughout a three-year followup.

References

Butler, A. M., Wilson, J. L., and Farber, S.: Dehydration and acidosis with calcification at renal tubules. J. Pediat., *8*:489, 1936.
Edelmann, C. M., Jr. et al.: Bicarbonate reabsorption and hydrogen ion excretion in normal infants. J. Clin. Invest., *46*:1309, 1967.
Hartman, A. F.: Clinical studies of acidosis and alkalosis. Ann. Intern. Med., *13*:940, 1939.
Latner, A. L., and Burnard, E. D.: Idiopathic hyperchloremic renal acidosis. Quart. J. Med., *19*:285, 1950.
Lightwood, R.: Calcium infarction of the kidneys in infants. Arch. Dis. Child., *10*:205, 1935.
Lightwood, R.: Idiopathic hypercalcemia in infants with failure to thrive. Arch. Dis. Child., *27*:302, 1952.
Lightwood, R., and Butler, N.: Decline in primary infantile renal acidosis. Brit. Med. J., *1*:*855*:1963.

Lightwood, R., Payne, W. W., and Black, J. A.: Infantile renal acidosis. Pediatrics, *12*:628, 1953.

York, S. E., and Yendt, E. R., Jr.: Osteomalacia associated with renal bicarbonate loss. Canad. Med. Assoc. J., *94*:1329, 1966.

25. Persistent Tubular Acidosis (The Fanconi Syndromes)

JOSEPH H. MAGEE

Causes: Not certain.

Results: Defective high capacity, low gradient (proximal) renal cortical hydrion secretion ("rate defect") with massive episodic bicarbonate wasting accompanying phosphogluco-aminoaciduria.

Secondary aldosteronism and non-osmotic vasopressinism due to decreased circulating volume.

K wasting despite low [K]s.

P wasting due to intrinsic tubular defect with bone disease.

Early Manifestations: Sodium-wasting syndromes.
(*a.*) Low arterial and venous pressure.
(*b.*) Pre-renal azotemia.
(*c.*) Anorexia, vomiting, weight loss.
(*d.*) Raised aldosterone secretion and excretion.
(*e.*) Raised plasma renin activity and concentration.
Hyperchloremic acidosis.
(*a.*) Blood: Low blood pH and [HCO$_3$]s, raised [Cl]s.
(*b.*) Urine: Inappropriate (paradoxic) alkaluria with urine pH seldom below 6.0 to 7.1, at [HCO$_3$]s 18 to 22 mM/l.; with profounder systemic acidosis and no bicarbonaturia weak acid excretion and titration of urine to normal minima may then occur.
(*c.*) Hyperpnea, anorexia, intermittent nausea and/or vomiting.
Hypokalemia with periodic paralyses, ileus, cardiac arrhythmias.
Nephrocalcinosis is characteristically absent in the Fanconi syndrome, without a bicarbonate rate defect but, as in Lightwood's syndrome, may occur when this is present.
Bone pain and skeletal deformities, resistant to vitamin D, due to hypophosphatemia and acidosis.

Treatment: Treatment of acidosis may require doses of NaHCO$_3$ or other salts of the same order as in Lightwood's syndrome and maintenance of urine pH 7.4 rather than 7.0 which suffices in Butler-Albright syndrome.

Oral neutral isotonic phosphate solution* up to 150 ml./day in divided doses, and vitamin D 50,000 to 300,000 μ/day may be required for active rickets, depending upon magnitude of phosphaturia following correction of acidosis.

Edathamil calcium (EDTA) treatment of lead intoxication where this is evident.

Penicillamine treatment of Wilson's disease.

Treatment of dysproteinemias.

Possible Dire Consequences without Treatment: Oligemic circulatory failure. Rickets, late rickets, or osteomalacia. Nephrocalcinosis.

---

* To 1 quart water add 1 teaspoon each of monosodium and disodium phosphate plus another 2 tablespoons disodium phosphate.

References

Albright, F., et al.: Metabolic studies in a case of nephrocalcinosis with rickets and dwarfism. Bull. Johns Hopkins Hosp., *66*:7, 1940.

Baines, G. H., Barclay, J. A., and Cooke, W. T.: Nephrocalcinosis associated with hyperchloremia and low plasma bicarbonate. Quart. J. Med., *14*:113, 1945.

Boyd, J. D.: Endogenous rickets. Proc. Soc. Exper. Biol. Med., *26*:181, 1928.

Brown, M. R., Currens, J. H., and Marshand, F.: Muscular paralysis and electrocardiographic abnormalities. J.A.M.A., *124*:545, 1944.

Eastham, R. D., and McElligott, M.: Potassium-losing pyelonephritis. Brit. Med. J., *1*:898, 1956.

Pines, K. L., and Mudge, G. H.: Renal tubular acidosis with osteomalacia. Am. J. Med., *11*:302, 1951.

Rule, C., and Grollman, A.: Osteonephropathy. Ann. Intern. Med., *20*:63, 1944.

26. Heritable Tubular Acidosis: Butler-Albright Syndrome

JOSEPH H. MAGEE

Synonyms: Nephrocalcinosis with rickets and dwarfism: Albright, 1940.
Osteonephropathy (hyperchloremic type): Rule and Grollman, 1944.
Tubular insufficiency without glomerular insufficiency: Albright, 1948.
Lower nephron insufficiency: Greenspan, 1949.
Renal anacidogenesis: Lundback, 1951.
Renal tubular acidosis: Mudge and Pine, 1951.
Incomplete renal tubular acidosis: Wrong and Davies, 1959.

Causes: Renal inborn errors.
(*a.*) Autosomal dominant trait, variably expressed, with greater penetrance in females, occurring in successive generations with large sibships and with related parents, age of onset one month to middle age, but extremely rare before two years of age.
(*b.*) Probably recessive trait ("medullary sponge kidney"), in which involvement in siblings and in successive generations is exceptional.
(*c.*) Accompanying non-renal inborn errors with dominant inheritance: Ehlers-Danlos syndrome, hereditary elliptocytosis, Fabry's disease.
Non-renal inborn errors.
(*a.*) Galactosemia.
(*b.*) Hereditary fructose intolerance.
Exogenous agents: Amphotericin therapy.
Hypercalciuric states.
Hypokalemic states.
Hypergammaglobulinemic states.

Results: Defective low capacity, high gradient (distal) renal hydrion secretion ("gradient defect").
Decreased urine weak acid formation due to above.
Reciprocally increased urine ammoniation dependent upon adequate corticol pNH_3.
Hyperchloremic acidosis unless above is adequate.
Increased urine mineral cation excretion.

Decreased [K]s and [Ca]s and decreased [Na]s with decreased circulatory volume, due to above.

Secondary aldosteronism and non-osmotic vasopressinism due to decreased circulatory volume.

Secondary parathormonism due to low [Ca]s.

Early Manifestations: Onset from two years to middle age with females predominating 2:1 and with history of occurrence in previous generation frequently obtainable. Sodium-wasting syndrome.
  (*a.*) Low arterial and venous pressure.
  (*b.*) Prerenal azotemia.
  (*c.*) Anorexia, vomiting, weight loss.
  (*d.*) Raised aldosterone secretion and excretion.
  (*e.*) Raised plasma renin activity and concentration.
Hyperchloremic acidosis.
  (*a.*) Blood: low pH and [HCO_3]s with reciprocally raised [Cl]s prior to azotemia.
  (*b.*) Urine: Inappropriate alkaluria with urine pH minimum 5.5 at low blood pH or at 8 hours after ammonium chloride loading (0.5 gm./kg.).
  (*c.*) Hyperpnea, anorexia, intermittent nausea and/or vomiting.
Azotemia (preventable) follows nephrocalcinosis and/or lithiasis; cryptogenic nephrocalcinosis merits search for incomplete renal tubular acidosis (Wrong-Davies).

Low [K]s with periodic paralysis, ileus, or cardiac arrhythmias.

Metabolic bone disease.

Treatment: Same as Chapter XII, Section 25.

Possible Dire Consequences without Treatment: Same as Chapter XII, Section 25.

References

Buckalew, V. M., et al.: Incomplete renal tubular acidosis. Am. J. Med., *45*:32, 1968.

Clarke, E., et al.: Acidosis in experimental electrolyte depletion. Clin. Sci., *14*:421, 1955.

Dent, C. E., Harper, C. M., and Parfitt, A. M.: The effect of cellulose phosphate on calcium metabolism in patients with hypercalciuria. Clin. Sci., 27:417, 1964.

Eales, L., and Linder, G. C.: Primary aldosteronism. Quart. J. Med., *25*:539, 1956.

Ferris,, T. F., et al.: Renal tubular acidosis and renal potassium wasting acquired as a result of hypercalcemic nephropathy. New Eng. J. Med., *265*:924, 1961.

Fourman, P., Smith, J. W. G., and McConkey, B. M.: Defect of water reabsorption and of hydrogen-ion excretion by the renal tubules in hyperparathyroidism. Lancet, *1*:619, 1960.

Ghose, R. R., and Harrison, A. R.: Nephrocalcinosis. Proc. Roy. Soc. Med., *56*:925, 1963.

McCurdy, D. K., Frederic, M., Jr., and Elkinton, J. R.: Renal tubular acidosis due to amphotericin. New Eng. J. Med., *278*:124, 1968.

Morgan, H. G., et al.: Metabolic studies on two infants with idiopathic hypercalcemia. Lancet, *1*:925, 1956.

Morris, R. C., and Fudenberg, H. H.: Impaired renal acidification in patients with hyper-gammaglobulinemia. Med., *46*:57, 1967.

Morris, R. C., et al.: Medullary sponge kidney. Am. J. Med., *38*:883, 1965.

Parfitt, A. M., et al.: Metabolic studies in patients with hypercalciuria. Clin. Sci., *27*:463, 1964.

Wertlake, P. T., et al.: Nephrotoxic tubular damage following amphotericin therapy. Am. J. Path., *43*:449, 1963.

Wrong, O.: Urinary hydrogen excretion. J. Clin. Path., *18*:520, 1965.

27. Transient Tubular Salt Loss: Payne's Syndrome

Joseph H. Magee

Cause: Biochemical immaturity of distal renal tubules.

Synonyms: Infantile salt-losing nephropathy.
Pseudohypoadrenocorticism (Donnel, 1959).
Saline diabetes (Lelong, 1960).

Early Manifestations: Onset of failure to thrive at age one to seven months.
Salt supplementation necessary until age fifteen to twenty months.
All cases males.
Subsequent growth in 10 to 50 percentile range for age.
No history in previous generations.

Treatment: Salt supplementation.

Possible Dire Consequences without Treatment: Circulatory failure, prerenal azotemia.

References

Cheek, D. B., and Perry, J. W.: A salt-wasting syndrome in infancy. Arch. Dis. Child., *33*:252, 1958.

Donnell, G. N., Hitman, N., and Roldan, M.: Pseudohypo-Adrenocorticism Renal sodium loss, hyponatremia and hyperkalemia due to renal tubular insensitivity to mineralocorticoid. Am. J. Dis. Child., *97*:813, 1959.

Lelong, M., et al.: Diabete salin par insensibilite congenital du tubule a l'aldosterone Pseudo-hypoadrenocorticism. Rev. Franc. Etude. Clin. Biol., *5*:558, 1960.

Payne, W. W.: Inborn defects of the renal tubule. Postgrad. Med. J., *30*:476, 1954.

Raine, D. N., and Ray, J.: A salt-losing syndrome in infancy. Pseudohypoadreno-corticism. Arch. Dis. Child., *37*:548, 1960.

Roger, P., Habib, R., and Mathieu, H.: Problemes Actuals de Nephrologic Infantile. Paris, Flammarion, 1963.

28. Recurrent Tubular Salt Loss

Joseph H. Magee

Cause: Postobstructive syndrome.

Early Manifestations: Polyuria. Arterial and valveless vein hypotension. Azotemia. Natriuresis and low [Na]s.

Treatment: Gradual decompression of vesical obstruction. Salt and water repletion monitored by arterial and venous pressures.

Possible Dire Consequences without Treatment: Continued symptoms, azotemia, death.

The postobstructive diuresis, or natriuresis, syndrome may be defined as a sustained increase in the absolute amount of salt and water excretion following release of chronic urinary tract obstruction. The initial case reports drew attention to the development of clinical shock following sudden relief of urinary tract obstruction, but it was the studies of Bricker and coworkers in 1957 which emphasized the prolonged salt wasting defect as critical to understanding the correct therapeutic approach.

Postobstructive diuresis has been likened to that observed during an osmotic diuresis. However, it is clear that the two entities are not comparable, although they are similar in certain respects. In the course of passage of glomerular filtrate along the proximal tubule, all of the valuable non-electrolyte constituents (*e.g.* glucose, amino acids) are absorbed and approximately 80% (4/5) of the Na, Cl, and HCO_3 are reabsorbed. This provides the osmotic force to reabsorb about 80% of filtered water. By virtue of water reabsorption, excretory products, such as uric acid and urea are concentrated but total osmolar concentration remains unchanged, and the proximal tubular fluid remains isosmotic with plasma. The ability of the kidney to convert the remaining filtrate to a highly concentrated urine, some four times the osmolar concentration of plasma, with a sodium content approximately 1% that of the filtered load requires the interplay of two endocrine, and a complex hemodynamic-transport, systems. Sodium extraction from the loop of Henle coupled with the hemodynamic properties of this counter-current-multiplier system initiate the development and maintenance of the high medullary interstitial osmotic gradient. Antidiuretic hormone allows distal tubular influx of tubular water to occur while aldosterone influences reabsorption of the remaining sodium.

The water removed in this final concentrating process within the medullary collecting ducts is "solute-free" water, since tubular osmotically-active particles are not required for its passage. The volume of water reabsorbed (T_w^c) in the collecting duct concentrating segment is somewhere between 4 to 10 ml./min.

When a non-reabsorbed osmotically-active particle is added to the glomerular filtrate, marked changes in intratubular dynamics occur. Water reabsorption in the proximal segment is restricted due to its obligation to the non-reabsorbable solute. The retained tubular water acts to dilute tubular Na concentration, and development of a blood-urine concentration gradient slows and ultimately limits Na reabsorption. Thus, water is retained in the tubule not only by the added solute, but also by electrolyte. Since the concentrating process is limited to values less than 10 ml./min. (T_{mw}^c), the effect of increasing urinary solids is a disproportionate increase in urine flow. If excess flow from the proximal tubule and past the distal tubule is 10 ml./min. and T_w^c is 6, the urine flow is 4 ml./min. If excess doubles to 20 and T_w^c approaches its maximum of 8, urine flow is 12 ml./min., or trebled. Thus, urine flow rates may rise to high values proportional to the excretion rate of solids. With increases in urine flow rates sodium excretion increases proportionally and urine osmolality decreases and approaches plasma osmolality as a limit.

In chronic urinary tract obstruction, ureteral pressures in excess of at least 15 mm. Hg are required to produce renal functional change. The initial, and obvious, but not most important, functional change is a reduction in GFR. This reduction can be highly variable depending upon the duration of the obstruction, ranging anywhere from 10 to 80% of normal. During sustained chronic bladder outlet obstruction, there is retention of fluid, salts, urea, and acid with a concomitant reduction in blood buffer base (total CO_2 content). This salt and water retention may be of such a magnitude as to produce clinical signs and symptoms of circulatory overload with peripheral and pulmonary edema, hepatomegaly, and cardiac gallop rhythm. This state of volume expansion sets the stage for the initial phases of the syndrome which is frequently characterized by a massive diuresis of up to 8 to 10 liters per twenty-four hours and a solute loss principally of urea and NaCl.

TABLE XII-1. COMPARATIVE RENAL FUNCTIONAL DATA ON POST-OBSTRUCTIVE DIURESIS SYNDROME.

Renal Functional Parameter	Bricker et al. (4 cases)	Maher et al. (1 case)	Capelli (1 case)
Creatinine Clearance ml./min.	16–50	80–100	9–20
Urea Clearance ml./min.	—	75–85	6–19
Osmolar Clearance ml./min.	2–9	18–30	2–4
Urine Na Concentration mEq./L.	55–160	60–80	50–115
Fraction of Filtered Na Excreted %	6–20	9–13	5–31
Fraction of Urine Osmolality %			
Urea	25–35	37–68	15–20
Na	50–75	15–20	35–45

References

Bricker, N. S., et al.: Abnormality in renal function resulting from urinary tract obstruction. Am. J. Med., *23*:554, 1957.

Easley, L. E.: Extreme polyuria in obstructive uropathy. New Eng. J. Med., *255*:600, 1956.

Maher, J. F., Schreiner, G. E., and Waters, T. J.: Osmotic diuresis due to retained urea after release of obstructive uropathy. New Eng. J. Med., *268*:1099, 1963.

Parsons, F. M.: Chemical imbalance in chronic prostatic obstruction. Brit. J. Urol., *26*:7, 1954.

Persky, L., et al.: Metabolic alterations in surgical patients. Surgery, *42*:290, 1957.

Pierce, J. M., Jr.: Sodium losing nephropathy in urologic patient. J. Urol., *81*:609, 1959.

Wilson, B., Riseman, D. D., and Moyer, C. A.: Fluid balance in the urologic patient. J. Urol., *66*:805, 1951.

Witte, M. H., Short, F. A., and Hollander, W., Jr.: Massive polyuria and natriuresis following relief of urinary tract obstruction. Am. J. Med., *37*:320, 1964.

29. Transient Tubular Salt Loss: Postnecrotic Syndrome

JOSEPH H. MAGEE

Cause: Recovery phase of ischemic tubular necrosis.

Early Manifestations: Persistently elevated [urea] and [Cr]s. Improvements with increased intake of salt-containing foods and salt supplementations.

Treatment: Increased dietary NaCl.

Possible Dire Consequences without Treatment: Fatigue, anorexia. Falsely pessimistic prognostic assessment.

References

Bull, G. M., Joeckes, A. M., and Lowe, K. G.: Renal function studies in acute tubular necrosis. Lancet, 2:229, 1949.
Hunter, R. B., and Muirhead, E. E.: Prolonged renal salt wastage in "lower nephron nephrosis." Ann. Intern. Med., 36:1297, 1952.
Swan, R. C., and Merrill, J. P.: The clinical course of acute renal failure. Med. 32:215, 1953.

30. Reversible Tubular Salt Loss: Burnett's Syndrome

JOSEPH H. MAGEE

Cause: Nephrocalcinosis due to milk and or calcium carbonate therapy of peptic ulcer. Systemic alkalosis due to volume depletion, potassium depletion and absorbable alkali ingestion.

Synonyms: Milk-Alkali syndrome. Milk Poisoning. Milk Drinker's syndrome.

Early Manifestations: Dilute or salt-wasting polyuria.
Alkalosis and high serum calciums, up to 14 mg./100 ml. despite azotemia.
Low calcium excretion paralleling azotemia: rising to hyperparathyroid levels as azotemia improves.
Serum phosphorus and alkaline phosphatase levels normal in presence of osteosclerosis and metastatic calcifications of soft tissue (vessels, cornea, conjunctiva, etc.).

Treatment: Discontinue milk and alkali.

Possible Dire Consequences without Treatment: Nephrocalcinosis

References

Cheyne, A. J., and Whitehead, T. P.: Thorn's syndrome following ingestion of alkali. Lancet, *1*:550, 1954.
Frank, A., and Greenspan, G.: Milk-alkali syndrome complicated by salt-losing nephritis. New Eng. J. Med., *260*:210, 1959.
Peterson, V. P.: Renal function and electrolyte metabolism in "salt-losing" nephritis. Acta Med. Scand., *154*:187, 1956.

31. Reversible Tubular Salt Loss: Analgesic Syndrome

JOSEPH H. MAGEE

Cause: Acetophenetidin in high doses.

Early Manifestations: History of headache.
   Evidence of renal disease.
   (*a.*) Non-dilute polyuria without glycosuria.
   (*b.*) Azotemia, anemia, metabolic acidosis.
   (*c.*) Intermittently abnormal urine sediment, which may contain macroscopic bits of papillary tissue.
   (*d.*) Scant proteinuria.
   Renal salt loss.
   (*a.*) Absence of edema and hypertension.
   (*b.*) Low [Na]s.
   (*c.*) Absence of hypopigmentation and [K]s elevation.
   (*d.*) Faintness and fatigue, benefitted by salt replacement.
   Improvement with cessation of analgesic abuse and taking supplemental salt.

Treatment: High fluid intake. NaCl 5–10 gm./day added to diet. NaHCO$_3$, 2 to 3 gm./day. Abdominal pain following correction of desalted state may represent papillary shedding with ureteral colic.

Possible Dire Consequences without Treatment: Confusion with other causes of polyuria, headache, renal, disease, and hypotensive episodes.

References

Schreiner, G. E.: The nephrotoxicity of analgesic abuse. Ann. Intern. Med., *57*:1047, 1962.
Schreiner, G. E. and Maher, J. F.: Toxic nephropathy. Amer. J. Med., *38*:409, 1965.

32. Heritable Tubular Salt Loss (Thorn's Syndrome)

Joseph H. Magee

Cause: Defective renal morphogenesis, heritable as an autosomal recessive trait, variable in expression and with greater penetrance in the male, with tubular ectasia and eventual cystic replacement of the renal pyramids.
Progressive renal cortical atrophy.
Renal salt loss.
Secondary parathormonism.
Secondary aldosteronism and vasopressinism.
Tubular unresponsiveness to hormonal effects: Aldosterone is ineffective in sodium conservation but exceptionally potassium excretion may be greatly augmented.

Synonyms: Salt-losing nephritis. Saline diabetes. Medullary cystic disease. Familial juvenile nephronophthisis. Combined renal and prerenal azotemia.

Early Manifestations: Evidence of renal disease.
(*a.*) Polyuria may precede azotemia by months to years.
(*b.*) Azotemia may precede proteinuria and urine sediment abnormalities.
(*c.*) Anemia may become a prominent feature concurrently with azotemia.
(*d.*) Hypertension and circulatory congestion may occur preterminally only or never.
Renal salt loss.
(*a.*) Low [Na]s.
(*b.*) Low arterial and venous pressures.
(*c.*) Impaired circulatory reflexes; exaggerated postural hypotension.
(*d.*) Fatigue, weakness, leg cramps, salt-craving.
(*e.*) Anorexia, nausea, vomiting, epigastric pain.
(*f.*) DOC and 5 to 8 gm. NaCl (105 to 135 mM)/day fail to correct.
(*g.*) 10 to 20 gm. NaCl (175 to 350 mM.)/day required to correct.
Evidence of renal disease persists after salt repletion.
Plasma cortisol and ACTH, urine 17-OHCS and 17-KS normal.
Aldosterone excretion (raised) up to 10 times normal.
Other studies.
(*a.*) [Glucose]s normal.
(*b.*) [Ca]s and [HCO$_3$]s low, [P]s high.
(*c.*) [K]s may be high paralleling acidosis; exceptionally it may be low.
Predilection for males (2/3) and for blonde and red-haired persons.
(*a.*) Hyperpigmentation present with established disease.
(*b.*) Onset from infancy to age forty (average about twenty-seven), and occasionally older.

Treatment: NaCl 10 to 20 gm./day. NaHCO$_3$ 3 to 4 gm./day.

Possible Dire Consequences without Treatment: Increasing azotemia. Fatal circulatory collapse.

Thorn encountered a case of azotemic renal disease in whom hypertension and urinary abnormalities were strikingly absent, with a resemblance to Addison's disease so striking as to have occasional referral to Johns Hopkins, because of the availability of potent adrenocortical extract. Soon after, in 1943, Smith and Graham consulted Dr. Longcope by phone with respect to a case of renal disease, with a similar dissociation of findings, disclosed during a workup for anemia.   On the basis of similarity to some of the cases seen by himself and by Thorn, he correctly predicted the existence of cysts, which were found at autopsy.   Cases have been reported at a rate of about 1 per year in adults for the past thirty years.   One of the most intensively studied cases was encountered by Earle and co-workers in 1948.

In many entities characterized by renal potassium wasting, there is reciprocal sodium saving with the patients hypertensive and edematous, or both.   But in the tubular acidosis syndromes, there may be concomitant potassium and sodium losses with the patients characteristically normotensive.   Instances both of inordinate potassium retention, and of wasting, have been seen in Thorn's syndrome.

The case of Earle and co-workers was a forty-one-year-old male with a history of muscle weakness, periodic paralyses, cardiac irregularities, postural hypotension, and polyuria.   Blood pressure was low and remained so after repletion of the 2 gm. salt/day needed to maintain balance.   There was history of onset of a similar malady at the same age in his mother.   He was slightly anemic, with urinary sediment abnormal, and inulin clearances 41 to 68 ml./min.   In addition to salt repletion, 450 mM. potassium/day was needed to maintain balance; and on intake of 650 mM./day, [K]s did not exceed 4 mM/l.   In 1963, when he had been maintained on supplementation of this order for sixteen years, urine aldosterone excretion at low [K]s levels was high, and rose further with both potassium loading and sodium restriction.   Similar findings have been obtained in other cases of Thorn's syndrome.

Infantile cases were first reported by Fanconi and colleagues in 1952.   In an analysis of adult cases in 1962, Strauss found a two-fold preponderance in males and an average onset at age twenty-seven (eight to fifty-six years).   In 1967 he and Sommers pointed out the probable identity of the cases studied by Fanconi and others, in consanguineous families, with sporadic medullary cystic disease in adults.

References

Earle, D. P., et al.:   Low potassium syndrome due to defective renal tubular mechanisms for handling potassium.   Am. J. Med., *11*:283, 1951.
Entnikap, J. B.:   Condition of the kidneys in salt-losing nephritis.   Lancet, *2*:454, 1952.
Fanconi, G., et al.:   Die familiare juvenile nephronophthisis.   Helvet Ped. Acta, *246*:289, 1952.
Hagness, J. R., and Burnell, J. M.:   Medullary cysts of the kidneys.   Arch. Intern. Med., *93*:355, 1954.
Hughes, J. M.:   Salt-losing nephritis.   Arch. Intern. Med., *114*:190, 1964.
Levere, A. H., and Wesson, L. G., Jr.:   Salt-losing nephritis.   New Eng. J. Med., *255*:373, 1956.
Smith, C. H., and Graham, J. B.:   Congenital medullary cysts with severe refractory anemia.   Am. J. Dis. Child., *69*:369, 1945.
Stanbury, S. W., and Mahler, R. F.:   Salt wasting renal disease.   Quart. J. Med., *28*:425, 1959.
Strauss, M. B.:   Clinical and pathologic aspects of cystic disease of the renal medulla.   Arch. Intern. Med., *57*:373, 1962.
Strauss, M. B., and Sommers, S. C.:   Medullary cystic disease and familial juvenile nephronophthisis.   New Eng. J. Med., *277*:863, 1967.
Thorn, G. W., et al.:   Hormonal studies in salt-losing nephritis.   Med. Clin. N. A., *22*:158, 1960.

33. Salt-Saving Nephropathy (Liddle's Syndrome)

Joseph H. Magee

Cause: Heritable dysregulation of renal tubular and/or ductular ion permeability despite normal or suppressed aldosterone secretion.

Early Manifestations: Low [K]s
Raised urine K excretion (730 mM/day) despite low [K]s in patient and 5 of 16 relatives who also had low [K]s.
Low aldosterone excretion despite liberal NaCl intake (2 to 15 mg./day vs. 30 to 250 mg./day in controls).
High salivary Na/K ratios unaffected by spironolactone.
Hypertension in 8 of 23 relatives.

Treatment: Triamterene 50 mg. b.i.d.

Possible Dire Consequences without Treatment: Confusion with primary aldosteronism.

References

Kjerulf-Jensen, K., Krarup, N. B., and Warming-Larsen, A.: Persistent hypokalemia requiring constant potassium therapy. Lancet *1*:372, 1951.
Liddle, G. W., Bledsoe, T., and Coppage, W. S., Jr.: A familial renal disorder simulating primary aldosteronism but with negligible aldosterone secretion. Tr. Am. Assn. Phys., *74*:199, 1963.

15

34. Potassium-Saving Nephropathy

Joseph H. Magee

Cause: Heritable dysregulation of renal tubular and/or ductular ion permeability despite normal or suppressed aldosterone secretion.

Early Manifestations: Raised [K]s in the presence of normal renal function, normal plasma aldosterone and secretory rate and normal 17-KS and 17-OHCS excretion. Slight hyperchloremic acidosis with [HCO$_3$]s 18 to 22 mM/l. and minimum urine pH 4.95.
Arterial hypertension.
Postexertional muscle weakness.
Beneficial effect of lowered [K]s on above.

Treatment: Saluretic agents: Chlorothiazide. Potassium removal: Sodium polystyrene sulfonate resin.

Possible Dire Consequences without Treatment: According to Arnold and Healy their patient's presenting difficulty, arterial hypertension with diastolics up to 140 mm. Hg in a fifteen-year-old boy, was favorably affected by measures restoring his usual [K]s values (7 to 8 mM/l.) to normal range. Hence, evaluation of new young hypertensive patients ideally should include [K]s, among other blood chemical studies, with respect to possible high values as well as the well recognized significance of low ones.

References

Arnold, J. E., and Healy, J. K.: Hyperkalemia, hypertension and systemic acidosis without renal failure associated with a tubular defect in potassium excretion. Am. J. Med., 47:461, 1969.
Luke, R. G., Allison, M., and Davidson, J.: Hyperkalemia and renal tubular acidosis due to renal amyloidosis. Ann. Intern. Med., 70:1211, 1969.

35. Reversible Tubular Potassium Loss

JOSEPH H. MAGEE

Cause: Pyelonephritis.

Early Manifestations: Low [K]s: 1.4 to 2.8 mM/l.
Raised [HCO_3]s: 30–39 mM/l.
Areflexia, muscle weakness, lethargy, confusion.
Urine specific gravity fixed at 1.010, rising to 1.024 after K repletion.
Average K excretion during hypokalemia 25 mM/day, with aldosterone excretion rate 3.0 mg./day; after recovery K excretion 21 mM/day on K restricted diet, with aldosterone excretion rate 6.0 mg./day.
Associated flank pain, pyuria, positive urine cultures.

Treatment: Prolonged antibiotic therapy. Oral liquid KCl 2 mM/kg./day.

Possible Dire Consequences without Treatment: Areflexia, muscle weakness, confusion, respiratory paralysis.

Reference

Jones, N. F., and Mills, I. H.: Reversible renal potassium loss with urinary tract infection. Am. J. Med., *37*:305, 1964.

Introduction: Bystanding Mineralotrophs

At least four mineralotrophic systems are capable of enhancing the initial step in aldosterone biosynthesis, the conversion in appropriate cells of cholesterol to Δ^5 pregnenolone. These are ACTH, potassium ions, serotonin and angiotensin II. The last, as the principal agency effecting aldosterone secretion in response to orthostasis and other physiologic or pathologic circulatory stresses, is perhaps most important. Its presence is not, however, an invariant condition to aldosterone secretion in the conditions considered in the final seven sections of the chapter, marked disparity in the respective productions of angiotensin II and of aldosteronism (1) occurs and (2) may be of assistance in diagnosis.

That this combination of events might occur and be diagnostically useful was foretold earlier in considering lesions, productive of hypertension with aldosteronism, confined to one kidney. Angiotensin II production, as conventionally measured by the renin activity of peripheral blood, may be high early in such lesions. The amounts of renin produced may both be high absolutely and secreted essentially without variation throughout the course of the day. As a consequence of the pressor effect of angiotensin II, baroreceptor control of renin release is reset. Diagnostic amounts of renin may no longer be found by peripheral sampling. Differential sampling reveals that the renin output of the unaffected kidney is absolutely low. This may be true even in a setting wherein secondary aldosteronism persists due to continued unphysiologic renin output by the affected kidney. The finding of a renin that is low in terms of the known aldosterone production, in the one case from only one kidney and in the second from both kidneys, is crucial to diagnostic certainty in the two forms of hypertension most amenable to surgical relief. Having considered lateralized kidney disease previously, we next proceed to Conn's syndrome.

36. Primary Aldosteronism: Conn's Syndrome

Joseph H. Magee and George Ross Fisher, III

Cause: Functioning endocrine neoplasm: Solitary adenomas, usually small (0.8 to 3.0 cm.; 1 to 6 gm.) slightly more prevalent on the left and sometimes (10%) bilateral; rarely a carcinoma, rarely extra-adrenal.
Contiguous and contralateral zona glomerulosa tissue hypofunctional.

Early Manifestations: (*a.*) Principal secretion is aldosterone accompanied by deoxy-corticosterone, corticosterone, and cortisol.
(*b.*) Urine 17-OHCS and 17-KS excretions are normal.
(*c.*) Urine excretions, and the secretory rates of aldosterone and corticosterone are elevated.
Low plasma renin and angiotensin 2°.
Sodium retention 2°.
(*a.*) Na$_e$, [Na]s, PV and ECFV values are raised.
(*b.*) Edema usually is absent.
(*c.*) Augmenting PV and/or ECFV, acutely, provokes "exaggerated natriuresis."
(*d.*) Ratios Na$_e$/K$_e$ and [Na]s/[K]s are *increased.*
(*e.*) Ratios [Na/K] in urine, sweat, saliva and gut fluids are *decreased.*
Potassium and magnesium wasting.
(*a.*) High [K]u/ [K]s ratios despite low absolute [K]s values.
(*b.*) Daily potassium excretions over 25 mM/day in contrast to gut losses occasioning similarly low [K]s.
(*c*). Resistance to potassium repletion in contrast to uncomplicated diuretic use, occasioning similarly low [K]s.
Effects 2°.
(*a.*) Muscle weakness (75%), paralyses (25%), fatigability (20%) and pain (15%).
(*b.*) Neuromuscular irritability: Paresthesias (25%), Trousseau (15%) and Chvostek (20%) signs, tetany (10%).
(*c.*) Vasopressin-resistant dilute polyuria and nocturia (75%), polydipsia (50%).
(*d.*) Impaired urine pH minimum and titratable acidity.
(*e.*) Reciprocally increased urine ammoniation permits sufficient net hydrion excretion to maintain plasma alkalosis.
(*f.*) Impaired glucose tolerance (50%).
Impaired Circulatory Reflexes.
(*a.*) Postural hypotension may be present.
(*b.*) Hypertensive phase ("overshoot") may not follow primary response (hypotension, bradycardia) to Valsalva maneuver.
(*c.*) Improvement may follow correction of potassium and magnesium wasting without sodium retention.

Treatment: Unilateral adrenalectomy for single tumor; bilateral adrenalectomy is sometimes required for hyperplasia.

Possible Dire Consequences without Treatment: Congestive heart failure, uremia or cerebrovascular disease as in essential hypertension. Hypokalemia may be the most dangerous problem.

References

Biglieri, E. G., and Forsham, P. H.: Studies on expanded extracellular fluid and the response to various stimuli in primary aldosteronism. Am. J. Med., *30*:564, 1961.

Brown, J. J., et al. Plasma renin in a case of Conn's syndrome with fibrinoid lesions. Brit. Med. J., *2*:1636, 1964.

Conn, J. W.: Hypertension, the potassium ion and impaired glucose tolerance. New Eng. J. Med., *273*:1135, 1965.

Conn, J. W.: Primary aldosteronism, a new clinical syndrome. J. Lab. and Clin. Med., *45*:6, 1955.

Conn, J. W., Knoff, R. F., and Nesbit, R. M.: Clinical characteristics of primary aldosteronism from an analysis of 145 cases. Am. J. Surg., *107*:159, 1964.

Crane, M. G., Harris, J. J., and Herber, R.: Primary aldosteronism due to adrenal carcinoma. Ann. Intern. Med., *63*:494, 1965.

Kaplan, N. M.: Primary aldosteronism with malignant hypertension. New Eng. J. Med., *269*:1282, 1963.

Milne, M. D.: Potassium losing nephritis and primary aldosteronism. Proc. Roy. Soc. Med., *48*:780, 1955.

Moder, I. J., and Iseri, L. T.: Spontaneous hypopotassemia, hypomagnesemia, alkalosis and tetany due to hypersecretion of corticosterone and mineralocorticoid. Am. J. Med., *19*:976, 1955.

Russell, G. F. M., Marshall, J., and Stanton, J. B.: Potassium losing nephritis. Scottish Med. J., *1*:122, 1956.

Smithwick, R. H.: Surgical treatment of aldosteronism. Am. J. Surg., *107*:178, 1964.

37. Non-Tumorous Primary Aldosteronism

Joseph H. Magee

Cause: Bilateral diffuse hyperplasia of adrenal cortex generally on a zona glomerulosa, or bilateral multinodular hyperplasia ("microadenomatosis") of adrenal cortex. Rarely may be caused by renin-producing renal tumor.

Synonyms: Idiopathic primary aldosteronism. Pseudoprimary aldosteronism.

Early Manifestations: Age: generally older than in Conn's syndrome.
Blood Pressure: Generally higher ($>200/120$) than in Conn's syndrome.
Aldosterone excretion about a third lower (24 vs. 36 μg/day) than in Conn's syndrome (normal 4 to 17 μg/day) with preservation of diurnal rhythm.
Plasma renin concentration about 4 times as high (3.0 vs. 0.7 mg./ml./hr.) as in Conn's syndrome though still low or subnormal (normal 2.5–12.5 mg./ml./hr.), but very high when caused by renin-producing tumor of kidney.
Sodium: [Na]s slightly lower.
Potassium: [K]s slightly higher (3.3 vs 2.7 mM/l.).
Bicarbonate: [HCO_3] slightly lower.

Treatment: Bilateral adrenalectomy, or nephrectomy for renal tumor as above.

Possible Dire Consequences without Treatment: Renal tumors are very prone to spontaneous hemorrhage, other consequences are the same as Section 36.

References

Aitchison, J., et al.: Quadric analysis in the preoperative distinction between patients with and without adrenocortical tumors in hypertension with aldosterone excess and low plasma renin. Am. Heart J., *82*:660, 1971.

Baer, L., et al.: Pseudoprimary aldosteronism. Circ. Res., *26,27* Suppl 1:203, 1970.

Biglieri, E. G., et al.: The intercurrent hypertension of primary aldosteronism. Circ. Res., *26,27* Suppl 1:195, 1970.

Biglieri, E. G., Stockigt, J. R., and Schambelan, M.: Adrenal mineralocorticoids causing hypertension. Am. J. Med., *52*:623, 1972.

Conn, J. W.: Aldosterone and hypertension. Arch. Intern. Med., *107*:813, 1961.

Coppers, T. H., and Race, G. J.: Primary aldosteronism without adrenal adenomata. Arch. Path., *69*:142, 1960..

Davis, W. W., et al.: Bilateral adrenal hyperplasia as a cause of primary aldosteronism with hypertension, hypokalemia and suppressed renin activity. Am. J. Med., *42*:642, 1967.

Ferriss, J. B., et al.: Hypertension with aldosterone excess and low plasma-renin preoperative distinction between patients with and without adrenocortical tumor. Lancet, *2*:995, 1970.

Hilton, J. G., et al.: Syndrome of mineralcorticoid excess due to bilateral adrenocortical hyperplasia. New Eng. J. Med., *260*:202, 1959.

Katz, F. H.: Primary aldosteronism with suppressed plasma renin activity due to bilateral nodular hyperplasia. Ann. Intern. Med., *67*:1035, 1967.

38. Redundant Aldosteronism (Glucocorticoid Suppressible Aldosteronism)

Joseph H. Magee

Cause: Non-tumorous primary aldosteronism.

Early Manifestations: Occurs primarily in children. Low [K]s and raised [HCO_3]s. Hypertension. Both hypokalemic alkalosis and hypertension respond to glucocorticoid therapy.

Treatment: Dexamethasone 10 μg./kg./day.

Possible Dire Consequences without Treatment: Continued symptoms and results of hypertension.

Aldosterone secretion is not autonomous here, and appears to reflect unusual sensitivity to prevailing levels of ACTH incident to glucocortex stimulation. ACTH is also one of several "AGTHs" catalyzing initial steps in aldosterone biosynthesis. In some patients reflex suppression of aldosterone secretion, and/or release, by volume expansion and other negative feedback elements fails at usual ambient ACTH levels, but is resumed when the latter are reflexly suppressed by exogenous glucocorticoid (dexamethasone) administration.

References

Salt, I. S., et al.: Non-tumorous "primary" aldosteronism. Canad. Med. Ass. J., *101*:11, 1969.
Sutherland, D. J. A., Ruse, J. L., Laidlaw, J. C.: Hypertension, increased aldosterone secretion, and low plasma renin activity relieved by hexamethasone. Canad. Med. Assoc. J., *95*:1109, 1966.

39. Reset Aldosteronism (Mineralocorticoid Suppressible Aldosteronism)

JOSEPH H. MAGEE

Cause: Non-tumorous primary aldosteronism.

Synonyms: Normokalemic primary aldosteronism. Indeterminate primary aldosteronism.

Early Manifestations: Arterial hypertension.
Hypokalemic alkalosis may be absent.
Screening for hypertension discloses low plasma renin activity and/or concentration.
Screening of low renin hypertensives discloses increased aldosterone excretion.
Administration of DOC 20 mg./day × three days suppressed aldosterone excretion into the normal range.

Treatment: Spironolactone 200 to 400 mg./day.

Possible Dire Consequences without Treatment: Continued symptoms and results of hypertension.

References

Biglieri, E. G., et al.: Diagnosis of an aldosterone-producing adenoma in primary aldosteronism: an evaluative maneuver. J.A.M.A., *201*:510, 1967.
Biglieri, E. G., et al.: Primary aldosteronism with unusual secretory pattern. J. Clin. Endocr., *27*:715, 1967.

40. Idiopathic Edema

Joseph H. Magee

Cause: Tumorous or non-tumorous primary aldosteronism, plus failure of usual tubular "escape" so that presentation is with edema, or occult heart failure, occult plasma volume contraction, or *other undiscovered* appropriate cause of secondary aldosteronism.

Early Manifestations: Most patients are women.

Many are obese, often with family history of diabetes.

Condition persists after menopause and is uncorrelated with menstrual cycle.

Diurnal variation in weight is exaggerated even when not detected as edema.

Postural salt retention is exaggerated even when not detected as edema.

Edema fluid with high protein content may occur.

Measured plasma volume may be contracted.

Hypertension and low renin activity and/or concentration bespeak primary aldosteronism despite unusual presence of edema.

Increased sympathetic, renin, and aldosterone activity suggest some stimulus such as low exercising cardiac output and/or primary plasma volume contraction.

Treatment: Spironolactone 200 mg./day.

Possible Dire Consequences without Treatment: Tertiary aldosteronism, with or without adenoma; thereafter unresponsive to measures which decrease sympathetic and renin activity, though probably still responsive to spironolactone.

References

Emerson, K., Jr., and Armstrong, S. H., Jr.: High protein edema due to diffuse abnormality of capillary permeability. Tr. Am. Clin. and Clim. Assoc., *67*:59, 1955.

Gill, J. R., Jr., Mason, D. T., and Bartter, F. C.: Adrenergic nervous system in sodium metabolism. J. Clin. Invest., *43*:177, 1964.

Gill, J. R., Jr., and Bartter, F. C.: Idiopathic edema resulting from occult cardiomyopathy. Am. J. Med., *38*:475, 1965.

Gill, J. R., Jr., Waldman, T. A., and Bartter, F. C.: Idiopathic edema I. Am. J. Med., *52*:444, 1972.

Greenough, W. B., III, et al.: Correction of hypoaldosteronism and of massive fluid retention of unknown cause by sympathomimetic agents. Am. J. Med., *33*:603, 1962.

Mach, R. S., et al.: Oedemes par retention de chlorure de sodium avec hyperaldosteronuria. Schweig Med. Woch., *85*:1229, 1955.

Sims, E. A. H., McKay, R. R., and Shirai, T.: The relation of capillary angiopathy and diabetes mellitus to idiopathic edema. Ann. Intern. Med., *63*:972, 1965.

Speller, P. J., and Streeten, D. H. P.: Mechanism of the diuretic action of d-amphetamine. Metabolism, *13*:453, 1964.

41. Analdosteronism: Surrogate Hormones: Licorice Ingestion

Joseph H. Magee

Causes: Unknown factor in a subset of essential hypertension causing suppression of renin secretion, presumably reflexly due to salt-retaining activity.

Mineralocorticoid excess syndrome due to isolated desoxycorticosterone excess.

Mineralocorticoid excess syndrome with paradoxically low aldosterone secretion and excretion due to licorice ingestion.

Early Manifestations: Low plasma renin activity or concentration with or without serum electrolyte abnormalities encountered in work-up of hypertension.

Low [K] and raised [HCO$_3$] in hypertensive patient.

Polyuria may be present.

Periodic paralyses, muscular weakness, myopathy, myoglobinuria especially in licorice ingestion.

Treatment: Spironolactone 200 to 400 mg./day. Identification and cessation of licorice habit.

Possible Dire Consequences without Treatment: Continued and exaggerated symptoms. Death.

References

Biglieri, E. G.: Hypokalemic alkalosis, edema and increased desoxycorticosterone secretion. J. Clin. Endo., *25*:884, 1965.

Brown, J. J., et al.: Apparently isolated excess desoxycorticosterone in hypertension. Lancet, *2*:243, 1972.

Channick, B. J., Adlin, E. V., and Marks, A. D.: Suppressed plasma renin activity in hypertension. Arch. Intern. Med., *123*:131, 1969.

Creditor, M. C., and Loschky, W. K.: Plasma renin activity in hypertension. Am. J. Med., *43*:371, 1967.

Fishman, L. M. et al.: Incidence of primary aldosteronism in uncomplicated "essential hypertension." J.A.M.A., *205*:497, 1968.

Helmer, O. M.: Metabolic studies with suppressed plasma renin activity not due to hyperaldosteronism. Circulation, *38*:965, 1968.

Helmer, O. M.: Renin activity in blood from patients with hypertension. Canad. Med. Assoc. J., *90*:221, 1964.

Kanako, Y., et al.: Renin release in patients with benign hypertension. Circulation, *38*:353, 1968.

Ledingham, J. G. G., Bull, M. H., and Laragh, J. H.: The meaning of aldosterone in hypertension disease. Circ. Res., *20,21*:Suppl. 2:177, 1967.

Spark, R. F., and Melby, J. C.: Hypertension and low plasma renin activity. Ann. Intern. Med., *75*:831, 1971.

Weinberger, M. H., et al.: Plasma renin activity and aldosterone secretion in hypertensive patients during high and low sodium intake and administration of diuretics. J.C.E.M., *28*:359, 1968.

Woods, G., et al.: Effect of an adrenal inhibitor in hypertensive patients with suppressed renin. Arch. Intern. Med., *123*:366, 1969.

42. Analdosteronism: Unsent Signals

Joseph H. Magee

Causes: Mineralocortex unstimulated by oligemia, due to autonomic areflexia. Mineralocortex unstimulated by oligemia and/or potassium excess, due to renin deficiency in renal disease.

Early Manifestations: Postural hypotension, decreased plasma and urine catecholamine response to standing, decreased renin activity and concentration, decreased aldosterone secretion and excretion, intolerance to salt deprivation.

Raised [K]s, disproportionately to creatininemia and acidemia, episodes of periodic paralysis or Adam-Stokes attacks; may tolerate salt restriction and have some hypertension, decreased renin activity and concentration, decreased aldosterone secretion and excretion.

Treatment: Fluorohydrocortisone 1 mg./day, reduced to 1 mg. every two or three days if edema develops.

Possible Dire Consequences without Treatment: Ventricular escape rhythm or asystole.

Hyperkalemia ultimately develops in renal disease when no amount of exertion by remaining nephrons can suffice to maintain potassium balance. Some uremic patients, however, who develop disproportionate dysfunction of their juxtaglomerular cells, are unable to produce renin and develop hyperkalemia at a much earlier stage in their nephropathy than would be the case if kaliuresis mediated by secondary aldosteronism could occur. Patients with this condition are often elderly, with renal failure seemingly mild, the presenting problem is cardiac arrhythmia, and their serum potassium is found to be high. The treatment is fluorohydrocortisone in physiological rather than pharmacological doses.

References

Gerstein, A. R., et al.: Aldosterone deficiency in chronic renal failure. Nephron, 5:9, 1968.

Jose, A., Crout, J. R., and Kaplan, N. M.: Suppressed plasma renin activity in essential hypertension. Ann. Intern. Med., 72:9, 1970.

Jose, A., and Kaplan, N. M.: Plasma renin activity in the diagnosis of primary aldosteronism. Arch. Intern. Med., 123:141, 1969.

Kramer, H. J., Goldman, R., and Gonick, H. C.: Salt-losing syndromes following renal transplantation. Am. J. Med., 53:368, 1972.

Kramer, H. J., Siegel, L., and Schreiner, G. E.: Selective hypoaldosteronism with hyperkalemia. Ann. Intern. Med., 76:757, 1972.

Luft, R., and Von Euler, U. S.: Two cases of postural hypotension showing a deficiency in release of norepinephrine and epinephrine. J. Clin. Invest., 32:1065, 1953.

Melby, J. C., Wilson, T. E., and Dale, S. L.: Secretion of 18-hydroxydesoxycorticosterone in human hypertensive disease. J. Clin. Invest., 62:204, 1970.

Perez, G., Siegel, L., and Schreiner, G. E.: Selective hypoaldosteronism with hyperkalemia. Ann. Intern. Med., 76:757, 1972.

Seaton, P. E., and Biglieri, E. G.: Reduction of aldosterone in patients with autonomic insufficiency. J. Clin. Endocrin., 27:37, 1967.

Wagner, H. N., Jr.: Orthostatic hypotension. Bull. Johns Hopkins Hosp., 105:322, 1959.

Weidman, P., et al.: Failure of renin-angiotensin system and selective hypoaldosteronism causing hyperkalemia in chronic renal disease. Clin. Res., 20:249, 1972.

Williams, G. H., et al.: Abnormal responsiveness of the renin-aldosterone system to acute stimulation in patients with essential hypertension. Ann. Intern. Med., 72:317, 1970.

Chapter XIII

Hypertension and Nephritis

Introduction: High Arterial Pressure

Recounting the story of hypertension research, Wakerlin observes "of course the story does not begin with Richard Bright." However, as a result of his influence the largely unsuspected entity of arterial hypertension emerges into clinical awareness, despite the paucity of Bright's written comment upon the subject, which totals one sentence.

Bright had come upon it by an impulse to divide dropsy into classes. In 1813 he had noted "the altered structure of the kidney in a patient who had died dropsical" and had made a sketch of it. Blackall's book on coagulable urine had just appeared. Bright began to boil urine in 1825 and thereafter did so compulsively.

He now had a triad of dropsy, coagulable urine and granulated kidneys.

Later he observed that "a great deal of derangement of the system" may result from "decreased action of the kidneys" and that "the blood becomes impregnated with" urea.

His new triad was coagulable urine, altered kidneys, and urea retention. Dropsy might or might not also be present.

In 1836 in the second of two articles by Bright in Guy's Medical Journal are listed 100 autopsied cases that had granular and mottled kidneys. Whether or not they had proteinuria is not actually tabulated; 52 had enlarged hearts, 22 without conventional reason. Hypertension seems a likely cause of this. Bright's one comment upon arterial hypertension reads: "Without any probable cause for the marked hypertrophy generally affecting the left ventricle . . . the two most ready solutions appear to be either that the altered quality of the blood affords irregular and unwonted stimulus to the organ immediately; or, that it affects the minute and capillary circulation, so as to render greater action necessary to force the blood through the distant subdivisions of the vascular system."

Heart Hypertrophy.   Overloading the heart in systole with a volume load (preload) raises arterial pressure. If the semilunar valves close competently, ventricular pressure falls back toward normal, and arterial pressure falls according to whatever runoff the arterioles allow. To whatever extent arterial pressure still is raised at the end of diastole a pressure load (afterload) is imposed upon ventricular systole. The extent of preload and afterload may vary during the natural history of hypertension as reactivity of vascular beds is regulated by the vasomotor centers which at the same time are able to vary ventricular performance by the inotropic and chronotropic effects of adrenergic agonists.   Ultimately, however, the effects of afterload assume significance and are recognized as ventricular hypertrophy.

Salt.   Salt is part of the circulation rather than of protoplasm which notoriously excludes it.   The ordinary agency by which it is acquired is diet; more immediately determinant of the salt available to fill the circulation is the kidney, by far the most important agency for its loss.   With its own partition between nutrient circulation and protoplasm and its own stake in this and other excretory functions, the kidney's handling of salt is nonetheless under exceptionally firm extrarenal control.   The changes in circulatory filling brought about by changing salt balance are monitored insensitively by pressure changes in accessible areas of a circulation in which capacitance is inhomogeneously distributed. Half the blood volume resides in systemic veins constituting the reactive venous reservoir, in which usual pressures are 6 to 8 mm. Hg (80 to 100 mm HOH).   There is a gradient of 3 to 4 mm. Hg (40 to 50 mm. HOH) between this reservoir and the next 17.5% of blood volume forming the central venous conduit, where conventional "venous pressure" determinations are made, averaging 3 to 4 mm. Hg (40 to 50 mm. HOH).   Adjustments in the reactive venous reservoir can adjust this decrement or "intravenous gradient" upward to 5 to 10 mm. Hg (60 to 130 mm. HOH) in the interest of enhanced flow.   The remaining 32.5% of blood volume is contained outside systemic veins.   In diastole 10% of this is in the pulmonary vasculature, 7.5% in the cardiac chambers, with 15% in the high pressure system (arteries) beyond the aortic valve.   This is not a static distribution based on volume, and considerable more than 85% of a 1 liter blood volume augmentation would go into the low pressure system ($\Delta V/\Delta P = 200$ ml./mm. Hg).   Considerably less would go into arteries ($\Delta V/\Delta P = 1$ ml./mm. Hg), but some would, and diastolic pressure would rise perceptibly, perhaps 5 to 10 mm. Hg.   Some hypertension, therefore, must be salt dependent.

Models.   A population with an incidence of hypertension may include a proportion of cases in which the hypertension is salt dependent.   This trait is itself a heterogeneous one, evolving from diverse faults in the excretion mechanism for salt or its hierarchical control.   Since the various faults also have varying degrees of gain, populations with the highest incidence of hypertension may likewise demonstrate the largest number of traits with hypertensive potential that have found expression.   Populations do vary markedly in their incidences of hypertension, and Dahl found this to be highly correlated with salt intake in five diverse populations.

Dahl, Heine and Tassinari have identified in the Sprague-Dawley rat a variety of hypertension coupled to salt intolerance.   Without salt challenge they remain normotensive into adulthood.   Rapp and Dahl have found their salt intolerance to be associated with decreased output of corticosterone. This hormone has a dual role, occurring in the adrenal zone glomerulosa as an intermediate in the synthesis of the mineralocorticoid hormone aldosterone. In the zona fasciculata its principal role appears to be as a glucocorticoid, in man secondary in importance to cortisol.   It arises from 11-B-hydroxylation of its immediate precursor DOC (desoxycorticosterone).   In the salt sensitive rat there appears instead to be preferential hydroxylation of the 18 position, forming a potent mineralocorticoid compound, 18-hydroxy-DOC.   The production of aldosterone in the zona glomerulosa appears to be unimpaired and to be suppressible by high salt intake. However 18-hydroxy-DOC is unsuppressed, hence salt accumulation, hence hypertension.

Neural Regulation. A one liter augmentation of blood volume will raise arterial pressure during diastole, depending upon the capacitance of the reactive venous reservoir. If the addition has been made in repair of an acute deficit, the only increase may be during systole, the principal effect having been to raise both reservoir pressure and the intravenous gradient, with enhanced atrial filling and stroke volume. The capacitance of the venous reservoir depends upon increases or relaxations of tone in response to baroreflexes. Contemporary treatment of hypertension implies that a large subset of essential hypertension is salt dependent (most patients receive saluretic agents). It next implies dependence to an important degree upon the liberation of agonists (many patients receive in addition adrenergic neuron blocking agents). As versatility in salt conservation is acquired, any cybernetic fault in controlling this capability commits the organism to limited salt tolerance. The threshold to salt dependent hypertension then may be crossed with the complicity of adrenergic mechanisms.

Baroreflexes. Mean arterial pressure at temporal artery level is $70 \pm$ 5 mm. Hg in giraffe, cow and man, despite (Figure XIII–1) widely differing pressures, respectively 220 ± 40, 140 ± 30, and 90 ± 20 mm. Hg, at heart level. Hypotension between these two points is detected by carotid baroceptors which undoubtedly are representative of others from aortic to brain level. The vasomotor center response to carotid hypotension is increased sympathetic and decreased vagal tone (most sympathetic neurons are adrenergic, all vagal neurons are cholinergic). The reverse response prevails in the absence of baroreceptor impulses or where they are blocked by drugs such as protoveratrine (Fig. XIII–2). Increased sympathetic flow to arteriolar effectors can be obviated by direct vasodilators such as hydralazine and diazoxide. The response of other structures remains unimpeded, per

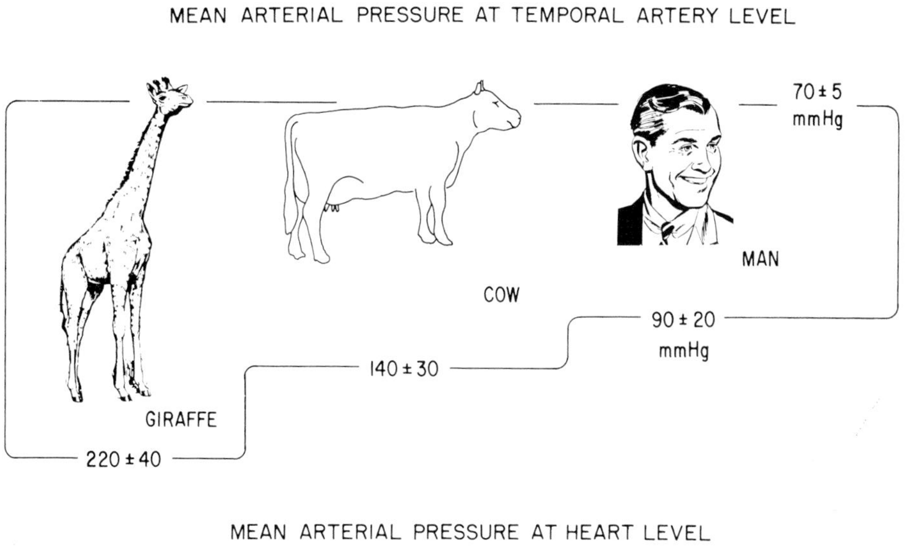

MEAN ARTERIAL PRESSURE AT TEMPORAL ARTERY LEVEL

MEAN ARTERIAL PRESSURE AT HEART LEVEL

Fig. XIII–1. Illustrating relationship between mean arterial pressure at heart level and at temporal artery level.

ARTERIAL PRESSURE : NEURAL AND AUTOREGULATION

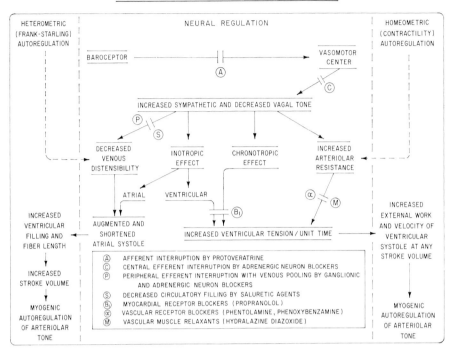

Fig. XIII–2. Neural and autoregulation of arterial pressure.

mitting reflex tachycardia with increased cardiac output, despite lowered arterial pressure. Other effects of increased vasomotor center activity in essential hypertension include increased lability of the reactive venous reservoir. To afterload hypertension from resistant arterioles is added preload hypertension, as seen in the exaggerated overshoot of arterial pressure (with bradycardia) following the Valsalva maneuver. This is lost early in the advent of left ventricular failure, but it also may be diminished with a still competent ventricular myocardium by venous pooling agents (Fig. XIII–3) or by agents (saluretics) which reduce venous volume.

Early Manifestations. Although many early manifestations of hypertension are mentioned below, it must be recognized that in all but a very small percentage of cases only one early manifestation really exists; namely, AN INCREASED BLOOD PRESSURE READING BY THE SPHYGMO-MANOMETER.

References

Gull, W. W.: Chronic Bright's disease with contracted kidney (arteriocapillary fibrosis). Brit. Med. J., *2*:673, 1872.

Mahomed, F. A.: Some of the clinical aspects of chronic Bright's disease. Guy's Hosp. Reports, *39*:363, 1879.

Mahomed, F. A.: On chronic Bright's disease and its essential symptoms. Lancet, *1*:46, 1879.

Rapp, J. P., and Dahl, L. K.: Mendelian inheritance of 18- and 11-B-steroid hydroxylase activities in the adrenals of rats genetically susceptible or resistant to hypertension. Endocrinology, *90*:1435, 1972.

Wakerlin, G. E.: From Bright toward light: the story of hypertension research. Circulation, *11*:131, 1962.

1. High Arterial Pressure (Big Pulse)

Joseph H. Magee

Cause: Big Pulse

INCREASED STROKE VOLUME:

Sinus bradycardia, A–V block, aortic insufficiency

INCREASED CARDIAC OUTPUT (STROKE VOLUME × RATE):
Anoxic (anemia, beriberi, cor pulmonale)
Hypermetabolic (hyperthyroidism)
Hyperkinetic (adrenergic receptor hypersensitivity)
A–V communications (traumatic fistulas, Paget's disease, hepatic cirrhosis, pregnancy, carcinoid syndrome, diffuse erythrodermas)
Congestive (oliguric or low filtration renal disease)

Preload (volume overload) systolic hypertension.

Early Manifestations: Arterial systolic and pulse pressures raised.   Venous pressure may be raised.   Circulation time not prolonged.   A–V oxygen difference normal or low.   Plasma volume may be increased with or without RBC volume increase. Edema may be present.

Treatment: Increased stroke volume: Measures which decrease stroke volume will decrease pulse pressure.
Increased cardiac output
(*a.*) Decrease the need for increased cardiac output in anoxic and hypermetabolic states and in A–V communications.
(*b.*) Digitalis for nocturnal dyspnea and nocturnal angina if present.
(*c.*) Decrease volume overload with salt restriction and saluretic agents in cardiac and hepatic congestive states.
(*d.*) Decrease volume overload, with fluid and salt restriction and/or dialysis, in renal congestive states.
(*e.*) Venous pooling (adrenergic neuron or ganglionic blocking) agents may be indicated where venous pressure is raised.
(*f.*) Adrenergic receptor blocking agents may be indicated for tachycardia and/or angina of effort where present.

Possible Dire Consequences without Treatment: Left ventricular failure, pulmonary edema, right ventricular failure, passive circulatory congestion, thromboembolic complications.

References

Bartels, E. C.: Anemia as the cause of severe congestive heart failure. Ann. Intern. Med., *11*:400, 1937.

Davies, C. E.: Heart failure in acute nephritis. Quart. J. Med., *20*:163, 1951.

Eichna, L. W.: Circulatory congestion and heart failure. Circulation, *22*:864, 1960.

Keefer, C. S.: The beriberi heart. Arch. Intern. Med., *45*:1, 1930.

Kontos, H. A.: General and regional circulatory alterations in cirrhosis of the liver. Am. J. Med., *37*:526, 1964.

Wintrobe, M. M.: The cardiovascular system in anemia. Blood, *1*:121, 1946.

2. High Systolic Pressure (Arteriosclerotic Hypertension)

Robert J. Gill

Cause: Arteriosclerosis with loss of vascular elasticity.

Early Manifestations: Elevated systolic blood pressure with mild, if any, diastolic elevation occurring primarily after the age of sixty.
Usually asymptomatic.
Symptoms of headache, throbbing sensation in the head, momentary giddiness, blurring of vision, motor instability, momentary loss of speech or thought processes are more likely due to cerebrovascular insufficiency than to the elevated blood pressure. However, moderate and gradual reduction of the elevated blood pressure may be followed by improvement of these symptoms. There is usually evidence of atherosclerosis on physical examination and radiologic study.

Treatment: Gradual and moderate reduction of blood pressure by mild antihypertensive agents, sedation, and removal of the removable burdens such as excessive salt intake, obesity, excessive use of stimulants and tobacco, anemia and thyrotoxicosis. Gentleness in handling the elderly vascular system is the key. Abrupt or severe drops in blood pressure are to be assiduously avoided but some reduction is essential.
Improvement in control of angina, congestive heart failure, and improved prognosis in relation to development of stroke may be anticipated by obtaining satisfactory blood pressure levels in a careful manner. The mildest effective drugs should be used in conjunction with the general measures above listed. Thiazide diuretics and sedation with barbiturates are most useful. Methyl-dopa may be employed in more refractory cases. Reserpine, though a mild antihypertensive, is more likely to produce side effects, particularly depression, in this older population than in the younger groups and is probably best avoided.
Guanethidine should be avoided because of the possibility of abrupt postural drop of blood pressure and the consequent dangers thereof. Hydralazine with its attendant production of tachycardia and increased cardiac output may precipitate angina or congestive heart failure and should be avoided, unless combined with propanolol.
Propanolol for tachycardia and/or angina pectoris, if no heart failure is present or imminent.

Possible Dire Consequences without Treatment: Stroke and other vascular complications (renal, cardiac, ocular).   The Framingham Study shows "No diminishing impact of systolic pressure with advancing age."   The old concept that systolic blood pressure elevations in the aged are innocuous and do not need treatment must be revised.   Treatment of essential hypertension has reduced mortality and the incidence of stroke, renal failure and congestive heart failure but not coronary disease, which seems to progress independently.   We cannot simply assume that the same will prove true in the older population with mainly systolic arteriosclerotic hypertension.   Until means are at hand to determine in advance who will or will not be seriously injured by elevated blood pressure we are duty bound to lower it in all, remembering the caveat "Primum non Nocere."

References

Kannel, W. B., Gordon, T., and Schwartz, M. J.:   Systolic versus diastolic blood pressure and risk of coronary disease.   The Framingham Study.   Am. J. Cardiol., *27*:335, 1971.

Kannel, W. B., et al.:   Epidemiologic assessment of the role of blood pressure in stroke: The Framingham Study.   J.A.M.A., *214*:301, 1970.

Sellers, A. M.:   Significance and management of systolic hypertension.   Am. J. Cardiol., *17*:648, 1966.

Statistical Bulletin (Metropolitan Life Insurance Company), May, 1972.

3. High Arterial Pressure (Aortic Coarctation)

ROBERT J. GILL AND JOSEPH H. MAGEE

Cause: Incomplete prenatal development of left 4th aortic arch.

Result: Hypoplastic descending aorta (stenosis, coarctation). Aortic collaterals. Diastolic hypertension. Afterload (pressure overload) systolic hypertension.

Associated Abnormalities: Regurgitant bicuspid aortic valve 30%
Stenotic bicuspid aortic valve 15%
Intracranial aneurysm 10%
Patent ductus arteriosus 7%
Ventricular septal defect 3%
Turner's syndrome 3%

Early Manifestations: Five times as common in males as in females.
Bounding neck, suprasternal and wrist pulses.
Widened right arm and usually left arm pulse pressure with raised diastolic and mean pressures.
Diminished femoral pulses and palpably delayed pulse summit compared to wrist pulse.
Absent popliteal and diminished pedal pulses, possibly with history of intermittent claudications in young individuals.
Lower pulse, mean and diastolic pressures below the coarctation.
Visible, audible and palpable collateral vessels between and below the shoulder blades.
Lower posterior rib notchings on PA chest radiographs.
Hypoplastic descending aorta with diminished shadow anterior to T6–8 vertebrae on ALO chest radiographs.
E-sign of the left border of the barium-filled esophagus.
Absence of rib notching and of the E sign in women may indicate general, rather than segmental, hypoplasia (coarctation) of the descending aorta, which should be verified by aortography.

Treatment: Excision of usual coarcted segments of about 1 cm. length, with primary anastomosis.
Aortic homografts or prostheses for long coarcted segments, inadequate proximal aortic caliber, poststenotic dilatations, and aorto-intercostal aneurysms.

Possible 'Dire Consequences without Treatment: Precocious death of related cause in 75%: Prior to age thirty in 40%, age thirty to fifty in 30%, and age fifty to seventy in only 5%.
(*a.*) Rupture, at average age nineteen, of stenotic site, in 5%.
(*b.*) Infection, at average age twenty-two, of stenotic site, in 5%.
(*c.*) Intracranial hemorrhage, at average age twenty-eight, in 10%.
(*d.*) Rupture, at average age thirty, of ascending aorta, in 20%.
(*e.*) Bacterial endocarditis, at average age thirty-one, in 15%; a fourth with normal and three-fourths with bicuspid aortic valves.
(*f.*) Cardiac circulatory failure, at average age thirty-nine, in 20%.
Death an average of twelve years later of unrelated causes in 25%, having a one-third loss incidence of bicuspid aortic valves: Prior to age thirty in 5%, age thirty to fifty in 10%, and age fifty to ninety in 10%.
The 55% of patients operated upon after age fifteen have only a 45% remission of hypertension to normal valves compared to 80% with operation prior to this age.
Surgical mortality is 33% after age fifty and 16% after occurrence of heart failure, 6% for ages thirty-five to fifty, less than 5% under age thirty-five, 2.1% for coarctation without heart lesions and 1.6% for such patients under age twenty.

References

Bailey, C. P., Lemmon, W. M., and Musser, B. G.: Experiences with coarctation of the aorta. Am. J. Cardiol., *4*:775, 1959.

Campbell, M., and Bayliss, J. H.: The course and prognosis of coarctation of the aorta. Brit. Heart J., *18*:475, 1956.

Campbell, M., and Polanzi, P. E.: The etiology of coarctation of the aorta. Lancet, *1*:463, 1961.

Cleland, W. B., et al.: Coarctation of the aorta. Brit. Med. J., *2*:379, 1956.

Cooley, D. A., Hallman, G. L., and Hamman, A. S.: Congenital cardiovascular anomalies in adults. Am. J. Cardiol., *17*:303, 1966.

Counihan, T. B.: Changes in the blood pressure following resection of coarctation of the aortic arch. Clin. Sci., *15*:149, 1956.

Morris, G. C., Jr.: Coarctation of the aorta with particular emphasis upon improved techniques of surgical repair. J. Thorac. Cardiovas. Surg., *40*:705, 1960.

Reifenstein, G. H., Levine, S. A., and Gross, R. E.: Coarctation of the aorta. Am. Heart J., *33*:146, 1947.

Rumel, W. R., et al.: Surgical treatment of coarctation of aorta. J.A.M.A., *164*:5, 1957.

Schuster, S. R., and Gross, R. E.: Surgery for coarctation of the aorta. J. Thorac. Cardiovasc. Surg., *43*:54, 1962.

Sellors, T. H.: Hypertension and coarctation of the aorta. Brit. J. Surg., *51*:726, 1964.

Introduction:

Hypertension is adrenergic (1) if there is increased liberation of adrenergic transmitter substances centrally or peripherally or both (2) if this is the primary or only abnormality present, and (3) it is causing hypertension. The common or primary or essential form of hypertension to which most propositi ultimately are allocated is included, because an increased firing rate by brain stem neurons is an ingredient essential to maintenance of their raised pressures. Stimulus is coupled to secretion, so that increased amounts of epinephrine (E) are liberated centrally. Since the rate of stimulation also increases peripherally, increased liberation of norepinephrine (NE) should be evident as well. This expectation is unfulfilled because a remarkable regulation of peripheral NE synthesis by negative feedback obscures this evidence of the increased stimulation peripherally. The absolute amounts of catecholamines, mostly NE, that are released in hypertension are either unincreased or increased insufficiently to identify hypertensives, by their individual excesses of blood or urine amines or metabolites, in population studies.

Despite this, a versatile array of drugs exploiting the principle of decreased synthesis, storage and release of transmitter substances, centrally or peripherally or both, plays a fundamental role in available hypertensive therapy. Reserpine and methyldopa are most extensively used; both cross perivascular glial cells constituting the blood-brain barrier and so affect the functioning of central as well as peripheral transmitters.

Both NE and E originate from neuronal uptake (Fig. XIII-3) from blood or tyrosine, an amino acid whose immediate precursor is phenylalanine. Three enzymatic steps are required to form NE. The first two, producing dihydroxyphenylalanine (DOPA) and subsequently dopamine, are accomplished by soluble enzymes of the cytoplasm or axoplasm. Entry into specialized storage vesicles precedes the third step, B-hydroxylation of dopamine's side chain to form NE. Vesicles arising within neurons of the sympathetic nerves migrate down neurotubules of the axons to within ready access of synaptic clefts, adjacent to receptors. In neurons of the adrenal medulla (Fig. XIII-3), which are without axons, the vesicles attain greater size. Some of their content is discharged periodically into cytoplasm, where a fourth enzyme, catechol N-methyltransferase (CNMT) methylates NE to form E; which is then restored to vesicles storing E only. CNMT requires perfusion by adrenal steroids directly from the enveloping cortex for its action; unlike the fetal enzyme originally present in all sympathetic neurons, which sometimes reappears in extra-adrenal tumors that are able to produce E.

Discharge of NE (or E) differs as well in neurons of the adrenal medulla. As neuron action potentials tranverse sympathetic axons, liberation of acetylcholine depolarizes their membranes, whereupon entering calcium ions induce exocytosis of

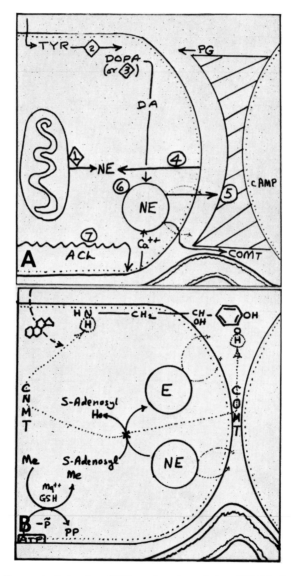

Fig. XIII–3. Free catecholamine (NE) and metanephrine (NME) form a higher proportion of free amine plus metabolites with tumor production. Ratio of free amine to VMA, 1:80 normally, may become 1:20.

vesicular contents into synaptic clefts. In neurons of the adrenal medulla, which are not adjacent to their receptors, exocytosis occurs directly into venous blood, transducing nerve impulses into hormonal ones, comprised of blood-borne E or NE. There is little accession of NE from synaptic clefts into blood, because of the *in situ* constriction induced in vessels activated by alpha receptors. This is not the case, however, in these tributaries supplying heart muscles, where beta receptors may predominate and into which considerable vicarious hormonal input from neuronal discharge may occur.

Along with NE or E, other storage vesicle contents may gain access to blood in equivalent proportions, including a binding protein (chromogranin), ATP, and the enzyme dopamine-B-hydroxylase. Assays of the last may prove useful as an index of adrenergic neuron activity, especially afferents of the myocardium and adrenal medulla. Studies of hypertensive populations suggest the existence of potentially important subgroups with low enzyme levels. Widespread application of the test might also result in the fortuitous earlier identification of chromaffin tumors in individuals prior to the emergence of characteristic symptoms.

Drugs used in hypertension may affect circulatory filling (saluretics) or vascular smooth muscle (hydralazine, diazoxide) directly, without interference with the neural mechanism of circulatory reflexes (Fig. XIII-3). There may be interruption of the afferent limb (veratrum) of such reflexes, or of the efferent limb by a nicotinic effect upon autonomic ganglia generally (trimethaphan, pentolinium). The latter have the disadvantage of blocking adrenergic and cholinergic autonomic afferents indiscriminately; such ganglionic blockers retain usefulness in hypertensive emergencies. Drugs that selectively block autonomic neurons or effectors however are obviously sought and preferred for long-term use.

Drugs that Block Adrenergic Neurons. The diverse modes of action of drugs used to blockade autonomic neurons are shown in Figure XIII-3. Ordinarily little NE is found in cytoplasm outside the sanctuary of specialized storage vesicles, due to the action of monoamine oxidase, abundantly present in mitochondria. Accordingly there is insufficient NE accumulation to effect endproduct inhibition of the initial (tyrosine hydroxylation) step in NE synthesis. Giving MAO inhibitors to hypertensives permits sufficient NE accumulation for inhibition of tyrosine hydroxylase to occur. Since MAO also is blocked in other tissues, the patient becomes at greater risk from ingested than from native amines, and may on the latter account suffer hypertensive crises. An agent for competitive rather than endproduct inhibition of a-methyl-p-tyrosine has been developed but not adopted therapeutically. In the next cytoplasmic step in NE synthesis, α-methyl-DOPA (Aldomet) acts as a false substrate for DOPA decarboxylase, ordinarily the agency for conversion of DOPA to dopamine, without necessarily diminishing its reaction rate. The dopamine produced ordinarily enters storage vesicles for hydroxylation to NE; other amines available for uptake competitively inhibit NE storage.

NE discharged into synaptic clefts from vesicle storage, if it does not escape into the circulation, is subject to one of two fates. One is reuptake into the axoplasm ("Uptake I") and restorage in vesicles, a step blocked by cocaine and the tricyclic antidepressants. The other is uptake by the receptor ("Uptake II"). Blockers of the receptor are discussed below.

Storage inhibition of NE re-entering axoplasm may be brought about noncompetitively by reserpine which blocks entry of E and NE into vesicles of sympathetic axons as well as in neurons of the adrenal medulla. It also may deplete amine storage in central adrenergic neurons relaying to the pons from limbus, thalamus, hypothalamus and cortex.

Release block may occur, even though the vesicles store NE, if liberation of acetylcholine by the neuron action potential is prevented with bretylium, effecting decreased membrane depolarization, calcium influx and exocytosis of vesicles near synaptic sites. Guanethidine, which does not gain access to central sites, has the attributes peripherally of both reserpine and bretylium, blocking both exocytosis and reuptake of amines into vesicles.

Drugs that Block Adrenergic Receptors. Amines in the synaptic clefts subject neither to Uptake I nor to Uptake II usually are methoxylated by catechol-O-methyltransferase, (COMT), prior to escape into the circulation. Those bound by the receptor release an hormonal deputy or second messenger in the form of cyclic adenosine monophosphate (CAMP), and at the same time direct a feedback element, in the form of prostaglandins (PG), as an additional regulator of NE synthesis. Drugs which block Uptake II (receptor uptake) differ according to the type of receptor involved. Alpha receptors of the microvasculature are muscle stimulating and hence constrictor in effect; both NE, via nerve transmission, and blood-borne E and NE are potential agonists; but E has so much more affinity for beta receptors that there is little alpha effect in low doses. Alpha blockers of E and NE, such as dibenzyline, are much more useful in managing hypertension due to increases in circulating catecholamines than that maintained neurogenically. The former includes the uninhibited and uncoupled states plus those where there is delayed excretion of agonists, as in uremia.

The beta-1 receptors of cardiac muscle also are muscle stimulating, their effect being inotropic and chronotropic. Both E and NE are agonists; and blockers such as propranolol ameliorate the cardiac stimulation of catecholamine excess, particularly including neurogenic excesses that produce reflex tachycardia that often accompanies direct vasodilator therapy such as with hydralazine. Since the beta-2 receptors are inherently vasodilator and bronchodilator, their blockade with agents more specific than propranolol is not desired, and hence is not at issue in hypertensive diseases.

4. Essential Hypertension (Hypertensive Vascular Disease, Hypertensive Cardiovascular Disease, Primary Hypertension)

Robert J. Gill

Cause: Unknown. Genetic factors are strongly implicated.

Early Manifestations: Usually none except for the elevated blood pressure. Hypertension is a silent disease until vascular damage occurs. Symptoms of morning headaches, visual blurring, nervousness, sweating, palpitations, nose bleed, excessive fatigue, and decreasing sexual performance are commonly elicited from hypertensive patients; although they may be ameliorated during successful antihypertensive therapy, they do not really correlate very well with early hypertension. Hypertensive patients tend to be asymptomatic for about three fourths of the duration of the disease, commonly fifteen to twenty years.
Symptoms and complications come much earlier in the black race, especially black males who have a shorter, more severe course of the disease.
Renal, central nervous system, and cardiac findings are really complications of hypertension and not primary manifestations thereof.

Treatment: See below.

Possible Dire Consequences without Treatment: Vascular damage affecting primarily heart, eyes, kidneys, brain, and acceleration of the atherosclerotic process. The vascular damage is manifested as renal failure, hypertensive retinopathy, cardiac enlargement, congestive heart failure, myocardial infarction, and stroke.

About twenty-six million Americans have high blood pressure of whom only half are diagnosed and only one half of those diagnosed are under treatment. Even fewer are under satisfactory and sustained treatment. Hypertension begins early; the trends are established by ages twenty-four to thirty-six. The best predictor of future development of essential hypertension is the early adulthood casual blood pressure determination.

There is no such thing as "benign hypertension." Even systolic elevation of blood pressure is bad. The Framingham Study indicates "no diminishing impact of systolic pressure with advancing age," that hypertension is no less dangerous in women than in men, and that the greatest preventive of stroke is the control of hypertension. Renal disease and congestive heart failure are also decreased by antihypertensive measures. Coronary disease seems to progress independently probably because of the genetic trait and its own set of factors that make up the risk profile.

Blood pressure is related to peripheral resistance as exemplified by the formula: BP = Cardiac Output $\times$ Peripheral Resistance. Cardiac Output = Stroke Volume $\times$ Heart Rate so the formula becomes: BP = SV $\times$ HR $\times$ PR. In labile hypertension the cardiac output tends to be elevated owing to an increased heart rate. Stroke volume and peripheral resistance are normal in labile hypertension which is primarily systolic in nature and seen mostly in young adults. In essential hypertension, the peripheral resistance is increased. The problem has been to determine what causes this increase in peripheral resistance and to find ways to diminish it. It is clear that treatment of the moderate and severe grades of hypertension is accompanied by decreased morbidity and mortality. It is still somewhat unclear whether treating mild hypertensives will have the same salubrious effect on the patient's future course. Unfortunately, we have no good way to determine in advance which hypertensive patients will or will not get into trouble in the future. Thus, since we have adequate tools at hand to lower the blood pressure and since it appears that simply lowering the blood pressure is a major determinant in reduction of hypertensive complications, it seems that we should treat all hypertensive patients. The hope is to prevent the appearance of complications. At this point there is no foreseeable cut-off date for treatment. Medications control, but do not cure, hypertension.

Philosophical and socioeconomic questions still to be decided are whether funds should be expended on in-depth study of hypertensives to search out the rare and specific cause of the disease which may be surgically correctable or to screen very large numbers of people in an effort to turn up the millions of undiagnosed hypertensives and get them into a treatment program. Seventy to 80% of this large mass of hypertensive patients will be controllable by relatively inexpensive simple regimens with thiazide as the base and one or two other antihypertensives added to it. Certain features will indicate which patients should be studied in depth: age of onset under thirty years; nonaccelerated hypertension enters the accelerated phase at any age; the patient under age fifty with abdominal bruit; a clinical syndrome of aldosteronism or pheochromocytoma; history suggests a possibility of unilateral renal involvement; de novo appearance of hypertension beyond age fifty. All hypertensive patients should have a certain basic study to include a thorough history and physical examination, urinalysis, SMA-12 series, serum electrolytes, electrocardiogram, chest film for heart size, and should probably have an IVP with rapid sequence films before therapy is undertaken. For most of them at this point therapy may be started unless there is a high suspicion of a specific etiology. If therapy results in good control of the hypertension, and continued observation fails to indicate any suspicion of a specific lesion, more complex and in-depth studies for correctable lesions may be deferred. If medical therapy is unsatisfactory or there is clinical suspicion or appearance of signs of one of the specific etiologies, further studies should be undertaken including catecholamine, renin studies, and arteriography as indicated in sections elsewhere in this chapter.

Therapy: We have many useful drugs today that will reduce high blood pressure and the trick is to apply them judiciously and effectively to attain optimal blood pressure reduction with the least discommoding of the patient. There are some serious problems with drug management. All the drugs have some unpleasant side effects and especially so if applied in adequate doses. The drop-out problem from hypertensive management is partially due to these factors. Therefore, before and during the application of drug therapy there should be a definite program of patient education to emphasize dangers of neglected hypertension, the demonstrated benefits from therapy, the necessity for prolonged therapy and the expected or possible symptoms that may accrue from the treatments themselves. The diabetologists for many years have been engaged in education of their patients and are in this regard

far ahead of those of us working with hypertensives. Patient cooperation and understanding are as essential in the management of hypertension as in diabetes. What is
optimal blood pressure reduction? It is the lowest level that does not produce hypotensive symptoms and is to be achieved at a rate that the patient can tolerate. The
physician who discontinues therapy when the pressure is brought down, or the
patient who drops out of therapy make future problems. Sooner or later the blood
pressure almost always rises again, time is lost in attempting to prevent or arrest
complications and the blood pressure may not be so easily controlled on subsequent
attempts.

The patient with cerebrovascular disease with or without stroke has always presented a special problem in hypertensive management. It used to be considered
dangerous to reduce the blood pressure significantly in these patients for fear of decreasing their central perfusion of blood. Hypertension is associated with an increased risk of stroke. Blood pressure control is crucial to the prevention of stroke.
The hypertensive patient has an increased cerebrovascular resistance. Reduction of
blood pressure has been shown to reduce cerebrovascular resistance and often to
increase the cerebral blood flow. Thus, the presence of known cerebrovascular disease is no contraindication to reducing high blood pressure. This should be done
judiciously and gradually, avoiding abrupt and large postural drops in blood pressure.
It is better to avoid the use of ganglionic and adrenergic blockade in these cases or,
if such must be used, to exercise extreme caution in dosage titration. The patient
with renal damage is another instance in which controversy has been present regarding lowering of blood pressure. Moyer and others have shown that reducing high
blood pressure can arrest the renal deterioration. In the malignant phase of hypertension, lowering the blood pressure will be accompanied by the healing of arteriolar
necrosis which is characteristic of the accelerated phase. Sometimes, if the renal
damage has not gone too far, reduction of the blood pressure is accompanied by some
improvement in renal function. In patients with severe renal damage the blood
pressure reduction may be accompanied by some further decline in renal function
as indicated by an increasing urea nitrogen, but after several months of control this
tends to stabilize. As in the case of cerebrovascular disease, the key phrase is judicious, gradual, slow reduction of the blood pressure to prevent worsening of the
renal state.

Aside from applying drug therapy alone, there are several general measures to be
applied to all patients. They include correcting overweight, decreasing the tempo
of living, promotion of fair balance of work, play and rest, reduction in the use of
coffee, tobacco and other stimulants, reduction of sodium intake, correction of
anemia, thyrotoxicosis, urinary tract infection if present.

At this time there is no ideal anti-hypertensive agent. All have advantages and
drawbacks with no real evidence that any particular drug or combination of drugs
per se is superior. What counts is to get the blood pressure down. The superior
drug is the one that does this in the given individual. Very often drugs used in
combinations allow for smaller doses for each individual agent so that adequate
effects can be attained with less chance of side reactions. This does not mean fixed
dose combinations because they lack flexibility in dosage regulation. A place for
fixed dose combination is where the therapist has determined by titration with
separate drugs which combination of medications works best for the patient and, if
individual dosages work out properly, an appropriate fixed dose combination tablet
may finally be utilized. This has the advantage that the patient will not mix up

TABLE XIII-1.   ANTIHYPERTENSIVE AGENTS

	X1	X2	X5	X6	X7	X8	Hours	Dose (mg.)	
*Chlorthalidone	C—CL	C—SO$_2$NH$_2$	C—OH	N—H	C=O	C—H	48–72	50–100	(Hygroton)
Polythiazide	C—CL	C—SO$_2$NH$_2$	S—O$_2$	N—CH$_3$	C—R	N—H	24–48	2–4	(Renese)
Trichlormethiazide	C—CL	C—SO$_2$NH$_2$	S—O$_2$	N—H	C—R	N—H	24	4–8	(Naqua, Methahydrin)
Methychlorthiazide	C—CL	C—SO$_2$NH$_2$	S—O$_2$	N—H	C—R	N—H	24	5–10	(Enduron)
Flumethiazide	C—CF$_3$	C—SO$_2$NH$_2$	S—O$_2$	N=	C—H	N—H	18–24	0.25–0.50	(Ademol)
Cyclothiazide	C—CL	C—SO$_2$NH$_2$	S—O$_2$	N—H	C—R	N—H	18–24	1–2	(Anhydron)
Bendioflumethiazide	C—CF$_3$	C—SO$_2$NH$_2$	S—O$_2$	N—H	C—R	N—H	18–24	5–10	(Natriueretin)
Hydroflumethiazide	C—CF$_3$	C—SO$_2$NH$_2$	S—O$_2$	N—H	C—H	N—H	18–24	50–100	(Saluron)
*Quinethasone	C—CL	C—SO$_2$NH$_2$	C=O	N—H	C—R	N—H	18–24	50–100	(Hydromox)
Benzthiazide	C—CL	C—SO$_2$NH$_2$	S—O$_2$	N—H	C—R	N=	12–18	50–100	(Aquatage, Edemex, Exna)
Hydrochlorothiazide	C—CL	C—SO$_2$NH$_2$	S—O$_2$	N—H	C—H	N—H	6–12	50–100	(Hydro-Diuril, Esidrix, Oretic)
Chlorothiazide	C—CL	C—SO$_2$NH$_2$	S—O$_2$	N—H	C—H	N=	6–12	50–100	(Diuril)
*Furosemide	C—CL	C—SO$_2$NH$_2$	COOH	NH—R	—	—	6–8	40 plus	(Lasix)
Diazoxide	C—H	C—CL	S—O$_2$	N—H	C—R	N=	None	———	(Hyperstat)

his various medications or dosage levels. It is usually unwise however, to start therapy with a fixed dose combination of drugs.

Initial therapy is best started with one of the diuretic agents and although many of these are available they all seem about similar in their action except for some difference in dosage size and duration in action (see Table XIII–1). This group of drugs is best exemplified by chlorothiazide which is the original. The initial effect is to reduce blood volume, total body sodium, and cardiac output, and thus blood pressure. After several weeks these return toward normal and the peripheral vascular resistance has decreased by a mechanism still unclear, but which may be associated with change in electrolyte ratios and water content within the arteriolar walls. The unwanted effects from these agents include elevation of uric acid with occasional precipitation of an attack of gout, occasional development of hyperglycemia, and a not infrequent development of hypokalemia. These situations, if anticipated, can be prevented or easily corrected and the agents need not be discontinued. Perhaps forty or fifty percent of the hypertensive patients can be controlled over a long period of time with thiazide agents alone. They are never satisfactory by themselves, however, in the accelerated phase. It is worth giving as much as two months' trial to these agents used alone before adding other drugs unless the clinical situation prevents that long a wait. The use of dietary salt restriction should be continued to allow the saluretic agents their fullest effect. The *rauwolfia* family best exemplified by reserpine seems to be having a decreased use in recent years. Rauwolfia depletes catecholamine stores at the neurochemical transducer presumably by upsetting the pump mechanism. Many patients develop an insidious onset of depression which may pass unnoticed by the patient or the physician until it is in full bloom, particularly among the elderly. Other side effects such as increase in stomach acid with development of peptic ulcer, stuffy nose, parkinsonian tremor, bad dreams, loose stools have all contributed to the decreased use of these agents. Adding *barbiturates* to the thiazide diuretic therapy has proved useful and helps one avoid the use of rauwolfia. Prolonged use of reserpine in the female seems to be accompanied by a three to four fold increase in the incidence of breast cancer, but this report needs confirmation. At this time it is not recommended that reserpine be discontinued in females. *Hydralazine* used alone causes the blood pressure to become more labile and widens the pulse pressure. Headache, tachycardia, and, in those with heart disease, angina or congestive heart failure may appear. Combining hydralazine with rauwolfia or propranolol prevents these unpleasant actions. By keeping the doses of hydralazine at 200 mg. daily or less, one can avoid the development of rheumatoid arthritis and the lupus erythematosus syndromes. The action of hydralazine appears to be a relaxing effect on the smooth muscle of the arteriolar walls.

α-Methyl-dopa has come into wide use as an antihypertensive agent which may or may not act by the formation of a false neuro-transmitter. *In vitro*, it inhibits the biosynthesis of catecholamines, but this is not the method by which it reduces blood pressure. Whatever its basic mechanism, it does produce a decrease of peripheral vascular resistance. It does not affect the cardiac output; it does not reduce renal blood flow or glomerular filtration rate. There is often a postural effect from this drug as well as somnolence and sometimes a salt and water retention. A diuretic agent should be used with it. It is not widely appreciated that depressive reactions may develop with methyl-dopa just as they may with the use of rauwolfia. About 20% of the patients will develop a positive Coombs test, but only rarely has there been any difficulty from this. Rarely hemolysis will occur and at times one sees abnormalities in the liver enzymes. Very often the dosage level used with methyl-dopa is too small. Usually a minimum of 750 mg. daily is required.

Guanethidine is a potent antihypertensive agent which acts by preventing the release of catecholamines from the postganglionic adrenergic stores. It also depletes the storage sites. Guanethidine also has a fairly marked postural effect on blood pressure and decreases heart rate, and cardiac output which features may be more marked after heavy exercise. Some decrease in renal blood flow may be seen, and salt and water retention may be noted. Failure of ejaculation is a distressing complaint in males taking this drug. There are some potentially serious drug interactions to be considered when using guanethidine. Propranolol decreases myocardial contractility and cardiac output and should probably not be used concurrently with guanethidine. The tricyclic anti-depressants such as imipramine, desipramine, and protriptyline effectively block the anti-hypertensive action of guanethidine resulting in a rise of blood pressure. Patients with reduced cardiac reserve should be carefully watched for the development of congestive heart failure when given guanethidine. If congestive heart failure or renal insufficiency are present, the drug is best avoided. *Monamine oxidase inhibitors* exemplified by pargyline, a drug of moderate potency, should not be used in antihypertensive therapy because of the hypertensive reactions that occur when combined with foods and beverages that contain tyramine. These include certain wines, cheeses, and beer. The older *ganglionic blocking agents* such as hexamethonium and pentolinium and mecamylamine have pretty much fallen by the wayside as drugs with more specific sites of action have been introduced. A large array of problems arising from ganglionic blockade such as constipation, failure of ejaculation, postural hypotension, dry mouth, and diminished renal function make these drugs only rarely indicated. An exception to this pertains to use of trimethaphan camsylate, an intravenously given short acting form of a ganglionic blocking agent, which still has a role to play in the initial control of hypertensive crises.

Propranolol is coming to use as an antihypertensive agent by virtue of its beta adrenergic blocking action. It also suppresses renin. Its best role appears to be when combined with hydralazine. It is not to be used in patients with A–V conduction defect or with marked brachycardia or in those with incipient or overt congestive heart failure. Its dosage level ranges from 40 to 160 mg. per day and occasionally slightly higher.

Clonidine has recently become available for clinical use in this country. It is an imidazoline derivative which appears to have its action in the central nervous system as a central alpha adrenergic stimulant. It does not deplete catecholamine stores. There is no great likelihood of postural hypotension. When given orally the blood pressure falls, the heart and stroke volume decrease somewhat. When given intravenously, an initial hypertensive response may be seen followed then by a decrease in the blood pressure. It also tends to produce some sodium retention. It appears to be useful in moderate to severe hypertension. Usual doses are 0.1 to 0.2 mg. twice daily. Caution should be exhibited in discontinuing the drug because occasional severe hypertension rebounds have occurred when it has been stopped abruptly. It should be tapered off.

Spironolactone. This is an aldosterone antagonist with saluretic-diuretic effects and potassium retaining properties. In the case of renal failure or added potassium, hyperkalemia may ensue. Twenty % of hypertensives generally will have a blood pressure lowering from spironolactone in the usual doses of 100 mg. per day, presumably from the osmotic effects. A much higher percentage of the low renin hypertensive group respond to it presumably by a suppressant effect on mineralocorticoids. If given in large doses of 400 mg. daily not all who respond in this manner have primary aldosteronism, however; but if they do not respond one can be fairly certain that they do not have primary aldosteronism. Genest has found that many non-malignant hypertensives have elevated plasma aldosterone, but normal secretion and excretion rates which he feels indicate decreased metabolic clearance by the liver. It may be that the spironolactone alone or combined with thiazide may assume a larger role in blood pressure management. The side effects are not usually great, but increasing potassium, lassitude, epigastric distress, gynecomastia, rash, confusion, headache, and ataxia have been reported.

TABLE XIII–2. WORK SHEET FOR STUDY OF HYPERTENSIVE PATIENT

Routine Studies	
History and physical exam	Routine studies may indicate etiology of the hypertension
Funduscopic evaluation	
Complete blood count	
Urinalysis	Necessary for the evaluation of severity and progress of the disease, results of therapy, and prognosis
Blood urea nitrogen	
Chest roentgenogram or orthodiagram	
Electrocardiogram	
Intravenous pyelogram	
Special Diagnostic Studies	
Urine Culture	Asymptomatic pyelonephritis may be cause of hypertension
Catecholamines (blood, urine)	Chemical tests—best screening tests for pheochromocytoma
Vanillylmandelic Acid (VMA—urine)	
Regitine test Histamine test	Pharmacologic tests may be performed jointly with chemical test to increase accuracy of diagnosis
Tyramine test	
Renal arteriogram; perirenal CO_2 study	To localize pheochromocytoma
Electrolytes Na, K, CO_2 (blood)	May indicate aldosteronism (primary or secondary)
Electrolytes (urine)	Often abnormal secondary to thiazide therapy
Aldosterone (urine)	
Renal arteriogram	Diagnosis of renovascular hypertension
Differential renal function	Diagnosis of branch renal artery lesion; helpful in bilateral renal artery stenosis
Radioactive renogram	Possible value as screening tests for renovascular hypertension, but not definitive
Scanning tests	
Renal biopsy	Occult pyelonephritis, juxtaglomerular granularity; histologic evidence of prognostic significance
Renin in peripheral venous blood	Separate primary from secondary hyperaldosteronism
Differential renal venous renin or angiotensin	Determine functional nature of anatomic renal artery stenosis

(From *Cardiac and Vascular Disease*, H. L. Conn, and O. Horwitz, Philadelphia, Lea & Febiger, 1971.)

In summary regarding the drug therapy of essential hypertension, one starts therapy in the mild to moderate hypertensive with thiazide diuretic. After several weeks or two months if adequate control is not attained, addition of either reserpine or a barbiturate may prove helpful. It would be worth giving spironolactone if the response to thiazide is poor, particularly if one determines that the patient has a suppressed renin level. The next step would be to add hydralazine or methyl-dopa to the reserpine or thiazide barbiturate combination. If the use of all of these together still fail to adequately control blood pressure, guanethidine and thiazide and hydralazine may be used.

The role of clonidine is still to be further clarified, but at present appears to be helpful for moderate to severe hypertensive situations. In those patients with high renin levels, propranolol has been useful in lowering the blood pressure and at the same time lowering the renin level. Excessive slowing of the heart rate can be avoided with the concomitant use of hydralazine. Laragh reports marked blood pressure reduction in patients with malignant hypertension and lowering of elevated renin levels by the use of propanolol.

References

Alarcon-Segovia, D., et al.: Clinical and experimental studies on the hydralazine syndrome and its relationship to systemic lupus erythematosus. Med., *46*:1, 1967.
Azcest, R., Gilmore, E., and Koch-Weser, J.: Treatment of hypertension with combined vasodilation and beta-adrenergic blockade. New Eng. J. Med., *286*:617, 1972.
Brechenridge, A., et al.: Positive direct Coombs tests and antinuclear factors in patients treated with methyldopa. Lancet, 2:1265, 1967.
Brunner, H. R., et al.: Essential hypertension: Renin and aldosterone, heart attack and stroke. New Eng. J. Med., *286*:441, 1972.
Buhler, F., et al.: Propranolol inhibition of renin secretion. New Eng. J. Med., *287*:1210, 1972.
Chasis, H.: Appraisal of antihypertensive drug therapy. Circulation, *50*:4, 1974.
Comens, P., and Schroeder, H. A.: L. E. cell as a manifestation of delayed hydralazine (phthalazine derivative) intoxication. J.A.M.A., *160*:1134, 1956.
Frank, E.: Bestehen Begiehungen zurschen chromaffinen System und der chronischen Hypertonie des Menschen? Deutsch. Arch. Klin. Med., *103*:397, 1911.
Freis, E. D.: Hypertension, 1973. An expert draws the line on whom to treat. Patient Care, *1*:63, 1973.
Freis, E. D.: Rebuttal: Appraisal of antihypertensive drug therapy. Circulation, *50*:9, 1974.
Frolich, E. D., et al.: Evaluation of the initial care of hypertensive patients. J.A.M.A., *218*:1036, 1971.
Hypertension Study Group (Report of inter-society commission for heart disease resources). Circ., *42*:A-39, 1970.
Janeway, T. C.: A clinical study of hypertensive cardiovascular disease. Arch. Intern. Med., *12*:755, 1913.
Kuchel, O., et al.: Effect of diazoxide on plasma renin activity in hypertensive patients. Ann. Intern. Med., *67*:791, 1967.
LeBriglio, A. F., and Jandl, J. H.: The nature of the alpha-methyldopa red cell antibody. New Eng. J. Med., *276*:658, 1967.
Manku, M. S., Nassar, B. A., and Horribin, D. F.: Furosemide as inhibitor of prolactin action. Lancet, 2:1261, 1973.
Mrocyzek, W. J., Finnerty, F. A., and Catt, K. J.: Lack of association between plasma-renin and history of heart attack or stroke in patients with essential hypertension. Lancet, 2:464, 1973.
Palmer, R. S., and Muench, H.: Cause and prognosis of essential hypertension. J.A.M.A., *153*:1, 1953.

Parfitt, A. M.: Chlorothiazide-induced hypercalcemia in juvenile osteoporosis and hyperparathyroidism. New Eng. J. Med., *281*:55, 1969.

Sellars, A. M., Itskovitz, H. and Lindauer, A.: Cardiac and Vascular Diseases, Chapter 32, p. 882, Conn, H. L. and Horwitz, O. (eds.). Philadelphia, Lea & Febiger, 1971.

Ueda, H., Yogi, S., and Kaneko, Y.: Hydralazine and plasma renin activity. Arch. Intern. Med., *122*:387, 1968.

Ulvilda, J. M., et al.: Blood pressure in chronic renal failure. J.A.M.A., *220*:233, 1972.

Warlledge, S. M., Carstairs, K. C., and Dacie, J. V.: Autoimmune hemolytic anemia associated with α-methyldopa therapy. Lancet, 2:133, 1966.

5. Vascular Crises: Established Hypertension

Joseph H. Magee

Synonyms: Malignant nephrosclerosis (1914). Malignant hypertension (1928). Accelerated form of hypertension (1958).

Cause: Vasospasm, with secondary vasonecrosis and impaired function of target organs, especially eyes, brain and kidneys in:

Primary hypertension	40%
Pregnancy hypertension	3%
Endocrine hypertension	3%
Multiple systems disease	7%
Primary renal disease (unilateral)	7%
Primary renal disease (bilateral)	40%

Early Manifestations: "I should like to say how we diagnose malignant hypertension in my department. We do not think that our criteria have any absolute value, but they usually are: diastolic blood pressure higher than 130, retinal changes grade III or IV, and marked alteration of the general condition. I think this last criterion is very important. Most patients lose weight. Even if they were obese, they lose weight, the general condition is altered, the central nervous system often shows signs of involvement. . . . I would not agree that azotemia is a very early sign. However, I have never seen normal renal function in a patient with malignant hypertension" (Reubi).

"No useful differences were seen between patients showing grade III and grade IV changes in their optic fundi. Consequently, it was decided that hemorrhage and exudates were as ominous as papilledema" (Hagans).

Papilledema which may be evanescent or even unilateral, was not seen in a fourth of patients with primary hypertension dying in renal failure.

Death follows initial observation of papilledema by three months in about half of untreated patients. Two-thirds are dead by one year, 95% by four years, 99% by five years.

Death follows initial observation of papilledema *plus azotemia* within three months, in all patients with primary hypertension, but half with primary renal disease survive three months to two years.

"Kimmelstiel and I found that about 3 percent of all cases of left ventricular hypertrophy at autopsy showed the histological features of malignant hypertension. This was obviously a selected series and I think essential hypertension becomes malignant in less than 0.1 percent of cases. On the other hand, in our series of chronic glomerular nephritis, 50 percent of patients developed malignant hypertension. . . .

Furthermore, papilledema seems to be reversible by hypotensive therapy much more easily in renal than in essential hypertension" (Wilson).

"Neuro-retinopathy indistinguishable from that of the malignant phase of hypertension may occur in severe anemia, particularly that following severe gastrointestinal hemorrhage, in subacute bacterial endocarditis, disseminated lupus polyarteritis nodosa, temporal arteritis and scleroderma. In all of these arterial pressure may be normal" (Pickering).

Twice as common in men, reversing the female predominance in primary hypertension. Generally preceding duration of primary hypertension averages seven years.

Visual impairment is first symptom in 80%; convulsions occur prior to uremia (pseudouremia) in 6% and following it in 12%. Headache nearly always occurs but has little specificity prospectively.

Proteinuria is heavy regardless of etiology.

Hematuria may be gross as well as microscopic and from lower tract ("urethral apoplexy") as well as upper.

Treatment: Ideally the treatment of vasospastic target organ damage, as evidenced by vasospastic retinopathy, is (whether this is due to hypercapnia, to hemorrhagic hypotension, or to hypertensive crisis) relief of the underlying cause. This is seldom possible in hypertensive crisis unless there is already amassed evidence for pheochromocytoma, or for a kidney lesion of only one kidney; or unless with little remaining renal function removal of both kidneys is to be undertaken. The alternative is drug therapies, which interrupt the mechanism of vasospasm at various points. All of the direct vasodilators induce reflex sodium retention which is combatted with chloruretic sulfonamides; any of them is satisfactory with good renal function, with furosemide preferred where this is greatly decreased. Oral hypoglycemic agents may be required for the hyperglycemic effect elicited.

Possible Dire Consequences without Treatment: The course of malignant hypertension continues remorselessly until the patient dies in uremic coma with or without heart failure. More rarely the course of the disease is suddenly interrupted by a neurological episode, but excessively rarely by a heart attack. Spontaneous regression of malignant hypertension is exceptional.

TABLE XIII–3.   ADULT PARENTERAL DOSES OF ANTIHYPERTENSIVE AGENTS USED TO TREAT HYPERTENSIVE EMERGENCIES (mg)

Drug	Intramuscular	Intravenous (Inject over 15–30 Minutes)	Intravenous (Continuous in 5% Dextrose in Water)
Diazoxide	—	300* q 2–12 h	
Reserpine	2.5(1.0–10.0) q 8–12 h	—	—
α-methyldopa	—	250(100–1000) q 6 h	—
Hydralazine	20(10.0–50.0) q 4–6 h	20(5.0–50.0) q 4–6 h	50–100/L
Pentolinium	5(2.5–50.0) q 6–8 h	5 q 6–8 h	50–100/L
Trimethaphan			
Camphorsulphonate	—	—	250–500/L
Sodium nitroprusside	—	—	60.0/L

* Inject rapidly within 15 seconds.

(From Cardiac and Vascular Disease, H. L. Conn and O. Horwitz, Philadelphia, Lea & Febiger, 1971).

References

Goldring, W., and Chasis, H.: Hypertension and Hypertensive Disease. New York, Commonwealth Fund, 1944.

Hagans, J. A., and Brust, A. A.: The natural history of hypertension. Am. J. Med., *28*:905, 1960.

Keith, N. M., Wagener, A. P., and Barker, N. W.: Some different types of essential hypertension: Their course and prognosis. Am. J. Med. Sci., *197*:332, 1939.

Perera, G. A.: Hypertensive vascular disease: Description and natural history. J. Chron. Dis., *7*:33, 1955.

Pickering, G. W.: High Blood Pressure. p. 345. New York, Grune & Stratton, 1968.

Reubi, F.: Discussion in Essential Hypertension: An International Symposium. Berne, June 7th to 10th, 1960, Bock, K. D., and Cottier, P. J. (eds.). Berlin, Springer-Verlag, 1960, p. 231.

Schottstaedt, M. F., and Sokolow, M.: The natural history and course of hypertension with papilledema (malignant hypertension). Am. Heart J., *45*:331, 1953.

6. Vascular Crises: Toxemia of Pregnancy Hypertension

Joseph H. Magee

Causes: Specific hypertensive disease of pregnancy in 70%. Pregnancy incidental to hypertension in 30%.

Early Manifestations: Hypertension with onset at five, and more often six, months of pregnancy means either of two things:
(*a.*) Amelioration of pre-existing hypertension during mid-trimester with return during last trimester, possible in patients in whom previous medical information is lacking, or
(*b.*) Specific hypertensive disease of pregnancy, in which case coexistent proteinuria and/or edema routinely are present also.
Earlier onset of hypertension means either of two things:
(*a.*) Pre-existing hypertension, or
(*b.*) Trophoblastic disease, the likelihood enhanced by definite information showing that the patient has hitherto been normotensive
Specific pregnancy hypertension is more common in teenagers, primigravida, closely spaced pregnancies, Rh incompatibilities, malnutrition, prediabetes, diabetes, postmaturity, and in women who give birth to boys. Fetal mortality is 25% and maternal mortality 5%.
Convulsions, which may occur antepartum, intrapartum, and up to two days postpartum, are correlated with height of arterial pressure; and usually preceded by central nervous system irritability (headache, alternate drowsiness and restlessness, hyperreflexia, nausea, vomiting), worsened proteinuria, and fluid accumulation (weight gain, pulmonary congestion). Differential diagnosis includes cerebral hemorrhage as well as cryptic epilepsy if untreated arterial pressure level is discordant.
Entire clinical picture is ameliorated by delivery of fetus and placenta, and persistence of hypertension more than seven weeks postpartum indicates coexistent established hypertension.

16

Treatment: Admit patients (a) with more than trace proteinuria, (b) arterial pressure 160/110 on one occasion and again six hours later, (c) decreased urine volume and (d) central nervous system irritability, to hospital for complete bed rest.

If blood pressure does not respond to bed rest, begin drug therapy and make plans for delivery.

Reserpine 0.25 mg. q. 8h may be used for about forty-eight hours before somnolence, nasal congestion, and pseudoparkinsonism limit use. Barbiturate premedication should be omitted and anesthetist informed of drugs already given.

Induction and vaginal delivery usually are preferred to cesarean section. Infant may have nasal congestion and bronchorrhea from reserpine if used.

Furosemide 80 mg. potentiates reserpine if longer use is necessitated; may be repeated in two hours if no diuretic effect is evident.

If one and one-half to two hour delay in hypotenisve effect of reserpine effect is not advisable, 5 mg./kg. diazoxide rapidly intravenously will reduce pressure promptly with persistence of effect for up to twelve hours.

Possible Dire Consequences without Treatment: Consumption coagulopathy. Adrenal cortical necrosis. Renal cortical necrosis. Hypertensive encephalopathy. Maternal death. Fetal death.

References

Gray, M. J.: Use and abuse of thiazides in pregnancy. Clin. Obstet. Gynec., *11*:568, 1968.
Finnerty, F. A., and Bepho, F. J.: Lowering the perinatal mortality and prematurity rate. J.A.M.A., *195*:429, 1966.
Kraus, G. W.: Prophylactic use of hydrochlorothiazide in pregnancy. J.A.M.A., *198*:1150, 1966.
Sarles, H. E., et al.: Sodium excretion patterns during and following intravenous sodium chloride loads in normal and hypertensive pregnancies. Am. J. Obst. Gynec., *102*:1, 1968.

7. Vascular Crises: Oral Contraceptive Hypertension

J. EDWIN WOOD AND JOSEPH H. MAGEE

Cause: Pills containing:

(*a.*) 0.05 to 0.1 mg. mestranol or ethinyl estradiol plus
(*b.*) 10 to 250 times as much progestogen simultaneously or sequentially.

Early Manifestations: Headache which may be preceded by scotomata and/or visual field defects. Vertigo. Epistaxes. Hypertension.

Treatment: The treatment is to discontinue oral contraceptives. If blood pressure has not returned to normal after six months or more, the patient should receive hypotensive agents; for diastolic blood pressures greater than 120 mm., hypotensive medication should be instituted at once.

Possible Dire Consequences without Treatment: Established hypertension, hypertensive complications.

It is certain that a patient with hypertension may have the disorder aggravated by oral contraceptives. Furthermore, young women who have not previously had hypertension may experience it for the first time following the use of oral contraceptives. In both instances, blood pressures will return to original levels with discontinuance of the agent; however, the fall is not immediate and usually requires at least four to five weeks.

The mechanism appears to involve mediation by the renin-angiotensin-aldosterone system. The most striking alteration is uniformly increased levels of renin substrate (angiotensinogen).

Regardless of the concomitant renin increase if any, reaction rate is increased over and above that caused by increased concentrations of the reactants. The increased formation of angiotensin causes increased aldosterone levels and between the two effects blood pressure is increased. The first manifestations of increased blood pressure may appear as early as two to three months after beginning use of the drug.

For this reason it is important to have some sort of base line study of the patient's blood pressure before starting oral contraceptive therapy. If a young woman has been on medication for more than a year without change in blood pressure, it becomes unlikely that such will occur, but blood pressure should be followed as long as medication is continued.

Most investigators in this field have concluded that it is unwise to allow patients already known to have intermittent or fixed hypertension to begin this medication because the likelihood of increased blood pressure is so great.

References

Laugh, J. H., et al.: Oral contraceptives. Renin, aldosterone and high blood pressure. J.A.M.A., *201*:918, 1967.

Skinner, S. L., Lumbers, E. L., and Symonds, E. M.: Alterations by oral contraceptives of normal menstrual changes in plasma renin activity, concentration and substrate. Clin. Sci., *36*:36, 1969.

Wood, J. E.: The cardiovascular effects of oral contraceptives. Mod. Concepts Cardiovasc. Dis., *51*:37, 1972.

Woods, J. W.: Oral contraceptives and hypertension. Lancet, *2*:653, 1967.

8. Vascular Crises: Reflexogenic from Hypercapnia

Joseph H. Magee

Cause: Hypercapnia.

Early Manifestations: Respiratory failure simulating cardiac failure.
Hypertension may ameliorate with ventilatory assistance, and not with oxygen therapy, at flow rates that do not induce apnea.
Raised pCO_2; compensatorily raised $[HCO_3]$s; low pO_2
A–V oxygen difference, circulation time, and venous pressure may be normal.
Low diaphragms, prolonged audible expiratory phase.

Treatment: Ventilatory assistance. Defer therapy of hypertension until effect of ventilatory assistance is observed.

Possible Dire Consequences without Treatment: Vascular collapse due to direct peripheral vasodilator effect of unchecked hypercapnia. Uncompensated respiratory acidosis. Carbon dioxide narcosis.

The initial effect of carbon dioxide accumulation is cerebral vasodilation. If sustained this can occasion papilledema and consideration of cerebral space occupying lesions, prior to the next effect, which is in effect a vascular crisis. As a late manifestation and part of an "alarm reaction," there is neurogenic peripheral vasoconstriction, which predominates over an ultimate direct peripheral vasodilator effect of carbon dioxide. The stage where hypertension is superimposed upon previous papilledema can sway diagnostic impressions dangerously if the primary respiratory problem is insufficiently recognized.

References

Sieker, H. O., and Hickam, J. B.: Carbon dioxide intoxication. Medicine, *35*:389, 1956.
Westlake, E. K., Simpson, T., and Kaye, M.: Carbon dioxide narcosis in emphysema. Quart. J. Med., *24*:155, 1955.

9. Vascular Crises: Reflexogenic from Low Output

JOSEPH H. MAGEE

Cause: Low cardiac output.

Early Manifestations: "During certain types of cardiac failure a diastolic hypertension may appear, the pressure returning to normal as improvement in cardiac function is achieved. Among these types may be mentioned those due to constrictive pericarditis or pericardial effusion, and that occurring occasionally in the early stages of myocardial infarction . . . rapidly progressive cardiac dilatation . . . is commonly associated with dome diastolic arterial hypertension. It seems quite paradoxical that a dilated failing heart with low output should maintain an elevated diastolic arterial pressure, and there is no ready explanation in physiological terms for this stiuation. The relation of the hypertension to the cardiac dilatation and failure can be seen clinically in some cases when they appear and disappear simultaneously" (Newman).

Treatment: Evaluate need for hypotensive agents after effect of bed rest, oxygen, inotropic and saluretic agents upon contemporaneous congestive phenomena is apparent.

Possible Dire Consequences without Treatment: Overzealous use of hypotensive agents, congestive failure, death.

Reference

Newman, E. V.: Heart Failure: Illustrative case, p. 66. In Differential Diagnosis, The Interpretation of Clinical Evidence. Harvery, A. M. and Bordley, J., III (eds.). Philadelphia, W. B. Saunders Co., 1956.

10. Vascular Crises: Cantrogenic (Cushing Effect)

Joseph H. Magee

Cause: Diencephalic stimulation by intracranial space occupying lesions.

Early Manifestations: "Only rarely is a brain tumor accompanied by hypertension. A high blood pressure, 175 mm. and above, therefore always places the burden of proof upon the diagnosis of a tumor, but it is by no means an absolute criterion. I recall two distressing instances in which I assumed the absence of a tumor because of the high grade of hypertension, 250 mm. in each, and several months later, operable dural endotheliomas were found" (Cushing).

Wider pulse pressures and greater lability of pressures is found than in vascular crises of established hypertension.

More marked peripheral sudomotor and vasomotor phenomena, with alternating or mixed skin flushing and blanching, may occur.

Localizing neurologic signs, behavioral change, or high index of suspicion, may occasion diagnostic skull films, scintiscan, ultrasound, air, or arteriographic studies.

Treatment: Surgery.

Possible Dire Consequences without Treatment: Medullary compression.

References

Cushing, H.: The blood pressure reaction of acute cerebral concussion illustrated by cases of intracranial hemorrhage. Am. J. Med. Sci., *125*:1017, 1903.

Cushing, H.: Neurohypophyseal mechanisms, Lancet, 2:119, 1930.

Dandy, W. E.: The Brain. New York, Hoeber Reprints, 1969, p. 440.

Page, I. H.: A syndrome simulating diencephalic stimulation occurring in patients with essential hypertension. Am. J. Med. Sci., *190*:9, 1935.

Schroeder, H. A., and Goldman, M. L.: A test for the presence of the "hypertensive diencephalic syndrome" rising histamine. Am. J. Med., *6*:162, 1949.

Zulch, K. J.: Diskussion uber das subdurale hamatom. Zbl. Neurosurg., *10*:305, 1950.

11. Vascular Crises: Buffer Nerve Section

Joseph H. Magee

Cause: Ninth cranial nerve injury due to acute intermittent porphyria. Diphtheria. Kanamycin toxicity.

Early Manifestations: Hypertension is labile, accompanied by tachycardia; history of previously normal pressures may be obtainable.

With kanamycin and similar drugs, accompanying eighth cranial nerve damage (vestibular, auditory) may also be present.

Treatment: Propranolol 1 to 3 mg. intravenously with electrocardiographic monitoring for acute life-threatening elevations.

Propranolol 10 to 30 mg. orally daily in divided doses for persistent hypertension.

Possible Dire Consequences without Treatment: Hypertensive encephalopathy. Intracranial hemorrhage.

References

Corcoran, A. C., Jr., Imperial, E. S., and Smith, H. E.: Neurogenic hypertension: A sequel of kanamycin intoxication. J.A.M.A., *174*:1838, 1960.

Kedzi, P.: Neurogenic hypertension in man in porphyria. Arch. Intern. Med., *94*:122, 1954.

Rosenbaum, I., Jr.: Hypertension in diphtheria. J. Pediat., *77*:210, 1940.

12. Vascular Crises from Bulb and Cord Section

Joseph H. Magee

Causes: Bulbar tabes, bulbar polio, platybasia, syringomyelia, traumatic spinal cord injury with lesion above fourth thoracic segment.

Early Manifestations: Paroxysmal hypertension.
Paroxysmal headache.
Cutaneous blush of dermatomes innervated by cord segments above injury level.
Pallor, piloerection of dermatomes innervated by cord segments below injury level.
Provocation by bowel or bladder distention.

Treatment: Prevention: Regitine 50 mg. orally 4 to 6 times/day.
Attacks: Regitine 5 mg. intravenously.
Ascertain causes such as blocked catheter, etc.

Possible Dire Consequences without Treatment: Intracranial hemorrhage.

References

Bennett, I. L., Jr., and Heyman, A.: Paroxysmal hypertension associated with tabes dorsalis. Am. J. Med., *5*:729, 1948.

Bors, E. and French, J. D.: Management of paroxysmal hypertension following injuries to cervical and upper thoracic segments of the spinal cord. Arch. Surg., *64*:803, 1952.

Hodgson, W. B., and Wood, J. A.: Studies of the nature of paroxysmal hypertension in paraplegics. J. Urol., *79*:719, 1958.

Koster, K., and Bethlem, J.: Paroxysmal hypertension caused by spinal cord lesions. Acta Psychial. Scand., *36*:346, 1961.

Mc Dowell, F. H., and Plum, F.: Arterial hypertension associated with acute anterior poliomyelitis. New Eng. J. Med., *245*:241, 1951.

Sizemore, G. W., and Winternitz, W. W.: Autonomic hyper-reflexia: Suppression with alpha adrenergic blocking agents. New Eng. J. Med., *282*, 795, 1970.

Introduction:

Access of norepinephrine (NE) to receptors is controlled quantitatively by nerve action potentials which regulate the access of calcium ions to exoplasm, whereupon exocytosis of storage vesicles delivers NE into synaptic clefts. There is little free amine in axoplasm outside vesicles because of the scavenging effect of monoamine oxidase. The relationship is changed where this action is inhibited in nerve and elsewhere, and endogenous and exogenous amines may gain uncoordinated access to receptors. A similar risk arises with NE or epinephrine production by neoplastic chromaffin tissue. The next three sections deal with the consequence of this adrenergic uncoupling.

13. Vascular Crises: Metabolic Inhibitors

Joseph H. Magee

Cause: Concomitant administration of

Monoamine Oxidase Inhibitors
- (*a.*) Furagolidone (Furoxone, Eaton 072) brown scored tablets
- (*b.*) Isocarboxazide (Marplan, Roche) peach scored tablets
- (*c.*) Nialamide (Niamid, Pfizer 532, 533) red or peach tablets
- Pargyline (Eutonyl, Abbott) red, peach or gray tablets
- Phenylzine (Nardil, Warner) red coated tablets
- Tranylcypromine (Parnete, SKF-N71) purple coated tablets.

and any of the following:

Bronchodilator Monoamines:
  Epinephrine (Asmolin Epicar, Medihaler, Susphrine)
  Ephedrine (Bronkolixir, Duovent, Mudrane, Quadrinal, Tedral).
Decongestant Monoamines:
  Hydroxyamphetamine (Paredrine, Vasocort)
  Naphthazoline (Privine, Vasocon)
  Oxymetazoline (Abrin)
  Phenylephrine (Dimetane, Dimetapp, Hostaspan, Hycomine, Neo-Synephrine, Novahestine, Robitussin, Vasocort)
  Pseudoephedrine (Actifad, Sudafed)
  Tetrahydrozoline (Tyzine, Visine)
  Xylometozoline (Otrivin)
Anorexiant Monoamines:
  Benzphetamine (Didrex)
  Dextroamphetamine (Amodex, Daprisol, Dimacol, Eskatrol, Obotan, Robitussin, Tussagesic)
  Diethylpropion (Tepanil, Tenuate)
  Leroamphetamine (Amodril, Cudril, Pedestal)
  Methamphetamine (Desbutal, Desoxyn, Fetamin, Obedrin)
  Racemic Amphetamine (Benzedrine, Edrisol, Obetral)
Levodopa (Dopar, Larodopa)
Methyldopa (Aldochlor, Aldomet, Aldoril)
Tyramine-containing foods: Beer, cheese, Chianti, chicken livers, chocolate, canned figs, pickled herrings, sour cream, string beans, yeast.
Tricyclic Antidepressants
  Amitryptyline (Elavil, Etrafon, Triavil)
  Desimipramine (Norpramin)
  Doxepin (Sinequan)
  Imipramine (Topanil)
  Nortryptyline (Aventyl)
  Protryptyline (Vivactyl)

Early Manifestations: Headache, nausea, vomiting, sweating, photophobia, dilated pupils, chest and neck pain, elevated blood pressure.

Treatment: Phentolamine. See Pheochromocytoma.

Possible Dire Consequences without Treatment: Increased symptoms, cerebrovascular accident.

References

Krikler, D. M., and Lewis, B.: Danger of natural foodstuffs. Lancet, *1*:1166, 1965.
Lewis, R. G., and Young, A.: A long-term study with pargyline in the treatment of hypertension. Med. J. Austral., *1*:339, 1967.

14. Vascular Crises: Pheochromocytoma

JOSEPH H. MAGEE

Cause: Neoplastic

Early Manifestations: They should be sought about two decades earlier than essential hypertension. If not recognized in these years, the patient incurs increasing risk of confusion with essential hypertension; and of exposure to such risks as anesthesia, delivery, surgery, trauma and unintentionally provocative procedures common to hypertensive work-ups. Compared to the patient with essential hypertension the patient is thinner, less often female and subject to pathogenetic mechanisms apart from raised arterial pressure and vasoconstriction. He thus becomes subject to paroxysmal events which may variously be painful (headache especially, 80%), sweating (70%), cardioregulatory (65%), vasomotor (50%), mental (40%), motor (35%), gastrointestinal (35%, mostly nausea, sometimes ileus), and respiratory (dyspnea chiefly, 15%). Because of greater heat production, these patients sweat more, and if metabolism testing is available their oxygen consumption is higher (65%); hyperglycemia is present in 40% and glycosuria in 35%. In contrast to the exaggerated circulatory reflexes of essential hypertensive (cold pressure response, overshoot post-Valsalva) theirs are depressed; they may manifest postural hypotension (45%) and postural tachycardia (55%) in part occasioned by decreased blood volume. Because of the still high surgical risk once the diagnosis is made, a preliminary period of treatment with receptor blocking drugs is indicated, with restoration of blood volume if low, and a reduced occurrence of paroxysms, as endpoints.

The diagnosis of pheochromocytoma is primarily dependent upon urine assays for catecholamines and metabolites. The excretion of unchanged catecholamines normally amounts to about 100 mg. a day, half being from the adrenal medullae, equally divided between E (epinephrine) and NE; the remainder being NE from nerve endings. About 99% of liberated catecholamines are excreted in inactivated form, 9% by methoxylation alone and the remaining 90% both by methoxylation and subsequent deamination. The absolute amounts excreted can be increased from 100 to 200 fold in tumors with rapid turnover rates, but amounts scarcely above the diagnostic threshold can result from relatively large tumors with slow turnover rates. Release rates can be augmented by tilting stress and by pharmacological agents, including histamine, tyramine, glucagon, nicotinic agonists bradykinin, and angiotensin. These maneuvers are potentially most useful in conjunction with blood rather than urine assays. In collecting blood for assay, the requirements for preserving and shipping the blood must be ascertained where not done locally.

Treatment: Preoperatively propranolol 10 mg., plus phentolamine 50 mg., q 4h around clock; omitting dose during hours of sleep if free of paroxysms soon after awakening. Surgery.

Possible Dire Consequences without Treatment: Paroxysmal hypertension due to inadvertent provocation by operative stress. Stroke, congestive heart failure, angina, coronary occlusion, sustained hypertension, and death.

Although a definitive diagnosis does depend on laboratory studies, a large percentage of these lesions can and are diagnosed by eliciting a proper history, with particular reference to paroxysmal sweating, headaches, hypertension and arrhythmia in younger individuals.

References

Harrison, T. S., Bartlett, J. D., Jr., and Seaton, J. F.: Current evaluation and management of pheochromocytoma. Ann. Surg., *168*:701, 1968.

Harrison, T. S., et al.: Adrenal medulla; some basic and clinical considerations with special reference to pheochromocytoma, Chapter 47, p. 1314 in Cardiac and Vascular Disease, Vol. II, Conn. H. L., Jr. and Horwitz, O. (eds.). Philadelphia, Lea & Febiger, 1971.

Ludwig, G. D.: Carcinoid heart disease, Chapter 47, p. 1309 in Cardiac and Vascular Disease, Vol. II, Conn, H. L., Jr. and Horwitz, O. (eds.). Philadelphia, Lea & Febiger, 1971.

Sjoerdsma, A.: Conjoint clinic on serotonin; norepinephrine and tyramine. The Chronic Diseases, *18*:429, 1965.

Wurtman, R. J.: Catecholamines. Boston, Little, Brown and Co., 1966.

15. Familial Pheochromocytoma

JOSEPH H. MAGEE

Cause: Neoplastic.

Early Manifestations: Episodic hypertension.

Treatment: Surgery.

Possible Dire Consequences without Treatment: Cerebral hemorrhage.
Episodic hypertension.
Fifty% of the cases are bilateral.
Onset is a decade earlier (age twenty-six) than in sporadic pheochromocytoma or essential hypertension.
Five% have von Recklinghausen's disease (multiple neurofibromatosis).
Should be expected where hypertensive or other paroxysms coexist with thyroid carcinoma, congenital heart disease, von Recklinghausen's or other neurocutaneous syndromes.

References

Cushman, P.: Familial endocrine tumors. Am. J. Med., *32*:352, 1962.

Hume, D. M.: Pheochromocytoma in the adult and in the child. Am. J. Surg., *99*:458, 1960.

Introduction: Nephrogenic Hypertension

In acute renal failure, hypertension may be in large measure due to ventricular preloading with the cardiac output (stroke volume times rate) raised as in other high output states with or without congestive phenomena. The hypertension of acute renal failure is volume and salt dependent, prevention of salt surfeits is a principal concern of therapy, and management is eased when and if oliguria wanes.

In chronic renal failure hypertension may be present due to low filtration renal disease without oliguria. If the salt retention, still hormone responsive, which mediates hypertension is overcome, hypertension may be relieved. In Thorn's syndrome no amount of salt eventuates in hypertension until preterminally, because kidney structures continue to leak it, unresponsive to astronomical levels of mineralocorticoid hormone. In oliguric chronic renal failure, however, hypertension becomes a regular finding but with the relative participation of salt retention and of other hormonal effects increasingly moot. A discriminant function is supplied, however, by the advent of modern dialysis procedures, and also frequently by the performance of bilateral nephrectomies. Removal of the kidneys corrects hypertension in some patients in whom salt removal has not. There is a further small subset in whom hypertension persists after both procedures and then is corrected by some other homeostatic link that a successfully functioning graft supplies.

Reference

Davies, D. L., et al.: Abnormal relation between exchangeable sodium and the renin-angiotensin system in malignant hypertension and in hypertension with chronic renal failure. Lancet, *1*:683, 1973.

16. Uremic Hypertension (Salt Dependent)

Joseph H. Magee

Cause: Low filtration renal disease without oliguria.

Early Manifestations: "Not all patients with chronic renal disease develop hypertension from ingestion of sodium . . . at one end of the spectrum are the true salt wasters. This type of patient almost never becomes hypertensive and usually requires supplementation of sodium intake. At the other are those patients in whom . . . getting rid of even 40 to 50 mEq. of sodium per day is impossible without the development of severe hypertension."
Weight may be stable and hypertension manageable with little in the way of drug therapy on 20 mEq./day sodium intake where hypertension has been present with unsupervised diet.
"Successful control of hypertension with dietary sodium restriction often requires impractical limitations on dietary sodium intake because as sodium intake and blood pressure fall, so does sodium excretion . . . long-term administration of furosemide can help solve this problem. . . . Muth has shown that furosemide can cause a consistent sabiresis in patients with a GFR as low as 0.5 ml./min."

Treatment: Instruct non-oliguric patients with serum creatinines 5 to 10 mg./100 ml. in fifty day dietary sodium restriction.
Follow daily weight record, circulatory reflexes, venous filling, arterial pressure.
With maintained or increasing weight, add 80–240 mg. furosemide, as single evening rather than divided dose.
Liberalize intake to 120 mEq./day (7 gm./day) in furosemide responsive patients.

Possible Dire Consequences without Treatment: High methyldopa or guanethidine doses may otherwise be required to reduce arterial pressure elevation.

References

Coodley, E. L., et al.: Nondialytic management of chronic uremia. J.A.M.A., *224*:864, 1973.

Levin, D. M., and Cade, R.: Influence of dietary sodium on renal function in patients with chronic renal disease. Ann. Intern. Med., *62*:231, 1965.

Muth, R. G.: Diuretic properties of furosemide in renal disease. Ann. Intern. Med., *69*:261, 1968.

Ulvila, J. M., et al.: Blood pressure in chronic renal failure. J.A.M.A., *220*:233, 1972.

17. Abdominal Coarctation

JOSEPH H. MAGEE

Result: Hypoperfusion affecting the renal circulation disproportionately. Renin dependent hypertension.

Cause: Aortic obstructions with inadequate collateral reentry above the kidneys.

Early Manifestations: Congenital abdominal coarctation: Precocious upper arm hypertension with low (abdominal or lumbar) continuous bruit, absent aortic notching and esophageal E signs of hypoplastic aorta and rib notching on chest radiogram, reduced or absent femoral or pedal pulses, coldness and exercise pains of lower extremities.

Intimal (nodular) arteriosclerosis *in situ*, or ascending Leriche syndrome: Onset of hypertension after age sixty, especially in males; intermittent claudications and easy fatigability of thighs and hips, decreased pulsation of abdominal aorta and femorals, bruit usually present anteriorly and posteriorly, impotence, abdominal angina postprandially and relieved by change of position.

Arteritis, *in situ*; or descending Takayusu syndrome: Precocious hypertension, especially in females, claudications of left shoulder and neck, masticatory muscles, weakness of orbital and shoulder muscles, septal perforation, convulsive disorders, carotid sinus syncope, decreased pulsation of radials and carotids compared to legs (reverse coarctation), bruit heard at base of neck, superficial thoracic collaterals, rib notching, esophageal E sign of hypoplastic aortic arch and thoracic aorta.

Treatment: Because of proximity of coeliac and superior mesenteric arteries, bypass graft of narrowed segment is preferred to excision and grafting.

Possible Dire Consequences without Treatment: Accelerated hypertension: which does not occur in proximal correlation occurs in a sixth of cases. Inadequate tributary flow to spinal cord, pelvic organs and extremities.

References

Daimon, S., and Kitamura, K.: Coarctation of the abdominal aorta. Jap. Heart J., *5*:562, 1964.

Kittredge, R. D., and Anderson, J. W.: Coarctation of the lower thoracic and abdominal aorta. Radiology, *79*:799, 1962.

Kondo, B., et al.: Congenital coarctation of the abdominal aorta. Am. Heart J., *39*:306, 1950.

Maycock, W. D.: Congenital stenosis of the abdominal aorta. Am. Heart J., *13*:633, 1937.

Pyorala, K., et al.: Coarctation of the abdominal aorta. Am. J. Cardiol., *6*:650, 1960.

Robicsek, F., Sanger, P. W., and Daugherty, H. K.: Coarctation of the abdominal aorta, diagnosed by aortography. Ann. Surg., *158*:6, 1965.

Schuster, R.: Coarctation of the abdominal aorta. Am. Surg., *158*:6, 1963.
Sondergaard, T., and Ottosen, P.: Coarctation of the abdominal aorta. Acta Chir. Scand., *125*: Suppl 283; 194, 1963.

Introduction: Segmental Reninism

If a patient is azotemic, and creatininemic as well, he or she has bilateral renal disease. Even this may be benefitted by treatment of congestive heart failure and control of accelerated progress of the hypertension. Without nitrogen retention, the possibility exists that the patient may have unilateral renal disease. Smith and colleagues reviewed early evidence that removal of the offending kidney relieved hypertension in 1943. Only 7 of 76, 59 with one year follow-up data, yielded this desired result, an incidence of 9%. In 1948, in 47 of 242 patients, hypertension was relieved for a 19% success rate; 22 had unilateral pyelonephritis. Thompson and Smithwick added 26 more successes out of 57, a 46% rate, raising the cumulative success rate to 24%. In Smith's 1948 review this was up only to 26% with success attending 149 of 575 additional cases. In Kincaid-Smith's 1961 review 130 of 326 more patients had relief, raising the success rate to 37%. Sixty-five percent of these were renal artery lesions, 19% pyelonephritis, 6% hydronephrosis, and 10% other entities.

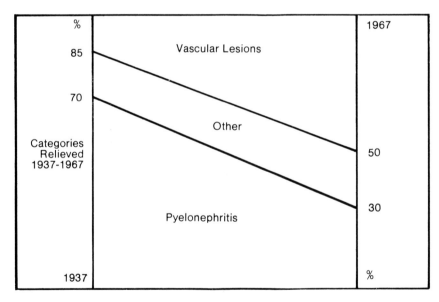

Fig. XIII–4. During the first 3 decades of remediable renal surgery for hypertension the therapeutic successes associated with vascular lesions rather than pyelonephritic, usually contracted kidneys, increased from 15 to 50% of the total.

References

Kincaid-Smith, P.: Renal ischemia and hypertension. Austral. Ann. Med., *10*:166, 1961.
Smith, H. W.: Hypertension and urologic disease. Am. J. Med., *4*:724, 1948.
Smith, H. W.: Unilateral nephrectomy in hypertensive disease. J. Urol., *76*:685, 1956.
Smith, H. W., Goldring, W., and Chasis, H.: Role of the kidney in the genesis of hypertension. Bull. N.Y. Acad. Med., *19*:449, 1943.
Thompson, R. H., and Smithwick, R. H.: Hypertension due to unilateral renal disease with special reference to renal artery lesions. Angiology, *3*:493, 1952.

18. Renal A-V Fistula

Joseph H. Magee

Cause: Congenital. Hypernephroma.
Traumatic (bullets, knives, biopsy needles, blunt trauma, postnephrectomy).

Early Manifestations: Hypertension. Onset before age thirty or after age fifty. History of trauma. Bruit is invariably present. Communication is usually aneurysmal, causing filling defects on pyelography, blush on arteriography, with early visualization of vena cava.

Treatment: Surgical closure.

Possible Dire Consequences without Treatment: Renal parenchymal compression. High output circulatory failure.

References

Maldonado, J. E., et al.: Renal arteriovenous fistula. Am. J. Med., *37*:499, 1964.
Naffah, P., Najafi, H., and DeWall, R. A.: Arteriovenous fistula involving the renal vessels. Minn. Med., *49*:227, 1966.
Scheifley, C. H., et al.: Arteriovenous fistula of the kidney. Circ., *19*:662, 1958.

19. Hypertension due to Non-Uremic Pyelonephritis (Butler-Longcope Effect)

Joseph H. Magee

Cause: Pyogenic pyelonephritis.

Early Manifestations: Back pain with costovertebral angle tenderness. Fever, usually spiking, without accompanying tachycardia, Pyuria.

Treatment: Success of this nature follows in only about one out of three instances of nephrectomy, which should be based upon urologic indication primarily; or demonstration of unilateral reninism by separate renal vein blood collections. Treatment of infection if active.

Possible Dire Consequences without Treatment: Progressive renal damage. Hypertension and its results.

Hypertension as a consequence of pyelonephritis progressing to bilateral renal contraction was convincingly documented by Lohlein in 1917. In 1937, Longcope wrote "Both Jacoby and Haslinger report instances of unilateral 'Shrumpfniere' due to chronic pyelonephritis and the condition does not seem to be extremely rare. It may occur in individual in whom a chronic infection of the kidney occurs in relation to a renal calculus imbedded in the calyces of the kidneys. One such case has come under my observation. In this patient pyelonephritis was associated with hypertension . . . there was no evidence of renal insufficiency . . . the question naturally arises, however, as to whether disease, such as this could produce a persistent elevation of blood pressure in man."

Butler had made some blood pressure observations beginning in 1935, indicating that hypertension *had preceded* uremia in 4 of 20 pyelonephritic children, and occurred without it in 9 more, 2 of whom died in congestive heart failure. In 1937 he reported a twenty-month remission of hypertension in a seven-year-old boy, and for five months in a ten-year-old girl, after nephrectomy for unilateral pyelonephritis. In the former, pyelonephritis had followed calculous disease, answering Longcope's query affirmatively in almost every respect.

References

Butler, A. M.: Chronic pyelonephritis and arterial hypertension. J. Clin. Invest., *16*:889, 1937.

Longcope, W. T.: Chronic bilateral pyelonephritis. Its origin and association with hypertension. Ann. Intern. Med., *11*:149, 1937.

20. Renovascular Hypertension (Low Pressure Kidney) (Goldblatt Effect)

Joseph H. Magee

Causes: Anomalous renal arteries.
   (*a.*) Accessory.
   (*b.*) Hypoplastic.
   (*c.*) Aneurysmal.
   Acquired stenoses.
   (*a.*) Simple or nodular intimal arteriosclerosis of proximal one-third of main renal arteries, usually after age fifty, and predominantly (8:1) in men.
   (*b.*) Fibromuscular narrowing of distal 2/3 of main renal arteries and their branches, usually before age fifty, and predominantly (3:1) in women.

Arteritis.
(*a.*) Takayusu's.
(*b.*) Buerger's.
(*c.*) Polyarteritis nodosa.

Early Manifestations: Index of suspicion is raised by atypical age of onset and by severity. In a retrospective series (Kincaid-Smith), operative relief was twice as likely for age less than twenty than for age twenty to forty years, and twice as likely for presentation with papilledema as without.

Renal size: Disparity in pole-to-pole length may be revealed by plain, body section and contrast radiography or by Hg^{203} scintiscans. Low grade disparity of less than 2 cm. correlates with (Smithwicks grade I) weight for the smaller kidney of 120 gm. (83 to 135), disparity of greater than 2 cm. (group II) with weight of 62.5 gm. (52 to 160), and the same with failure of the smaller kidney to excrete dye (group III) with weight of 55.5 gm. (28 to 83). Disparity is accordingly an available and somewhat late indicator of a kidney reduced in size, as well as of one containing less blood in diastole.

Hypoperfusion: When a kidney is hypoperfused it looks smaller, and less easy to ascertain, has a lower rate of urine flow per minute. Setting it apart from other small kidneys is that the low rate of urine flow in part derives from reabsorbing a very high percentage of the glomerular filtrate (of the order that both kidneys do in shock) compared to the unaffected kidney. A way of ascertaining this is use of a marker that gets into tubular fluid (at the time of filtration or by tubular secretion) and is subject to minimal reabsorption. Kidneys forming urine at different rates, but with the same fractional reabsorption, would put out marker at like concentrations per ml. urine. But a kidney with high fractional reabsorption would put out the marker in high concentration, a mirror image of the raised reabsorption. The kidney has received larger dose of marker than would otherwise be suspected from its flow rate. Since the flow rate is slow for the dose carried, cumulative excretion by this kidney will be slow compared to the opposite kidney. The ureters have to be individually catheterized to compare their concentrations of already colored (PSP) or chromogenic markers (creatinine, inulin, PAH), The principle of the I^{131} renogram is that external gamma detector curves over the kidney approximate cumulative marker excretion curves derived by urine collection. If excretion of half an isotope dose requires 3.5 to 6.5 minutes normally, it takes about twice this long by a hypoperfused kidney (Fig. XIII–5).

Rapid sequence pyelography is also based upon a slower rate of urine flow into the pelves, where appearance of marker normally is detected in two or three minutes and is also delayed when the kidney is hypoperfused. Since concentration is greater, density of the fluid should be greater, though this is not easily quantitated radiographically.

Tests based on above detect about 70% of lesions producing hypoperfusion compared to about 80% for aortography.

Hypokalemic alkalosis due to renin-induced secondary aldosteronism.

Nocturnal polyuria without evidence of congestive circulatory failure, possibly due to reninism.

Postural hypotension possibly due to renin-dependent vascular tone and impaired postural circulatory reflexes.

Treatment: The finding of unilateral oliguria (Fig. XIII–6) is a criterion favoring renal artery surgery and is about 70% successful in predicting the existence of renin-dependent hypertension.

Possible Dire Consequences without Treatment: Loss of renal parenchyms due to ischemic tubular atrophy. Drug resistance. Drug complications. Overlooking curable hypertension.

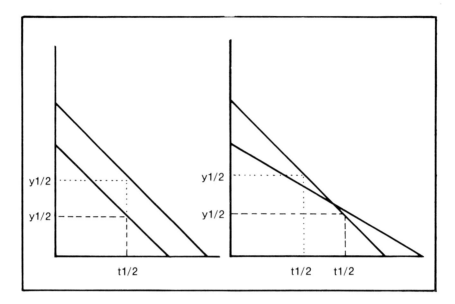

Fig. XIII–5. If kidneys disparate in size accumulate $(Y\frac{1}{2})$ different radioisotope doses, but fractional excretion per minute is the same, slope $(T\frac{1}{2})$ will be unchanged. If fractional excretion of the same accumulated dose is slower, slope $(T\frac{1}{2})$ will be prolonged. The lower dose accumulation $(Y\frac{1}{2})$ may indicate an underperfused rather than smaller organ in such instances.

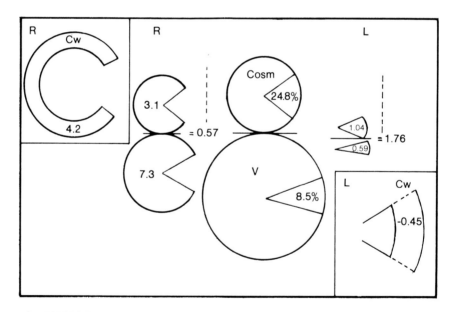

Fig. XIII–6. A patient with unilateral oliguria. V is urine flow rate, the patient's left kidney contributing but 7.5%. However 3.1 ml./min. of the total 7.3 ml./min. recorded as V is due to solute, labeled Cosm or osmolar clearance, and the left kidney is responsible for 24.8% of this. As a consequence, during water load sufficient to permit dilute urine on the right, with Cw or free water clearance 4.2 ml./min., there was water reabsorption on the left further accentuating the unilateral oliguria. Hypertension remitted with left nephrectomy; inulin clearance of right kidney increased from 70 to 83 ml./min.

References

Bookstein, J. J., et al.: Radiologic aspects of hypertension I. J.A.M.A., *220*:1218, 1972.

Bookstein, J. J., et al.: Radiologic aspects of renovascular hypertension II. J.A.M.A., *220*: 1225, 1972.

Bookstein, J. J., et al.: Radiologic aspects of hypertension III. J.A.M.A., *221*:368, 1972.

Goldman, A. G., Varady, P. D., and Franklin, S. S.: Body habits and serum cholesterol in essential hypertension and renovascular hypertension. J.A.M.A., *221*:378, 1972.

Maxwell, M. H., et al.: Demographic analysis of the study. J.A.M.A., *220*:1193, 1972.

Reiss, M. D., Bookstein, J. J., and Belifer, K. H.: Radiologic aspects of renovascular hypertension 4. J.A.M.A., *221*:374, 1972.

Simon, N., et al.: Clinical characteristics of renovascular hypertension. J.A.M.A., *220*:1209, 1972.

Varady, P. D., and Maxwell, M. H.: Assessment of statistically significant changes in diastolic pressure. J.A.M.A., *221*:365, 1972.

21. Renal Hypertension (Hydronephrosis)

Joseph H. Magee

Causes: Bilateral hydronephrosis.
Urethral stricture.
Prostatic hypertrophy.
Periureteral fibrosis.
Intraureteral obstruction.
Nephrolithiasis
Ureteral trauma
Papillary necrosis
Extraureteral obstruction.
Ectopic vessels
Ectopic ureter

Early Manifestations: Flank pain. Flank enlargement. Ureteral colic. Hematuria. Infected hydronephroses with fever, leukocytosis, and pyuria.

Treatment: Surgical relief of obstruction, indicated whether or not hypertension is present.

Possible Dire Consequences without Treatment: Pressure atrophy, loss of renal function.

References

McCann, W. S., and Romansky, M. J.: Hypertension from kidney ptosis. Tr. Am. Assn. Phys., *55*:239, 1940.

Oster, J.: Arterial hypertension in a child cured by nephrectomy. Acta Med. Scand., *128*:42, 1947.

22. Renal Hypertension

JOSEPH H. MAGEE

Causes: Congenital (constricting bands).
Neoplastic (Wilm's tumor).
Traumatic (hematoma, hygroma, perinephritis).
Infectious (perinephritis).
Radiation perinephritis, with symmetric or asymmetric involvement depending upon portals used.

Early Manifestations: Hypertension, onset within six months of radiation, or with decades delay after trauma; onset often before or after thirty to fifty age range, but typically in this range when postirradiation for seminoma.
Severe hypertension with retinopathy and early heart failure is common.
Proteinuria may be disproportionate to erythrocyturia and may be unilateral.
Radiographic shadows may be asymmetric or without border contrast on one side; collecting systems may be displaced.
Palpable mass and/or bruit may be present.
Severe anemia with or without azotemia may be present in postradiation perinephritis.

Treatment: Surgical decompression or decortication.

Possible Dire Consequences without Treatment: Drug resistant hypertension. Drug complications. Curable hypertension is overlooked.

References

Braasch, W. F., and Wood, W. W., Jr.: Clinical perinephritis and blood pressure. Proc. Staff Meet. Mayo Clin., *17*:52, 1942.
Cogan, S. R., and Ritler, I. I.: Radiation nephritis (Left nephrectomy cured infantile hypertension occurring after radiation for neuroblastoma). Am. J. Med., *24*:531, 1958.
Dean, A. L., and Abels, J. C.: Study by the newer function tests of an unusual case of hypertension following irradiation of one kidney and the relief of the patient by nephrectomy. J. Urol., *52*:497, 1944.
Engel, W. J.: The association of unilateral kidney disease with hypertension. Cleveland Clin. Quart., *7*:290, 1940.
Farrell, J. I., and Young, R. H.: Hypertension caused by unilateral renal compression. J.A.M.A., *118*:711, 1942.
Levitt, W. M., and Oram, S.: Irradiation-induced malignant hypertension cured by nephrectomy. Brit. Med. J., *2*:910, 1956.
Luxton, R. W.: Radiation nephritis. Lancet, *2*:1221, 1961.
Luxton, R. W.: Radiation nephritis. Quart. J. Med., *22*:215, 1953.
Schmock, C. L.: Hypertension associated with traumatic perinephritis. Am. J. Cardiol., *11*:557, 1963.
Semans, J. H.: Nephrectomy for hypertension in a two-and-a-half-year old child with apparent cure. Bull. Johns Hopkins Hosp., *75*:184, 1944.
Sobel, I. P.: So-called essential hypertension in childhood. Am. J. Dis. Child., *61*:280, 1941.
Wilson, C., Ledingham, J. M., and Cohen, M.: Hypertension following X-irradiation of the kidneys. Lancet, *1*:9, 1958.

23. Renal Embolism and Infarction

Joseph H. Magee

Causes: Paradoxic emboli from veins.
Paradoxic emboli from marrow.
Cardiac emboli (ventricular, valvular, atrial).
Aortic (atheromatous) emboli.
Narrowing of renal artery ostiae by aortic dissection or aortic thrombosis (ascending Leriche or descending Takayusu syndrome).
Thrombosis of renal artery.

Early Manifestations: De novo or worsened hypertension.
Flank pain.
Fever, leukocytosis, increased sedimentation rate.
Hematuria.
Evidence of extrarenal embolization.
Condition predisposing to embolization such as heart disease, recent aortic surgery.

Treatment: Dependent upon source: aggressive if source is cardiac, because of accompanying risk of brain embolization.
Obtain adequate baseline films for serial estimation of renal size.
Direct vasodilators (diazoxide, hydralazine) for severe acute hypertension.

Possible Dire Consequences without Treatment: Atrophy of kidney. Hypertension. In some cases no dire consequences.

References

Arnold, M. W., Goodwin, W. E., and Colston, J. A. C.: Renal infarction and its relation to hypertension. Urol. Survey, 1:191, 1951.
Bellman, S., and Oden, B.: An unusual case of renal embolism. Acta Chir. Scand., 120:276, 1960.
Fishberg, A. M.: Hypertension due to renal embolism. J.A.M.A., 119:551, 1942.
Halpern, M.: Acute renal artery embolus. J. Urol., 98:552, 1967.

24. Primary Reninism

Joseph H. Magee

Causes: Wilm's tumor. Juxtamedullary hemangiopericytoma.

Early Manifestations: Severe hypertension associated with hypokalemia, polyuria, polydypsia.
Aldosteronism is shown to be secondary, accompanied by raised plasma renin activity and concentrations.
Renal artery disease is not demonstrable by angiography.
Aldosteronism is unresponsive to antihypertensive therapy that controls blood pressure well.
Separate renal venous renin determinations localize renin excess to one kidney; only a 25% difference in concentration may be significant.
In some cases concentration from contralateral kidney is lower than in peripheral veins.
Tumors which are only 0.8 to 4.0 cm. in diameter may demonstrate slightly earlier washout in early nephrogram phase done with selective injection and body section technique.

Treatment: Total or partial nephrectomy.

Possible Dire Consequences without Treatment: Severe hypertension with secondary aldosteronism refractory to usual drug therapy.

References

Bonnin, J. M., Hodge, R. L., and Lumbers, E. R.: A renin-secreting renal tumor associated with hypertension. Austr. N. Z. J. Med., 2:178, 1972.
Conn, J. W., et al.: The syndrome of hypertension, hyperreninemia and secondary aldosteronism associated with renal juxtaglomerular cell tumor (primary reninism). Arch. Intern. Med., 130:682, 1972.
Eddy, R. L., and Sanchez, S. A.: Renin-secreting renal neoplasm and hypertension with hypokalemia. Ann. Intern. Med., 75:725, 1971.
Hirose, M., et al.: Primary reninism with renal hamartomatous alteration. J.A.M.A., 230:1288, 1974.
Kihare, I., et al.: A hitherto unreported vascular tumor of the kidney. Acta Path. Japan, 18:197, 1968.
Mitchell, J. D., et al.: Renin levels in nephroblastoma (Wilm's tumor). Arch. Dis. Child., 45:376, 1970.
Robertson, T. W., et al.: Hypertension due to a renin-secreting tumor. Am. J. Med., 43:963, 1967.
Schambelan, M., et al.: Role of renin and aldosterone in hypertension due to a renin-secreting tumor. Am. J. Med., 55:86, 1973.
Voute, P. A., Jr., van der Meer, J., and Staugaard-Koozerziel, W.: Plasma renin activity in Wilm's tumor. Acta End., 67:197, 1971.

*Aldosteronism

(Discussed in Chapter XII, Sections 12–23.)

Chapter XIV

Vascular Diseases

Introduction

There are twenty-one conditions listed as treatable in this chapter which represents about a 2,000% increase in the last twenty-five years. One of the conditions did not even exist (pill phlebitis). About 1946 I explained to a patient that one of the important arteries to his leg had been occluded. Since he was a plumber, he suggested that a new section of pipe be installed. I told him in a pitying way that such things were possible for plumbers but not for medical men. The fact that medical men have heeded his advice must be responsible for many of our advances in this field, particularly, in arterial disease.

1. Peripheral Arterial Occlusive Disease

ORVILLE HORWITZ

Cause: Atherosclerosis, thromboangiitis obliterans, arterial emboli, collagen disease, necrotizing angiitides, other arteritides, arterial thrombosis. Occasionally trauma.

Early Manifestations: Usually intermittent claudication, sometimes pain.

Treatment: Diet, abstinence from tobacco, removal of aneurysm, arterial grafting, sympathectomy, removal of angiomata, corticosteroids in some necrotizing angiitides. Possibly fibrinolytic agents. Most often prophylactic measures emphasizing lack of *dirt* and trauma. Possibly vitamin E.

Possible Dire Consequences without Treatment: Continued intermittent claudication, ischemic ulcers, gangrene, amputation.

The commonest of the diseases leading to peripheral ischemia are listed in Table XIV–1.

TABLE XIV–1. DIAGNOSTIC POINTS OF FOUR PERIPHERAL ARTERIAL DISEASES

	Arteriosclerotic Occlusion	Thromboangiitis Obliterans (Buerger's Disease)	Arterial Embolism	Raynaud's Disease
Sex distribution	Male more frequent	98% male	About equal	90% female
Age at onset	Usually over 50. Often earlier in diabetes	Under 35	Any age	15–50, but usually 25–30
Order of incidence	1	4	2	3
Cause	Probably multiple factors.	Probably tobacco	Most frequently mitral stenosis, valve prosthesis, myocardial infarction, arterial plaque, aneurysm	Unknown
Symmetry	Generally asymmetrical unless aorta is involved	Generally asymmetrical	Asymmetrical unless aorta is involved	Symmetrical
Onset	Usually insidious	May be acute and preceded by migratory phlebitis	Sudden	Often in cold weather and often following psychic trauma
Migratory phlebitis	Coincidental	Frequent. Varies in different series from 30–70%	Coincidental	Coincidental
Intermittent claudication	Common	Common	May be present later	Absent
Conspicuous vasospasm	Not remarkable	Almost invariable in involved limb	Not infrequent in acute stages	Invariably symmetrical
Absent pulses	Infrequent in upper and common in lower extremities	Common in upper and lower extremities	In involved artery	Occurs only in late and extreme cases

472

Edema	Only with infection or prolonged dependency	With inflammatory reactions and prolonged dependency	Rare	Rare
Skin (if involved)	Thin, often hairless	Thin, atrophic, and red or cyanotic	Normal	Normal except in spasm
Rubor on dependence	If ischemia severe and prolonged	If ischemia severe and prolonged	May be late sign	Absent
Ulcers (if any)	Dry and usually superficial	Moist, deep, inflamed and invasive	May occur later	Dry, fingertip
Presence of aneurysm	Not infrequent	Extremely rare	Rare except when embolus arises from aneurysm	Coincidental
Plain roentgenograms of extremities	Often calcification of artery	Normal	Usually normal	Often atrophy of phalanges
Arteriogram findings	Arteries often frayed. Segmental blocks frequent. Collaterals established.	Tree root configurations	Occlusion demonstrated. Well localized. Minimal collateral flow.	Absence of dye in peripheral digits. May be relieved by Priscoline intra-arterially.
Cholesterol	301*	225*	Depends on cause	Not remarkable
Presence of coronary or cerebral disease	Common	Rare early in disease	Common	Coincidental
Capacity for blood flow as measured by skin temperature studies	Decreased in involved extremity	Decreased in involved extremity	Decreased in involved extremity	Normal except in late and extreme cases

* Statistics of the Hospital of the University of Pennsylvania.

The procession of events in acute arterial occlusion is as follows:

0–15 minutes	Absent pulses, pain on walking (intermittent claudication), pallor, coldness, pain at rest
2–6 hours	Hypesthesia, paresthesia, cyanosis (local), mottled cyanosis
8 hours	Motor paralysis, anesthesia
24 hours or more	Visible dehydration of toes, bleb formation, ecchymosis
Finally	Gangrene

This process may occur over a number of years as well as in the time mentioned above. Any signs or symptoms further advanced than absent pulses or intermittent claudication are serious. Nerves have a low metabolism and indicate a severe degree of deprivation when they emit symptoms such as pain at rest and paresthesias.

The laboratory and x-ray studies involved in peripheral arterial disease are few. The ultra-sound flow meter and oscillometer are of some use. But by far the most rewarding study, when indicated, is the arteriogram. This should be performed only when arterial surgery is contemplated. Surgery should in turn be contemplated almost always when the leg is in danger and sometimes to aid the patient's locomotion.

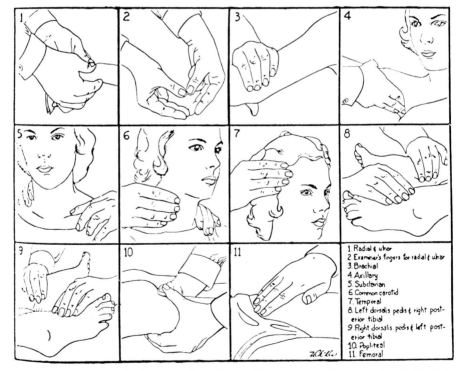

Fig. XIV–1.   Methods of palpating pulses. (From Montgomery, H.: Pennsylvania Medicine. *57*:59, 1954.)

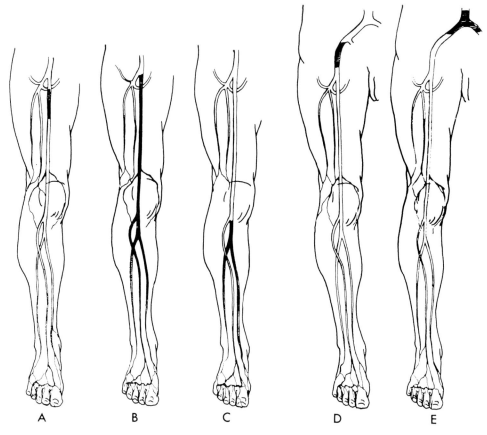

Fig. XIV–2. Relationship of site of arterial obstruction to considerations about surgical treatment. A, Segmental block of femoral artery; suitable for direct arterial surgery. B, Block of femoral artery without patency of major distal vessel; unsuitable for arterial surgery. C, Block of distal artery; unsuitable for direct arterial surgery. D, Segmental block of iliac artery; suitable for arterial surgery. E, Block of terminal part of aorta and common iliac arteries (Leriche syndrome); suitable for arterial surgery. (Horwitz, O., and Roberts, B.: General Practitioner, 17:26, 1958.)

The selection of the surgical procedure may be made as follows:

Pulses	Probable Location of Block	Radiographic Procedure Indicated
Good popliteal	Below knee	None: grafting usually impractical
Absent popliteal, present femoral	Superficial femoral	Femoral arteriogram
Absent femoral, opposite femoral present	Iliac	Aortogram
Both femorals absent	Aorta	Aortogram
Both femorals weak with bruits	Aorta	Aortogram

The main therapeutic tools are as follows:
1. *Suppression of infection,* and avoiding trauma.
2. *Abstinence from tobacco.*
3. *Cold.* Only as a pre-amputatory measure.
4. *Heat.* Keep the ischemic extremity as warm as possible short of causing pain. This will provide maximum oxygen tension and probably maximum nutrition.
5. *Position.* DEPENDENT. NEVER ELEVATE A TRULY ISCHEMIC EXTREMITY:
6. *Sympathectomy* almost always a last ditch procedure.
7. *Arterial Surgery.*

References

Allen, E. C., Barker, W. W., Hines, E. A., Jr.: Peripheral Vascular Diseases, 3rd Ed., Chapters I to XXI, Philadelphia, W. B. Saunders Co., 1962.
Conn, H. and Horwitz, O.: Cardiac and Vascular Diseases, Chapter 58, Vol. II. Philadelphia, Lea & Febiger, 1971.
Haeger, K.: Long-time treatment of intermittent claudication with vitamin E. Amer. J. Clin. Nutrition, 27:1179, 1974.
Holling, H. E.: Peripheral Vascular Diseases. Diagnosis and Management. Philadelphia, J. B. Lippincott Co., 1972.

2. Thromboangiitis Obliterans (Buerger's Disease)

ORVILLE HORWITZ

Cause: Not completely understood. Tobacco plays large part.

Early Manifestations: Migratory phlebitis in less than 50% of cases. Intermittent claudication of foot.

Treatment: Stop use of tobacco; pedal hygiene

Possible Dire Consequences without Treatment: Gangrene and loss of tissue.

This is a distinct pathophysiological entity featuring mild to severe ischemia of the upper extremity, as well as of the lower extremity. It is almost invariably accompanied by the use of tobacco which is probably the cause of the disease. Other features are the rarity of coronary artery involvement, frequent co-existence of migratory phlebitis, conspicuous early vasospasm, and normal cholesterol level. It involves only the small and medium sized vessels such as the posterior tibial dorsalis pedis, ulnar and radial arteries and their branches. It usually presents between the ages of twenty-five and forty and is more prevalent in males.

References

Horwitz, O.: Buerger's disease retrieved. Ann. Intern. Med., *55*:341, 1961.
Horwitz, O.: Diseases of the arteries of the extremities, p. 1517, Vol. II in Cardiac and
    Vascular Diseases. H. L. Conn, Jr. and O. Horwitz (Eds.), Philadelphia, Lea & Febiger,
    1971.
McKusick, V. A. *et al.*: Buerger's disease: A distinct clinical and pathological entity.
    J.A.M.A., *181*:5, 1962.

3. Occlusion of The Terminal Aorta

Edwin T. Long

Cause: Atherosclerotic stenosis or occlusion of the terminal aorta and iliac arteries.

Early Manifestations: Intermittent claudication, bruits over the femoral arteries.
Later diminished or absent femoral pulses, occasional impotence.

Treatment: Surgical restoration of arterial flow to the lower limbs.

Possible Dire Consequences without Treatment: Worsening of arterial insufficiency,
gangrene of the lower limbs and renal failure.

Rene Leriche first described in 1923 and later more completely in 1940 the clinical picture of "insidious thrombosis of the aortic bifurcation." Morel, in 1943,
proposed that this clinical picture as described by Leriche have the name of Leriche
syndrome. The syndrome consists of intermittent claudication, absent femoral
pulses and impotence, thus calling attention to the predominant occurrence of this
syndrome in males. A number of investigators have pointed out that impotence is
not as common as suggested by Leriche and that the syndrome does occur less frequently in females. The occlusion of the aortic bifurcation is of slow onset and frequently goes unrecognized. The prolonged course allows for development of collateral circulation. The condition is generally well tolerated by the patient. Approximately 50% of patients with this type of aortic occlusion are hypertensive. It occurs
primarily in older people, 90% in the seventh, eighth, ninth decades of life. In
my experience, those patients with Leriche syndrome under the age of seventy are
almost invariably smokers, whereas patients over the age of seventy may have had
no exposure to tobacco. This disease is thought to originate in the iliac arteries and
progress proximally. Once occlusion of both of the iliac arteries has taken place,
the occlusion propagates proximally and eventually may involve not only the inferior
mesenteric artery, but the renal arteries as well, producing first renal insufficiency
and then renal failure. Curiously enough these individuals seldom develop ischemia
of the toes as measured by skin temperature studies. Therefore, although intermittent claudication is invariably present, collateral circulation is nearly always
sufficient to allay the development of gangrene.

The predisposition of the terminal aorta and iliac vessels to this type of insidious thrombosis is presumably due to the traumatic effect of excessive blood flow in this major vessel to the lower extremities. It is known that the lower extremity during peaks of exercise can increase its demand for blood by 15 to 25 times resting flows. Surgical reconstruction of the circulation to the lower extremities in these patients restores over 90% of pedal pulses.

The treatment has been a direct attack on the occlusive disease with one of three techniques:

(*a*) Resection of the stenotic or occluded section with replacement using a prosthetic vessel.

(*b*) Thromboendarterectomy of the involved segment.

(*c*) Bypass of the involved segment using a prosthetic vessel.

There may be the necessity to combine one of these techniques with a thromboendarterectomy or graft reconstruction of renal arteries if they are involved with an occlusive or stenotic lesion.

Failure to restore normal circulation to the lower extremities is invariably accompanied by worsening of the situation.

The patient may present with intermittent claudication and yet have good femoral and pedal pulses. Under these circumstances a bruit will almost always be detected over the femoral artery.

References

DeBakey, M. et al: Surgical considerations of occlusive disease of the abdominal aorta and iliac and femoral arteries, analysis of 803 cases. Ann. Surg., *148*:306, 1958.
Leriche, R.: "Des obliterations arterielles hautes (obliteration de la terminaison de l'aorte) Comme cause des insuffisances circulatoires des membres inferieurs." Bull et Mem. de la Soc. de Chir., *49*:1404, 1923.
Leriche, R.: "De la resection du carrefour aortico-iliaque avec double sympathectomie lombaire pour thrombose arteritique de l'aorte, le syndrome de l'obliteration termino-aortique par arterite. Presse Med., *48*:601, 1940.
Roberts, B. and Johnson, L. L.: Diseases of the abdominal aorta and its major branches. Chapter 56, pp. 1505–1506, Vol. II, in Cardiac and Vascular Diseases, Conn, H. L., Jr. and Horwitz, O. (Eds.), Philadelphia, Lea & Febiger, 1971.

4. Aneurysm of the Abdominal Aorta

Edwin T. Long

Cause: Usually atherosclerosis.

Early Manifestations: Usually none, may be microemboli to lower extremity or toes (Fig. XIV–3). Later bruit, palpable pulsatile mass, pain and rupture.

Treatment: Resection and reconstruction usually with prosthetic material.

Possible Dire Consequences without Treatment: Peripheral emboli, rupture, sudden death.

Abdominal aneurysms of less than 5 cm. diameter tend to rupture infrequently, whereas, those of large diameter (over 7 cm.) have a 70% chance of rupture if neglected. Unfortunately, rupture may be the first symptom of an aneurysm. More commonly, however, the pattern of progress is divided into three parts. The first part is the asymptomatic state, the second part is the symptomatic period, and the the third part is the rupture. The mortality and morbidity increase as the symptoms increase.

Now that there is adequate surgical treatment for these lesions a much larger percentage are diagnosed, mostly by routine physical examination. Since the bifurcation of the aorta is approximately at the level of the umbilicus, the aneurysm presents as a wide pulsatile mass usually in the lower part of the left upper quadrant.

Abdominal films show calcification and a curvilinear deviation of the normal aortic margin. About 70% of abdominal aneurysms manifest themselves in the lateral views. Aortography has the disadvantage that laminated clots may only show a tubular lumen in spite of a largely expanded artery wall. However, the aortogram does serve to show the condition of the rest of the arterial tree which is of considerable importance in planning therapy. It is, for instance, vital to show

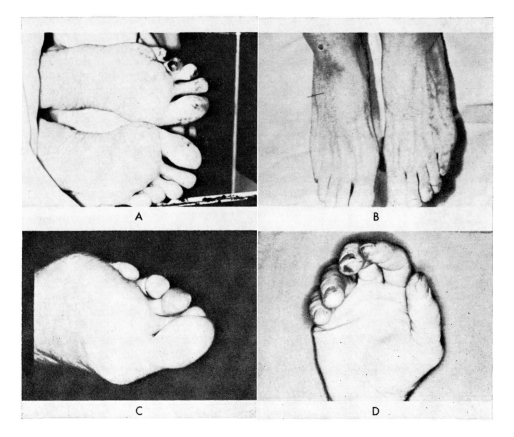

Fig. XIV–3. General appearance of digits in which micro-emboli, presumably from aneurysms in more proximal part of artery, have lodged. A, Bilateral micro-embolization from aneurysm of aorta. B, Embolus to left third toe from aneurysm of aorta. C, Emboli to left foot from popliteal aneurysm. D, Emboli to right hand from aneurysm of subclavian artery.

if the aneurysm of the abdominal aorta extends to or above the renal arteries and if renal artery stenosis is present which requires concomitant therapy.   Measurements by ultrasonic mapping of the aortic wall is becoming an accurate technique.

References

Crawford, E. Stanley et al.:   Surgical consideration of peripheral arterial aneurysms. AMA Arch. Surg., *78*:226, 1959.
DeBakey, M. E. *et al.*:   Aneurysm of the abdominal aorta. Ann. Surg., *160*:622, 1964.
Horwitz, Orville: In Cardiac and Vascular Disease. Conn, Hadley and Horwitz, Orville (Eds.), Vol. II, p. 1517, Chap. 58. Philadelphia, Lea & Febiger, 1971.
Roberts, B and Johnson L.:   In Cardiac and Vascular Disease. Conn, Hadley and Horwitz, Orville (Eds.), Vol. II, p. 1500, Chap. 56. Philadelphia, Lea & Febiger, 1971.

5. Superior Mesenteric Artery Syndrome

BROOKE ROBERTS

Condition: Symptomatic stenosis or occlusion of superior mesenteric artery. Intestinal angina.

Cause: Usually atherosclerosis. Occasionally arteritis, aneurysm, trauma, etc.

Early Manifestations: Postprandial, epigastric or peri-umbilical crampy pain, worse after large meals with a resultant reluctance to eat. An abdominal bruit is usually audible.

Treatment: Surgical restoration of vessel lumen or bypass graft.

Possible Dire Consequences without Treatment: Weight loss and cachexia or sudden development of gangrene of gut.

This condition is to be distinguished from compression of the duodenum by the superior mesenteric artery, which may also be referred to as "superior mesenteric artery syndrome."

This syndrome is almost always associated with other evidence of vascular disease such as ischemia of the legs, history of coronary occlusion, stroke, etc. Although there is no definite test for blood flow to the gut, postprandial pain and fear of eating suggest it.

Weight loss in these patients may be striking, as they often relate the degree of pain to the size of the meal which they have ingested. For this reason, they become afraid to eat normally. A sense of bloating is frequent and the patients sometimes get relief from assuming the elbow-knee position when they have pain. Abdominal bruits are usually present. Occult blood in the stool is common as is some degree of malabsorption. In retrospect, the majority of patients who develop gangrene of the gut have preceding attacks of pain, suggesting intestinal ischemia. On the other hand, many patients with ischemia of the gut can have symptoms for years without developing necrosis.

A definitive diagnosis usually depends on aortography. Lateral view of the aorta and roots of the mesenteric vessels are often essential in picking up the areas of occlusion or stenosis. Usually at least two of the three major vessels supplying the bowel are involved before symptoms develops. The pattern of collateral circulation may also clearly suggest a lesion in the superior mesenteric system. Routine gastro-intestinal roentgenograms may show mucosal edema but more often show normal appearing bowel.

As in the celiac artery, therapy consists in reconstruction of the stenotic or occluded area of the vessel or the use of a bypass graft around the lesion. This usually results in dramatic weight gain and relief of symptoms.

Reference

Boley, S. J., Schwartz, S. S. and Williams, L. F.: Vascular Disorders of the Intestine. New York, Appleton-Century-Crofts, Inc., 1971.

6. Celiac Artery Stenosis or Occlusion

Brooke Roberts

Cause: Usually arteriosclerosis with plaque formation at origin of the vessel or it may be related to external pressure from the arcuate ligament of the diaphragm. Occasional cases may arise on the basis of arteritis, aneurysm, or other lesions.

Early Manifestations. Bruit over upper abdomen associated with crampy abdominal pain, usually soon after eating and proportional to the size of the meal. May have associated fullness and vomiting.

Treatment: Direct operative relief of the stenosis or occlusion or bypass graft.

Possible Dire Consequences without Treatment: Continuing pain and weight loss and eventual cachexia.

This uncommon entity is still a bit controversial and some deny its existence pointing out that in some patients, the celiac and superior mesenteric arteries may be totally occluded without producing symptoms. While such is undoubtedly true, it is apparent that many patients cannot tolerate major reduction in the blood supply to areas in their bowel and they do develop symptoms which can be relieved by revascularization. Celiac artery syndrome is usually seen in elderly patients and it appears to be more common in women than in men. Mild symptoms are often misdiagnosed for long periods of time.

17

An aortogram is essential in confirming the diagnosis of this condition and usually the only view which will demonstrate the lesion is one taken in the lateral plane. It is unusual to have symptoms unless there is involvement of the superior mesenteric artery also.

The condition is often confused with biliary, pancreatic, or gastric disease and, when such is not found, patients are often labeled "functional." The presence of a bruit in association with postprandial pain should alert the physician to the possibility of the celiac artery syndrome. If total occlusion of the celiac artery occurs, a bruit will not normally be heard. Relief of symptoms can be anticipated from surgical correction in about 90% of the patients.

Reference

Boley, S. J., Schwartz, S. S. and Williams, L. F.: Vascular Disorders of the Intestine. New York, Appleton-Century-Crofts, Inc., 1971.

7. Traumatic Aneurysms of the Thoracic Aorta

ORVILLE HORWITZ

Cause: Blunt deceleration of fairly violent nature usually in vehicle.

Early Manifestations: Horizontal deceleration followed by chest pain, wide mediastinum, and soft systolic murmur to left of spine.

Treatment: Surgery.

Possible Dire Consequences without Treatment: Death.

Traumatic aneurysms of the aorta, although fundamentally surgical lesions, are mentioned here because successful operation on such lesions has become progressively more successful in the past few years. Cooley has reported over 60 cases without a death. Of course, this implies a prompt and proper diagnosis, which in turn depends on a high index of suspicion.

Blunt deceleration injuries of a fairly violent nature are responsible, such as those resulting from automobile and aircraft accidents. Multiple fractures, particularly of ribs, often co-exist. The favorite site is in the descending aorta (13 of 14 in one series) just distal to the subclavian artery at the ligamentum arteriosum. The tear is usually transverse and varies from incompletely to completely circumferential.

Once the condition is suspected, the history of horizontal deceleration and chest pain, particularly with injury, should be extremely suggestive. A widened mediastinum on roentgen study and the development of a soft systolic murmur to the left of the spine should be indications for angiography, which some observers advocate routinely in all cases of severe trauma to the chest.

Surgery is the treatment of choice.

Reference

Cooley, D. A.: In a discussion of Stoney, R. J. and Roe, B. B. Rupture of thoracic aorta due to closed chest trauma. Arch. Surg., *89*:846, 1964.

8. Aneurysm of the Subclavian Artery

EDWIN T. LONG

Cause: Atherosclerosis or poststenotic.

Early Manifestations: Transient ischemia of fingers of affected side. Bruit over area.

Treatment: Resection and graft.

Possible Dire Consequences without Treatment: Sometimes rupture and sometimes peripheral ischemia.

Aneurysm of the subclavian artery is not common. It is of interest that it was the site chosen for the first attempts at strengthening aneurysms by applying irritating cellophane wrapping. Aneurysms in this location share with other aneurysms the etiology of weakness of the arterial wall most often by atherosclerosis. The most common shape is fusiform and may be poststenotic.

The first symptom may be that of embolization of thrombotic material distally, resulting in transient ischemia of the fingers.

Surgical resection with reconstitution is the procedure of choice.

Reference

Crawford, E. Stanley, DeBakey, Michael E. and Cooley, Denton A.: Surgical consideration of peripheral arterial aneurysm. AMA Arch. Surg., *78*:226, 1959.

9. Popliteal Aneurysm

Edwin T. Long

Cause: Usually atherosclerosis; may be trauma.

Early Manifestations: Often none. May be transient ischemia of toes, or pain or pulsatile sensation. Later a palpable pulsatile mass in the popliteal area.

Treatment: Ideally resection with reconstruction using artery substitutes, possibly a neighboring vein.

Possible Dire Consequences without Treatment: Occlusion of vessel with gangrene and loss of limb.

These aneurysms seldom rupture but are a real menace to the extremity which lodges them, as they frequently result in arterial occlusion and gangrene.

They are usually bilateral, and often present as transient ischemia of toes from clots thrown peripherally. They may also present as pain or as a feeling of pulsation. Although some are completely innocuous, all such lesions should be detected and probably repaired as they frequently lead to amputation.

References

Crawford, E. Stanley, DeBakey, Michael E., and Cooley, Denton A.: Surgical consideration of peripheral arterial aneurysms. AMA Arch. Surg., *78*:226, 1959.
Horwitz, O. and Roberts, B.: The choice of treatment in peripheral and arterial disease. General Practitioner, *17*:126, 1958.

10. Raynaud's Phenomenon

Jay Coffman

Cause: Unknown in Raynaud's disease and collagen diseases.

Due to artery or nervous tissue compression or involvement (thoracic outlet syndromes, syringomyelia, spinal cord tumors), disease of a limb (postpoliomyelitis, strokes), sludging of blood (cryoproteins, macroglobulins, cold agglutinins), vasoconstriction (ergot and methysergide), trauma (pneumatic drills, piano playing, typing) or obstructive arterial diseases (thromboangiitis obliterans, arterial emboli, atherosclerosis).

Early Manifestations: Intermittent attacks of pallor and/or cyanosis of the digits (sometimes ears, nose) on exposure to cold; bright redness may occur as the attacks end.

Treatment: Raynaud's disease, collagen disease, neurogenic diseases, obstructive arterial diseases: reserpine, prolonged acting tolazoline if necessary.   Thoracic outlet syndromes: shoulder girdle exercises, surgery if necessary.   Drug toxicity: stop medication, anticoagulation if severe.   Trauma: avoid precipitating cause. Cryoproteinemias and macroglobulins: none successful if underlying disease cannot be treated.

Possible Dire Consequences without Treatment: In severe cases of Raynaud's disease but mostly in collagen diseases, painful ulcers or gangrene of the fingertips and sclerodactyly (thickening of the subcutaneous tissues, fixation of the joints, and sometimes subcutaneous calcifications) may develop.

Raynaud's phenomenon is a vasospastic syndrome affecting the digital arterie and producing intermittent ischemic episodes on cold exposure and sometime emotional stimulus.   Attacks last minutes to hours, the blanching or cyanosis of the digits often becoming bright red on warming.

When no secondary cause can be discovered, it is termed Raynaud's disease.   The disease occurs predominantly in young females in the third to fifth decades and is usually mild.   A local sensitivity of the blood vessels to cold or an overactivity of the sympathetic nervous system are the two main theories of etiology.   Manifestations may start in one or two fingers but later spread to all fingers symmetrically; the thumbs are often spared.   The toes are involved in about 40% of patients. Radial, ulnar, dorsalis pedis and posterior tibial pulses are present.   Only about one-third have progression of the disease and less than 10% of patients lose part of a digit.   Sclerodactyly and gangrene and ulcers of the fingers rarely occur.   The small areas of gangrene and ulcers may occur only on the fingertips but not elsewhere.

In order to diagnose Raynaud's disease, the secondary causes must be ruled out as best possible.   This involves a careful history for symptoms of systemic disease (arthritis, arthralgias, dysphagia, frequent heartburn, skin rashes or vitiligo, dyspnea) and drug or trauma exposure, a careful physical examination for loss of pulses, neurological deficits, and signs of collagen diseases; this should include maneuvers of the shoulder girdle and neck to test for the thoracic outlet syndrome.   A hematogram for leukopenia, sedimentation rate, and anemia; a urinalysis for red cell casts and proteins; a screening test for rheumatoid factor; antinuclear antibodies; protein electrophoresis; and a chest film for cervical ribs should all be done.   Plasma should also be stored overnight in a refrigerator to observe for cryoproteins (fibrinogen and globulin precipitate in plasma; globulins in serum). If pertinent symptoms, signs, or laboratory findings are found, secondary causes of Raynaud's phenomenon cannot be dismissed.

In mild cases, no treatment is necessary; the patient can be reassured that the idiopathic disease is benign and usually non-progressive with advice to avoid cold exposure of all parts of the body (because of reflex sympathetic nerve vasoconstriction) and tobacco smoking (a sympathetic nerve vasoconstrictor stimulus). In more severe cases, reserpine, starting with 0.25 mg. a day and then increasing the dose every other week by 0.125 mg. to tolerance (nasal stuffiness, lethargy, depression), produces remarkable palliation in some cases. Reserpine increases nutritional (capillary) blood flow which is decreased in the fingers of patients during cold exposure. Reserpine should not be used if there is a history of depressive episodes. If the response to reserpine is inadequate, tolazoline (prolonged action tablets, 80 mg. q. 12 hr.) may be added to the regimen. Usually these two drugs will control most cases of moderate to severe Raynaud's disease. In patients with recurrent painful ulcers, sympathectomy has been recommended but usually is of benefit for only six months to two years before symptoms recur. Only supportive treatment can be offered to patients with protein abnormalities, obstructive arterial disease, and collagen diseases if the above drugs fail. Sympathectomy is of no benefit in scleroderma.

In thoracic outlet syndromes, exercises to strengthen the shoulder girdle muscles are most successful but should they fail after a six-month trial, the scalenus anticus muscle must be severed or the cervical or first thoracic rib resected, depending on the anatomical defect (cervical rib; scalenus anticus, costoclavicular or hyperabduction syndrome). In ergot or methysergide vasoconstriction, the vessels will usually reopen in two to three days after the drug is stopped. In severe cases, anticoagulation may be indicated to prevent thromboses until normal flow is reestablished. In cases secondary to trauma, the syndrome usually disappears with cessation of the inciting activity.

References

Allen, E. C., Barker, N. W. and Hines, E. A., Jr.: Peripheral Vascular Diseases, 3rd Ed., Philadelphia, W. B. Saunders Co., 1962.
Coffman, J. D. and Cohen, A. S.: Total and capillary fingertip blood flow in Raynaud's phenomenon. New Eng. J. Med., *285*:259, 1971.

11. Complication of Angiography

John McClenahan

Cause: Sensitivity to iodides. Local trauma.

Early Manifestations: Extravasation of contrast agent, thromboembolism and arterial insufficiency, and possibly acute renal failure.

Treatment: Prevention and correction. Care in placement of needle or catheter, strict asepsis, local anesthesia, test injection, dilute agents when possible, vasodilators through catheter prior to injection, compression of puncture site after withdrawal of catheter, adequate hydration of patient, intravenous dextran before injection. Oxygen, epinephrine, anticoagulants, surgical endarterectomy.

Possible Dire Consequences without Treatment: Renal failure, sudden death, coronary thrombosis, ventricular fibrillation, asphasia, blindness, hemiplegia, hematoma with infection, gangrene of intestine or extremity.

The complications of angiography, mild or dramatic, vary with the experience of the operator, the age and debility of the patient, the nature of the contrast agent and the condition of the injected vessel. Diffuse atherosclerosis, general anesthesia and prolonged or repeated opacification of a vessel sharply increase the risk.

Side effects range from the relatively trifling (nausea, vomiting, urticaria and transient fall in blood pressure) to the catastrophic. The latter include shock, renal failure, respiratory or cardiac collapse, hemiplegia and death.

The speed of injection, which is essential for clear opacification, contributes to extravasations of contrast material, hematomas and sloughing at the site of injection. Renal failure can be late or acute when an iodide in high concentration is inadvertently directed into the renal artery on either side.

Serious neurological complications (paresthesias, convulsion, hemiplegia, blindness, coma) result when an atherosclerotic plaque is dislodged by a catheter tip or when highly concentrated medium perfuses an artery—most commonly an anterior radicular artery in the lumbar region. Such a reaction most commonly occurs when an old patient is examined under general anesthesia.

Obstruction of a major visceral artery is heralded by abdominal pain and digestive disorders. In an extremity ischemia is recognized by pallor, numbness or blueness of the part and by diminished or absent pulses.

Disorders of vision can be relieved to some degree with vasodilators, anticoagulants and stellate ganglion block. Temporary spasm of an artery usually responds to injection of a vasodilator through the catheter. As a rule prompt surgical endarterectomy is required to avert death and the loss of limb after arterial occlusion.

No system has yet been devised to eliminate clotting on a catheter. Heparinization of a patient after withdrawal of a catheter may diminish this risk while introducing the possibility of hemorrhage from an injured artery.

Complications can be reduced by carotid compression during retrograde injection and, when possible, the use of dilute rather than concentrated media. Hydration of the patient before examination diminishes the incidence of renal complications.

Low molecular weight dextran given intravenously immediately before angiography (a 10% solution in 5% glucose) appears to prevent sludging and reduce complications. There is experimental evidence that in dogs high doses of aspirin given by mouth will protect the animal from arterial thrombosis.

References

Abrams, H. L.: Radiological aspects of operable heart disease. The hazards of retrograde thoracic aortography: A survey. Radiology, *68*, 812, 1957.

Ansell, G.: A national survey of radiological complications: Interim report. Clin. Radiol., *19*, 175, 1968.

Formanek, G., Frech, R. S. and Amplatz, K.: Arterial thrombus formation during clinical percutaneous catheterization. Circulation, *41*, 833, 1970.

Haney, W. P. and Preston, R. E.: Ocular complications of carotid arteriography in carotid occlusive disease. Arch. Ophthalmol., *67*:127, 1962.

Lang, E. K.: A survey of the complications of percutaneous retrograde arteriography. Radiology, *81*:257, 1967.

Langsjoen, P. H. and Best, E. B.: Studies in the prevention of complications of angiography. Am. J. Roent., Rad. Ther. and Nuc. Med., *106*:425, 1961.

McAfee, J. G.: A survey of complications of abdominal aortography. Radiology, *68*:825, 1957.

Moldveen, G. and Merriam, J. C.: Cholesterol embolization from pathological curiosity to clinical entity. Circulation, *35*:946, 1967.

Reiss, M. D.: Radiologic aspects of renovascular hypertension. Arteriographic complications. J.A.M.A., *221*:374, 1972.

Sones, F. M. and Shirey, E. K.: Coronary arteriography. Mod. Concepts Cardiovasc. Dis., *31*:735, 1962.

Staal, A., Van Voorthuisen, A. E. and Van Dijk, L. M.: Neurological complications following arterial catheterization by the axillary approach. Brit. J. Rad., *39*:115, 1966.

Weiss, H. J. et al.: Prevention of experimentally induced arterial thrombosis by Aspirin (abst.). Fed. Proc., *29*:381, 1970.

12. Arterial Embolus to Extremity

ORVILLE HORWITZ

Cause: Mitral stenosis with or without atrial fibrillation. Postmyocardial infarction. Arterial plaque especially from embolus. Prosthetic heart valves. Bacterial endocarditis.

Early Manifestations: Intermittent claudication, pain in extremity involved.

Treatment: Preferably embolectomy, otherwise rest, dependency of limbs and anticoagulants.

Possible Dire Consequences without Treatment: From mild ischemia to gangrene.

When acute arterial occlusion of a major vessel of an extremity occurs, signs and symptoms are likely to develop in the order outlined in Chapter XV (p. 532).

The commonest lodging sites for emboli are at bifurcations of such arteries as femorals, carotids, popliteals, brachials, and aortas.

If surgery is feasible, the sooner after embolization the embolectomy is performed, the more satisfactory will be the result.

TABLE XIV–2. SITES OF EMBOLIZATION

Site	Warren	Luke (%)	Tyson (%)
Internal carotid	18		
Axillary	5	4.5	8
Brachial	9	9.1	
Mesenteric	7		
Aortic bifurcation . . .	9	9.1	12
Common iliac	8	16.6	16
Femoral	23	38.5	56
Popliteal	9	14.2	8

For discussion of hidden mitral stenosis see Conn. H. L. under Cardiac Disorders, p. 532.

References

Horwitz, O.: Disease of the arteries of the extremities. In Cardiac and Vascular Diseases. Conn, H. L., Jr. and Horwitz, O. (Eds.), Vol. II, p. 1525, Philadelphia, Lea & Febiger, 1971.

Luke, J. C.: Textbook of Surgery, St. Louis, C. V. Mosby Co., 1955.

Montgomery, H., Horwitz, O., and Roberts, B.: The signs of acute peripheral arterial occlusion. Penn. Med. J., *60*:877, 1957.

Tyson, R. R.: Arterial embolism. In Vascular Surgery. Springfield, Charles C Thomas, 1965.

Warren, R.: Surgery. Philadelphia, W. B. Saunders Co., 1963.

13. Temporal Arteritis, Cranial Arteritis, or Giant Cell Arteritis, Polymyalgia Rheumatica

ORVILLE HORWITZ

Cause: Unknown. Cranial arteries become inflamed and occluded.

Early Manifestations: Headaches, fever, tenderness over cranial arteries.

Treatment: Steroids.

Possible Dire Consequences without Treatment: Blindness, death and disability.

This definite clinical and pathologic entity occurs in elderly patients; the cause is unknown. Dire consequences including blindness and death may result from this disease if it is not properly treated. The arteries most frequently involved are the branches of the aortic arch, particularly the carotid artery. It occurs slightly more frequently in women than men. It is featured by tenderness over the scalp arteries resulting from inflammation of these vessels. Temporal arteritis, the commonest name for the disease, is probably not a good one. It does not properly convey the viciousness of the condition.

The lumen of an affected artery is usually greatly reduced in size due to intimal thickening. Inflammatory and giant cells are found in the intima and media as well as focal necrosis and granulomatous formation near the elastic lamellae. Small hemorrhages are not uncommon, but aneurysms as in periarteritis nodosum are rare.

If the disease is manifested, as it frequently is, as tenderness in the region of one of the arteries of the scalp, particularly the temporal artery, the diagnosis is relatively simple. Intermittent claudication of the masseter muscle may be a symptom. Almost invariably there is general malaise and fever. Unfortunately the most dreaded complication of the disease, blindness, may be the presenting symptom, as may fever of unknown cause or the more explosive onset of severe headaches. The arteries of the scalp may show signs of severe inflammatory disease by induration, rubor, and dolor. If the original symptoms are malaise, fever, and aching of the joints, it may be indistinguishable at this time from an affliction caused by the prevailing virus.

The diagnosis is, as are many other diagnoses, not difficult if one keeps the condition in mind as a diagnostic consideration. The picture of tenderness over the scalp arteries, tenderness over the cheek, intermittent claudication of the masseter, fever, grossly increased sedimentation rate, leukocytosis, and anemia is unique. Sometimes biopsy may be necessary to make a definitive diagnosis. Yet in 175 cases of temporal arteritis admitted to the Mayo Clinic and reported by Hollenhorst *et al.*, only 13 were diagnosed as temporal arteritis by their referring physicians. Of these 175 patients, 73 had visual defects, 21 had blindness of both eyes, and 25 others had blindness of one eye. Still another 27 had partial loss of vision. Nineteen of the 175 patients had neurologic lesions of which 13 were attributed to the temporal arteritis.

Because of the success of a prompt therapeutic program, and because a therapeutic diagnostic guess may be indicated, treatment is mentioned here. In the vast majority of cases the dreaded complications can be prevented. The notable therapeutic success is based on the use of corticosteroid drugs. The patient should be given relatively large doses particularly if the symptoms are severe. Sixty mg. of prednisone daily for the first four or five days may be used, followed by a tapering off process until one achieves the minimal dose needed to alleviate the symptoms and manifestations of the disease. The purpose of the treatment is to allay the occlusion of cranial arteritis until such time as the disease has worn itself out. This time may vary from three months to three years. Three years after the origin of her symptoms one patient is doing well on 2.5 mg. of prednisone daily, but her symptoms recur if she misses her daily dose for two consecutive days. This is the only form of arteritis that invariably responds well to steroid therapy. This is a vicious and successfully treatable disease. The diagnosis should be made early. The treatment should be adequate and should not be delayed.

References

Fairchild, P., Rygvold, O. and Oystese, B.: Temporal arteritis and polymyalgia rheumatica. Ann. Intern. Med., 77:845, 1972.

Waksman, B. H.: Auto-immunization and the lesions of auto-immunity. Med., *41*:93, 1962.

14. Glomus Tumor or Glomangioma

ORVILLE HORWITZ

Cause: Micro-arterio-venous anastomosis of the skin usually of an extremity, often under the nail. Exquisite tenderness in same area.

Early Manifestations: Sudden excruciating pain radiation from the extremity, short in duration. Small, often less than 1 mm. in diameter purplish spot in the extremity, frequently under the nail.

Treatment: Surgical excision denervation.

Possible Dire Consequences without Treatment: Continued symptoms.

This disease may proceed undiagnosed for years as the painful and often disabling symptoms precede the signs. The use of a pin to probe suspicious areas will often provoke the symptoms under the circumstances.

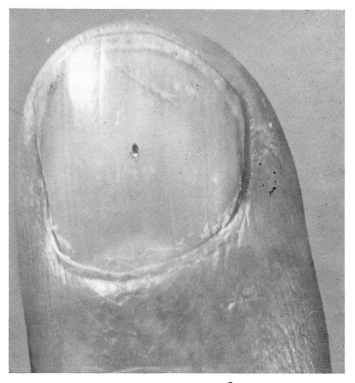

Fig. XIV–4. Glomus tumor under nail of right great toe.

Reference

Allen, E. V., Barker, N. W. and Hines, E. A., Jr.: Peripheral Vascular Diseases. 3rd ed., Chap. 26, Philadelphia, W. B. Saunders Co., 1962, p. 666.

15. Patent Ductus Arteriosus

Orville Horwitz

Cause: Not clearly understood but congenital.

Early Manifestations: Fatigue, machinery murmur.

Treatment: Generally surgery.

Possible Dire Consequences without Treatment: Pulmonary hypertension, subacute bacterial endocarditis, aneurysm with rupture.

Of the huge numbers of congenital heart lesions we have chosen only to mention patent ductus arteriosus. It accounts for about 10% of all such defects, usually is an isolated lesion, and may first be recognized in adult life. It was the first to be remedied surgically and is still the most easily corrected of the congenital heart lesions. It is often symptomless but is surely not signless, the murmur (Fig. XIV–5) is usually unmistakable. Surgical correction nearly always averts the above mentioned dire consequences.

Exact diagnosis of most other treatable congenital lesions is much more difficult, the surgery much more complicated, and less satisfactory and for these reasons is not discussed in this book.

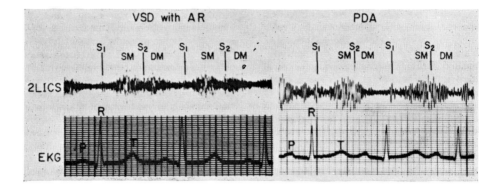

Fig. XIV–5. Phonocardiograms comparing the continuous murmur of patent ductus arteriosus (PDA, righthand panel) and the to-and-fro murmur of ventricular septal defect with aortic regurgitation (VSD with AR, lefthand panel). The murmur of PDA is of maximum intensity at or near the second heart sound, S_2, while the systolic murmur, SM, and the diastolic murmur, DM, of VSD with AR are maximal in midsystole and early diastole and the period surrounding S_2 is relatively quiet. (Plauth, W. H., Jr., et al.: Amer. J. Med., *39*:552, 1965.)

References

Danilowicz, D. A. and Ross, J. R., Jr.: Congenital heart disease, p. 624, Vol. I, in Cardiac and Vascular Diseases, Conn, H. L. Jr. and Horwitz, O. (eds.), Philadelphia, Lea & Febiger, 1971.

Plauth, W. H., Jr., *et al.*: Ventricular septal defect and aortic regurgitation. Amer. J. Med., *39*:552, 1965.

16. Acquired Arteriovenous Aneurysm

ORVILLE HORWITZ

Cause: Trauma causing A–V communication, disc operation.

Early Manifestations: Bruit over area, decreased diastolic pressure, slowing of pulse rate upon compressive occlusion.

Treatment: Surgical repair.

Possible Dire Consequences without Treatment: Danger to involved extremity, congestive failure, shock, death, if large enough.

Congenital A–V aneurysms are seldom amenable to operative correction because of the diffuse nature of the condition, with blood passing through large numbers of small vessels. The fistula may not be obvious at birth but only in childhood when the affected leg becomes larger and warmer. The lesion may be obvious early, presenting as a cavernous hemangioma. Bruits are generally absent. The volume of blood passing directly from the arterial to the venous side is usually too small to cause systemic circulatory embarrassment. Arteriograms probably should be performed routinely, since occasionally operable lesions will be revealed. Unfortunately, the usual management involves a palliative rearguard action with grudging acceptance of deformity, disability, and even in extreme cases, amputation.

Acquired fistulas may be formed by various types of wounds and occasionally by invasive diseases. Wounds may be traumatic (often among the military), or surgical. Surgical wounds are occasionally purposeful but more frequently inadvertent, as in intervertebral disc operations. The seriousness of these fistulas varies directly with the volume of blood flowing from the arterial to the venous side. The severe consequences may include greatly increased cardiac output, decreased diastolic pressure, greatly increased venous pressure locally, and congestive failure. Shock sometimes follows the acute development of large fistulas.

Undiagnosed and/or untreated acute acquired fistulas become chronic acquired fistulas. It is possible that they may never cause trouble, but generally the arterio-venous communication increases in size and symptoms ensue. Locally a systolic or machinery murmur is present.

Ideally in acquired fistulas surgical repair should be undertaken as promptly as possible.

Reference

Roberts, B. and Holling, H. E.: Arteriovenous fistulae, in Vascular Surgery. Springfield, Charles C Thomas, 1965.

17. Venous Thrombosis-Pulmonary Embolus Complex

ORVILLE HORWITZ

Cause: Unknown, immobility commonest precipitating factor. Others are: (1) Immobilization; flaccid as in: prolonged febrile illness, severe ischemia, carcinomatosis, congestive heart failure, chronic brain syndrome, postpartum period, period following severe trauma, period following operation. Spastic as in catatonia. (2) Chemical injury; intravenous injection of caustic substances. (3) Mechanical injury; direct trauma, muscular effort or strain, misuse of elastic bandage, venous surgery. (4) Varices. (5) Inflammatory or suppurative lesions. (6) Blood dyscrasias. (7) Dehydration, especially following diuretic therapy.

Early Manifestations: Numerous. Most common are *none*, unilateral or bilateral edema, dyspnea, leg pain, venous cord in leg, chest pain, hemoptysis, arrhythmia, and just sudden death.

Treatment: Heparin, leg elevation, oxygen, rest, mobilization, inferior vena cava ligation, pulmonary embolectomy.

Possible Dire Consequences without Treatment: Prolonged morbidity, chronic cor pulmonale, postphlebitis syndrome, death.

This disease may be more common, more lethal, more satisfactorily treatable, and more frequently undiagnosed than any other disease.

1. Venous thrombosis is a common disease and probably affects close to 100% of Americans to a greater or usually lesser extent.
2. All individuals who live long enough absorb at least one pulmonary embolus (fortunately small and few).
3. The cause is contained in one of the following or a combination of two or more of the following:
   (*a*) Plasma.
   (*b*) Cells in the plasma.
   (*c*) The vessel.
   (*d*) The velocity or acceleration of the blood through the vessel.
4. The precipitating factors are many but the main one is probably immobility.

Signs and Symptoms: 1. Although the presenting symptom or sign may be any of the above early manifestations, the cardinal sign or symptom of thrombosis of a deep vein is EDEMA, either obvious or measurable.

2. Dyspnea is the main symptom of pulmonary embolus and perhaps the only one that is relevant prognostically.

Laboratory Studies: 1. *Pulmonary function* studies may be particularly helpful in the early diagnosis of multiple and repeated small pulmonary emboli. It is usual to find a reduction of arterial blood pO_2 accompanied by an even greater reduction of arterial blood CO_2, as the ratio is increased. The poor gas exchange in the dead space also is reflected by a low CO_2 tension of the tidal air. Such changes may be exaggerated following exercise, affording an even more sensitive indication of multiple microembolic pulmonary disease.

494

2. *Electrocardiogram.* The electrocardiogram may well be the most helpful of all findings except for dyspnea in determining whether or not severe pulmonary embolization has occurred. In order to obtain ECG changes, pulmonary hypertension must be present. This is usually the result of multiple embolization or gross embolization by a large thrombus. Occasionally it can result from a small embolus with resultant pulmonary arterial constriction.

3. *Enzyme studies* are significant. In the absence of other known diseases affecting serum lactic dehydrogenase activity (LDH), and increase, coupled with a normal serum glutamic-oxalacetic transaminase (GOT) activity, has been considered highly specific for pulmonary embolism.

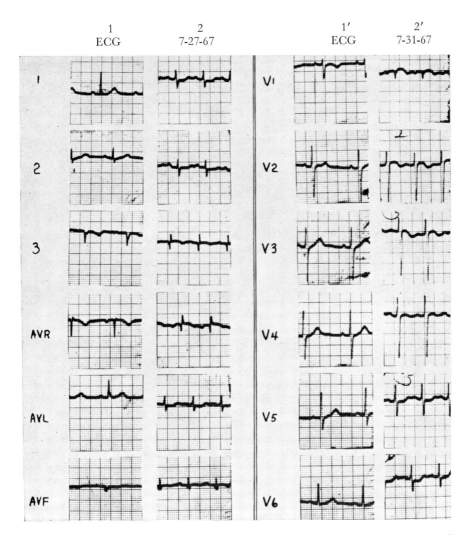

Fig. XIV–6. Electrocardiographic changes following massive pulmonary embolism. *1* and *1'*, Normal electrocardiogram. *2* and *2'*, Alterations shortly following acute massive pulmonary embolism in the same patient. Note depression of S–T segment in leads I and II, right axis deviation, prominent Q waves in lead III, and inverted T-waves in lead III and the right chest leads. (Conn and Horwitz, Cardiac and Vascular Diseases, Lea & Febiger.)

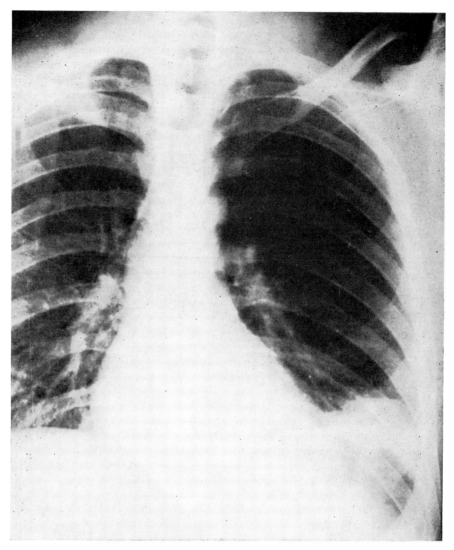

Fig. XIV–7. Pulmonary infarction at left costophrenic angle.
(Conn and Horwitz, Cardiac and Vascular Diseases, Lea & Febiger.)

4. *Radiographic findings.* If large pulmonary arteries are embolized, there may be persistent pleural effusion, patches of conspicuously reduced vascular markings, and signs of pulmonary infarction sometimes presenting as peripheral triangular opacities. However, such wedge-like shadows should not be counted on to make a diagnosis and, indeed, the usual pulmonary infarct does not bear this configuration. If the small arteries and arterioles only are involved in the thromboembolic process, there may be thin or even absent peripheral vascular markings. Regardless of the size of the involved arteries, evidence of dilatation of the pulmonary artery, right ventricle, and frequently the right atrium may be expected.

5. Radioisotope scanning following intravenous injection of either ^{131}I or ^{51}Cr labeled macroaggregated human serum albumin is now possible and is useful

TABLE XIV–3

ELECTROCARDIOGRAPHIC CHANGES IN PULMONARY EMBOLUS

Origin	Mechanism	The Change	Location	Frequency	Duration
Sinus Node	Sinus tachycardia	↑ Rate	Rhythm Strip	66%	Days
Atrium	Ectopic Mechanism	No P	Rhythm Strip	5%	Days
	Enlargement	↑ P	Rhythm Strip	5%	Days
Left Ventricle	Subepicardial ischemia	↓ T	Left Precordials	10%	Days
	Subepicardial ischemia	↓ T	III, aVF	10%	Days
Biventricle	Subendocardial ischemia	↓ T	Rt. Precord., aVR	50%	Days
	Subendocardial ischemia	↑ T	Lt. Precord., aVF	50%	Days
Biventricle	Subendocardial injury	↑ T	Rt. Precord., aVR	25%	Weeks
	Subendocardial injury	↓ ST	Lt. Precord., aVF	25%	Weeks
Enlarged Left Ventricle	Verticalization	$S_1 Q_3 T_3$	Bipolar leads	50%	Weeks
	Verticalization	AVF $V_{5,6}$	Unipolar leads	50%	Weeks
	Rotation	Transition $\longrightarrow$	Precordial leads	33%	Weeks
	Rotation	R	aVR	33%	Weeks
	Conduction	LBBB or $S_1 S_2 S_3$	Bipolar leads	10%	Weeks

in detecting spaces in the lungs where there is a lack of blood flow. Certain pulmonary emboli which may otherwise defy recognition, may be detected and localized by this method.

6. *Ultrasonic scanning* is another method of detecting pulmonary emboli.

Diagnosis: Diagnosis of pulmonary embolic disease depends on a high index of suspicion on the part of the physician. Since its treatment and that of deep venous thrombosis are so similar, except in extreme circumstances, little can be lost by actually assuming that these two conditions coexist until proven otherwise. A common pitfall is mistaking such symptoms as hemoptysis and pleuritic pain for those of primary pneumonic disease. Another is to attribute rapidly developing dyspnea to congestive heart failure rather than to multiple and remorseless microemboli, which may masquerade under the guise of hysterical dyspnea, episodes of syncope, or a gradually falling blood pressure. The symptoms of myocardial infarction may be indistinguishable from those of pulmonary embolus. Constant vigilance is of the essence. Once the possibility has been planted in the examiner's mind, a more extensive history, proper examination and mensuration of the extremities, and review

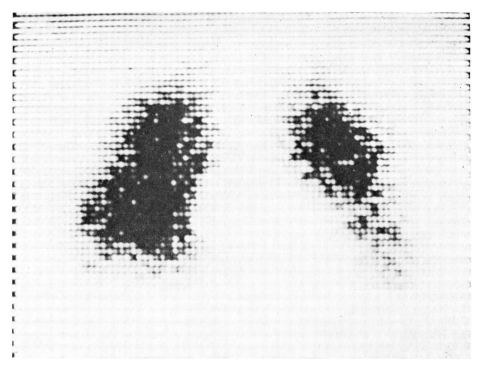

Fig. XIV–8.   Lung scan showing bilateral pulmonary emboli.
(Conn and Horwitz, Cardiac and Vascular Diseases, Lea & Febiger.)

of the chest roentgenogram, the electrocardiogram, and pulmonary function studies should be sufficient to lead to the correct diagnosis.   It is conceivable that another reason for missed diagnosis is that the examiner contentedly attaches his mind to a condition he considers to be a more common cause of the patient's symptoms.   This should not be.   Pulmonary embolism is a common disease.

Treatment: It has been attempted to establish the concept that deep venous thrombosis and pulmonary embolus almost invariably coexist.   It follows that the treatment must be almost identical.   As in prophylaxis, the keystones of treatment are anticoagulant drugs and discouragement of vascular stasis by exercise, elevation of the legs, and elastic stockings.   Contrary to the problem of prophylaxis, once the disease is established, bed rest (or immobilization) is considered to be mandatory in the acute states of severe venous thrombosis and pulmonary embolism.   This is dichotomous, since immobility has been established as a factor predisposing to venous stasis.

It has been our policy to mobilize these patients as soon as they are (1) adequately anticoagulated with heparin, (2) without pain or edema in the extremities, and (3) completely devoid of respiratory embarrassment as judged by absence of dyspnea and normal pO_2 and pCO_2.

Adequate anticoagulant therapy with heparin is by far the most potent weapon in our therapeutic arsenal and, unless otherwise contraindicated should be instituted immediately by intravenous injection if necessary.   The word "adequate" is used advisedly.   In no other condition is it so imperative to maintain the clotting time at a uniformly high level of over twenty-five minutes five hours after previous injection.

This may be achieved by as little as 15,000 units (150 mg.) daily, but in patients with massive thrombotic processes, over 60,000 (600 mg.) may be needed daily. It has been suggested by some investigators that heparin therapy be controlled by determination of Activated (Kaolin) Partial Thromboplastin Time (PTT). There appears to be a straight line relationship between PTT and Lee White Clotting time, a PTT of one hundred seconds corresponding approximately to an LW of thirty minutes. In venous thrombosis and pulmonary embolus heparin therapy may be expected to be more successful than in any other condition. It is our practice to continue heparin for two weeks or until the manifestations have either disappeared or have become stabilized.

Mechanical methods for minimizing venous stasis as outlined under prophylaxis are also valid in treatment.

Constipation should be avoided if necessary by the use of laxatives and enemas.

Fibrinolytic agents, such as streptokinase, have been used in severe thrombotic conditions, but streptokinase causes severe antigen-antibody reactions which may render the patient even more prone to thrombotic episodes. More purified preparations in larger doses have shown more promise. Urokinase is even more promising in this respect, but clinical trial seems to indicate that both streptokinase and urokinase decrease the morbidity but not the mortality.

Pulmonary emboli, and especially infarctions, may become secondarily infected by the flora of the respiratory tract. Also, septic emboli may result from pyophlebitis. Such conditions require the use of appropriate antibiotic drugs. These drugs are also often employed prophylactically against pneumonia in thromboembolic pulmonary disease.

Although it is probable that a majority of patients will recover with no treatment whatsoever, proper management undoubtedly will decrease the incidence of the post-phlebitic syndrome, of a pertinent pulmonary embolus, and of death.

TABLE XIV–4

COMPARISON OF THERAPEUTIC MEASURES USED IN MASSIVE PULMONARY EMBOLUS AND MYOCARDIAL INFARCTION.
(Conn and Horwitz, Cardiac and Vascular Diseases, Lea & Febiger.)

Therapeutic Measures	*Massive Pulmonary Embolus*	*Severe Acute Myocardial Infarction*
Position	Flat	Fowler's position
Application of warmth	Usually contraindicated	Usually indicated
Digitalis	Usually indicated	Usually not indicated
Morphine	Usually contraindicated	Usually indicated
Diuretics	Not indicated	Often indicated
Respiratory stimulants	Sometimes effective	Seldom employed
Atropine	Indicated	Generally not indicated
Pressors	Usually effective	Usually effective
Heparin	Strongly indicated, often in large dosage	Usually indicated
Inhalation of 100% oxygen	Indicated	Indicated
Aminophyllin 0.25 to 0.1 Gm	Indicated	May be indicated

References

Alpert, J. S. *et al.*: Experimental Pulmonary Embolism: Effect on Pulmonary Blood Volume and Vascular Compliance. Circulation, *49*:152, 1974.

Gray, Frank L.: Pulmonary Embolism, Philadelphia, Lea & Febiger, 1966.

Moses, D. C., Silver, T. M., and Bookstein, J. J.: The complementary roles of chest radiography, lung scanning, and selective pulmonary angiography in the diagnosis of pulmonary embolism. Circulation, *49*:179, 1974.

Horwitz, O.: Chapter 61, pp. 1577–1595, Vol. II, Cardiac and Vascular Diseases. Conn, H. L., Jr. and Horwitz, O. (eds.), Philadelphia, Lea & Febiger, 1971.

Sasahara, A. A.: Pulmonary Embolic Disease. Sasahara, A. A. and Stein, M. (Eds.), New York, Grune & Stratton, 1965.

Welch, W. H.: Thrombosis and Embolism. Reprinted from Allbutt's System of Medicine, 1899.

18. Post-Phlebitic Syndrome

Orville Horwitz

Cause: Destruction of valves and irritation of vessel wall by venous thrombosis.

Early Manifestations: Pain and edema following phlebitis.

Treatment: Antigravity measures, tetraethyl ammonium chloride.

Possible Dire Consequences without Treatment: Increased pain, edema, postphlebitic ulcers.

The diagnosis of postphlebitic syndrome is usually obvious, although in some instances it cannot be distinguished from lymphedema. In either case the therapy is almost identical, and, in the case of venous vascular incompetence, is to reduce or counteract the high venous pressure that is present when the patient is not lying down.

Only the patient can, for example, lose the unnecessary weight, arrange for periods of rest and of elevation of the legs, persist in obtaining and wearing well-fitted elastic stockings, and avoid constricting garters and abdominal girdles. The patient who has varicose veins should bear the responsibility for a considerable part of his own treatment.

Pain may be persistent in this condition. Often it is caused by the cycle of

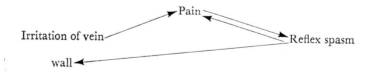

Sometimes the reflex spasm can be halted by a ganglionic blocking agent, such as tetraethyl ammonium chloride. In order to be effective this should be given slowly (100 mg. per minute intravenously) in doses of no more than 200 mg. Blood pressure should be monitored during the injection as rapid decreasing may occur, in which case the injection should be stopped.

Reference

Conn, H. L., Jr. and Horwitz, O.:   Cardiac and Vascular Diseases, Chapters 61, 62, and 63,
   Vol. II, Philadelphia, Lea & Febiger, 1971.

19. Varicose Veins

Hugh Montgomery

Causes: Inheritance, phlebitis, trauma, malignancies.

Early Manifestations:
Early   Usually visibly dilated veins, having retrograde flow of blood.
Late   Pain, edema, inflammation, dermatitis, ulceration.

Types: 1. Varices with incompetence of valves of superficial and communicat-
              ing veins.
           2. Varices with incompetence of valves of deep veins also.

Treatment: 1. Surgical removal.
               2. External support.

Possible Dire Consequences without Treatment: Severe pain, pulmonary embolism.

Varicose veins are veins of the lower extremities that have incompetent valves.
That is, the valves allow retrograde passage of venous blood.   Such venous valvular
incompetence causes little or no difficulty when the patient is reclining and the
venous pressure is slight, but when the patient is upright large volumes of blood pass
in a retrograde manner down into the veins of the legs.   This flow may be so great
as to overload the pumping action of that combination of deep veins and overlying
muscle called the "venous heart."   This is especially embarrassing when the valves
of the deep veins as well as those of the superficial and communicating veins are
incompetent.   The high venous pressure when the patient is standing is not relieved
by walking but is lessened somewhat by sitting and is completely relieved by lying
down.

Varicose veins may be present, with or without symptoms, in legs that look normal,
or—at the other extreme—may present as unsightly, tortuous and enlarged veins
accompanied by edema, ulceration and dermatitis.

The complications of varicose veins: pain, edema, ulceration, dermatitis, etc., are
largely a result of prolonged, unsupported venous pressure.   The evidence for this is
that these complications are lessened if the venous pressure is reduced by prolonged
bed rest, or by surgical removal—when feasible—of the veins that have incompetent
valves, or when the venous pressure is counterbalanced by supportive bandages,
stockings or boots.

The choice of treatment depends in part upon the severity of the symptoms.   It
also depends upon whether only the valves of the superficial and communicating
veins are involved or whether those of the deep veins are also involved.   The superficial and communicating veins are not part of the "venous heart," but they play a
subsidiary role by leading the blood into the deep veins.   Often the flow of venous
blood from varicose superficial and communicating veins is so large as to overburden

the capacity of the "venous heart" to eject it, and thus to cause troublesome symptoms even when the valves of deep veins themselves are intact.

In order to distinguish incompetence of valves of superficial veins only from that of valves of both superficial and deep veins, the following procedure is used: With the patient supine, raise a leg to empty all its veins. Then have the patient stand and carefully note the number of seconds required for the veins at the ankle to fill; if this is less than twenty seconds there are incompetent venous valves in the leg. Repeat the maneuver but when the leg is elevated, apply a venous tourniquet just below the knee and again note the filling time after the patient stands. If the veins fill in thirty or more seconds the valves of superficial (and probably communicating veins) are incompetent, but the valves of the deep veins are competent. However, if the veins fill in less than twenty seconds, valves of the deep veins are considered to be incompetent.

Varicose superficial and communicating veins may cause bothersome symptoms by contributing large retrograde flow to the deep veins of the leg. Ligation, section, and stripping of these superficial veins may relieve the symptoms.

Varicose deep veins, whether or not accompanied by varicose superficial and communicating veins, contribute retrograde flow of the blood throughout the whole venous system in the leg. This easily overwhelms the capacity of the failing "venous heart." In such a case, ligation or stripping out of superficial veins will not measurably improve the situation. Ligation and stripping of the deep veins is contraindicated because this would seriously obstruct the venous system and abolish any remaining function of the "heart." Medical measures are needed: bed rest, external support, and education of the patient.

Reference

Montgomery, Hugh: Varicose Veins, in Cardiac and Vascular Diseases, Vol. II, pp. 1597–1604. Conn, Hadley, Jr. and Horwitz, Orville (Eds.). Philadelphia, Lea & Febiger, 1971.

20. Thrombophlebitis and the Pill

J. Edwin Wood

Cause: Oral contraceptive agents.

Early Manifestations: Pain and tenderness of calf muscles, leg edema. Tenderness over veins. Blatant thrombosis of superficial veins.

Treatment: Intravenous heparin, discontinuation of oral contraceptive agent. In mild cases Butazolidin and discontinuation of oral contraceptive agent.

Possible Dire Consequences without Treatment: Pulmonary embolism, cor pulmonale, or sudden death.

It seems well established now that oral contraceptive agents containing estrogenic compounds as well as progestational compounds are associated with a definite increase in the incidence of thrombophlebitis and thromboembolism. This incidence is eight times greater than would be expected in a population of nonpregnant, normal, young women. The hazard of oral contraceptives is thromboembolism. This hazard in a nine-month period is probably not as great as the total risk of one pregnancy plus the postpartum period.

The mechanism is derived from the effect of oral contraceptives upon the velocity of blood flow in veins upon the clotting mechanism of blood, and possibly upon the blood vessels themselves. The veins of the human are dilated, particularly in the leg, by oral contraceptives. This has the effect of reducing the rate of flow in the veins, thus, causing stasis which in turn enhances the likelihood of thrombosis. Clotting is effected to some extent by oral contraceptives in the spheres of platelet function, fibrinolytic activity, and other clotting factors. The results of these various studies are somewhat contradictory so that exposition of their detail is probably not useful.

Young women taking oral contraceptives may have just begun taking them, or more often will have been taking them for three to six months or more, before noting the sudden onset of pain and tenderness in one or both calves. Unlike older individuals with thrombophlebitis, the presence of tenderness and soreness is quite specific and the patient is usually certain of the abnormality of the discomfort. Examination of the patient reveals redness, warmth, and edema, along with the "doughy" quality of the calf muscle. This, of course, is equally true of any form of thrombophlebitis. The patient may have symptoms of pulmonary embolism and accompanying findings.

Treatment of these patients should consist of elevation of the extremity. Discontinuation of oral contraceptives and the admonition to the patient that she not use these agents in the future is all important. If the thrombophlebitis is advanced, heparin therapy in the hospital is indicated. If the thrombophlebitis is early and little or no edema is present or if it primarily involves superficial veins, then the use of Butazolidin and temporary bed rest with discontinuation of oral contraceptive therapy is acceptable. Most patients have prompt relief of their phlebitis with these measures. It is unusual for the phlebitis to return if the patient does not recommence use of oral contraceptive agents.

Reference

Horwitz, O.: Venous thrombosis—Pulmonary embolus complex and other venous diseases—Chap. 61, p. 1577. In Cardiac and Vascular Diseases. H. L. Conn, Jr. and O Horwitz (Eds.), Philadelphia, Lea & Febiger, 1971.

21. Impotence Due to Deficient Circulation Through the Internal Iliac Arteries and their Branches

ORVILLE HORWITZ

Cause: Stenosis or occlusion of the above vessels usually due to arteriosclerosis. Congestive failure or severe cachexia may also be result by sympathectomy and certain antihypertension agents.

Early Manifestations: Complete inability to obtain complete and effective erection. Many or no pulses may be absent.

Treatment: Correction of cause, sometimes by arterial surgery, particularly by end-arterectomy of stenotic areas of the internal iliac arteries.

Possible Dire Consequences without Treatment: Continued impotence. Complications of a hidden aneurysm.

Patients who have the above early manifestations should have aortography. Not only can the patient's complaint be corrected in some instances, but also other correctable lesions of the terminal aorta and its branches, such as aneurysm and early stenosis may be detected.

Reference:

Horwitz, O.: Diseases of the arteries of the extremities. Chap. 58, p. 1517. In Cardiac and Vascular Diseases. H. L. Conn, Jr. and O. Horwitz (Eds.), Philadelphia, Lea & Febiger, 1971.

22. Hyperlipidemia (Hyperlipoproteinemia)

WILLIAM T. M. JOHNSON AND ORVILLE HORWITZ

Cause: Unknown, believed to be combination of genetic and environmental factors (diet, smoking, stress), resulting in elevated blood lipids and lipoproteins that are both endogenous and exogenous in origin.

Early Manifestations: None.

Late Manifestations: Creamy or turbid plasma, periodic abdominal pain, eruptive xanthomas, corneal arcus, premature atherosclerosis.

Treatment: Dietary: Diet low in fats (for hypercholesterolemia) and carbohydrates (for hypertriglyceridemia). Drugs: Anti-hyperlipidemic drugs such as Clofibrate or Atromid-S, in daily dosage of 1.5 to 2.25 gm. Small doses of intravenous heparin (2000 units) will temporarily clear serum triglycerides and this action may be beneficial to the patient.

Possible Dire Consequences without Treatment: Arterial occlusive disease, intermittent claudication, atherosclerosis, gangrene, stroke, myocardial infarction, death.

CORRELATION OF HYPERLIPIDEMIA WITH HYPERLIPOPROTEINEMIA; CLINICAL FEATURES

Hyper-lipopro-teinemia Types	*Hyper-lipidemia*	*Lipoprotein Pattern*	*Serum Lipids*		*Manifestations*
			Choles-terol	*Triglyc-eride*	
I	Exogenous or fat-induced lipidemia	Hyperchylomicronemia (chylomicron)	Normal range to 1+	4+	Creamy plasma; lipemia retinalis; hepatosplenomegaly; eruptive xanthomas; periodic abdominal "crisis"; acute pancreatitis
II	Essential familial hypercholesterolemia	Hyper-beta-lipoproteinemia (low-density lipoprotein)	2+ to 3+	Normal range to 1+	Corneal arcus; xanthelasmas; tendinous and tuberous xanthomas; premature atherosclerosis
III	Hypercholesterolemia and hypertrigylceridemia (familial hyperlipidemia)	Increase in "floating" beta-lipoprotein	Variable 2+ to 4+	Variable 1+ to 4+	Palmar and tuberous xanthomas; glucose intolerance; hyperuricemia; premature atherosclerosis
IV	Endogenous hypertriglyceridemia or "carbohydrate-induced" hyperlipidemia	Hyper-pre-beta-lipoproteinemia (very low-density lipoprotein)	Normal range to 2+	1+ to 4+	Turbid plasma; glucose intolerance; accelerated atherosclerosis
V	"Mix" hypertriglyceridemia (exogenous and endogenous)	Hyper-pre-beta-lipoprotein and hyperchylomicronemia (very low-density β-lipoprotein chylomicron)	1+ to 2+	3+ to 4+	Creamy or very turbid plasma; periodic abdominal pain; eruptive xanthomas

1. Elevated serum cholesterol does not always mean directly related intimal deposition of cholesterol or atherosclerosis. There is clinical and experimental evidence to support this conclusion.
2. However, the best single test for elevated blood lipids is serum cholesterol determination.
3. Individuals with low cholesterol are significantly less likely to acquire arterial occlusive disease.
4. Of the various hyperlipidemias, Type IV, hypertriglyceridemia, can best be controlled; the means is a low carbohydrate diet.

References

Benditt, E. P.: Evidence for a monoclonal origin of human atherosclerotic plaques and some implications. Circulation, *50*:650, 1974.
Dock, W.: Atherosclerosis, why do we pretend the pathogenesis is mysterious? Circulation, *50*:647, 1974.
Kuo, P. T.: Atherosclerosis in Man; Genetic and Metabolic Implications of Hyperlipidemia. Conn, H. L., Jr., and Horwitz, O.: Cardiac and Vascular Diseases, Philadelphia, Lea & Febiger, 1971, p. 978.

23. Retrolental Fibroplasia

Lois H. Johnson

Cause: Not completely understood. Basic lesion is one of retinal anoxia secondary to obliteration of retinal arterioles with subsequent neovascularization and invasion of the vitreous by retinal vessels. Pre-disposing conditions: *In utero;* unknown. *Ex utero;* of major importance is exposure of immature retinal vasculature to excessive oxygen tensions resulting in vasoconstriction and vaso-obliteration. Vitamin E deficiency seems also to play a role.

Early Manifestations: Recognizable only by serial examination with the indirect ophthalmoscope. Stage I—Neovascularization in peripheral retina (tufting and arcading of growing ends of arterioles). Stage II—Also edematous retinal detachment line. Stage III—Also hemorrhages and exudate.

Prevention and Management: Rigid monitoring of arterial oxygen tension after birth; treatment with vitamin E by best available preparation.

Possible Dire Consequences without Treatment: In severe cases, blindness. Increased visual morbidity in milder forms of the disease.

Retrolental fibroplasia is largely confined to the prematurely born infant in whom vascularization of the retina must proceed in an extra-uterine environment. This form of the disease has been found to be greatly increased, in incidence and severity, by exposure to excessive concentrations of oxygen. The resulting hyperoxemia causes vasoconstriction followed by vaso-obliteration of growing retinal arterioles. The resulting anoxia of the peripheral retina spurs an uncontrolled vascular overgrowth which invades the vitreous. These aberrant vessels subsequently retract into a mass of fibrous scar tissue. In severe forms of the disease there is associated retinal detachment and total loss of sight (stage 4 and 5).

Modern methods of controlling oxygen therapy have resulted in the virtual disappearance of this severe form of the disease. But milder forms still occur, especially in the very prematurely born, and result in an increased incidence of myopia, strabismus and amblyopia in early childhood and retinal degenerations with detachment in early adult life. This mild form of the disease is recognized in the newborn nursery only by means of examination with the indirect ophthalmoscope and occurs in spite of careful control of oxygen therapy. It occasionally occurs in the complete absence of supplemental oxygen. Therefore it is encouraging to note that treatment with vitamin E has been shown to decrease the incidence and severity of this persisting form of the disease.

Though not generally known, vitamin E is common in children with fibrocystic disease and in prematurely born infants, both of whom have impaired intestinal fat absorption. In the premature this is due to immaturity of the intestinal enzymes which persists until about a term gestational age. Synthetic oral E acetate, the only readily available form of the vitamin, is as poorly absorbed as the naturally occurring vitamin in food. The most well recognized manifestation of this E deficiency state in the premature is a self limited hemolytic anemia of varying degrees of severity.

Clear E sufficiency from birth onward, in sick as well as vigorous prematures, can best be achieved by treatment with a parenteral preparation, supplemented when feasible by the oral route. Unfortunately, parenteral E preparations are as yet available only on a research basis. One such preparation, dl-α-tocopherol acetate, is in the final stages of development by Hoffman LaRoche, Inc.

In a controlled clinical trial using this parenteral E acetate among infants weighing less than 2000 gm. at birth, treatment with vitamin E, as opposed to placebo, was associated with a significant reduction in the incidence and severity of retrolental fibroplasia when incidence and severity were considered as a combined index. (p 0.05, n = 18). Furthermore, among infants who developed some degree of RLF in the nursery, the number of deviations from the normal hyperopic state of the one year old among those who had received the vitamin was approximately half that of those treated with the placebo (N = 15, 10 placebo and 5 E treated). Serum E concentrations in the range of 1.0 to 1.5 mg.% were maintained until maturity of the retinal vasculature had been achieved or until regression of active disease occurred. While preliminary, these results are highly encouraging.

Therefore, at the present state of our knowledge, management of the premature infant with respect to retrolental fibroplasia consists of careful control of oxygen therapy and early provision of diets rich in vitamin E to optimize whatever intestinal absorption is available. As more effective preparations of vitamin E become available they should be included in the treatment regimen. It should be noted that iron by the oral route interferes with intestinal absorption of vitamin E and is not indicated in the nursery period; also that colostrum is remarkably rich in vitamin E and that breast milk and breast milk substitutes (in particular Enfamil) are considerably higher in E content than evaporated milk formulas.

References

DeLeon, A. S., Elliott, J. N. and Jones, D. B.: The resurgence of retrolental fibroplasia. Ped. Clin. N. A., *17*:309, 1970.

Johnson, L., Schaffer D., and Boggs, T. R.: The premature infant, Vitamin E deficiency and retrolental fibroplasia (RLF). Amer. J. Clin. Nutrition, *27*:1158, 1974.

Kinsey, V. E. and Chisholm, J. F.: Retrolental fibroplasia: Evaluation of several changes in dietary supplements of premature infants with respect to the incidence of the disease. Amer. J. Ophthal., *34*:1259, 1951.

Oski, F. A. and Barnes, L. A.: Vitamin E deficiency: a previously unrecognized cause of hemolytic anemia in the premature infant. J. Pediat., *70*:211, 1967.

Patz, A.: The role of oxygen in retrolental fibroplasia. Pediat., *19*:504, 1957.

Chapter XV

Cardiac Disorders

Introduction

Steady progress is being made in the treatment of cardiac diseases, and in certain specific spheres this progress has been substantial which is reflected in the size of some of the individual sections, particularly surgical correction of heart disease. However, the magnitude of the problem of atherosclerosis so dominates this field, and in particular myocardial infarction which is now the commonest cause of death in the U. S. A., that a considerable amount has been written about the specific therapies for this condition. The area of specific therapy for acute myocardial infarction has changed in one area suddenly; namely, the role of the mobile coronary care unit, or coronary ambulance, in treatment. This has forced the physician to look beyond the confines of the hospital when considering how to treat this condition. This area has been well studied by the originator of this concept, Dr. J. F. Pantridge. I have endeavored to put in words what I consider his present ideas to be on the pre-hospital phase of the specific treatment of myocardial infarction.

Sections 24 to 33 inclusive deal with cardiac conditions in which surgery is to be considered particularly. Most of these conditions are valvular diseases. Only the commonest congenital lesions are considered.

The efficacy of the surgical treatment for hyperlipidemia is still somewhat controversial but is fully discussed in Circulation Volume XLIX, No. 5, supplement number 1.

1. Angina Pectoris

Norman Makous

Cause: Impaired myocardial blood flow without myocardial necrosis usually due to coronary artery atherosclerosis.

Early Manifestations: Episodic discomfort usually of the chest, sometimes in the jaw, the arm, or epigastrium often accompanied by dyspnea, palpitation, sweating, pallor, and hypertension.

Treatment: *Medical.* Nitrates, activity control, abstinence from tobacco, beta adrenergic blocking agents, digitalis or diuretics and antihypertensives, when specifically indicated. Diet for weight control and alteration of lipoprotein profile.
Surgical. Coronary artery by-pass grafting, removal of aortic stenotic valve or ventricular aneurysm.

Possible Dire Consequences without Treatment: Sudden death, shock, congestive heart failure, myocardial infarction and incapacitating pain.

The clinical manifestations can be divided into four acute and three chronic syndromes. The acute syndromes consist of sudden death, acute myocardial infarction (p. 518), angina pectoris and the intermediate coronary insufficiency syndromes. The chronic syndromes are asymptomatic, postacute, recurrent acute and cardiomyopathic.

Tests of cardiac function are not diagnostic of coronary heart disease. Incipient CHD is strongly suggested by stress induced attenuation of cardiac performance measured during cardiac catheterization or indirectly, by such techniques as exercise electrocardiography or echocardiography. In general these tests are not specific enough to justify the certain diagnosis of coronary heart disease in the absence of other manifestations unless accompanied by coronary arteriographic evidence of significant obstructive arterial disease. Practically it often is most prudent to regard the isolated non-specific findings, not as evidence of incipient CHD, but as the "risk factors" or latent or pre-CHD, along with such high risk factors as hypertension, hypercholesterolemia, and smoking. Early recognition of non-specific and atypical syndromes may prove life saving. Mortality reduction seems feasible in that at least 25% of those dying suddenly had consulted a physician the preceding week. But the manifestations are non-specific, obscure and often go unrecognized. Just as CHD represents but a small visible portion of coronary artery disease iceberg, so too, the classical syndromes of angina pectoris and acute myocardial infarction represent but a small portion of the total CHD picture.

Diagnosis is reviewed first from the viewpoint of postulated pathophysiologic mechanisms and then from the viewpoint of the clinical problem.

PATHOPHYSIOLOGY OF ACUTE NON-NECROTIC CHD

Coronary artery atherosclerosis limits myocardial blood flow. This causes ischemia which in turn induces discomfort, acute myocardial power failure and arrhythmias. The power failure arising from the ischemic metabolic abnormality produces two major responses of left ventricular dysfunction. These may be characterized as forward and retrograde heart failure. The arrhythmias may be designated primary or secondary. The primary arrhythmias may initiate their own clinical manifestations such as ventricular fibrillation, the presumed cause of sudden death. These in turn may cause power failure. The secondary arrhythmias arise from power failure, but also in turn can contribute to it.

EFFECTS OF ISCHEMIA

Acute myocardial ischemia modifies cardiac function and causes circulatory responses that produce most of the clinical manifestations. Pain is a major response. Arrhythmias, retrograde failure and forward failure are the others.

Discomfort. Pain is considered the sine qua non of angina pectoris. The heart has two types of sensory nerves none of which contain pain fibers. A perivascular network encircles the coronary artery and paravascular fibers terminate between the cardiac muscle fibers in unmyelinated non-specific nerve endings. Transmission is through the eighth cervical and first five thoracic ganglia. Overflow spreads along the ganglionic chain and within the lateral ascending tract of the cord along which stimuli from other organs are transmitted. Information from the heart cannot be distinguished as such, but is projected to the body area supplied by the same spinal cord segments through somatic reference. Cardiac stimuli can summate with those from gastrointestinal or musculoskeletal sources. Thus pain is referred to the mid anterior chest, left shoulder, and down the arms especially the medial aspect, into the left lower interscapular area, to the neck, throat and lower jaw as well as to the epigastrium.

The exact mechanism of pain production remains unknown. A chemical stimulus has been postulated for years, but a neuromechanical explanation is more appealing.

Arrhythmias. Arrhythmias appear as a result of ischemia through several mechanisms. The sinus node is supplied in 55% of the hearts by a branch originating early in the course of the right coronary artery. The remaining 45% are supplied by the first branch of the left circumflex artery. Likewise the A–V node is usually supplied by a distal branch of the right circumflex artery. Variation in sinus node artery function can cause bradycardia, tachycardia, or a pacemaker shift. Likewise variable degrees of heart block can develop. Episodes of arrhythmia may be isolated manifestations of ischemia that are transient and reversible brought about by brief coronary "steal" mechanisms. Ventricular irritability is the most common arrhythmia of acute ischemia. Premature ventricular contractions, especially if coupled and multiple, can lead to tachycardia, fibrillation, and cardiocirculatory arrest.

Myocardial Dysfunction. Ischemia decreases contractility of the involved myocardium and impairs compliance. Force and velocity of contractions are slowed. Pressure and ejection rates and peaks are impaired and delayed. Residual systolic and end-diastolic volumes are increased along with pressures. Stroke volume is reduced which leads to an impaired cardiac output if uncompensated by adrenergic stimulation of the uninvolved myocardium or by an increased heart rate.

The myocardial impairment is accompanied by *clinical* signs. Involvement of the anterior myocardium can produce a palpable precordial bulge during systole or a filling impulse in diastole. A late systolic murmur from dysfunction of papillary muscle and the supporting left ventricular wall may be heard. With the change in compliance ventricular and atrial gallop sounds appear. The second heart sound can split paradoxically.

The manifestations of retrograde failure arise from increased pulmonary venous pressure, and pulmonary edema or from increased pulmonary vascular resistance. The right sided findings are related to venous distention in the mediastinum and neck, and to acute hepatic congestion.

Peripheral. Acute myocardial insufficiency evokes a positive sympathetic nervous system response. A rise in peripheral resistance accompanied by increased contractility of the non-ischemic myocardium is signaled by a rise in systolic blood pressure, tachycardia and insufficiency of diseased peripheral vascular beds. Compromise of the skin, cerebral, splanchnic and extremity blood flow causes pallor, cool skin, headache, giddiness, syncope, abdominal pain or claudication. Thus occasionally symptoms arising from peripheral sites may appear before the cardiac centered chest symptoms, and can dominate the clinical picture.

CLINICAL MANIFESTATIONS OF ISCHEMIA

Discomfort. Derivationally, angina pectoris means choking or strangling at the breast. Clinically it is interpreted as pain. Actually many equivalents are accepted, *i.e.* pressing, tightness, squeezing, heaviness, choking. These often are reinterpreted as pain by the physician when more appropriately they are equivalent to the original meaning of angina. Shortness of breath is a frequent descriptive equivalent often overlooked by the physician. The dyspnea of mild left sided failure or pulmonary insufficiency like the physiologic dyspnea of youth is usually identified by the patient as a light or puffy sensation. Many who first describe their discomfort as shortness of breath readily pick one of the more appropriate and acceptable synonyms of angina pectoris, and strongly deny that the sensation is anything like their physiologic dyspnea. Actually the most specific description is not a symptom but a sign where the clenched fist or more commonly open flat hand is held over the mid anterior chest. Pain localized with one or two fingers rarely is ischemic heart pain. Brief sharp shooting pain is not heart pain, as cardiac discomfort lasts for several minutes, at least.

Location and Radiation. The location and radiation of the discomfort is often diagnostically helpful. It usually begins or ends deep in the mid anterior chest. Sites of reference are the neck, throat or lower jaw. More commonly the discomfort radiates to the pectoral and subclavicular areas, shoulder, and arms, especially the medial aspect, but infrequently to the hand. This is to the left more often than the right. The lower left interscapular area is a consistent point of radiation in the back. The epigastric location especially when accompanied by indigestive discomfort is frequently mis-diagnosed as a gastrointestinal disorder. Pain of radicular distribution is not an isolated symptom of ischemic heart disease. Ischemic heart pain is referred to the left of the cardiac apex or to the left upper quadrant only when the heart is enlarged in my experience.

Associations. Angina pectoris often interacts with other conditions. Chronic recurrent discomfort from musculo-skeletal factors can interact with the heart. Costo-chondritis, cervical or dorsal arthritis, bursitis, tendonitis, and chest wall myositic and fibrositic trigger points make diagnosis difficult when associated with angina pectoris. The non-cardiac factors may initiate pain which provokes myocardial ischema. The non-cardiac pain pathways then respond to the ischemia. Interpretation is aided if the discomfort also spreads to other more typical areas of reference. But the appearance of dyspnea, sweating or pallor may be the only clues that the discomfort has become cardiac in origin. Angina pectoris can also appear initially in a typical pattern but then be followed by hours of discomfort at a referred site long after myocardial ischemia has subsided due to the chronic underlying non-cardiac problem.

An interrelationship between cardiac and gastrointestinal activity is well known. Angina pectoris may appear more readily after a meal. Altered blood viscosity is one reason, but increased splanchnic flow and decreased circulatory efficiency along with the non-specific dynamic metabolic stimulation by protein may also be important. The diagnostic confusion accompanying the association of gallbladder disease or hiatus hernia are notorious. Innumerable healthy teeth have been extracted when the pain first appears or is limited to the jaw and dental consultation obtained before medical. Deglutition angina, that with swallowing, is unpredictable and usually indicates very severe coronary artery disease.

Circumstances. The circumstances which precipitate the discomfort of angina pectoris are important diagnostically. Typically exertion of a relatively consistent degree produces the discomfort. It comes on more readily after meals and in the cold wind or air. Emotional upset is a well recognized precipitant even without exercise. Meals, the cold and emotion all appear to increase cardiac work through modification of peripheral circulatory responses, although a change in blood viscosity is probably an additional factor after meals.

Angina pectoris and coronary insufficiency syndromes are not well recognized under unusual circumstances. Warm up angina pectoris is relatively common; an activity such as shaving, bathing, or eating early in the A.M. often causes chest discomfort while greater activity later in the day does not. Pain appears on walking to the bus or from the parking lot to the office in the morning but not in the afternoon on return at a much faster pace. Temperature differences, meal time or emotional factors do not account for the difference in most instances.

Angina pectoris may also first arise paradoxically on the termination of exertion. This angina develops in one to two minutes from loss of myocardial efficiency through after-loading of the left ventricle by a rapidly rising peripheral resistance. The residual left ventricular volume enlarges; the ejection time prolongs; and the mean ejection pressure remains unchanged even though maximal systolic pressure falls. Thus myocardial oxygen demand rises at a time cardiac output and external work are falling.

Postural angina pectoris is precipitated by the same mechanism. Retiring for the night may precipitate chest discomfort. For some, preparation for bed involved more physical activity than any other of the day. The combination of postural change during exercise recovery decreases cardiac efficiency and can provoke ischemia and angina pectoris.

Nocturnal angina probably arises through several mechanisms. In those whose angina is stable and mainly exertional, cardiac stimulation and cardiocirculatory inefficiency associated with the REM phase of sleep is apparently responsible. When coronary disease is severe, the gradual increase in central and cardiac volume in part through shifting of extra cellular fluid and edema may be of major importance. The crescendo pre-infarction angina could be due to the same mechanisms in part, but local coronary vascular factors and the state of blood may prove more important in view of the different electrocardiographic changes observed. This angina is often walked off. The assumption of an upright posture reduces central volume and ventricular filling. Cardiac efficiency improves with the posture change and exertion.

Peripheral.   Peripheral vascular beds already compromised by arterial disease may give rise to local non-cardiac symptoms from cardiac insufficiency prior to the development of chest discomfort.

Arrhythmias.   Arrhythmias may be primary or secondary.   In the primary type the arrhythmia begins as the isolated manifestation of ischemia.   Then because of the arrhythmia, the myocardial load increases, coronary insufficiency develops and angina pectoris appears.   If the arrhythmia is prevented, so is the angina.

These are of atrial origin most often, and include paroxysmal atrial tachycardia, flutter and fibrillation.   Occasionally nodal and ventricular tachycardia are seen under these circumstances, as are bradycardias and heart block.

The secondary arrhythmias appear with or as a result of the angina pectoris and coronary insufficiency.   They are ventricular in origin most often, and arise from the more generalized coronary and myocardial functional inadequacy, but also contribute to it once they appear.

Diagnostic differentiation is often made by therapeutic trial.   For instance, anginal pain can sometimes be prevented by proper control of an arrhythmia and occasionally paroxysmal arrhythmias without angina pectoris can be prevented by the regular use of long acting nitrates.

Signs.   The signs of coronary insufficiency appear with changes in myocardial and cardiac function.   When isolated, they are non-specific, but in the appropriate circumstances the signs provide objective and often diagnostic evidence that the associated symptoms originate in the heart.

The cardiac findings are palpatory and auscultatory.   The ischemic hypodynamic area of the myocardium is detected as a palpable sustained systolic bulge or prominent diastolic impulse in the apical region.   Changes in myocardial compliance modify the first heart sound, and ventricular and atrial gallop sounds appear.   The second sound may split paradoxically.   Transient apical systolic murmurs of mitral regurgitation follow papillary muscle and the adjacent ventricular wall dysfunction. A bigeminal rhythm from ventricular premature beats is semispecific for coronary insufficiency.   Pallor and coolness of the digits, ears, and nose develop.   Initially the systolic blood pressure may rise.   Hypotension appears later.

Electrocardiography.   The resting ECG is normal in roughly one half of patients with angina pectoris.   Ventricular premature contractions arising from each preceding T wave in alternate or bigeminal rhythm is the most typical rhythm disturbance of coronary heart disease.   Any arrhythmia may appear but others are less characteristic.   Intraventricular conduction disturbances also may appear as a result of acute coronary insufficiency.

The most characteristic lesion involves the ST segment.   Occasionally at rest, and especially during the acute attack and on exercise the ST segment lengthens at the expense of the T wave and occupies a larger proportion of the QT interval.   ST depression below the isoelectric line is typically ischemic when horizontal, and almost diagnostic when it exceeds 0.1 mv. (1.0 mm.) and may be considered diagnostic when it reaches 0.3 mv. (3.0 mm.).   T waves in the same leads become inverted only when the ST depression is severe.   When the resting tracing is abnormal with T waves inverted, the polarity reverses, as usual.   The T waves now become more upright while typical ischemic ST depression develops or becomes more marked.

The post-exercise ECG shows the same ischemic ST changes.   The ST depression usually exceeds 0.1 mv. (1.0 mm.) if the exercise is adequate.   In over 90% the ECG response exceeds this if the exercise is continued to maximum.   Contrary to previous reports the change is less common during than after submaximal exercise. One half of those with positive post-exercise ECG changes are maximal after the first minute of recovery, apparently reflecting the left ventricular after loading phenomenon of recovery.

The ischemic ST depression of exercise is relatively specific for ischemia but it is not specific for coronary disease. Unless the ST depression exceeds 0.2 to 0.3 mv. (2 to 3 mm.) as an isolated clinical finding, it is probably best to regard the change as evidence of latent coronary heart disease at most and a factor of increased risk at the least. Ischemic ST depression from tachycardia is quite suggestive of a compromised myocardial oxygen supply, but again does not warrant a diagnosis of clinical coronary heart disease if this is the only finding. The junctional type of ST depression is of much less, if any, significance. With this depression the ST segment retains its concave normal upward sloping contour and only the beginning portion appears to be depressed below the isoelectric line or PR–QRS junction.

T wave inversion is less specific for coronary disease than is the ischemic ST depression. The inverted T waves from acute ischemic damage are usually symmetrical. If T waves invert as a result of angina pectoris, they return to the resting level within minutes; if due to coronary insufficiency syndrome, they resolve in days and if due to myocardial infarction the inversion persists for weeks.

EXERCISE TESTING

Exercise testing can be of considerable help in the evaluation of coronary heart disease. Information derived from symptoms, the cardiopulmonary auscultatory responses, and the blood pressure is often more informative than that from the ECG changes. In those at increased risk but asymptomatic and in those apparently normal, information concerning cardiocirculatory reserve is obtained from maximal exercise testing. In the symptomatic where etiology is not clear, testing helps clarify the complaint and the nature of physical and ECG findings. In those with known coronary heart disease objective information concerning performance is obtained, and the effect of therapy including exercise can be assessed.

The type of exercise is not of paramount importance, and may be by two steps, treadmill, or bicycle ergometer. Submaximal tests of a fixed type such as the Masters' double two-step have the disadvantage of not adequately testing many with early but significant coronary heart conditions. The stress is moderate at most and may be adequate only if the test is continued beyond the three minutes. The testing is safe if performed under the supervision of a physician.

CORONARY ARTERIOGRAPHY

Arteriography is a definitive diagnostic method. At present it is used principally in the evaluation of ischemic heart pain that has become so intolerable that surgical intervention is contemplated. The procedure is also useful in the differential diagnosis of atypical chest pain.

CLINICAL RECOGNITION

Coronary heart disease can be divided into three phases that are generally related to the severity of the CAD but exceptions are common. The pre-disease phase is asymptomatic, and the coronary artery disease is usually not advanced. Slight non-specific symptomatology is characteristic of incipient coronary heart disease which is usually associated with moderately advanced coronary artery disease. Overt coronary heart disease is associated with more severe coronary artery disease.

The type of clinical presentation varies. It can be typical or atypical, and is usually symptomatic. Occasionally the presentation is limited to signs, electro-cardiographic abnormalities or radiographic cardiomegaly.

LATENT CORONARY HEART DISEASE

The individual considers himself to be in usual and good health. The pre-disease concern often arises in conjunction with an annual industrial or preventive care health examination, or is initiated by anxiety over a family history of premature cardiovascular disease, or is initiated following the sudden death of an acquaintance. These examinations frequently reveal an accentuated awareness of trivial symptoms.

Here the so called "risk factors" are the dominant findings. The most important ones of greatest risk are smoking, hypertension, and hypercholesterolemia. Others, less significant are the family history of an immediate member developing coronary heart disease before the age of sixty, obesity with weight more than 10% above the individual's best or ideal weight, carbohydrate intolerance especially if there is overt diabetes mellitus, hypertriglyceridemia, uric acid elevation, premature ventricular contractions, nonspecific electrocardiographic abnormalities, an isolated positive electrocardiographic exercise test and sedentarism.

The risk associated with combinations of these findings is accumulative and graduated. Working men thirty to sixty-five years without these factors suffer first episodes of acute coronary heart disease at a rate of about 3 per thousand per year. Those who previously have had an acute episode, *i.e.* those with coronary heart disease, have an annual recurrence rate of approximately 100 per thousand. The incidence in those with risk factors exceeds 5 per thousand per year. It should be emphasized that the presence of a number of high risk factors alone does not justify a diagnosis of coronary heart disease.

Incipient Disease. In view of the dominance of non-specific complaints at this stage a high index of suspicion is required if coronary heart disease clues are to be recognized and the condition diagnosed. The patient's real motive for seeking medical attention should be sought behind the apparent one often masked by the chief complaint. A change in pattern of health concern often is a sign of incipient disease even though complaints are superficial or unchanged. The man who requests a health survey for the first time in years, but denies symptoms should be viewed with suspicion. The anxiety of such a denier may have been aroused by the unexpected death of an acquaintance or by the onset of depression which is often associated with the development of overt coronary heart disease. Unmasking the atypical or vague symptoms of heart disease in these patients offers considerable challenge.

One subgroup of deniers are exercise enthusiasts. Any vague feeling of ill-being is first attributed to lack of exercise conditioning so of course exercise is turned to as their first line of therapy. The physician has to be particularly wary when these people seek medical clearance for jogging. However, most do not; some of the past jogging deaths may have been preventable had cardiovascular clearance been sought first.

Cardiac symptoms frequently are atypical or masked in the early stages and puzzle both patient and physician. Single or infrequent episodes of pain and inconsistent pain under unusual circumstances are difficult to evaluate. The patient who experiences new and unusual shortness of breath or indigestion is often uncertain as to the symptoms' significance. The dyspnea and ease of fatigue often are attributed to "growing old" or physical unfitness, if not to recent weight gain. The unusually rapid deterioration in exercise tolerance in a six- to twelve-month period compared to similar periods over the preceding five years is abnormal. Also unusual exertional or paroxysmal tachycardia or palpitation may be an initial symptom.

Disturbance in sleep pattern may be due to cardiocirculatory insufficiency rather than depression. Paroxysmal nocturnal dyspnea can be an angina pectoris equivalent. Excessive nocturnal sweating or physical exhaustion on waking after a full night's sleep are other sleep related signs of cardiocirculatory stress.

The non-cardiac effects of coronary and cardiac insufficiency can be the dominant initial manifestation. The possibility that syncope is a Stokes-Adams attack should always be entertained. Headaches, especially in women, or giddiness on exertion may be early symptoms. Pain especially exertional atypically located in the teeth, throat, chest or back, shoulders or epigastrium may be referred from the heart. The recent onset of mild to moderately severe systemic hypertension relatively refractory to antihypertensive medication, but sensitive to the long acting nitrates is an occasional early sign of coronary heart disease. And exertion-induced lower abdominal or low back pain and intermittent claudication may be due to peripheral circulatory insufficiency, secondary to cardiac insufficiency.

References

Aronow, W. S. and Stemmer, E. A.: Bypass graft surgery versus medical therapy of angina pectoris. Amer. J. Card., *33*:415, 1974.

Blackburn, H.: Measurement in Exercise Electrocardiography, Springfield, Charles C Thomas, 1969.

Committee on exercise. Exercise testing and training of apparently healthy individuals. A hand book for Physicians, Am. Heart Assoc., New York, 1972.

Donald, K. W.: Hemodynamics in chronic conegstive heart failure. J. Chronic Dis., *9*:476, 1959.

Goot, V. L.: Outlook for patients after coronary artery revascularization. Amer. J. Card., *33*:431, 1974.

Hood, W. B.: Pathophysiology of ischemic heart disease. Prog. Cardiovasc. Dis., *14*:297, 1971.

Hurst, J. W. and Logue, R. B.: The Heart, New York, McGraw-Hill Book Co., 1970, p. 904.

Kuller, L.: Sudden death in arteriosclerotic heart disease. Am. J. Cardiol., *24*:617, 1969.

Makous, N., Gittleman, M. A. and Atencio, N. E. V.: The post two-step ECG and hemodynamic determinants of myocardial oxygen consumption. Malattie Cardiovasculari., *10*:1, 1969.

O'Rourke, R., Mann, O. and Harvery, W. P.: Control of coronary pain by prevention of tachycardia. J.A.M.A., *188*:1005, 1964.

Paul, O.: Coronary artery disease: Clinical aspects, *In* Cardiac and Vascular Diseases, pp. 1038–1155, Vol. II, Conn, H. L., Jr. and Horwitz, O. (Eds.), Philadelphia, Lea & Febiger, 1971.

Prinzmetal, M. *et al.*: Variant form of angina pectoris. J.A.M.A., *174*:1794, 1960.

Reeves, T. J., Oberman, A., Jones, W. B. and Sheffield, L. T.: Natural history of angina pectoris. Amer. J. Card. *33*:423, 1974.

Rowell, L. B.: Cardiovascular limitation to work capacity. *In* Physiology of Work Capacity and Fatigue, Simonson, E. (Ed.), Springfield, Charles C Thomas, 1971, p. 132.

Sampson, J. J. and Cheitlin, M. D.: Pathophysiology and differential diagnosis of cardiac pain. Prog. Cardiovascular Dis., *13*:507, 1971.

Schaper, W.:   Pathophysiology of coronary circulation. Prog. Cardiovasc. Dis., *14*:275, 1971.
Shappell, S. D. *et al.*:   Acute change in hemoglobin affinity for oxygen during angina pectoris.
New Eng. J. Med., *282*:1219, 1970.

2. Myocardial Infarction

PETER F. BINNION AND KENNETH L. KERSHBAUM

Cause: Impaired myocardial blood flow due to coronary artery atherosclerosis with
resultant myocardial necrosis.

Early Manifestations: Severe substernal pain or possibly jaw, shoulder, head or
epigastric discomfort; dyspnea, palpitation, pallor, sweating, syncope; one of the
commonest early manifestations is sudden death; some patients are asymptomatic.

Treatment:

Medical.   *General*
Early admission to Coronary Care Unit system, either hospital or Mobile
Coronary Care Unit.
Bed rest and sedation.
Analgesics.
Oxygen therapy.
Anticoagulants.
Polarizing solutions.
Complications
Arrhythmias (see also sections on arrhythmias and heart block).
Congestive heart failure—digitalis, diuretics, salt restriction.
Shock—plasma expanders, vasopressors, inotropic agents, *e.g.* digitalis,
dopamine, isoproterenol, glucagon.

Surgical.   Counterpulsation with intra-aortic balloon for cardiogenic shock.
Emergency coronary artery by-pass surgery, either saphenous vein or
internal mammary artery by-pass.
Surgical repair of specific complications, *i. e.* intraventricular septal rupture,
papillary muscle rupture, ventricular wall rupture.

Possible Dire Consequences without Treatment: Death, shock, congestive heart failure.

Myocardial infarction is, of course, a major clinical manifestation of coronary
atherosclerosis. The Framingham epidemiologic survey of coronary heart disease
has demonstrated that the initial clinical manifestation was myocardial infarction
(including 10% sudden death) in 55% of male subjects and 31% (including 6%
sudden deaths) of females under observation. In the remainder angina pectoris, or
in a relatively small percentage the intermediate syndrome (acute coronary insufficiency) was the earliest clinical manifestation. Furthermore, of men over forty-five
years of age presenting with angina approximately 50% develop myocardial infarction or sudden death within eight years following the onset.
Pathogenesis. Coronary atherosclerosis is the predominant pathologic process
underlying myocardial infarction. There are, however, exceptions as myocardial
infarction may develop in association with congenital anomalies of the coronary

arteries, coronary arterial emboli (such as in infective or marantic endocarditis, prosthetic cardiac valves), dissecting aneurysms, and syphilitic coronary ostial stenosis. Causes of non-atherosclerotic occlusions of the coronary artery include amyloidosis, tuberculosis, sickle cell disease, collagen vascular disease and thrombotic thrombocytopenic purpura. Furthermore there have been recent reports of typical myocardial infarction in patients with coronary arteries demonstrated by angiography to be entirely normal in origin and distribution and free of any occlusive disease. An as yet unanswered question concerns the possible role of disease of small (*i.e.* 0.1 to 1.0 mm.) coronary arteries in some instances of myocardial infarction.

Atherosclerotic lesions of the coronary arteries, present to a significant degree in the vast majority of instances of myocardial infarction, represent a complex interplay of local and metabolic factors. The pathologic process consists of intimal deposition of lipid-laden macrophages, degenerative changes of the internal elastic lamina and lipid accumulation in the media, accompanied by fibrotic reaction, varying degrees of calcium deposition and ingrowth of capillaries in the intimal and medial layers, along with surface ulceration of the atheromatous plaques. The luminal narrowing produced by the atheromatous lesions may be further compounded by intramural hemorrhage, intimal rupture, and intraarterial thrombosis in the segments of the coronary arteries involved with the primary process. Pathologic studies of the coronary arteries in fatal acute myocardial infarctions by Roberts have emphasized the diffuse nature of the atherosclerotic plaques, being present along practically every millimeter of the extramural coronary arteries. There was greater than 75% occlusion of at least 2 of the 3 major coronary arteries in the majority of patients dying with either transmural or subendocardial necrosis, or dying suddenly without evidence of necrosis. These investigations also explored the role of coronary arterial thrombi in the pathogenesis of myocardial infarction. Coronary thrombosis was found in only about 50% of transmural myocardial infarction and about 10% of instances of subendocardial infarction or sudden death without myocardial necrosis. These findings were consistent with earlier pathologic studies which demonstrated that the frequency of coronary thrombi increased with increasing intervals between the onset of symptoms of myocardial infarction and the time of death. Roberts also notes a close correlation between the finding of coronary arterial thrombi and the presence of myocardial pump failure in the patient's clinical course. It is concluded that thrombi in coronary arteries are usually a consequence, rather than the cause of acute myocardial infarction. This does not exclude, however, their possible importance in the pathogenesis of atherosclerotic plaques.

While myocardial infarction is usually associated with severe occlusions of the coronary arteries, the converse is often not true. Proudfit *et al.* in their cineangiographic studies of the coronary arteries in 1,000 patients found that about 85% of patients who had myocardial infarctions had luminal obstruction of 90% or more in at least one major coronary artery. By contrast, this same group reported that about half the patients demonstrated to have total occlusions of the right coronary artery or left circumflex artery and about one-third of patients with total occlusions of the left anterior descending artery had no evidence of myocardial infarction, either by electrocardiogram or by the demonstration of asynergic segments of myocardium by left ventriculography. The presence or absence of significant myocardial necrosis in association with severe occlusive coronary artery disease may well be related to the rate at which the occlusive lesions develop and the extent of collateral circulation.

Clinical Manifestations. The classic symptom of myocardial infarction is severe substernal chest pain which may radiate over the precordium and to the epigastrium, neck, jaw, shoulder, and arm. The pain most commonly is described as a constriction, tightness, heaviness, squeezing, or pressure-like sensation. It may occur only in one or more of the usual areas of radiation without chest involvement. It is unaffected by respiration, movement or positional changes, and is usually constant until relieved spontaneously after one or more hours or following parenteral administration of a narcotic agent. There is often associated pallor, diaphoresis, lightheadedness, nausea or vomiting as well as obvious anxiety and a sense of impending doom.

In a patient who has previously experienced angina pectoris the pain of myocardial infarction is usually distinctly unique from prior episodes. It may be differentiated from angina by its greater severity, longer duration, and absence of relief with nitroglycerin. There is more frequent association with diaphoresis, gastrointestinal symptoms, cerebral symptoms, including syncope, due to an abrupt fall in cardiac output sometimes associated with a transient arrhythmia, and dyspnea, due to acute left ventricular failure. Unlike angina, which usually occurs at times of physical or emotional stress, the onset of pain in myocardial infarction is more commonly during a period of rest or ordinary activity. In one study the initial symptoms of myocardial infarction developed during sleep in 22%, at rest or with mild activity in another 51% and with unusual or severe exertion in only 2% of attacks. Many earlier reports have suggested that acute myocardial infarction occurs without prior warning in the majority of instances. In a recent study, however, in which 100 consecutive patients admitted to a coronary care unit with acute myocardial infarction were interviewed in detail, there was a 65% incidence of prodromal symptoms. These prodromata consisted of new symptoms of cardiac origin (usually progressive chest pain) or significant worsening of pre-existing cardiac symptoms (*i.e.* angina) during the two months preceding the acute attack.

A significant proportion of myocardial infarctions may go entirely unrecognized clinically either due to absent or atypical symptoms. In the Framingham Study 23% of myocardial infarctions, as detected by new diagnostic changes appearing on sequential periodic electrocardiograms, were clinically "silent." Some instances of unrecognized infarction may be those occurring under general anesthesia and those in which the predominant manifestation is gastrointestinal, a syncopal episode or an associated cerebrovascular accident. They are also said to occur more frequently in diabetic patients.

There are no diagnostic physical findings in acute myocardial infarction. The patient's general appearance may be unremarkable or he may be cool, pale and diaphoretic. The pulse and blood pressure may or may not be normal. Atrial diastolic gallops are frequently present due to decreased left ventricular compliance. An ectopic precordial impulse may be palpable resulting from dyskinetic left ventricular contraction and there may be paradoxical splitting of the second heart sound. Often, particularly with inferior wall infarctions, an apical systolic murmur of papillary muscle dysfunction is heard. This represents mitral insufficiency, usually due to infarction of a papillary muscle and/or its adjacent left ventricular wall. The murmur is described typically as occurring in mid and late systole with a crescendo-decrescendo configuration, however, the timing and character of the murmur is actually highly variable. Of importance is the fact that papillary muscle dysfunction murmurs, as well as the other physical findings noted above are not pathognomonic of myocardial infarction and may all appear transiently during episodes of myocardial ischemia without infarction.

Laboratory Diagnosis. The typical electrocardiographic features of an acute myocardial infarction are well known. These consist of the appearance of abnormal Q waves (*i.e.* ≥0.04 seconds in duration), ST segment elevations with upward convexity, and T wave inversions, often deep and symmetrical. These changes all usually occur in the same group of leads, those which face the area of myocardial damage. In addition, "reciprocal" changes consisting of increased height of R waves, ST segment depression and tall upright T waves may appear in leads facing the opposite surface of the heart. Hence, the area of myocardial necrosis may be localized by the leads in which these typical changes are identified (*e.g.* inferior, anteroseptal, anterolateral), or, as in diagnosing infarction of the posterior wall of the left ventricle, solely from the appearance of "reciprocal" changes (*i.e.* broad, tall R waves and tall upright T waves in the right precordial leads, V1 and V2). Experimental studies in which coronary arteries are ligated in nonanesthetized closed-chest dogs, as well as human myocardial infarction when observed in its earliest clinical stages, have demonstrated that the initial recorded electrocardiographic change is often the appearance of tall, peaked, "hyperacute" T waves. This is usually followed within hours, or possibly a day or more, by transitory ST segment elevation and the appearance of Q waves, followed by progressive T wave inversion which persists for weeks to months. While the time sequence of the electrocardiographic changes is highly variable, the abnormal Q wave is ordinarily the only permanent indication of a myocardial scar. Even these may become smaller or even disappear with time. If the ST segment elevation persists for several weeks or more after onset of a myocardial infarction, a left ventricular aneurysm is suggested.

While these are the typical electrocardiographic findings of a myocardial infarction, they are present in only 50 to 70% of instances. When the necrosis is nontransmural (*e.g.* subendocardial), the QRS complex may remain unaltered with only ischemic nonspecific ST segment and/or T wave changes. Furthermore, in about 10% of cases there are no significant electrocardiographic changes. Additional pitfalls in relying upon the electrocardiogram are the frequent absence of diagnostic changes in the presence of previous myocardial infarction and left bundle branch block (the characteristic changes usually are seen in the presence of right bundle block). Conversely, a false positive diagnosis of myocardial infarction may be made on the basis of abnormal Q waves in Wolff-Parkinson-White syndrome, cardiomyopathy, idiopathic hypertrophic subaortic stenosis and left ventricular hypertrophy.

Another useful adjunct in diagnosing myocardial necrosis is recognition of elevation in serum levels of certain enzymes present in myocardial cells which are released as a result of heart damage. Experimental studies have demonstrated that there is a close correlation between the depletion of myocardial enzymes and the rise in serum enzyme levels over a wide range of infarct sizes. The serum glutamic oxalacetic transaminase (SGOT) becomes elevated within eight to twelve hours following the onset of myocardial infarction, reaching peak levels in twenty-four to thirty-six hours and declining to the normal range within four to six days. SGOT has its greatest concentration in myocardial tissue but substantial amounts are present in liver and skeletal muscle, and to a lesser degree brain, kidney, testes, lung, and spleen. Hence, elevations frequently occur with hepatic dysfunction (including that due to congestive failure or shock without myocardial infarction), skeletal myopathies and, on occasion, with pulmonary infarction. The lactic acid dehydrogenase (LDH) usually becomes elevated in the serum twenty-four to forty-eight hours following myocardial infarction, reaches peak elevation in three to six days and returns to normal range within eight to fourteen days.   LDH is extremely nonspecific, being present in large concentration in liver, skeletal muscle, erythrocytes, kidney and brain tissue, with marked elevations in serum levels occurring with hemolysis, megaloblastic anemias (ineffective erythropoiesis), hepatic dysfunction, skeletal muscle injury, renal infarction and in a variety of neoplastic diseases.   The creatinine phosphokinase (CPK) is a sensitive and relatively specific myocardial enzyme, as significant concentration is also present only in skeletal muscle and brain.   In acute myocardial infarction the serum CPK activity usually exceeds normal within the first six to eight hours, reaches its peak around twenty-four hours and returns to normal by three days.   Noncardiac elevations in CPK are primarily due to skeletal muscle disease such as myositis, muscular dystrophy, and following convulsions or intramuscular injections.   Alpha-hydroxy-butyric acid dehydrogenase (αHBD) is also relatively specific representing the fraction of LDH which is primarily concentrated in the heart.   It, also, may increase with hemolysis, megaloblastic anemias or renal infarction.   The CPK and αHBD are therefore useful in differentiating serum enzyme elevations of hepatic or skeletal muscle origin which may accompany shock, congestive heart failure, recent surgery or direct-current countershock from those due to myocardial necrosis.   In addition to transmural myocardial infarction, elevations of serum enzyme activity of cardiac origin have been described in some instances of subendocardial infarction, typical angina pectoris, myocarditis, and following tachyarrhythmias.

In addition to being of value in diagnosing and timing the onset of myocardial infarction, serum enzyme levels, as a correlate of the extent of myocardial necrosis, may be of prognostic value as well.   In a study of 125 patients with acute myocardial infarction a direct relationship was demonstrated between the magnitude of serum enzyme elevation (particularly SGOT and CPK) and the appearance of ventricular arrhythmias, congestive heart failure and cardiogenic shock, as well as overall mortality.

Most recently, a newly developed technique of cardiac scintiscanning with radio-isotope labeled tetracycline, which selectively binds to necrotic cardiac muscle, has been demonstrated to be a potentially effective method of diagnosing, localizing and quantitating acute myocardial infarction.

Treatment.   The treatment of myocardial infarction can be divided into a pre-hospital phase, hospital phase and post-hospital phase.   Within the hospital phase are included general measures, such as oxygen therapy, analgesics, rest, sedation, polarizing solutions, and anticoagulants, and treatment of complications, including arrhythmias, myocardial pump failure and surgical complications.

Pre-Hospital Phase.   When all the deaths due to coronary artery disease in a certain area are studied, it becomes apparent that a large proportion of these patients die outside hospitals without adequate medical attention and that most of these deaths occur within the first hour after onset of symptoms.   The figures quoted vary but over 50% of all patients with acute myocardial infarction die outside a hospital and it was for this reason that the concept arose of a mobile coronary care unit (M.C.C.U.) or coronary ambulance which provided definitive therapy for those patients before they reach a hospital.   The two commonest complications which cause rapid death appear to be bradyarrhythmias (for which atropine I.V. is effective) or ventricular fibrillation (which requires direct current cardioversion).   Using such a mobile system with specific therapy undoubtedly prevents a number of deaths from acute myocardial infarction and represents a definite step forward in the treatment of this dangerous disease.

Hospital Phase. The treatment here includes the general medical measures mentioned above, and, of course, recognition and management of any complications that may occur.

With the advent of careful patient monitoring, advances in electrical and pharmacologic therapy, and coronary care units, there has been substantial reduction in the mortality resulting from arrhythmias complicating acute myocardial infarction. Recognition and treatment of specific cardiac rhythm disorders is outlined in the sections on arrhythmias and heart block; however certain principles apply particularly in the setting of acute myocardial infarction:

1. Ventricular premature beats are often premonitory of ventricular tachycardia or ventricular fibrillation and prompt treatment is indicated. This is particularly true if they occur greater than 5 per minute, in salvos of 2 or more, with close coupling to the preceding sinus beat or with multiform configuration. Intravenous lidocaine is usually effective in suppressing VPB's and is the treatment of choice.

2. Bradyarrhythmias (sinus or A–V junctional bradycardia, 2° or complete A–V nodal block) occur relatively frequently early in the course of, particularly, inferior wall myocardial infarction. These slow rhythms may significantly compromise cardiac output or may predispose to dangerous ventricular arrhythmias. They often respond to the administration of atropine 0.5 to 1.0 mg. intravenously.

3. Supraventricular arrhythmias (*e.g.* atrial tachycardia, fibrillation or flutter) are often a manifestation of pump failure in acute myocardial infarction. Rapid digitalization is usually indicated both for its inotropic effects and for control of the ventricular rate response.

4. The appearance of intraventricular conduction disturbances in the course of acute myocardial infarction, particularly when there is evidence of "bilateral bundle branch block" (*e.g.* right bundle branch block with left anterior or posterior division block, alternating right and left bundle branch block, Mobitz type II second degree A–V block) often is followed by the development of complete heart block, and the prophylactic placement of a temporary demand pacemaker electrode may be indicated.

Congestive heart failure or shock associated with acute myocardial infarction must be recognized and treated promptly. However, in contrast to the successes in treating arrhythmic complications, results in management of power failure are usually poor, with overall mortality in cardiogenic shock uniformly 80 to 90% despite any mode of therapy currently available. Elevated blood pressure should be reduced to normal levels with antihypertensive medication and a regular exercise regimen, such as walking, should be encouraged as a form of therapy, during the post-hospital phase.

References

Alderman, E. L. *et al.*: Hemodynamic effects of morphine and pentazocine differ in cardiac patients. New Eng. J. Med., *287*:623, 1972.

Cobbs, B. W., Hatcher, C. R., and Robinson, P. H.: Cardiac rupture: Three operations with two long-term survivals. J.A.M.A., *223*:532, 1973.

Coodley, E. L.: Prognostic value of enzymes in myocardial infarction. Circulation, *46*: II–46, 1971.

Cotton, S. G. *et al.*: Factors discriminating men with coronary heart disease from healthy controls. Brit. Heart J., *34*:458, 1972.

Donkman, W. B. *et al.*: Effects of intra-aortic balloon pumping for cardiogenic shock. Circulation, *44*:II–103, 1971.

Drapkin, A. and Mersky, C.: Anticoagulant therapy after acute myocardial infarction. J.A.M.A., *222*:541, 1972.

Ebert, R. V.: The use of anticoagulants in acute myocardial infarction. Circulation, *45*: 903, 1972.

Fox, S. M., Naughton, J. P. and Gorman, P. A.: Physical activity and cardiovascular health. Mod. Concepts Cardiovasc. Dis., *41*:17, 1972.

Friedberg, C. K.: General treatment of acute myocardial infarction. Circulation, *40*: (Supp. IV), 252, 1969.

Fulton, M., Julian, D. G., and Oliver, M. F.: Sudden death and myocardial infarction. Circulation, *40*, Supp. 4:182–193, 1969.

Holman, B. L. et al.: Detection and sizing of acute myocardial infarcts with ^{99m} Tc (Sn) Tetracycline. New Eng. J. Med., *291*:159, 1974.

Josephson, M. E. *et al.*: Electrophysiologic properties of procainamide in man. Amer. J. Cardiol., *33*:596, 1974.

Kannel, W. B. and Feinleib, M.: Natural history of angina pectoris in the Framingham Study. Am. J. Cardiol., *29*:154, 1972.

Lal, S., Savidge, R. S. and Chabbra, G. P.: Cardiovascular and respiratory effects of morphine and pentazocine in patients with myocardial infarction. Lancet, *1*:379, 1969.

Levine, H. D., Young, E. and Williams, R. A.: Electrocardiogram and vectorcardiogram in myocardial infarction. Circulation, *45*:457, 1972.

Lown, B., Klein, M. D. and Hershberg, P. I.: Coronary and precoronary care. Am. J. Med., *46*:705, 1969.

Maroko, R. R. *et al.*: Effects of glucose-insulin-potassium infusion on myocardial infarction following experimental coronary artery occlusion. Circulation, *45*:1160, 1972.

Master, A. M., Dack, S. and Jaffee, H. L.: Activities associated with the onset of acute coronary artery occlusion. Am. Heart J., *18*:434, 1939.

Mittra, B.: Potassium, glucose and insulin in treatment of myocardial infarction. Lancet, *2*:607, 1965.

Mundth, E. D. *et al.*: Surgery for complications of acute myocardial infarction. Circulation, *45*:1279, 1972.

Pantridge, J. F. and Adgey, A. A. J.: Pre-hospital coronary care: Mobile coronary care unit. Am. J. Cardiol., *24*:666, 1969.

Paul, O.: Coronary artery diseases: Clinical aspects. *In* Cardiac and Vascular Diseases. Conn, H. L., Jr. and Horwitz, O. (Eds.), Vol. II, p. 1043, Philadelphia, Lea & Febiger, 1971.

Proudfit, W. L., Shirey, E. K. and Sones, F. M.: Distribution of arterial lesions demonstrated by selective cinecoronary arteriography. Circulation, *36*:54, 1967.

Report by the Medical Research Council Working-Party on the treatment of myocardial infarction: Potassium, glucose and insulin treatment for acute myocardial infarction. Lancet, *2*:1355, 1968.

Roberts, W. C.: Coronary arteries in fatal acute myocardial infarction. Circulation, *45*:215, 1972.

Scott, M. E. and Orr, R.: Effects of diamorphine, methadone, morphine and pentazocine in patients with suspected acute myocardial infarction. Lancet, *1*:1065, 1969.

Sobel, B. E. and Shell, W. E.: Serum enzyme determinations in the diagnosis and assessment of myocardial infarction. Circulation, *45*:471, 1972.

Sodi-Pallares, D. *et al.*: Potassium, glucose and insulin in myocardial infarction. Lancet, *1*: 315, 1969.

Solomon, H. A., Edwards, A. L. and Killip, T.: Prodromata in acute myocardial infarction. Circulation, *40*:463, 1969.

Spain, D. M. and Bradess, V. A.: Frequency of coronary thrombosis as related to duration of survival from onset of acute fatal episodes of myocardial ischemia. Circulation, *22*: 816, 1960.

Stamler, J.: Acute myocardial infarction—progress in primary prevention. Brit. Heart J., *33*:145, 1971.

Swan, H. J. C. *et al.*: Power failure in acute myocardial infarction. Prog. Cardiovasc. Dis., *12*:568, 1970.

Walsh, J. H. *et al.*: Mobile coronary care. Brit. Heart J., *34*:701, 1972.

Wasserman, A. J.: Anticoagulants in acute myocardial infarction. Ann. Intern. Med., *71*: 855, 1969.

Welch, C. C. *et al.*: Cinecoronary arteriography in young men. Circulation, *42*:647, 1970.

Working Party on Anticoagulant Therapy in Coronary Thrombosis: Assessment of short-term anticoagulant administration after cardiac infarction. Brit. Med. J., *1*:355, 1969.

Wyman, M. G. and Hammersmith, L.: Comprehensive treatment plan for the prevention of primary ventricular fibrillation in acute myocardial infarction. Amer. J. Cardiol., *33*:661, 1974.

Yu, P. N.: Pre-hospital care of acute myocardial infarction, Circulation *45*:189, 1972.

3. Pericarditis

F. Tremaine Billings, Jr.

Cause: Infection, trauma, neoplasm, metabolic disorders.

Early Manifestations: Sharp anterior and/or posterior chest pain exaggerated by respiration or cough, often lessened by sitting up or leaning forward; most frequently pericardial friction rub with or without pain; when pericardial effusion is collecting, increasing weakness, shortness of breath, tachycardia, hypotension, decreased pulse pressure with pulsus paradoxus, and distended neck veins.

Treatment: Management of specific cause when etiology has been discovered. Pericardiocentesis may be life saving.

Possible Dire Consequences without Treatment: Seriousness of this disorder depends upon underlying disease. So called acute benign pericarditis though painful, usually needs only general symptomatic treatment, but failure to recognize pericarditis due to infection, for example tuberculous, neoplastic or purulent, may lead rapidly to cardiac tamponade and death.

Pericarditis is a disorder the basic lesion of which is an acute inflammatory process involving the pericardium. It is most frequently manifested by pain, precordial in location but which may have the same distribution as the pain of myocardial infarction. This pain may vary in intensity. It frequently varies with respiration and may be exaggerated in the supine position and relieved by leaning forward. Pericardial inflammation may occasionally be near enough to the esophagus to cause dysphasia. Unless significant myocardial disease, arrhythmia or pericardial tamponade is present, there is no impairment of circulatory dynamics. A pericardial friction rub is the most common and most frequent sign. It may vary in intensity from time to time, may change with respiration and change of position and is often described as "to and fro" in character. Heart sounds are normal but when pericardial fluid develops they may become muffled.

While the leukocyte count may or may not be increased and serum enzymes are only elevated when there is significant myocardial involvement, the electrocardiogram is usually diagnostically revealing. Early there is concordant elevation of S–T segments without change of T wave. Later T waves may be diffusely inverted. These findings appearing sequentially can usually be differentiated from the changes of myocardial infarction or digitalis intoxication.

Roentgenographic Studies.   Especially when obtained serially will reveal increased size of the cardiac shadow if there is myocardial dilatation or pericardial effusion. Differentiation can be accomplished by intravenous injection of carbon dioxide, cardiac radioisotope scanning, ultrasound examination or cardiac catheterization with angiocardiography.

Pericardial Effusion.   Percardial effusion with tamponade is the most serious consequence of pericarditis.   Rapid onset of this condition must be recognized quickly and pericardiocentesis accomplished.   The xiphoid or apical approaches with the patient in the sitting position are preferable.   Electrocardiographic monitoring should accompany the procedure.   The needle may be used as an exploring unipolar electrode.   When it touches the myocardium, gross injury currents are detectable in the specific lead.   It is safest to carry out pericardiocentesis in a laboratory where resuscitative equipment is present.

Constrictive Pericarditis.   Constrictive pericarditis occurs when chronic pericardial disease leads to interference with the heart's action and congestive circulatory failure results.   The onset is insidious, there is fluid retention, and characteristic signs of right heart failure.   Differential diagnostic consideration must be given to diffuse myocardial disease, nephrosis and cirrhosis of the liver.   Early appropriate diagnosis and treatment of acute pericarditis are important to prevent the development of chronic constrictive pericarditis.   But when it is fully developed, surgery offers hope of benefit in the majority of patients.

References

Bishop, L. H., Jr., Estes, E. H., Jr., and McIntosh, H. D.:   The electrocardiograms as a safeguard in pericardiocentesis.   J.A.M.A., *162*:264, 1956.

McKusick, V. A. and Harvey, A., McG.:   Disease of the Pericardium, p. 157.   *In* Advances in Internal Medicine, Dock, W. and Snapper, I (Eds.), Chicago, Year Book Medical Publishers, 1955.

Winters, W. L. Jr. and Cortex, F. M.:   Pericardial disease.   In Cardiac and Vascular Diseases. Vol. II.   Chap. 48, p. 1326.   Conn, H. L. and Horwitz, O. (eds.).   Philadelphia, Lea & Febiger, 1971.

4. Anemic Heart Disease

Joseph A. Wagner

Cause: Anemia, with or without underlying heart disease.

Early Manifestations: Shock, *i.e.*, dyspnea, tachypnea, weakness, and dizziness in acute blood loss; and angina pectoris if there is underlying coronary artery disease. Chronic anemia may be well tolerated or cause weakness, dyspnea, palpitation, and precordial pain.

Treatment: The correction of anemia, in acute or severe blood loss, by transfusion. If there is underlying heart disease, it is usually wise to digitalize the patient and give transfusions of packed cells rather than whole blood transfusions.

Possible Dire Consequences without Treatment: In the absence of underlying heart disease the response of the heart to anemia is well tolerated, but in the presence of arteriosclerotic heart disease the failure to treat the anemia may lead to myocardial ischemia, myocardial infarction and death.

An increased cardiac output with exercise, if not at rest, has been recognized and associated with anemia.

The cause of the high cardiac output and decreased circulation time in anemia is unknown, but was thought due to decreased viscosity of blood and to decreased peripheral resistance, thereby serving the tissues with adequate amounts of oxygen even in the presence of decreased concentrations of hemoglobin. Animal experiments have suggested that high cardiac output occurs before decreased peripheral resistance develops. The increased cardiac output is due mainly to increased stroke volume for beta-adrenergic blockade reduces heart rate without reducing cardiac output. Edema of the lower extremities develops as evidence of congestive failure, possibly secondary to reduced renal blood flow and subsequent salt and water retention.

The so-called "high output" response of the heart depends on the rate of development of the anemia, its duration, and the presence or absence of underlying heart disease. Acute blood loss may cause weakness, dsypnea, and palpitation. Tachycardia, induced by exercise may persist for a prolonged period following the exercise. The patient is hypovolemic, hypotensive, and often in "shock." Treatment with whole blood transfusion relieves the problem, whereas the failure to treat the condition may lead to coma and death.

Chronic blood loss over a long period of time may be well tolerated and cause little or no distress. The cardiac output may be increased at rest or by exercise. The heart may be dilated. There may be soft systolic murmurs over the precordium together with mid-diastolic gallop sounds or murmurs. Systolic bruits are often heard over the great vessels in the neck. The chest films may show cardiac enlargement.

Frequently, either with acute blood loss or in chronic anemia of long duration, there is coexisting heart disease aggravated by the anemia. If the patient has chronic valvular heart disease, congestive failure is precipitated or aggravated by the anemia. If there is arteriosclerotic heart disease, then anginal syndrome is made worse by the anemia.

Although digitalis is not specific for anemic heart disease, it is usually wise to digitalize the patient with anemia who has, or probably has, underlying heart disease. If digitalis can be administered before transfusion, it may be helpful; otherwise, it can be done concurrently. Transfusion of packed red cells may be preferred to whole blood causing less volume load on the circulation. It is sometimes remarkable how exquisite a slight increase in hemoglobin may be on the patient's symptoms. A patient with a hemoglobin of 8 gm.% may be complaining of severe and frequent chest pain which is totally relieved following a transfusion and elevation of hemoglobin to but 9.5 gm.%. This observation has been made many times in different patients suggesting that each of the many such patients has his or her own critical level where symptoms are produced.

References

Conn, Hadley L., Jr. and Horwitz, Orville: Cardiac and Vascular Diseases. Vol. II. Philadelphia, Lea & Febiger, 1971.
Duke, M. and Abelman, W. H.: The hemodynamic response to chronic anemia. Circulation, *39*:503, 1969.
Escobar, E. *et al.*: Ventricular performance in acute normovolemic and effects of beta blockade. Amer. J. Physiol., *211*:877, 1966.

5. Heart Disease: Beriberi

Joseph A. Wagner

Cause: Thiamine deficiency.

Early Manifestations: Tachycardia, warm flushed skin, bounding pulses, right ventricular failure.

Treatment: Thiamine chloride parenterally and orally.

Possible Dire Consequences without Treatment: Progressive myocardiopathy with low output failure.

Background. In beriberi and in those with nutritional deficiency with or without alcoholism, there is often observed a hyperkinetic circulatory response, *i.e.* a warmed flushed skin, an increased pulse pressure due to elevation of systolic pressure and decrease in diastolic pressure, a rapid collapsing pulse together with signs of right-sided failure, i.e. neck vein elevation, hepatomegaly, and ankle edema. If alcoholism is unchecked, the patient may develop a myocardiopathy with low output failure which, unlike that seen early in the course, is unresponsive to thiamine chloride.

History and Physical Examination. The patient may complain of exertional dyspnea or rapid heart beat. Examination of the heart reveals tachycardias, a diffuse apical impulse with gallop sound and soft murmurs. These signs are associated with a dilated heart revealed as cardiomegaly on chest roentgenogram. The circulation time is short to normal, despite overt and congestive heart failure.

Laboratory. Laboratory and EKG lack specificity and may be normal.

Metabolic Aspect. Thiamine deficiency blocks carbohydrate utilization. Myocardial extraction of lactate and pyruvate is reduced leading to an elevation of these substances in the arterial blood.

Hemodynamic Changes. The cardiac output in beriberi is usually increased. There is peripheral vasodilatation with decreased peripheral resistance. This change may be the primary one due to the altered peripheral metabolism. Later, with the development of congestive failure the skin vessels become constricted and pallor replaces the flushed appearance.

Experimental studies in thiamine-depleted rats showed a decreased myocardial contractility, which after three weeks responded to thiamine, but later was unresponsive. There was also a decreased vascular responsiveness to vasopressor drugs (Methoxamine). There is marked increase in skeletal muscle blood flow, hepatic and splenic blood flow. Renal blood flow is decreased. There is sodium retention and increased blood and plasma volume.

Pathology. Dilatation and hypertrophy of the heart is noted grossly. Nonspecific swelling, fatty degeneration and fragmentation of fibers are seen microscopically, especially in subendocardial layers. Mural thrombi in the ventricles have been noted.

Treatment and Progress. Thiamine replacement in the diet is the specific treatment for beriberi. Improvement in hemodynamic response may occur within an hour of parenteral administration of thiamine, and signs of congestive heart failure may clear within a week following diuresis.

Digitalis is usually given concomitantly. Its effects are difficult to assess but no harmful effect has been described. The protracted use of alcohol may lead to irreversible alteration in structure and progressive difficulty in treatment.

References

Aalsmeer, W. C., and Wenkeback, K. F.: Herz und kreislauf bei der Beriberi-Krankheit. Wien, Arch. Int. Med., *16*:193, 1929.

Akberian, M., Youkopoaloas, N. A. and Abelmann, W. H.: Hemodynamic studies in beriberi heart disease. Am. J. Med., *41*:197, 1966.

Blacket, R. B. and Palmer, A. J.: Hemodynamic studies in high output beriberi. Brit. Heart J., *22*:483, 1960.

Keefer, C. S.: The beriberi heart. Arch. Intern. Med., *45*:1, 1930.

6. Embolization from Hidden Mitral Stenosis

ORVILLE HORWITZ

Cause: Mitral stenosis without usual signs.

Early Manifestations: Those of arterial emboli.   Peripheral ischemia, visceral ischemia, or major or minor stroke.   No murmur.

Treatment: Embolectomy or prophylaxis (below).

Possible Dire Consequences without Treatment: Various degrees of peripheral ischemia, visceral ischemia, and stroke.

Mitral stenosis should always be suspected following embolus or following unexplained acute arterial occlusion especially in younger patients with or without atrial fibrillation.

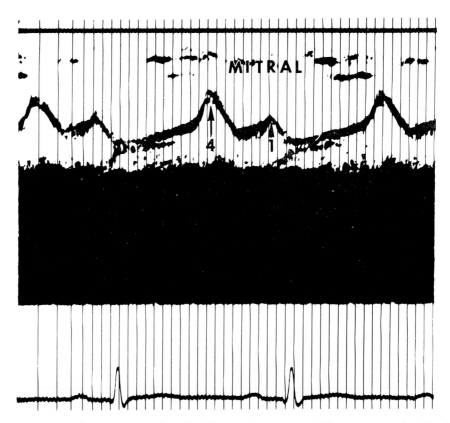

Fig. XV–1.   The normal anterior mitral leaflet echo pattern.   Movement anteriorly in the chest is represented by movement toward the top of the figure, and movement posteriorly is recorded as movement toward the bottom of the record.   (Joyner, C. R. *et al.*: Amer. J. Cardiol., *19*:66, 1967.)

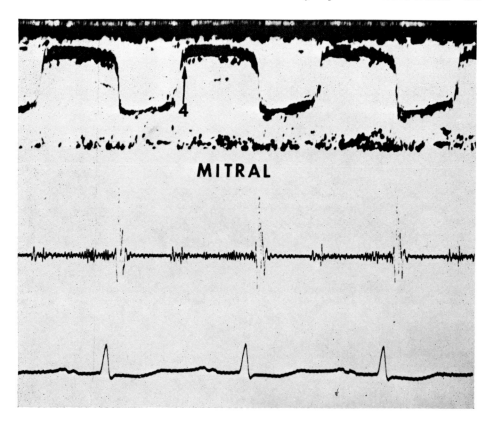

Fig. XV–2. Ultrasound pattern of the mitral valve in the presence of mitral stenosis. The descent from Peak 4 is delayed as the anterior leaflet is maintained in an open position in the left ventricle during all of diastole. (Joyner, C. R. *et al.*: Amer. J. Cardiol., *19*:66, 1967.)

The classical signs including an apical diastolic murmur may be absent. Under these circumstances ultrasound may be helpful diagnostically.

Cardiac catheterization is also helpful.

Once the diagnosis of mitral stenosis is established, decision as to the proper therapeutic or prophylactic procedure can be considered. Presently the thought is that surgery should be considered only if congestive failure and/or atrial enlargement are prominent. Otherwise long-term anticoagulant therapy has been expedient in conspicuously reducing the incidence of arterial embolization.

References

Bannister, R. B.: The risks of deferring valvulotomy in patients with moderate mitral stenosis. Lancet, 2:329, 1960.

Joyner, C. R.: Experience with ultrasound in the study of heart disease and the production of intracardiac sound. *In* Diagnostic Ultrasound, Grossman, C. C. *et al.* (Eds.), New York, Plenum Press, 1966.

7. Hidden Mitral Stenosis Resulting in Atrial Fibrillation and Congestive Failure

Hadley Conn, Jr.

Cause: Rheumatic fever.

Early Manifestations: Congestive failure and/or emboli.

Treatment: Treatment of congestive failure. Mitral valve surgery.

Possible Dire Consequences without Treatment: Deeper congestive failure, peripheral emboli, death.

One of the often unsuspected causes of atrial fibrillation and of congestive heart failure in individuals over fifty years of age is rheumatic mitral stenosis. In one review covering a ten-year period of the Hospital of the University of Pennsylvania, 13 such cases were identified. The problems complicating the diagnosis seem to be (a) onset of atrial fibrillation with disappearance of the pre-systolic apical murmur, (b) reduction in cardiac output so that intensity of mitral murmurs is diminished, (c) increased chest dimensions, particularly in older males, which reduces intensity of all cardiac sounds and murmurs, (d) a modest degree of left atrial enlargement and changing cardiac-pulmonary anatomic relationships with increasing age which tend to minimize some of the QRS axis shifts and P wave notching considered to be characteristic electrocardiographic changes, (e) failure to take oblique views (left lateral) in the chest roentgenogram, following a barium swallow, designed to show left atrial size; failure to use image intensification fluoroscopy which is the best tool for identifying calcium deposits in the mitral valve.

In any case in which the etiologic diagnosis is obscure in the presence of atrial fibrillation and/or congestive heart failure, a few diagnostic measures should be taken. Even the most complex of these should be available at most community hospitals. First, the physician should auscult the area of the cardiac apex immediately after the patient has exercised and then assumed the left lateral recumbent position. Many previously unheard or minimally detected diastolic bruits become grade $\frac{2}{6}$ or $\frac{3}{6}$ in intensity as a consequence of increased cardiac output. Second, image intensification fluoroscopic examination followed by PA, lateral, and oblique chest roentgenograms taken during and after barium swallow should be routine. Third, the mitral valve should be studied by echocardiography. Echocardiograph findings, if appropriate, are diagnostic. The echocardiogram is obtained by a non-invasive, simple technique and can easily be repeated. It is this last technique which has made possible the accurate diagnosis of mitral stenosis, once the defect is suspected, on the outpatient, non-invasive basis. Even the degree of stenosis, mobility of the valve, and involvement of the chorda tendinae can be semi-quantitated so that it is possible to select out pre-operatively with considerable accuracy not only those patients who may benefit from operation, but also one group of patients who will require a valve prosthetic replacement rather than some form of valvuloplasty.

In summary, unsuspected mitral stenosis is a lesser but still surprisingly frequent cause of heart failure, atrial arrhythmia or peripheral arterial emboli in older age. It has special complications, and is susceptible to surgical correction. Therefore it is important that this diagnosis always be among those considered in such patients presenting with heart failure and/or arrhythmia. If an uncertainty exists after initial examination, appropriate radiographic studies and echocardiography are mandatory. Reliable and accurate diagnosis can be made with these non-invasive methods. Long-term follow-up of operative results generally supports the view that valve correction in selected cases should not be importantly influenced by the advanced age of the patient.

References

Bannister, R. B.: The risks of deferring valvulotomy in patients with moderate mitral stenosis. Lancet, 2:329, 1960.

Joyner, C. R.: Experience with ultrasound in the study of heart disease and the production of intracardiac sound. *In* Diagnostic Ultrasound, Grossman, C. C. *et al.* (Eds.), New York, Plenum Press, 1966.

Joyner, C. R.: Diagnostic ultrasound, p. 1654. *In* Cardiac and Vascular Diseases, Conn, H. L., Jr. and Horwitz, O. (Eds.), Philadelphia, Lea & Febiger, 1971.

8. Digitalis Toxicity

Peter Binnion

Cause: Digitalis preparations especially in conjunction with strong diuretics.

Early Manifestations: Premature ventricular contractions, bigeminy paroxysmal atrial tachycardia.

Treatment: Stop digitalis and correct electrolyte imbalance.

Possible Dire Consequences without Treatment: Atrioventricular block, ventricular tachycardia, ventricular fibrillation and death.

An idea of the effect of digitalis glycosides can be obtained from simple bedside observations such as the presence of well-known side effects or slowing of the ventricular rate in atrial fibrillation and more recently by measuring the duration of the rate-connected left ventricular ejection time before and after giving digitalis to the patient.

Digitalis can be measured in the laboratory by a variety of techniques but until recently these were of insufficient sensitivity to permit measurement of plasma digoxin levels (the variety of available tests is given in Table XV–1). The most common one today is radioimmunoassay system in which radioactive labeled digoxin competes with unlabeled digoxin in the patient's plasma for antibody binding sites. Other useful modern methods are based on the inhibition of labeled rubidium uptake by

TABLE XV–1.   ESTIMATION OF DIGITALIS

Biological Effect on Man
Withering (1785)—side effects in man
Gold (1929)—blocking effects of digitalis in atrial fibrillation
Acetyl strophanthidin test; titrate additional glycoside until 3 ventricular extrasystoles
  occur together

Chemical
a.	reaction of sugar moiety of the glycoside	
b.	based on chemistry of the lactone ring	
c.	reactions of steroid nucleus and the best one is a fluorimetric method (16 ng)	
	i) paper	(500 mg.)
	ii) thin-layer	(100 ng.)
	iii) gas	(1 ng.)

Biological
Embryo duck heart assay of Friedman	(5 ng.)
Embryonic chick heart	(12000 ng.)
Papillary muscle preparation	(10 ng.)

Enzymatic methods
Inhibition of ATPase	(12 ng.)
Enzymatic isotopic displacement	(0.5 ng.)

Radiochemical
Radioimmunoassay	(0.1 ng.)
Double isotopic dilution technique	(10 ng.)
^{86}Rb uptake by red cells	(0.1 ng.)
	(approx. sensitivity of system in brackets)

---

red cells in the presence of digoxin or the displacement of tritiated ouabain from the enzyme, ATPase, by digitalis glycosides.   All the last three methods are suitable for chemical laboratory use and the one employed depends on how rapidly a result has to be produced and whether all forms of digitalis glycosides have to be measured simultaneously or just digoxin.

Method.   The method of assay in commonest use is the radiommunoassay.   Tritiated digoxin, added *in vitro*, competes with the unlabeled digoxin in the patient's plasma for digoxin-specific antibodies (Schwartz-Mann, Orangeburg, N.Y.).   A calibration curve has to be prepared for each daily batch of patient plasmas which are to be processed using plasma to which known amounts of digoxin have been added.   Tritium is counted in a liquid scintillation counter with quench correction by the channels ratio method from a previously prepared quench correction curve. From the calibration curve (Fig. XV–3) the digoxin in any patient's plasma can be measured and duplicate estimations agree extremely well; the method takes approximately two hours from start to final graphing of the calibration curve and analysis of the first few patients' samples.   As about 16 calibration mixtures are needed for an accurate curve, the method is relatively inefficient when only one sample a day is to be processed.   In our laboratory blood drawn from patients into heparinized tubes before breakfast (and the morning digoxin dose) is analyzed in the afternoon and the results reported by 5 P.M. on the same day.

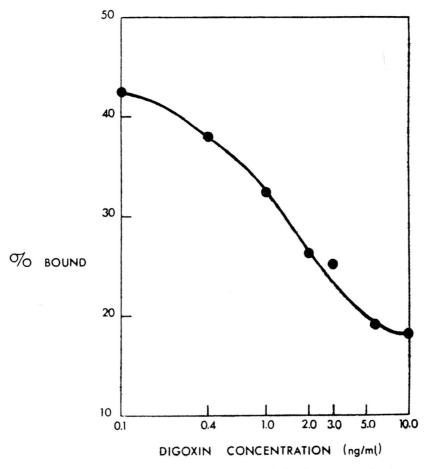

Fig. XV–3.   Calibration curve for measurement of digoxin concentration in plasma using the radioimmunoassay method.

Clinical Studies.   The presence of digitalis intoxication has been assessed electro-cardiographically and most studies to date are based on the ECG criteria given below:

(*a.*) Supraventricular tachycardia with atrioventricular block.

(*b.*) Frequent or multifocal premature ventricular beats, ventricular bigeminy or ventricular tachycardia.

(*c.*) Sinus rhythm with second or third degree atrioventricular block.

(*d.*) Atrial fibrillation with ventricular response less than 50/min. and premature ventricular beats.   These criteria have been extended by certain workers to include other ECG abnormalities.

(*e.*) First degree heart block.

(*f.*) Nodal premature contractions.

Many of these ECG changes have been considered specific for digitalis overdosage on clinical grounds, the most common one being abolition or marked improvement of the above changes following withdrawal of digitalis (with or without other forms of therapy).

The most radical suggestion is that practically every known cardiac arrhythmia and/or conduction disturbance can be due to digitalis but, of course, this applies to

TABLE XV–2.   OVERDOSE OF DIGITALIS IN HEALTHY PERSONS

Supraventricular tachycardia with second degree atrioventricular block
Sino-atrial block
First degree A–V block
Atrioventricular dissociation leading to asystolic arrest and death
Atrioventricular dissociation leading to ventricular fibrillation and recovery
Atrioventricular dissociation with atrial fibrillation

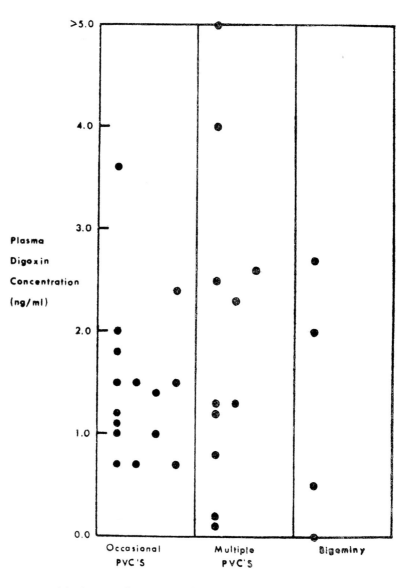

Fig. XV–4.   Plasma digoxin concentration in patients with
various ventricular arrhythmias.

cardiac disease in general. However, in healthy people taking an overdose of digoxin the ECG disorders produced tend to be different, especially with regard to ectopic rhythms (Table XV–2).

Using these clinical and ECG criteria for digitalis overdosage, a number of studies have been done relating the serum or plasma digitalis concentrations to the incidence of these disorders. In two series the nontoxic patients had a mean level of 1.1 ng./ml. and 1.4 ng./ml. respectively, and toxic patients had an average level of 3.3 and 3.4 ng./ml., though there was overlap in individual patients. The implications are that a high plasma digoxin level is associated frequently with a so-called digitalis-induced arrhythmia.

However, if one takes the approach that previous electrocardiographic work on these arrhythmias is not completely accurate in that it represents a clinical impression, and that true digitalis-produced disorders should be associated with high plasma digitalis levels, then the picture becomes more confused. So far we have been unable to associate plasma digoxin levels with specific ECG disorders apart possibly from atrial tachycardia with block and even the classical ventricular dysrhythmias, including bigeminy, were not apparently related to high plasma levels (Fig. XV–4).

Conclusion. The problem of the relationship of plasma digoxin concentration to ECG abnormalities has not yet been solved in spite of some work to the contrary. The most logical reason for this is that many factors, other than plasma digoxin concentration, are related to the induction of arrhythmias such as the basic cardiac lesion and its site, the cell membrane potassium gradient and the state of the membrane ATPase enzyme system which is probably sensitive to many changes in the blood. It is not surprising that a clearcut association between arrhythmias and plasma digoxin concentrations has not really been demonstrated yet. However, measurement of plasma glycoside concentration is an essential requirement for logical and safe digitalis administration, and allows use of this drug in therapy where the arrhythmia would superficially contraindicate its use.

References

Asplund, J. *et al.*: Four cases of massive digitalis poisoning. Acta Med. Scand., *189*:293, 1971.

Binnion, P. F.: The plasma-digoxin controversy. Lancet, *1*:535, 1972.

Binnion, P. F. *et al.*: Plasma and myocardial digoxin concentrations in patients on oral therapy. Brit. Heart J., *31*:636, 1969.

Brooker, G. and Jelliffe, R. W.: Serum cardiac glycoside assay based upon displacement of 3H-ouabain from Na-K ATPase. Circulation, *45*:20, 1972.

Chung, E. K.: Digitalis Intoxication. Baltimore, The Williams & Wilkins Co., 1969.

Evered, D. C. and Chapman, C.: Plasma digoxin concentrations and digoxin toxicity in hospital patients. Brit. Heart J., *33*:540, 1971.

Fisch, C. and Knoebel, S. B.: Recognition and therapy of digitalis toxicity. Prog. Cardiovasc. Dis., *13*:71, 1970.

Gold, H. *et al.*: Behavior of synthetic esters of strophanthidin, the acetate, proprionate, butyrate, and benzoate, in man. J. Pharmacol. Exptl. Therap., *86*:301, 1946.

Irons, G. V. and Orgain, E. S.: Digitalis-induced arrhythmias and their management. Prog. Cardiovasc. Dis., *8*:539, 1966.

Lowenstein, J. M. and Corrill, E. M.: An improved method for measuring plasma and tissue concentration of digitalis glycosides. J. Lab. Clin. Med., *67*:1048, 1966.

Rodensky, P. L. and Wasserman, F.: Observations on digitalis intoxication. Arch. Int. Med., *108*:61, 1961.

Smith, T. W. and Haber, E.: Digoxin intoxication: the relationship of clinical presentation to serum digoxin concentration, J. Clin. Invest., *49*:2377, 1970.

Smith, T. W. and Wilkerson, J. T.: Suicidal and accidental digoxin ingestion. Circulation, *44*:29, 1971.

Smith, T. W., Butler, V. P. and Haber, E.: Determination of therapeutic and toxic serum digoxin concentration by radioimmunoassay. New Eng. J. Med., *287*:1212, 1969.

Weissler, A. M. *et al.*: The effect of digitalis on ventricular ejection in normal human subjects. Circulation, *29*:721, 1964.

Withering, W.: An Account of the Foxglove and Some of its Medical Uses with Practical Remarks on Dropsy and Other Diseases. London, G. G. J. & J. Robinson, 1785.

Introductory Remarks Concerning the Arrhythmias

CARDIAC ARRHYTHMIAS

A classification based on etiology is impractical, for identical rhythm disorders can result from widely varying causes. Most rhythm disorders result from disturbances of impulse formation and/or impulse conduction, and these are usually subdivided, when practicable, into anatomical subdivisions (atrial junctional, ventricular.)

DISTURBANCES OF IMPULSE FORMATION

The heart may be activated by a pacemaker other than the sinus node (ectopic beats or rhythms) which fall into two groups:

   (*a*.) Escape beats which occur when there is a pause in the dominant rhythm (originate in subsidiary cardiac pacemaker); a "passive" phenomenon.

   (*b*.) Extrasystoles and ectopic tachycardias are "active" phenomena; must be faster than sinus rate in the case of atrial ectopics but not otherwise. They arise in abnormal pacemaker tissue.

   (*c*.) Occasionally, ectopic focus discharges slowly but is protected from dominant pacemaker (parasystole).

DISTURBANCES OF IMPULSE CONDUCTION

Physiological

   i) AV node unable to conduct all impulses, *e.g.* in rapid atrial tachycardia.

   ii) Impulse blocked because it encounters tissue in a normal refractory phase.

   iii) Ectopic ventricular impulse entering AV node retrograde and blocks passage of next atrial impulse from sinus node (interference).

Pathological

   i) Anatomical lesion of some part of conduction pathways.

ECTOPICAL ATRIAL TACHYCARDIAS

They include atrial extrasystoles, atrial tachycardia (with or without AV block), atrial flutter and atrial fibrillation, and may occur in paroxysmal or chronic form. In most instances these are probably due to an ectopic focus in one of the internodal tracts (between SA and AV node). Although many authors consider these tachycardias are always due to rapidly discharging ectopic focus, more recent work suggests that many are due to re-entry mechanisms via the AV junction (atrial discharge travels down one part of junctional tissue and returns via another ascending pathway to discharge atria again) or within the atria themselves.

9. Escape Beats

PETER BINNION

Cause: When sinus node fails to produce impulse, heart protected from asystole by subsidiary pacemaker, usually in AV junction. When AV block suddenly occurs, idioventricular escape rhythm may occur. Common in sinus bradycardia, *e.g.* early phase of inferior wall myocardial infarction and also in the otherwise fit elderly patient with sinus bradycardia; variety of cardiac diseases treated with digitalis, *e.g.* atrial fibrillation when AV conduction depressed by digitalis.

Early Manifestations: Often none, sometimes thumping in chest, often anxiety.

Treatment: Speed up sinus rate with I.V. Atropine, 0.5 mg. or stop digitalis. No specific treatment for the escape beats themselves (suppressing them could be dangerous, resulting in asystole).

Possible Dire Consequences without Treatment: Usually none.

Reference

Stock, J. P.: Diagnosis and Treatment of Cardiac Arrhythmias. Escape beats and escape rhythms. Chap. 4. London, Butterworths, 1969.

10. Ventricular Premature Contractions

PETER BINNION

Cause: Damage to ventricular musculature but may be benign or sign of serious myocardial disease, and best guide to this is the clinical circumstances in which they occur. Acute myocardial infarction, cardiomyopathy, digitalis intoxication, myocardial ischemia due to coronary artery disease. Ventricular extrasystoles also caused by pregnancy, hypokalemia.

Early Manifestations: Dropped beat or extra beat felt at radial pulse; in bigeminy an extra beat follows each beat of the dominant rhythm; wide QRS complex often of considerable amplitude, premature occurrence and no preceding P wave. If ectopic beat has L.B.B.B. pattern most likely ventricular in origin (if R.B.B.B. pattern most likely supraventricular ectopic with aberrant conduction). May be multifocal in origin (must have different QRS contour and different coupling times to the initiating beat).

Treatment: If asymptomatic, no specific therapy but eliminate smoking, excessive coffee intake, ephedrine and epinephrine, thyroid hormone. If symptomatic or in presence of known cardiac disease, should try antiarrhythmic drugs:
1. Quinidine sulfate 200 to 300 mg. q. 4 h.; quinidine polygalacturonate tablets 1 to 2 B.I.D.
2. Procainamide 250 to 500 mg. q 4 h.
3. Lidocaine 50 to 100 mg. I.V. and 1 to 4 mg./min. IV drip.
4. Propranolol, usually orally, in dose up to 80 mg. T.I.D. when heart failure controlled and no bronchospasm present.
5. Diphenylhydantoin 400 to 1000 mg. IV over twenty-four hours during first day, then 100 mg. q. 6 h. orally.
6. Stop digitalis (if considered cause of the ventricular extrasystoles).

Possible Dire Consequences without Treatment: Usually none. May be preamble to ventricular tachycardia.

References

Bellet, S.: Clinical Disorder of the Heart Beat. Chap. 9. Philadelphia, Lea & Febiger, 1971.
Stock, J. P.: Diagnosis and Treatment of Cardiac Arrhythmias, London, Butterworths, 1969.
Yattean, R. F. and Wallace, A. G.: Clinical pharmacology of antiarrhythmic agents in acute myocardial infarction. *In* Progress in Cardiology. Chap. 4, p. 95. Yu and Goodwin, (Eds.), Philadelphia, Lea & Febiger, 1972.

11. Atrial Premature Contractions

PETER BINNION

Cause: An ectopic pacemaker in same part of the heart as the dominant pacemaker which is often prematurely discharged. May occur in normal heart; when frequent may herald atrial fibrillation, *e.g.* rheumatic mitral valve disease, acute myocardial infarction; common in association with chronic lung disease.

Early Manifestations: Usually none, but patient or physician may detect missed pulse beat. Electrocardiographically usually premature beat has normal QRS contour and is preceded by a P wave.

Treatment: If heart normal, careful reassurance, reduce excessive consumption of coffee, alcohol, tobacco; if great anxiety and introspection try propranolol 10 to 40 mg. Q.I.D. If propranolol ineffective try quinidine sulfate 200 to 300 mg. Q.I.D. or procainamide 500 mg. Q.I.D.; with heart disease treat underlying condition and they often disappear with digitalization.

Possible Dire Consequences without Treatment: Usually none.

Reference

Zipes, D. P. and McIntosh, H. D.: Cardiac Arrhythmias. Chap. 17, p. 301. *In* Cardiac and Vascular Disease. Conn, H. L., Jr. and Horwitz, O. (Eds.), Philadelphia, Lea & Febiger, 1971.

12. Junctional Premature Contractions

PETER BINNION

Cause: Usually secondary to effect of disease or drugs on AV junction, *e.g.* digitalis toxicity, myocarditis.

Early Manifestations: Occasional palpitation; dropped beats; either no visible P, or retrograde P wave after normal QRS complex; normal sequence of P waves and post-extrasystolic pause is usually compensatory, so that the normal sequence of P waves is not interfered with.

Treatment: Directed to the underlying clinical state.

Possible Dire Consequences without Treatment: Usually none.

Reference

Zipes, D. P. and McIntosh, H. D.: Cardiac Arrhythmias. Chap. 17, p. 301. *In* Cardiac and Vascular Disease. Conn, H. L., Jr. and Horwitz, O. (Eds.), Philadelphia, Lea & Febiger, 1971.

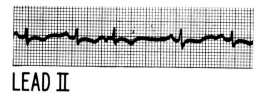

LEAD II

Fig. XV–5. Premature A–V junctional beat. The negative P wave preceding the third QRS complex suggests that the premature beat arose from a low atrial or A–V junctional focus and had slightly delayed antegrade conduction. The pause after the premature systole is only slightly longer than fully compensatory, suggesting that the sinus node was not discharged by retrograde conduction from the premature beat. It is also possible that the premature systole discharged the sinus node prematurely, suppressing and delaying the return cycle. (Conn and Horwitz, Cardiac and Vascular Diseases, Lea & Febiger.)

13. Parasystole

PETER BINNION

Cause: Independent ventricular pacemaker which is protected from dominant pacemaker. Third type of ectopic beat (in addition to escape beats and extrasystoles) usually from the ventricle (from an idioventricular pacemaker protected from discharge by entrance block).

Early Manifestations: Extra beat or dropped beat felt in arterial pulse. Diagnosed by ECG criteria:

(*a.*) As ectopic beat independent of dominant rhythm there is wide variation in coupling time to preceding beat.

(*b.*) Time interval between ectopic beats have nearly precise simple arithmetical relationship to each other.

(*c.*) Can cause fusion beat intermediate in contour between beat of dominant rhythm and parasystolic beat.

Possible Dire Consequences without Treatment: Usually none.

Reference

Stock, J. P.: Diagnosis and Treatment of Cardiac Arrhythmias Parasystole. London, Butterworths, 1969, p. 73 et seq.

14. The Wolff-Parkinson-White Syndrome

PETER BINNION

Cause: Usually no evidence of heart disease, but can appear for first time in acute rheumatic carditis, thyrotoxicosis and myocardial infarction. Sometimes seen in association with congenital heart disease. Due to accelerated conduction from atria to ventricles, most likely due to accessory conduction pathway by-passing the atrioventricular node.

Early Manifestations: Episodes of paroxysmal tachycardia; short (less than 0.12 sec.) PR interval and wide QRS complex (at least 0.12 sec.) with slurred upstroke (delta wave) on the electrocardiogram.   In one variant form the QRS appears normal, but patient still subject to ectopic tachycardia; ECG changes may be transient.   Signs are due to rate of tachycardia and state of myocardium *e.g.* palpitations, faintness, etc.

Treatment: Tachycardia is supraventricular in origin and patient should be informed of cause of disease and reassured if attacks infrequent (try breath-holding to abort an attack).   For drug therapy use oral quinidine, or better use propranolol 10 to 40 mg. T.I.D. or Q.I.D.).

If ectopic tachycardia persists, use direct current cardioversion.

If ectopic tachycardia resistant to drug treatment and symptoms are severe, then open heart surgery to transect accessory conducting pathway can be used. Also, fixed-rate atrial or ventricular pacemaker impulses may succeed in terminating the tachycardias.

Possible Dire Consequences without Treatment: Usually none.

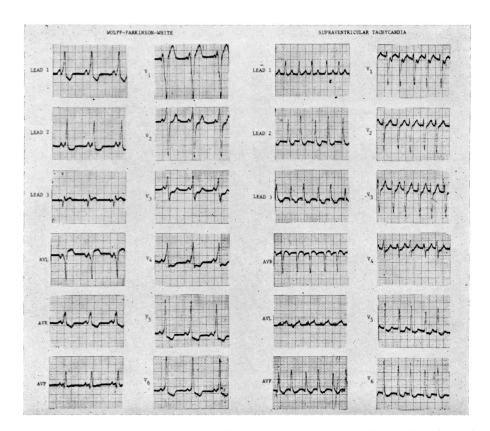

Fig. XV–6.   Pre-excitation syndrome.   During normal sinus rhythm, the short P–R interval, QRS prolongation, and secondary ST–T wave changes are seen.   The delta wave producing the QRS prolongation is negative in V_1, biphasic in V_2, and positive in V_{3-6} (type B).   A regular paroxysmal supraventricular tachycardia (probably A–V junctional) alternating between 158 and 176 beats/minute is seen in the 12 lead tracing to the right.   The slight change in the morphology, rate, and P–R interval (the latter seen best in V_1) of every other beat suggests alternating changes of conduction in the re-entrant pathway.   Note the absence of the delta wave during the tachycardia. (Coff, F. R., *et al.*: Circulation, *38*:1018, 1968.)

Reference

Conn, H. L., Jr. and Luchi, R. J.:   Cardiac structure, metabolism and mechanics, Chap. 13, p. 214.   *In* Cardiac and Vascular Diseases.   H. L. Conn and O. Horwitz (Eds.), Philadelphia, Lea & Febiger, 1971.

15. Ectopic Atrial Tachycardia– Atrial Fibrillation

PETER BINNION

Cause: Due to rapid depolarization of diseased atrium (450 to 600 times/min). Irregularity of slower ventricular response due to blocking by A–V junction where concealed conduction occurs.   Rheumatic, atherosclerotic or hypertensive heart disease; thyrotoxicosis, particularly in the older patient; may occur after acute myocardial infarction; after thoracic operations; constrictive pericarditis.   Rarely no heart disease is discovered.

Early Manifestations: Irregularly irregular pulse.   Second most common arrhythmia (after premature beats).   May be paroxysmal or chronic.   Palpitations or overt cardiac failure may occur (*e.g.* acute pulmonary edema in patient with mitral stenosis).

Treatment: 1. Initial treatment digitalis to control ventricular rate (oral digoxin 0.75 mg. stat, 0.5 mg. q. 6 h. until ventricular rate falls then 0.25 mg. O.D. or B.I.D. depending on age and renal function).
  2. If of recent onset direct current cardioversion; also electrical conversion useful after removal of cause (*e.g.* after mitral valvotomy in mitral stenosis).
  3. Before and after cardioversion give oral quinidine.
  4. When present with mitral valve disease, especially mitral stenosis, which is not treated surgically then long-term oral anticoagulant therapy necessary to reduce risk of arterial embolism.
  5. Can try chemical cardioversion with quinidine sulfate; 0.3 gm. q. 2 h. for twelve hours in absence of congestive heart failure or renal insufficiency until cardioversion occurs or toxic side-effects noted; maintenance dose 0.2 to 0.3 gm. Q.I.D.   Always give preliminary small dose to check for idiosyncrasy.
  6. If digitalis will not reduce ventricular rate to around 80/min. without toxic blood levels (over 2.0 ng. digoxin per ml.) can add propranolol 10 mg. Q.I.D.
  7. For paroxysmal atrial fibrillation use digoxin orally on maintenance dosage.

Possible Dire Consequences without Treatment: Congestive failure and/or myocardial ischemia.

References

Bellet, S.:   Clinical Disorders of the Heart Beat, 3rd Ed., Chap. 8, Atrial Fibrillation (clinical manifestations).   Philadelphia, Lea & Febiger, 1971.
Conn. H. L., Jr. and Horwitz, O.:   Cardiac Arrhythmias, Chap. 17.   *In* Cardiac and Vascular Diseases, Philadelphia, Lea & Febiger, 1971.

16. Ectopic Tachycardias— Junctional Tachycardia

Peter Binnion

Cause: In non-paroxysmal form probably increased automaticity of AV junction; the paroxysmal form may be due to A–V nodal re-entry. In both instances suppression of sinus automaticity may be initiating factor. Paroxysmal form often occurs in normal hearts but other causative factors are similar to those causing paroxysmal atrial tachycardia; nonparoxysmal type generally manifestation of organic heart disease (*e.g.* rheumatic and other forms of myocarditis, recent inferior wall myocardial infarction) and especially digitalis overdosage (in presence of hypokalemia).

Early Manifestations: Rate of 60 to 110/min. without abrupt onset or cessation is called nonparoxysmal junctional tachycardia to distinguish it from the paroxysmal form where rate is 140 to 220 beats/minute. Patient conscious of palpitations, and signs of cerebral or coronary insufficiency may occur; cannon waves in jugular venous pulse are common. On ECG the QRS complexes usually normal in duration with retrograde P wave visible in the ST segment.

Treatment: *Paroxysmal form:* Therapy of underlying cause as in any paroxysmal tachycardia.
Nonparoxysmal form: Stop digitalis (commonest cause—approximately 45% patients) and give oral potassium salts. Propranolol particularly efficacious if, when digitalis is withdrawn, a rapid atrial mechanism occurs. Treatment of other underlying causes.

Possible Dire Consequences without Treatment: Congestive failure.

Reference

Zipes, D. P. and McIntosh, H. D.: Cardiac Arrhythmias, Chap. 17, p. 301. *In* Cardiac and Vascular Diseases, H. L. Conn, Jr. and O Horwitz (Eds.). Philadelphia, Lea & Febiger, 1971.

19

17. Atrial Tachycardia

PETER BINNION

Cause: Ectopic pacemaker focus in atrium with rate of discharge faster than sinus rate; also can be due to reciprocating tachycardia (excitation wave, having reached the ventricles via the normal AV conduction pathways, returns to the atria via an accessory pathway to redischarge atria). Unknown, but in one series 34% had no heart disease, 34% had rheumatic heart disease, 14% had atherosclerotic heart disease, and in 18% it occured in association with other diseases (hypertension, thyrotoxicosis, etc.). Seen in digitalis intoxication in association with AV block.

Early Manifestations: Rapid heart action, often of abrupt onset and cessation with symptoms similar to those produced by any rapid ectopic rhythm which depend largely on the state of the heart muscle. Pulse rate rapid, regular and weak (rate 140 to 220 per minute); blood pressure may fall; angina or heart failure may be produced. Pulse rate usually halved by application of carotid sinus pressure.

Treatment: if brief and not distressing, reassurance only (plus trying holding breath for as long as possible or eyeball pressure when attack starts). When prolonged or associated with distressing symptoms (dyspnea, angina, syncope), try these methods of treating the acute attack in order:
1. Self imposed pressure on eyeballs or carotid area, Valsalva maneuver.
2. Edrophonium (tensilon) 10 mg. I.V.
3. Digoxin I.V. 0.5 to 1.0 mg.
4. Direct current cardioversion (if rhythm not due to digitalis toxicity).
5. Quinidine sulfate or procainamide may be used orally when treatment is not urgent.
6. Propranolol is particularly effective for preventing attacks which are provoked by exertion or emotion.
7. When the tachycardia is associated with the Wolff-Parkinson-White syndrome, oral propranolol 40 mg. T.I.D. (or more) is the treatment of choice.
8. Sometimes when the systemic pressure is reduced by the tachycardia an intravenous infusion of phenylephrine will increase the blood pressure and often abolish the attack.
9. In the presence of acute myocardial infarction atrial tachycardia is probably best treated by direct current shock.

In rare instances where none of the above work a fixed rate cardiac pacemaker will stop the tachycardia (when due to re-entry through the AV node, *i.e.*, impulse goes from atrium through AV node and back retrograde through AV node temporarily). Rarely intra-atrial pacing at rapid rate to produce atrial fibrillation and then digoxin therapy will produce a good result. Between attacks prophylaxis of paroxysmal atrial tachycardia is done with digitalis, preferably digoxin. Quinidine can be used, either alone or with digoxin (the latter is preferable). Propranolol may be the best prophylactic therapy of all. When the rhythm is associated with AV block, digitalis therapy should be stopped.

Possible Dire Consequences without Treatment: Congestive failure, death.

References

Stock, J. P.: Diagnosis and Treatment of Cardiac Arrhythmias. London, Butterworth, 1969.

Bellet, S.: Clinical Disorders of the Heart Beat, Chap. 10. Paroxysmal Atrial Tachycardia, Philadelphia, Lea & Febiger, 1971.

Bigger, J. T. and Goldreyer, B. N.: The mechanism of supraventricular tachycardia. Circulation, *42*:673, 1970.

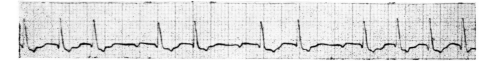

Fig. XV–7. Atrial tachycardia with A–V block. Monitor lead. Carotid sinus stimulation after the third QRS complex produced Mobitz type I (Wenckebach) second-degree A–V block with a 3:2 conduction ratio. Note the P–R prolongation in the complex preceding the nonconducted P wave. The P–P intervals vary slightly, but the rate of atrial discharge (158 beats/minute) does not slow during carotid sinus massage. (Conn and Horwitz, Cardiac and Vascular Diseases, Lea & Febiger.)

18. Ectopic Tachycardias– Ventricular Tachycardia

Peter Binnion

Cause: Either an ectopic focus in ventricle going at a rapid rate or re-entry phenomenon due to inhomogeneity of ventricular tissue. In 12 to 15% no serious heart disease present. Commonest cause is coronary artery disease (71 to 74%); about 8% seen in rheumatic heart disease. It commonly occurs transiently during cardiac catheterization. Up to 60% of patients with recent myocardial infarction have ventricular tachycardia at some time during their illness. Occasionally may be precipitated by digitalis therapy.

Early Manifestations: May be paroxysmal or sustained; may be almost symptomless but often can cause cardiogenic shock or angina; jugular venous 'a' wave less rapid than ventricular rate; in half there is changing intensity of first heart sound; not influenced by carotid sinus pressure. Wide QRS complexes (over 0.12 sec) with T wave written in opposite direction.

Treatment: *During attacks:* Depending on patient's condition use either direct current cardioversion or lidocaine therapy. Lidocaine 50 to 100 mg. I.V. bolus, then I.V. drip of 1 to 4 mg./min., or quinidine or procainamide I.M. Sometimes propranolol works well. If no response to drugs, use blow to chest (but can produce ventricular fibrillation so only use when patient in extremis and no cardioversion equipment available).
  To prevent attacks: Avoid known precipitating factor (exercise, emotion, etc.). Oral quinidine or procainamide, oral propranolol can be used.

Possible Dire Consequences without Treatment: Ventricular fibrillation, death.

Reference

Bellet, S.: Clinical Disorders of the Heart Beat, Chapter 15, Paroxysmal Ventricular Tachycardia, Philadelphia, Lea & Febiger, 1971.

19. Ventricular Flutter and Fibrillation

PETER BINNION

Cause: Irritable ventricular foci discharging in partially or completely incoordinate fashion. Ventricular fibrillation is most common in ischemic heart disease especially myocardial infarction where it probably causes the majority of deaths; other causes are digitalis toxicity, electric shock and lightning; during emergency conditions seen with chloroform anesthesia and epinephrine; may occur in complete heart block in paroxysmal form (also in children as familial condition associated with greatly prolonged Q–T interval). Hypoxia due to different causes appears to be a precipitating factor quite frequently. Open heart surgery.

Early Manifestations: Large, rapid fluctuations in ECG voltage without discernible separate QRS complexes is called ventricular flutter while in ventricular fibrillation there is no coordinated mechanical contraction of ventricles, *i.e.* cardiac arrest. No palpable pulse, no heart sounds, blood pressure unobtainable, pupils small if of recent onset or patient given morphine previously, dilated pupils if cardiac arrest has lasted over about one to two minutes. Ventricular flutter can cause Stokes-Adams attacks in patients with complete heart block.

Treatment: Prophylaxis: Treatment of premature ventricular beats and ventricular tachycardia. Removal of hypoxic stimulus. Prevent toxic drug reactions and electrolyte imbalance. *Active Therapy:* Treat cardiac arrest with artificial ventilation and external cardiac message until direct current cardioversion possible. Occasionally external blow to precordium will work. During external cardiac massage give intravenous sodium bicarbonate (to treat metabolic acidosis), and after cardioversion use lidocaine drip.

Possible Dire Consequences without Treatment: Death.

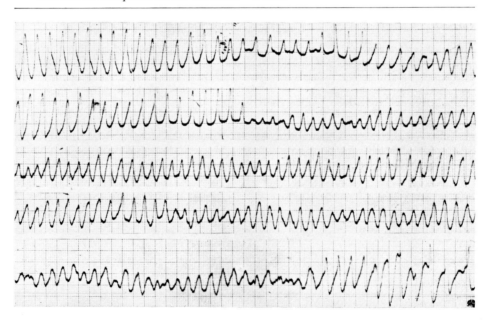

Fig. XV–8. Ventricular tachycardia, flutter, fibrillation. A continuous tracing demonstrates ventricular tachycardia deteriorating into ventricular flutter (middle tracings) and ventricular fibrillation (lower tracing). (Conn and Horwitz, Cardiac and Vascular Diseases, Lea & Febiger.)

Reference

Bellet, S.: Ventricular flutter and fibrillation, Chapter 16. Clinical Disorders of the Heart Beat, 3rd Ed., Philadelphia, Lea & Febiger, 1971.

20. Ventricular Asystole

Peter Binnion

Cause: No synchronized depolarization of heart muscle due to severe muscle damage or absence of a subsidiary pacemaker. Often follows untreated ventricular fibrillation due to myocardial infarction; sudden onset of complete heart block (Stokes-Adams attack); end phase of severe muscle damage in acute myocardial infarction, end stage of many severe electrolyte and acidotic disorders; failure of a pacemaker (*e.g.* forgetting to replace batteries).

Early Manifestations: Cardiac arrest with similar clinical picture to ventricular fibrillation.

Treatment: *External cardiac massage* and *artificial ventilation is first* essential before methods used below (usually five chest compressions to one breath in mouth-to-mouth technique). If due to *complete heart block* need to increase ventricular response so give Isoproterenol drip (1 to 2 mg. in 250 ml. 5% dextrose solution) and titrate to produce satisfactory ventricular rate.

As soon as possible insert right ventricular demand pacemaker; if due to battery failure of implanted pacemaker put in new pacemaker battery pack.

If due to *acute myocardial infarction:* Give 1 ml. 1:1000 epinephrine solution IV and commence external cardiac compression; if ventricular fibrillation produced, as one hopes, then defibrillate with direct current (non-synchronized) cardioverter. If no response repeat and set up isoproterenol drip to try and produce ventricular fibrillation; the last desperate measure is to give intracardiac epinephrine (long needle via sub-xiphoid approach).

If due to severe systemic disease producing acidosis, try to reverse situation (*e.g.* artificial ventilation) while proceeding as above.

If due to hyperkalemia give 50 gm. glucose, 10 units regular insulin and sodium bicarbonate, IV; repeat as needed, while proceeding as above; when improved can try oral ion exchange resins.

Possible Dire Consequences without Treatment: Death.

Reference

Bilitch, M.: Manual of Cardial Arrhythmias. Chapter 6. Cardiac Arrest, Mechanisms and Management, Boston, Little, Brown and Co., 1971.

21. Congestive Heart Failure—Unusual Manifestations

FRANK S. HARRISON, JR.

Cause: Myocardial and/or valvular disease.

Early Manifestations: Confusion, restlessness, apprehension, depression, weakness, apathy, cough on exertion or on assuming supine position, trepopnea, hoarseness, atrial fibrillation, diaphoresis, unstable anginal pattern, anorexia, weight change.

Treatment: Bed rest, digitalis, diuretics.

Possible Dire Consequences without Treatment: More severe failure, death.

Congestive heart failure can be a subtle, difficult diagnosis. The patient may manifest virtually none of the expected signs and symptoms so frequently encountered in clinical practice. Early indicators of cardiac dysfunction may be missed and therapy, therefore, withheld. Long-standing complaints, especially in the elderly, not recognized as associated with chronic congestive failure, may be disregarded by even the most concerned physician. Atypical clinical and roengtenographic signs may guide the clinician to inappropriate diagnostic study and therapy.

Obtaining a history from an irritable elderly patient is a frequent and often difficult chore. What may not be appreciated is that impairment of cardiac output may masquerade as a primary central nervous system disturbance. Confusion, restlessness, dizziness, insomnia, Cheyne-Stokes respirations, and even coma may be principally manifestations of cardiac dysfunction. Emotional disorder, such as severe apprehension, or depression, may dominate the scene. Psychotic behavior may occur. Central nervous system symptoms are, of course, influenced by the degree of cerebral vascular disease and drug effects.

Weakness, apathy, and fatigue may be a clue to the myocardial insufficiency. A weary patient with poor exercise tolerance may limit exertion and not readily admit to dyspnea. Cardiac fatigue has been an especially prominent feature of severe mitral and pulmonic valvular stenosis.

Cough is more commonly associated with pulmonary disease. However, this symptom may be the sole manifestation of congestive heart failure. Usually dry and irritating, the cough may occur on exertion or assuming the supine position. The chronic bronchitis of the elderly is often in reality congestive heart failure. Wheezing may likewise be misinterpreted as related to primary pulmonary disease. Marked airway resistance responsive to bronchodilaters may be recurrent for months before cardiac genesis is suspected. Most commonly associated with hypertension, coronary disease, or aortic valvular disease, cardiac asthma tends to occur after one to two hours of recumbency. Orthopnea noted in one recumbent position and not another has been observed. Termed trepopnea, this unusual complaint should indicate congestive heart failure to the examiner. Hoarseness, likely related to distended pulmonary vessels affecting the recurrent laryngeal nerve, has also been described with congestive heart failure.

In addition to clinical pulmonary symptoms, knowledge of atypical roentgeno-graphic features of congestive heart failure gives the physician a useful lead to the resolution of diagnostic problems. Logue and associates reviewed 114 cases of pulmonary edema. Twenty-five per cent of these cases were diagnosed by the radiologist being unsuspected clinically. Rosenau and Harrison demonstrated numerous cases of congestive failure mimicking primary pulmonary conditions, such as neoplasm and pneumonitis. Roentgen changes depend on duration, location, and distribution of edema. Increased heart size, although a frequent finding in congestive heart failure, need not be present.

Ventricular decompensation increases sympathetic activity and at times subsequent diaphoresis. A frequent finding in infants with congestive failure, adults may mention unexplained perspiration as a subtle clue to this diagnosis, as well. Extrasystoles and atrial fibrillation may prompt complaints of palpitation. Either of these arrhythmias may be caused by ventricular decompensation, and should receive therapeutic attention. On occasion, patients complain of forceful beating of the heart with the onset of congestive failure. Tricuspid regurgitation may produce a throbbing sensation in the neck. An unstable anginal pattern, especially with increased episodes at rest, should indicate a concern for congestive failure. Pulsus alternans is a reliable clinical observation favoring this diagnosis. An abnormal cardiovascular response to the Valsalva maneuver has also been described.

Gastrointestinal complaints have a wide range and can easily be misinterpreted. Right upper quadrant tenderness, sometimes exertional, occurs commonly with hepatic congestion. Hyperbilirubinemia, liver enzyme abnormalities, and increased BSP retention, are other indications of hepatic dysfunction, possibly misinterpreted as relating to primary liver disease. Anorexia, nausea, vomiting, and the sense of abdominal fullness may occur. Inactivity is a contributing factor to the common complaint of constipation. Weight loss, hypoproteinemia, and at times hypoglycemia, are features of cardiac cachexia. Patients may needlessly be subjected to multiple diagnostic tests for a neoplastic disease when improvement in myocardial function is their critical need. Rarely, cardiac failure may contribute to mesenteric insufficiency with resulting abdominal pain, vomiting, fever, and bloody diarrhea. Severe mesenteric venous engorgement with edematous bowel and patent mesenteric arteries are the usual anatomic findings. Dysphagia, associated with a distended pulmonary vein, has been reported in recent radiologic literature.

Congestive failure may also first manifest itself by an unexplained increase in weight, signifying fluid accumulation.

In conclusion, the heart on occasion gives few and only subtle signs of failing to function as a pump. Awareness of the unusual or obscure indicators of congestive heart failure is the responsibility of all clinicians.

References

Berkowitz, B., Croll, M. N. and Likoff, W.: Malabsorption as a complication of congestive heart failure. Am. J. Cardiol., *11*:43, 1963.
Conn, H. L. and Horwitz, O.: Cardiac and Vascular Diseases, Philadelphia, Lea & Febiger, 1971.
Friedberg, C. K.: Disease of the Heart, Philadelphia, W. B. Saunders Co., 1966.
Hurst, J. W. and Logue, R. B.: The Heart. New York, McGraw-Hill Book Co., 1970.
Jacobs, R. C. and Gershengorn, K., and Chait, A.: Dysphagia associated with a distended pulmonary vein. Brit. J. Radiol., *45*:225, 1972.

Logue, R. B. and Robinson, P. H.: Differential diagnosis of congestive heart failure. J. Prog. Cardiovasc. Dis., *12*:55, 1970.

Logue, R. B., Rogers, J. V. and Gay, B. B.: Subtle roentgenographic signs of left heart failure. Am. Heart J., *65*:464, 1963.

Losowsky, M. S., Ikram, H., and Snow, H. M.: Liver function in advanced heart disease. Brit. Heart J., *27*:578, 1965.

Rosenau, E. C. and Harrison, E. C.: Congestive heart failure masquerading as primary pulmonary disease. Chest, *58*:28, 1970.

Stapleton, J. F.: Cardiac failure incognito. G. P., *28*:78, 1963.

Wood, F. C. and Wolferth, C. C.: The tolerance of certain cardiac patients for various recumbent positions (trepopnea). Am. J. Med. Sci., *193*:354, 1937.

22. Heart Block

WAYNE W. KELLER

Cause: Damage to AV or intraventricular conduction system.

Early Manifestations: Bradycardia, prolonged P–R interval, widened QRS complex.

Treatment: Atropine, Isoproterenol, pacemaker, digitalis.

Possible Dire Consequences without Treatment: Stokes-Adams attack, death.

The development of intracardiac recordings, specifically His bundle electrocardiography, has added much information about the various types of heart block, their relative significance, and their early manifestations. From this understanding has come clearer indications for specific treatment and its timing.

First degree heart block is defined arbitrarily, as prolongation of the P–R interval greater than 0.20 seconds. Such lengthening occurs as a normal aging phenomenon to some degree. It may result from delay in conduction through the atria, AV node or infranodal (but supraventricular) conduction system. Prolonged intra-atrial conduction is characterized by a broad, prolonged P wave. The most common site of delay in first degree block is the AV node itself and is generally associated with a normal P wave and QRS complex. Prolongation of the infranodal conduction time (His bundle to Ventricle, H–V) usually occurs in the presence of diffuse myocardial and conduction system disease, and a widened, abnormal QRS complex is generally seen. When the block is in this latter area, the P–R interval rarely exceeds 0.28 seconds in duration. While first degree block has little risk, causative factors such as digitalis or quinidine excess or increased vagal tone should be sought. Conduction delay of the infranodal variety, especially when associated with a widened QRS suggests diffuse, organic involvement and should alert the physician to seek other areas of myocardial difficulty.

Second degree heart block or intermittent AV conduction is generally classified into two types according to the anatomic area of block. Mobitz Type I, or the Wenckebach phenomenon is a progressive lengthening of the P–R interval followed by a transient loss of AV conduction. This block has been shown to occur between the atria and the His bundle (A–H interval) and infranodal and intraventricular conduction are generally normal. The area of block is vagally innervated; hence, increased vagal tone frequently contributes to the production of Mobitz Type I block. Digitalis, by its known effect on AV conduction and vagal tone, can produce or worsen this abnormality. Type I block occurs frequently with acute inferior myocardial infarction, in part because of the common blood supply of the AV node and inferior wall by the right coronary artery.

For several reasons, Mobitz Type I second degree block frequently requires treatment. Repetitive episodes can result in a slow, ineffective heart rate and resultant poor perfusion. Also the block may progress from transient to complete block at the level of the AV node with loss of an adequate cardiac output. Atropine (0.3 to 1.0 mg. IV or IM) generally will eliminate this kind of block by removal of vagal suppression of the AV node. Oral anticholinergics, such as Probanthine 15 mg. Q.I.D. are generally less effective but may be a significant aid. The chronotropic effect of isoproterenol IV or sublingually may reverse the Wenckebach phenomenon but side effects of ventricular irritability limit its use.

Atropine occasionally is not effective or produces disabling side effects (dry mouth, urinary retention, GI atony, etc.) . Then the risks and difficulties of ventricular pacing must be balanced against the severity of the block. If the effective heart rate is slow, perfusion poor and pacemaking easily and efficiently available, it should be instituted. If the episodes are infrequent and without hemodynamic significance, the patient may be safely observed without therapy but frequent checks for progression of the block must be made.

Mobitz Type II block, the second type of second degree block, is characterized by a sudden failure of AV conduction and has a more ominous significance. As the block occurs in the infranodal region (H–V), rather than in the AV node, preceding H–V conduction is prolonged but there is no progressive P–R lengthening. This block can produce a slow, ineffective rate but the more dangerous aspects are the frequent progression to third degree block, the lack of response to atropine because of the infranodal, non-vagally innervated location of the block, and the slow ineffective escape rhythms associated with it. Mobitz Type II block occurs most frequently with ischemic heart disease, and suggests organic conduction system disease, occurring often with QRS widening.

Because of its propensity to third degree block with a slow, idioventricular rate, Mobitz Type II block requires prompt treatment. Chronotropic stimulants such as isoproterenol may increase the escape rhythm rate but no drug has been shown to effectively accelerate H–V (infranodal) conduction in the face of intermittent block. Temporary pacing seems the only effective means of treatment. Because this block generally occurs in the presence of diffuse coronary artery disease and ischemia, treatment with a pacemaker may not improve the ultimate survival statistics.

A 2 : 1 AV block should not be considered a separate entity but as a more severe variant of either Type I or Type II second degree block. If every other impulse is blocked at the AV nodal level, and the variety of block is Type I, it responds similarly to anticholinergics and occurs most frequently in the presence of excess digitalis or inferior infarction. The QRS is narrow as ventricular conduction is generally normal and the same treatment principles apply as described above for Wenckebach Type I. If a 2 : 1 block occurs with a wide QRS, very slow rate or in the presence of severe myocardial ischemia or anterior infarction, the block is more likely in the infranodal region and analogous to Type II.   It should be treated in the same fashion as outlined for Mobitz Type II block.

Third degree block can also be divided into two types depending on the area of block and corresponding to the two types of second degree block.   If complete block follows progression of Type I second degree block, the area of block is still in the AV nodal region and escape rhythms originate from the lower junctional region. The escape rhythm rate is generally adequate to maintain perfusion and is between 50 to 70 beats per minute.   The QRS is narrow as ventricular conduction is normal, the rate may be responsive to atropine to some extent, and the block is more likely to be transient.   The need for pacing depends on the response to atropine.   If an adequate rate can be maintained without treatment or on acceptable doses of anti-cholinergics, the patient may simply be observed, especially if digitalis excess is the main cause and the situation is thus likely to be temporary.   Transvenous pacing should be undertaken if an adequate rate can not be maintained.   Congenital heart block is nearly always of this type and is usually well tolerated for years until the appearance of other types of heart disease complicate the situation.

Third degree block that occurs as a sequela to Mobitz Type II second degree block is generally not hemodynamically satisfactory.   The escape rhythm must come from the ventricle and is very slow, generally below 35/minute. The QRS is broad, the rate is not responsive to atropine, the block is less likely to be transient, and the associated presence of severe myocardial disease frequently further depresses left ventricular function.   Chronotropic agents such as isoproterenol may increase the rate somewhat but are likely to produce dangerous ventricular rhythms and increased oxygen consumption.   The only effective means of treatment again is transvenous pacing which should be instituted as early and as quickly as possible.

Early recognition of the presence, types and degrees of heart block is of great importance as the course of progression is usually predictable and early treatment can do much to prevent disastrous complications of inadequate heart rates.

References

Damato, A. N. *et al*.:   A study of heart block in man using His bundle recordings. Circulation, *39*:297, 1969.
Goldreyer, B. N.:   Intracardiac electrocardiography in the analysis and understanding of cardiac arrhythmias. Ann. Intern. Med., 77:117, 1972.
Hoffman, B. R. *et al*.:   Functional properties of the atrioventricular conduction system. Circulation Research, *13*:308, 1963.
Langendorf, R. and Pick, A.:   Atrioventricular block type II (Mobitz): its nature and clinical significance. Circulation, *38*:819, 1968.
Narula, O. S. *et al*.:   Significance of His and left bundle recordings from the left heart in man. Circulation, *42*:385, 1970.
Parsonnet, V., Furman, S. and Smyth, N. P. D.:   Implantable cardiac pacemakers: Status report and resource guideline. Amer. J. Card., *34*:487, 1974.

23. Mitral Stenosis

John A. Kastor

Cause: Rheumatic fever.

Early Manifestations: Dyspnea on effort, orthopnea, paroxysmal nocturnal dyspnea, hemoptysis, palpitations. Apical diastolic rumbling murmur, opening snap of mitral valve, loud first heart sound.

Treatment: Mitral commissurotomy or mitral valve replacement.

Possible Dire Consequences without Treatment: Peripheral emboli, congestive heart failure, death.

Rheumatic mitral stenosis was the first valvular lesion to be successfully and consistently relieved by operation in a large number of patients. Almost twenty-five years have elapsed since the first commissurotomy procedures were performed and the indications for this operation are fairly well established. In general, mitral stenosis should be relieved by surgery when: (1) symptoms from the obstruction interfere significantly with the patient's way of life; (2) systemic emboli have occurred which are thought to originate in the left atrium of a patient with significant mitral stenosis.

When troublesome symptoms of pulmonary congestion develop in a patient with mitral stenosis and sinus rhythm, there is little advantage in administering digitalis since the basic problem derives from anatomical obstruction within the heart, not from myocardial failure. Although fluid retention may be relieved with diuretic drugs, it is more physiologically appropriate and clinically advantageous to relieve the primary obstructive difficulty.

If a patient who is otherwise asymptomatic decompensates with the development of *atrial fibrillation*, two therapeutic options are reasonable to consider. The patient may be anticoagulated (to prevent the development of arterial emboli), and digitalis administered to decrease the ventricular rate. If the patient then becomes asymptomatic, she may be left in controlled atrial fibrillation for the time being. Electrical cardioversion to sinus rhythm with the addition of anti-arrhythmic drugs is also sometimes carried out under these circumstances. However, if control of the ventricular response and/or cardioversion does not produce a relatively asymptomatic state, mitral surgery should be performed. When mitral valve surgery is postponed under these circumstances, the patient is left with the continuing obstruction plus the necessity of taking digitalis, anticoagulants and possibly anti-arrhythmic drugs. The development of atrial fibrillation in the presence of mitral stenosis is associated in a significant number of cases with arterial emboli which may leave the patient with important neurological deficits. Whether long-term anticoagulation is as effective as commissurotomy in preventing emboli has not been adequately settled.

When a patient with mitral stenosis begins to develop significant symptoms, certain factors unrelated directly to the obstruction itself must be considered. Recurrent rheumatic fever, thyrotoxicosis or anemia may be present, and if these disorders are successfully treated the symptoms may abate.

Mitral stenosis may be surgically treated by commissurotomy either with or without cardiopulmonary by-pass or by mitral valve replacement. Whether to perform commissurotomy without opening the heart or under direct vision on by-pass is a decision usually reached by the cardiac surgeon. Equally good therapeutic results have been reported by groups using either technique. As a general rule mitral valve replacement for mitral stenosis is required when the valve has been rendered particularly immobile by calcification or severe fibrosis or when significant mitral regurgitation is also present. The degree of calcification can often be estimated on examination by the absence of the opening snap of the mitral valve and a soft first sound which strongly suggest the presence of calcification in the anterior leaflet.

References

Bannister, R. G.:   The risks of deferring valvotomy in patients with moderate mitral stenosis. Lancet, *2*:329, 1960.

Campbell, M.:   The early operations for mitral stenosis. Brit. Heart J., *27*:670, 1965.

Editorial: When to Operate on the Rheumatic Mitral Valve. Lancet, *1*:279, 1970.

Higgs, L. M. *et al.*:   Mitral restenosis: An uncommon cause of recurrent symptoms following mitral commissurotomy. Am. J. Cardiol., *26*:34, 1970.

Litwak, R. S. *et al.*:   Factors associated with operative risk in mitral valve replacement. Am. J. Cardiol., *23*:335, 1969.

Selzer, A. *et al.*:   Immediate and long range results of valvuloplasty for mitral regurgitation due to ruptured chordae tendineae. Circulation, *45–46* (Supplement I) 1–52, 1972.

Winter, T. Q. *et al.*:   Current status of the Starr-Edwards cloth-covered prosthetic cardiac valves. Circulation *45–46*:(Supplement I) 1–14, 1972.

24. Mitral Insufficiency

JOHN A. KASTOR

Cause: Rheumatic fever, ruptured chordae tendineae, ruptured papillary muscle, bacterial endocarditis, previous "closed" mitral valve operation.

Early Manifestations: Weakness, dyspnea on effort, rapidly progressing signs of left ventricular failure upon development of new apical holosystolic murmur. Holosystolic murmur at the apex radiating to axilla or left sternal border, third heart sound, fourth heart sound (in acute regurgitation).

Treatment: Mitral valve replacement or valvuloplasty.

Possible Dire Consequences without Treatment: Congestive heart failure, death.

Mitral regurgitation is most frequently treated surgically by the replacement of the valve with a rigid mitral prosthesis or occasionally with a homograft. Successful annuloplasty and valvuloplasty without replacement of the valve have been performed in some patients with mitral insufficiency.

Mitral regurgitation may be present for decades without significant clinical decompensation. When symptoms do appear, it is quite acceptable to use medical treatment with digitalis and diuretic drugs as long as the patient continues to live a satisfactory full life. When following adequate medical therapy the symptoms prove to be significant, then surgery should be seriously considered.

In recent years we have become increasingly aware that pure mitral insufficiency is often due to causes other than rheumatic fever. Various conditions of uncertain type can produce elongation of the chordae tendineae and hooding of the valve leaflets. Again for unknown reasons chordae tendineae may suddenly rupture producing congestive failure from acute mitral insufficiency. The same general rules of therapy apply in these situations as with rheumatic mitral insufficiency. A medical trial should be first given and operation delayed until the physician is satisfied that drugs will not suffice. A patient with mitral insufficiency should not, however, be permitted to progress until signs of chronic right ventricular failure are present. Patients with this syndrome represent a significantly higher risk to cardiac surgery.

References

Bannister, R. G.: The risks of deferring valvotomy in patients with moderate mitral stenosis. Lancet, *2*:329, 1960.
Campbell, M.: The early operations for mitral stenosis. Brit. Heart J., *27*:670, 1965.
Editorial: When to Operate on the Rheumatic Mitral Valve. Lancet, *1*:279, 1970.
Higgs, L. M. *et al.*: Mitral restenosis: An uncommon cause of recurrent symptoms following mitral commissurotomy. Am. J. Cardiol., *26*:34, 1970.
Litwak, R. S. *et al.*: Factors associated with operative risk in mitral valve replacement. Am J. Cardiol., *23*:335, 1969.
Selzer, A. *et al.*: Immediate and long range results of valvuloplasty for mitral regurgitation due to ruptured chordae tendineae. Circulation, *45–46* (Supplement I) 1–52, 1972.
Winter, T. Q. *et al.*: Current status of the Starr-Edwards cloth-covered prosthetic cardiac valves. Circulation, *45–46*:(Supplement I) 1–14, 1972.

25. Valvular Aortic Stenosis

John A. Kastor

Cause: Congenital malformation, rheumatic fever, "calcific valvular degeneration."

Early Manifestations: Angina, dyspnea on effort, syncope. Mid-systolic ejection murmur in aortic area or apex, decreased intensity of aortic component of the second sound, narrow pulse pressure, aortic ejection sound (click) (when uncalcified), fourth heart sound, slow upstroke carotid pulses, thrill in aortic area.

Treatment: Aortic valve replacement with prosthesis or homograft.

Possible Dire Consequences without Treatment: Congestive heart failure, death.

Valvular aortic stenosis in the adult reveals itself with three general symptom complexes; left ventricular failure, syncope and angina. The presence of left ventricular failure is particularly ominous since many patients with aortic stenosis and left ventricular failure will be dead in less than a year unless the stenosis is relieved.

Significant valvular aortic stenosis may be easily overlooked because the murmur can be rather faint particularly in the presence of a decreased cardiac output or a large chest in an older patient. One can be especially misled when the mid-systolic murmur of aortic stenosis is heard maximally at the apex rather than the base. Furthermore, the electrocardiogram does not always reveal the expected left ventricular hypertrophy. Consequently, the examining physician should always consider this diagnosis in any patient who presents with left ventricular failure, angina or syncope.

The surgical treatment of valvular aortic stenosis may be considered like that of mitral stenosis in one important respect. Again the fundamental problem is obstruction to blood flow and not myocardial disease as such. Therefore, when symptoms of any significance develop, operation seems warranted. The valve is usually replaced by a mechanical prosthesis but in some centers homografts have been used with excellent results.

References

Barratt-Boyes, B. G. *et al.*: Aortic homograft valve replacement. A long-term follow-up of an intial series of 101 patients. Circulation, *40*:763, 1969.
Hutter, A. M. *et al.*: Aortic valve surgery as an emergency procedure. Circulation, *41*:623, 1970.
Midell, A. I. and DeBoer, A.: Multiple valve replacement. Arch. Surg., *104*:471, 1972.
Najafi, H.: Aortic insufficiency: Clinical manifestations and surgical treatment. Am. Heart J., *82*:120, 1971.
Pacifico, A. D., Karp, R. B. and Kirklin, J. W.: Homografts for replacement of the aortic valve. Circulation, *45–46* (Supplement I) 1–44, 1972.
Shean, F. C. *et al.*: Survival after Starr-Edwards aortic valve replacement. Circulation, *44*:1, 1971.
Wallace, R. B., Giuliani, E. R. and Titus, J. L.: Use of aortic valve homografts for aortic valve replacement. Circulation, *43*:365, 1971.

26. Aortic Insufficiency

John A. Kastor

Cause: Rheumatic fever, bacterial endocarditis, dissecting aortic aneurysm, congenital malformations, syphilis.

Early Manifestations: "Run-off" pulses, low diastolic pressure, decrescendo diastolic blowing murmur usually maximal at left sternal border, diastolic rumbling apical ("Austin Flint") murmur, normal to decreased intensity of first heart sound.

Treatment: Aortic valve replacement with prosthesis or homograft.

Possible Dire Consequences without Treatment: Congestive heart failure, death.

Aortic insufficiency producing significant symptoms is rarely overlooked because the physical findings are easily observed. The lesion can be missed when it is associated with another valvular problem which dominates the picture. Patients with aortic insufficiency who become mildly symptomatic may be treated successfully with digitalis and diuretics. If symptoms are thus relieved, the patient should be followed with regular examinations and review of chest roentgenograms. If symptoms of left ventricular failure or of chest pain then develop and the heart appears to increase in size, operative replacement of the valve with prosthesis or homograft is usually indicated.

Particular attention must be paid to patients who develop aortic insufficiency acutely, often from infective endocarditis. Unnecessary delay in operating can prove fatal. Vigorous medical treatment should be given in such cases, but if clinical deterioration persists, emergency valve replacement may be required.

References

Barratt-Boyes, B. G. *et al.*: Aortic homograft valve replacement. A long-term follow-up of an initial series of 101 patients. Circulation, *40*:763, 1969.

Hutter, A. M. *et al.*: Aortic valve surgery as an emergency procedure. Circulation, *41*:623, 1970.

Midell, A. I. and DeBoer, A.: Multiple valve replacement. Arch. Surg., *104*:471, 1972.

Najafi, H.: Aortic insufficiency: Clinical manifestations and surgical treatment. Am. Heart J., *82*:120, 1971.

Pacifico, A. D., Karp, R. B. and Kirklin, J. W.: Homografts for replacement of the aortic valve. Circulation, *45–46*: (Supplement I) 1–44, 1972.

Shean, F. C. *et al.*: Survival after Starr-Edwards aortic valve replacement. Circulation, *44*:1, 1971.

Wallace, R. B., Giuliani, E. R., and Titus, J. L.: Use of aortic valve homografts for aortic valve replacement. Circulation, *43*:365, 1971.

27. Tricuspid Stenosis

John A. Kastor

Cause: Rheumatic fever.

Early Manifestations: As seen with mitral stenosis plus in particular: diastolic murmur along sternum increasing with inspiration, elevated venous pressure with large A waves if the patient is in sinus rhythm, ascites, pleural effusions, edema.

Treatment: Usual treatment of congestive failure. In extreme cases: commissurotomy, valvuloplasty or prosthetic valve replacement.

Possible Dire Consequences without Treatment: Congestive heart failure, death.

Obstruction at the tricuspid orifice may be caused by certain congenital lesions including tricuspid atresia and patients with this abnormality may occasionally first present in young adult life. Tricuspid stenosis from rheumatic fever is virtually never isolated but occurs in association with lesions of the mitral and aortic valves. Significant tricuspid stenosis can be easily overlooked because one's attention is directed to the other valves. When right side failure dominates the clinical picture, then careful attention should be paid to the characteristic physical signs of tricuspid stenosis. The presence of atrial fibrillation makes recognition of tricuspid stenosis difficult by obscuring some of the abnormalities in the neck veins. The diagnosis can be confirmed at cardiac catheterization.

Surgeons repair tricuspid stenosis by either commissurotomy and valvuloplasty or by tricuspid valve replacement with a prosthesis. The decision about the type of surgery to be performed depends in part upon what the surgeon finds upon inspection of the valve at operation.

References

Braunwald, N. S., Ross, J., Jr. and Morrow, A. G.: Conservative management of tricuspid regurgitation in patients undergoing mitral valve replacement. Circulation, *35–36*: (Supplement I) 63, 1967.

Perloff, J. K. and Harvey, W. P.: Clinical recognition of tricuspid stenosis. Circulation, *22*:346, 1960.

Sanders, C. A. *et al.*: Tricuspid stenosis. A difficult diagnosis in the presence of atrial fibrillation. Circulation, *33*:26, 1966.

28. Tricuspid Insufficiency

John A. Kastor

> *Cause:* Rheumatic fever, pulmonary hypertension (from variety of causes), congenital, infectious endocarditis.
>
> *Early Manifestations:* Holosystolic murmur and third heart sound along left sternal border increasing with inspiration, edema, elevated venous pressure with systolic waves in neck veins, pulsatile liver.
>
> *Treatment:* Relief of associated mitral and/or aortic valve disease; occasionally tricuspid valve replacement or annuloplasty.
>
> *Possible Dire Consequences without Treatment:* Congestive heart failure, death.

Tricuspid insufficiency is most commonly produced by pulmonary hypertension and right ventricular failure. The etiologic problem may actually be mitral valve disease or myocardiopathy. Under these circumstances the tricuspid valve itself has not been specifically diseased and the regurgitation is functionally related to the state of the right ventricle. If the physical findings of tricuspid insufficiency decrease and cardiac compensation is improved by medical treatment, then it is likely that the tricuspid insufficiency is secondary and not primary. The surgeon decides upon inspection of the valve whether or not a secondarily affected tricuspid valve must be replaced. Some surgeons favor performing valvuloplasty or annuloplasty of the tricuspid valve under these circumstances and occasionally the valve may need to be replaced. At other times no operative procedure on the tricuspid valve is needed.

If rheumatic disease has affected the tricuspid valve directly, then the valve is often both stenotic and insufficient and direct surgical attention to the valve may be necessary.

References

Braunwald, N. S., Ross, J., Jr. and Morrow, A. G.:   Conservative management of tricuspid regurgitation in patients undergoing mitral valve replacement.   Circulation, *35–36*: (Supplement I) 63, 1967.

Perloff, J. K. and Harvey, W. P.:   Clinical recognition of tricuspid stenosis.   Circulation, *22*:346, 1960.

Sanders, C. A. *et al.*:   Tricuspid stenosis.   A difficult diagnosis in the presence of atrial fibrillation.   Circulation, *33*:26, 1966.

29. Angina Pectoris

John A. Kastor

Cause: Coronary artery disease from atherosclerosis.

Early Manifestations: Substernal pressing chest pain exacerbated by exercise and relieved by rest and nitroglycerine.   Fourth heart sound, occasional apical systolic murmur during attacks.   Positive exercise electrocardiographic test.   Significant narrowing of coronary arteries as visualized by coronary angiography.

Treatment: Coronary artery bypass graft with saphenous vein or internal mammary artery in selected cases.

Possible Dire Consequences without Treatment: Continuing angina, congestive heart failure, sudden death.

Operative intervention for the treatment of angina pectoris and for the complications of myocardial infarction is the most controversial subject in cardiac surgery today.

The operation most frequently performed for this condition is Coronary Artery Bypass Grafting (CABG) with saphenous veins or internal mammary artery.   The procedure was first performed in 1964 and the following results have been fairly well established: (1) the procedure relieves or markedly decreases the symptoms of angina pectoris in a sizable majority of patients; (2) the hospital mortality for the procedure is usually less than 6% and is highest in patients with congestive failure (Class IV, New York Heart Association), and 3 or 4 vessel obstructive disease; (3) up to 30% of the grafts may obstruct within the first two years. (Most graft obstruction develops within the first three months after operation and is more frequent when the flow within the graft at operation is low and when the coronary artery lumen is small.   These data probably exaggerated the incidence of this complication since patients who have postoperative coronary angiography tend to be those who have redeveloped symptoms which may be associated with occlusion of the grafts.)

The most important unsettled question is whether the mortality of patients with angina is changed by coronary artery bypass grafting when compared with patients treated by the more conventional medical means. In particular clinicians want to know whether patients with unstable angina, a condition variously known as acute coronary insufficiency or impending myocardial infarction will live a longer or better life with surgery or with medical treatment.

References

Anderson, R. P. et al.:   Direct revascularization of the heart. Early clinical experience with 200 patients. J. Thorac. Cardiovasc. Surg., *63*:353, 1972.

Aronow, W. S. and Stemmer, E. A.:   Bypass graft surgery versus medical therapy of angina pectoris. Am. J. Card., *33*:415, 1974.

Berger, R. L. and Stary, H. C.:   Anatomic assessment of operability by the Saphenous-Vein Bypass operation in coronary artery disease. New Eng. J. Med., *285*:252, 1971.

Ecker, R. R. et al.:   Control of intractable ventricular tachycardia by coronary revascularization. Circulation, *44*:666, 1971.

Effler, D. B. et al.   The simple approach to direct coronary artery surgery: Cleveland Clinic Experience. J. Thorac. Cardiovasc. Surg., *62*:503, 1971.

Fowler, N. O.:   "Preinfarctional" angina. A need for an objective definition and for a controlled clinical trial of its management. Circulation, *44*:755, 1971.

Gott, V. L.:   Outlook for patients after coronary artery revascularization. Am. J. Card., *33*:431, 1974.

Hill, J. D. et al.:   Emergency aortocoronary bypass for impending or extending myocardial infarction. Circulation, *43–44*, (Supplement I) I-105, 1971.

Kouchoukos, N. T., Kirklin, J. W., and Oberman, A.:   An appraisal of coronary bypass grafting. Circulation, *50*:11, 1974.

Krauss, K. R., Hutter, A. W., Jr., and DeSanctis, R. W.:   Acute coronary insufficiency: Course and follow-up. Circulation, *45–46* (Supplement I) I-66, 1972.

Loop, F. D.:   Ventricular aneurysmectomy. Surg. Clin. N.A., *51*:1071, 1971.

Morris, G. C. et al.:   Follow-up results of distal coronary artery bypass for ischemic heart disease. Am. J. Card., *29*:180, 1972.

Mundth, E. D. et al.:   Circulatory assistance and emergency direct coronary artery surgery for shock complicating acute myocardial infarction. New Eng. J. Med., *283*:1382, 1970.

Mundth, E. D. et al.:   Surgery for complications of acute myocardial infarction. Circulation, *45*:1279, 1972.

Reeves, T. J. et al.:   Natural history of angina pectoris. Am. J. Card., *33*:423, 1974.

Sanders, C. A. et al.:   Mechanical circulatory assistance. Circulation, *45*:1292, 1972.

Spencer, F. C.:   Bypass grafting for preinfarction angina. Circulation, *45*:1314, 1972.

Spencer, F. C. et al.:   Coronary bypass grafts for congestive heart failure. J. Thorac. Cardiovasc. Surg., *62*:529, 1971.

Walker, J. A. et al.:   Determinants of angiographic patency of aortocoronary vein bypass grafts. Circulation, *40–41* (Supplement I) I-86, 1972.

30. Ventricular Aneurysm

John A. Kastor

Cause: Fibrotic replacement of functioning myocardial tissue following myocardial infarction.

Early Manifestations: Left ventricular failure, systemic emboli, ventricular arrhythmias. Paradoxical precordial bulge, persistent ST segment elevation over Q waves of infarct on ECG.

Treatment: Ventricular aneurysmectomy.

Possible Dire Consequences without Treatment: Congestive heart failure, rupture of aneurysm, death.

References

See Section 29, p. 562.

31. Rupture of Ventricular Septum

John A. Kastor

Cause: Lysis of ventricular septal tissue following myocardial infarction.

Early Manifestations: Rapid development of decreased cardiac output with onset of new holosystolic murmur at left sternal border.

Treatment: Repair of defect (plus aneurysmectomy in some cases).

Possible Dire Consequences without Treatment: Congestive heart failure, sudden death.

Ventricular aneurysmectomy, surgical repair of a ventricular septal defect or mitral valve replacement for ruptured papillary muscle are best performed several weeks to months after onset of the myocardial infarction. A few patients have had successful surgery during the acute period after myocardial infarction for these complications, but the mortality under such circumstances is high.

References

See Section 29, p. 562.

32. Acute Mitral Regurgitation from Rupture of a Portion of the Left Ventricular Papillary Muscles

John A. Kastor

Cause: Infarction of the papillary muscles, usually the posterior muscle.

Early Manifestations: Similar to rupture of the ventricular septum; rapid development of congestive failure and hypotension with onset of a new holosystolic decrescendo murmur at the left ventricular apex.

Treatment: Mitral valve replacement.

Possible Dire Consequences without Treatment: More severe congestive failure, shock, sudden death.

References

See Section 29, p. 562.

*Bacterial Endocarditis

(Discussed in Chapter VII, INFECTIONS pp. 103–119).

Reference

Black, S., O'Rourke, R. A. and Karlimer, J. S.: Role of surgery in the treatment of primary infective endocarditis. Amer. J. Med., *56*:357, 1974.

Index

Page numbers followed by *t* refer to tables.